Clinical Trials in Hypertension

Clinical Trials in Hypertension

edited by
Henry R. Black
Rush-Presbyterian-St. Luke's Medical Center
Chicago, Illinois

MARCEL DEKKER, INC. NEW YORK • BASEL

ISBN: 0-8247-0270-0

This book is printed on acid-free paper.

Headquarters
Marcel Dekker, Inc.
270 Madison Avenue, New York, NY 10016
tel: 212-696-9000; fax: 212-685-4540

Eastern Hemisphere Distribution
Marcel Dekker AG
Hutgasse 4, Postfach 812, CH-4001 Basel, Switzerland
tel: 44-61-261-8482; fax: 44-61-261-8896

World Wide Web
http://www.dekker.com

The publisher offers discounts on this book when ordered in bulk quantities. For more information, write to Special Sales/Professional Marketing at the headquarters address above.

Current printing (last digit):
10 9 8 7 6 5 4 3 2 1

PRINTED IN THE UNITED STATES OF AMERICA

To Hallie, for all she does for me in so many ways and for her patience and forbearance with my zeal for work, which often neglects her and her needs.

To Matt and Dana, for providing me with so much joy and comfort.

And for all of my colleagues, near and far, who have made working in this field so exciting and rewarding.

Preface

In the past decade, we have entered an era of evidence-based medicine. Although many types of clinical, preclinical, and population-based studies constitute "evidence," the high priests of evidence-based medicine have spent much time and energy attempting to provide an acceptable hierarchy for the many types of evidence available to us for making clinical decisions.

In general, in vitro, animal, and observational studies in human or nonhuman populations are not viewed as particularly compelling. Prospective studies in non-randomly selected cohorts and retrospective case/control studies are valuable, but only slightly more useful than in vitro, animal, or epidemiological surveys. Clinical trials, especially if properly done, are considered the best evidence and remain the "gold standard" in our evidence-based era. Fortunately for those of us interested in hypertension and for the billion hypertensives worldwide, there is no shortage of clinical trials to help us decide how to treat our patients.

But clinical trials, too, are more or less useful if we are to make clinical decisions as accurately as possible. Studies that are short in duration and small in sample size are rarely helpful in deciding how best to treat a chronic condition such as hypertension. Studies focusing on surrogate endpoints, such as a reduction in blood pressure, do not necessarily provide reliable data, since reducing mortality and morbidity (clinical outcomes) is the objective of treatment. We do not treat hypertension simply to lower the blood pressure. We treat it to prevent strokes, heart attacks, heart failure, and chronic renal disease, conditions for which epidemiological and other studies have provided evidence of a direct relationship. Similarly, we do not treat hypercholesterolemia to lower the level of total or low-density lipoprotein cholesterol in the blood but rather to reduce episodes of coronary heart disease, which we feel are attributed to elevated levels of serum or low-density lipoprotein cholesterol.

This book is designed to provide a historical perspective on clinical trials in hypertension in which pharmacologic therapy was evaluated. There are 25 chapters. With the exception of the final chapter, each reviews in detail either a completed trial or an important trial that was still in progress as the book went to press, but would be completed soon. The final chapter reports on the prospective collaboration of the WHO/ISH Trialist Group that will pool data from the more than 30 large clinical trials in hypertension in progress. Some of the trials included here were not specifically for hypertensives, but included a large number of hypertensive participants. Those studies were designed to establish the efficacy of a treatment for a common complication of hypertension, such as heart failure or chronic renal disease, and, to this end, also tested drugs used as antihypertensives.

This book does not include all the clinical trials of pharmacologic therapy done for hypertension. The trials selected for inclusion have addressed an important question; have been of sufficient length and size to answer that question; and, with few exceptions, have had or will have an important impact on clinical practice. Mortality and morbidity are the primary outcomes of most of the studies, but some were designed to help clinicians decide which drug to use to treat hypertensive patients.

Most, but not all, of the studies detailed here were government sponsored (in the United States, the United Kingdom, Scandinavia, and elsewhere in western Europe). But several very important studies were wholly or partly sponsored by the pharmaceutical industry in partnership with academic investigators or governmental agencies. We cannot do large and long-term clinical trials without support from industry. If the studies were done and analyzed properly, the results are as valid and useful as the data from trials totally under the control of nonindustry personnel.

The chapters are presented in chronological order; when the book is read in sequence from Chapter 1 to Chapter 25, it presents a history of what has been accomplished over the past 35 years.

Some studies, such as the VA Trial (Chapter 1), the USPHS Trial (Chapter 2), the Australian National High Blood Pressure Study (Chapter 4), and the MRC Trial of the Treatment of Mild Hypertension (Chapter 5), established the value of treating younger hypertensives with diastolic blood pressure elevations. This now universally accepted evidence was in question until these trials were completed. The value of treating hypertension was not accepted by many on ''faith'' alone.

The Hypertension Detection and Follow-Up Program (Chapter 3) and the Hypertension Optimal Treatment Study (Chapter 15) evaluated the goal of treatment of diastolic hypertension. No study to date has been completed, or even planned, specifically to determine the treatment goal for systolic blood pressure.

Several studies compared available antihypertensive drugs. The studies completed in the 1980s, such as HAPPHY and MAPHY (Chapters 6 and 7), compared diuretics and β-adrenergic receptor blockers. Studies completed in the 1990s, such as TOMHS (Chapter 12) and VA Cooperative Study of Monotherapy (Chapter 13), compared those agents to ''new'' drugs: angiotensin-converting-enzyme inhibitors, α-adrenergic receptor blockers, and calcium antagonists.

This book also details the studies done in older hypertensives (≥60 years of age). Only one trial that was exclusively for the elderly—the European Working Party on Hypertension in the Elderly (Chapter 8)—was finished in the 1980s. Five more trials (Chapters 9, 10, 11, 14, and 20) were completed in the 1990s. All the participants in the European Working Party on Hypertension in the Elderly had an elevated diastolic blood pressure (≥90 mm Hg). These newer studies also randomized older individuals with both diastolic and systolic hypertension or with only isolated systolic hypertension.

Four chapters are devoted to studies either in heart failure (Chapters 17 and 19), in nephropathy (Chapter 18), or in the immediate postmyocardial infarction setting (Chapter 16).

Chapters 21 to 24 detail important studies still in progress. Hopefully, the report of the collaborative group (Chapter 25) will provide adequate detail about these trials.

The format of each chapter is relatively uniform, which makes it easy for the reader to compare studies. In each case, the author or authors were part of the study leadership. Each chapter contains details of inclusion and exclusion criteria, baseline characteristics of the enrolled subjects, the planned analyses and calculations used to interpret the results, the drug regimen used, and the primary and, in many cases, secondary results.

When possible, I have had the authors include a list of their collaborators, including those on study committees, those who helped enroll the cohort (the investigators), and those who were charged with evaluating and protecting the participants in the trial while it was still blinded (the Data and Safety Monitoring Boards).

There are many whom I could not specifically thank and credit:

- Innumerable study coordinators, recruiters, secretaries, data managers, and others who actually did much of the work and who almost never get recognition. Without their efforts, none of the data presented here could ever have been accrued. Many who participate in the design and implementation of clinical trials toil without recognition. I hope they derive satisfaction from knowing that their efforts are not in vain.
- Government and industry officials who provided the financial support needed for these trials. In each case, they chose to allocate scarce resources to answer the questions posed by the study rather than for other, equally important, problems.
- The hundreds of thousands of hypertensive participants who willingly gave their time and took the potential risks of treatment (or no treatment) to enroll in these and other studies. I wish I could personally thank them and include their names, but because of confidentiality requirements and space restrictions, this is impossible. They are the real unsung heroes of this story and of clinical research in general.

I would also like to acknowledge the invaluable assistance of the staff of Marcel Dekker, Inc., especially Graham Garratt, who invited me to write this book and who sadly is not with us to see if his faith in me was justified, and Sandra Beberman. Special thanks go to Norma Sandoval, who worked tirelessly for many months to see that this volume was done properly. Without her dedication, *Clinical Trials in Hypertension* would never have been completed successfully.

This volume will be a valuable resource for those in the field. As new trials are completed and new evidence is accumulated, it is especially important that we have the perspective of time. We can understand so much better where we need to go if we really understand how we got to where we are.

Henry R. Black

Contents

Clinical Trials in Hypertension

1

The Veterans Administration Cooperative Study on Antihypertensive Drugs

EDWARD D. FREIS

Veterans Administration Hospital, Washington, D.C.

I. INTRODUCTION

The first controlled trial concerning the effects of drug treatment on morbidity and mortality in hypertension was the Veterans Administration Cooperative Study (VA Trial) (1–3). In the early 1960s when the trial was initiated, the drug treatment of hypertension was not accepted by most physicians. Goldring and Chasis, two of the opinion leaders at the time, wrote, "There can be no doubt that the disabling and lethal agent in chronic hypertensive disease is not the blood pressure (BP) but the associated arterial and arteriolar disease" (4). They also emphasized that reducing the BP with drugs was of no therapeutic benefit because it did not affect the fundamental and unknown cause of the vascular disease. They argued that it was first necessary to find the cause or causes of hypertension before it could be treated effectively.

At the same time, a minority opinion asserted that although the fundamental cause for the hypertension was unknown, the increased intravascular pressure could have injurious effects in the arterial system. In the large arteries, the high pressure might aggravate and accelerate the development of atherosclerosis; in the arterioles, it might cause narrowing of the lumen because of the reactive arteriolosclerosis. The elevated BP could then be the determining factor in the development of such complications as heart attacks, strokes, congestive heart failure, and nephrosclerosis. If this hypothesis were correct, reducing the BP should arrest the progression of the vascular disease and prevent major complications. This controversy provided the stimulus for undertaking the VA trial.

Table 1 Inclusion and Exclusion Criteria

Inclusion Criteria Diastolic BP	
Average of last two baseline clinic visits	90–129 mm Hg
Severe group	115–129 mm Hg
Mild and moderate group	90–114 mm Hg
Exclusion Criteria (past or present)	
Hypertensive neuroretinopathy	
Cerebral hemorrhage	
Recent myocardial infarction	
Congestive heart failure	
Dissecting or ruptured aortic aneurysm	
Renal failure	
Secondary hypertension	
Unrelated fatal disease	
Normal BP when hospitalized	

II. DESIGN OF THE TRIAL

Because it was generally believed that drug treatment was of no benefit in essential hypertension, even if severe, the VA trial was designed to test the effects of drug treatment in both mild hypertension and essential hypertension of all degrees of severity. An exception was malignant hypertension (diastolic BP > 130 mm Hg with hypertensive neuroretinopathy), because several reports had indicated improvement using the drugs then available (5, 6). Therefore, patients with malignant hypertension were excluded from the trial. Patients with major complications or with unrelated life-threatening diseases such as cancer were also excluded. Other exclusion criteria are listed in Table 1.

The population admitted to the study was weighted more toward moderate to severe essential hypertension (1, 2) than was the case in subsequent trials. Although patients with mild hypertension were included, their number was too small to provide adequate statistical power. All patients were males whose BP at entry averaged 90 to 129 mm Hg (1). The patients were first admitted to the hospital for one week to rule out curable forms of hypertension and to identify ''white-coat'' hypertension. Patients whose BP fell to normal levels during hospitalization were excluded. The baseline blood pressure was taken as the average of three readings recorded during the first outpatient visit after the hospitalization.

Drug treatment consisted of a combination tablet containing 50 mg of hydrochlorothiazide and 0.1 mg of reserpine taken twice daily plus 25 mg of hydralazine three times daily (Table 2). The control group received matched placebos of these drugs. Compliance was tested during a 2-week prerandomization period. The patients received a placebo

Table 2 Active Drug Regimen

Drug	Dose	Frequency
Hydrochlorothiazide*	50 mg	2 times daily
Reserpine	0.1 mg	2 times daily
Hydralazine	25 mg	3 times daily

* Hydrochlorothiazide and reserpine were combined in a single tablet.

containing riboflavine, which caused the urine to fluoresce when viewed under ultraviolet light. Patients identified as being noncompliant by pill counts or the fluorescence test were excluded from the trial. Testing for compliance was continued postrandomization and the importance of adherence was repeatedly emphasized.

III. RESULTS

A. Severe Hypertension

Of the 523 patients randomized into the study, 143 had severe hypertension as defined by a baseline average diastolic BP in the range of 115 to 129 mm Hg (1). The mean age of these patients was 51 years and their average weight was 83.5 kg. Seventy-seven patients were black and 66 were white. There were no significant differences in major characteristics at the time of randomization between the treated patients and the placebo group (Table 3). The patients with severe hypertension were removed from the trial after only 18 months of follow-up because of the large number of morbid events occurring in the control group.

In the severe group, BP fell significantly among the drug-treated patients. The average diastolic BP decreased from 121 mm Hg before randomization to 91.6 mm Hg at 12 months afterward. There was no significant fall of BP in the placebo group. Four patients, all in the placebo group, died, three from ruptured aortic aneurysms and one from sudden death (Table 4). In the control group, 27 patients developed terminating events as compared with only 2 in the treated patients. The nonfatal events included progression to malignant hypertension, congestive heart failure, stroke, myocardial infarction, and impairment of renal function. The trial was then terminated by the oversight committee, a group of outside physicians who periodically reviewed the unblinded data. The only event in the treated group was a nondisabling stroke. The other termination was the result of an adverse drug reaction.

Table 3 Baseline Characteristics of Patients with Diastolic Hypertension (115–129 mm Hg)

Characteristics	Placebo number	Active drugs number
Total randomized	70	73
White	35	31
Black	35	42
Cardiac symptoms	22	21
Left ventricular hypertrophy (ECG)	22	24
Prior cerebrovascular thrombosis	5	6
Diabetes	5	8
	Mean	Mean
Age (yrs)	51	50
Weight (lb)	183	184
Systolic BP (mm Hg)	187	186
Diastolic BP (mm Hg)	121	121
Blood glucose, fasting (mg/100 ml)	96	97
Blood cholesterol (mg/100 ml)	251	242

Table 4 Morbid Events by Diagnostic Categories in Patients with Initial Severe Diastolic Hypertension (115–129 mm Hg)

	Total events		Terminating events	
Diagnosis	Control	Treated	Control	Treated
Deaths				
Aortic dissecting aneurysm	2	0	2	0
Ruptured abdominal aneurysm	1	0	1	0
Sudden death	1	0	1	0
Nonfatal Events				
''Accelerated''* hypertension	9	0	9	0
Diastolic BP >140 mm Hg	3	0	3	0
Progressive renal disease	2	0	2	0
Stroke	4	1	4	1
Transient ischemic attack	0	0	1	0
Myocardial infarction	2	0	0	0
Congestive heart failure	2	0	0	0
Adverse drug reactions†	0	0	0	1

* Diastolic BP > 130 mm Hg with hemorrhages, exudates, or papilledema in the optic fundi.
† Fasting blood glucose 450 mg/100 ml and serum potassium 2.5 mEq/L.

B. Mild and Moderate Hypertension

Three hundred eighty patients were randomized into the trial with entry diastolic BP ranging between 90 and 114 mm Hg (2, 3). The average follow-up was 3.3 years, although some were followed up for more than 5 years. Blacks comprised 42% of the control patients and 41% of the treatment group. The average ages were 52.0 years in the control group and 50.5 years in the treatment group. The two groups also were similar in other demographic characteristics (Table 5).

The effectiveness of the triple-drug regimen of thiazide-reserpine-hydralazine in reducing BP was demonstrated in the changes after randomization. Blood pressure in the placebo group rose slightly from a baseline average of 165/105 to 169/106 mm Hg at 4 months after randomization. In the treated group, the average BP had fallen significantly from 162/104 to 135/87 mm Hg. It is noteworthy that this combination of inexpensive older drugs lowered the BP of the majority of patients into the normal range. These drugs seemed to be just as effective or more effective in this regard than the newer, more expensive drugs.

During the average follow-up of 3.3 years, 56 patients (28.9%) in the placebo group had major cardiovascular events develop (Table 6). In the treatment group, only 22 (11.8%) had cardiovascular complications. Also, 20 additional patients, all in the control group, did not have a specific event but did develop an increase in the severity of their hypertension. Their diastolic BP increased to more than 125 mm Hg, requiring removal from the trial and institution of drug treatment. Many of these patients probably would have had cardiovascular complications develop if left untreated.

A direct relationship was seen between the level of diastolic BP at entry and the effectiveness of treatment. In patients with entry diastolic BP of 105 to 114 mm Hg, there were 75% fewer morbid events in the treatment group, as compared with the control group.

Table 5 Baseline Characteristics of Patients with Mild and Moderate Diastolic Hypertension (90–114 mm Hg)

Characteristic	Placebo	Active drugs
Total randomized	186	194
Black	76	110
White	110	113
	Mean	Mean
Age (yrs)	52.0	50.5
Body weight (kg)	81.8	80.1
Hospital systolic BP (mm Hg)	157.5	154.0
Hospital diastolic BP (mm Hg)	101.3	100.2
Clinic systolic BP (mm Hg)	165.1	162.1
Clinic diastolic BP (mm Hg)	104.7	103.8
Serum creatine (mg/100 ml)	1.26	1.24
BUN (mg/100 ml)	15.6	16.2
Serum potassium (mEq/1)	4.4	4.4
Fasting blood glucose (mg/100 ml)	96.5	100.4
Serum cholesterol (mg/100 ml)	250.1	245.0
Serum uric acid (mg/100 ml)	6.3	6.0

By contrast, in patients with entry diastolic BP of 90 to 104 mm Hg, only a 35% reduction in complications among the treated patients was noted.

There were 19 deaths from cardiovascular causes in the control group, compared with 8 among the treated patients. Seven of the deaths in the control group were the result of strokes. Only one patient died of stroke among the treated patients (Table 6). Fatal myocardial infarction or sudden death occurred in 11 patients in the control group and in 6 of the treated patients. When fatal and nonfatal coronary artery events were combined, however, the total events were nearly the same in the 2 groups, that is, 13 in the control group and 11 among the treated patients. This shortfall in the prevention of myocardial infarction has also been reported in many of the subsequent treatment trails with antihyper-

Table 6 Classification of Morbid Events by Diagnostic Categories in Patients with Initial Mild and Moderate Diastolic Hypertension (90–114 mm Hg)

	Total events	
Diagnosis	Control	Treated
Cerebrovascular accident	20	5
Coronary artery disease	13	11
Congestive heart failure	11	0
"Accelerated" hypertension	4	0
Renal damage	3	0
Other	5	6
Total	56	22

Source: Ref. 2.

tensive drugs (7). It may be related to the fact that risk factors other than hypertension, such as cigarette smoking or an elevated serum cholesterol level, also are important in the pathogenesis of myocardial infarction.

The development of stroke, on the other hand, which may be more BP dependent, occurred in 20 patients in the placebo group versus only 5 among the treated patients (Table 6). Even more striking was the association between treatment and prevention of congestive heart failure, a complication that occurred in 11 patients in the control group versus none in the treated patients. Left ventricular hypertrophy also was strikingly influenced by drug treatment, as judged by electrocardiographic evidence (8). Only one fourth as many treated patients had left ventricular hypertrophy develop during the trial as occurred among the placebo group.

Life-table analysis of morbid events during a 5-year follow-up period indicated a cumulative incidence rate of 55% for the control group as compared with 18% for the treated patients (Fig. 1). It can be estimated, therefore, that over a 5-year period, treatment prevented 37% of morbid events (the difference between control and treated groups). This represents an effectiveness of treatment of 67%, that is, the difference between control and treated groups divided by the percent of events in the control group. Figure 1 also

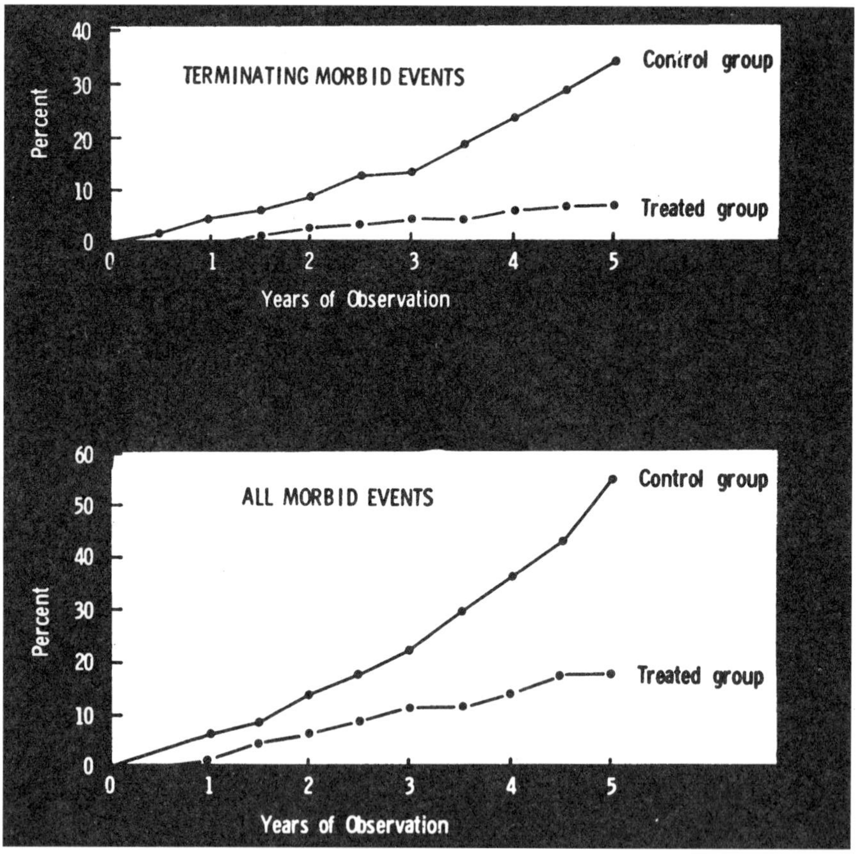

Fig. 1 Estimated cumulative incidence of morbidity over a 5-year period as calculated by the life table method. Terminating morbid events (*top*) and all morbid events (*bottom*). (From Ref. 2.)

shows that the spread between events in the treatment and control groups appears early and then widens, indicating increasing benefit with the passage of time.

Most of the patients in whom complications developed were older than the average age. In the control group, only 15 of the 56 patients in whom complications developed were younger than age 50. Nevertheless, the percentage difference in the effectiveness of treatment between control and treated patients was essentially the same in the two age groups.

Drug-related adverse effects occurred in 20% of the patients. Biochemical adverse effects included hypokalemia, elevated serum uric acid level, and increased blood sugar. Hypokalemia occurred in 20% of the treated patients. However, no cardiac arrhythmias were reported in any of these patients despite the 100 mg/day dose of hydrochlorothiazide. Serum uric acid levels were above the normal range in 16% of the control patients and 30% of the treated group. Acute gout developed in one treated patient. After 1 year of treatment, 15.6% of the control group and 20.8% of the treated patients had fasting blood glucose levels greater than 110 mg/100 ml.

Subjective complaints that might be drug related also were recorded. Adverse effects that occurred more frequently in the treated patients included lethargy and weakness, nasal stuffiness, and ulcer symptoms. However, the incidence of nightmares, arthritis, angina, and headache was greater in the control group, whereas complaints of depression, skin rash, and impotence were essentially the same in both groups. These results indicated that these older drugs in the doses used produced few drug-related subjective adverse effects.

IV. DISCUSSION

The VA trial was innovative in several ways. To this author's knowledge, it was the first multiclinic, long-term, controlled trial in any type of cardiovascular disease. The demonstrated success of the method, as demonstrated by the VA trial, provided a model for subsequent controlled trials of drug treatment in hypertension and other cardiovascular diseases. Long-term controlled trials have become the standard by which most treatments are evaluated.

The VA trial also was very important in clarifying the relationship between the pathological changes associated with hypertension and elevated BP. Before the VA trial, the prevailing opinion was that the high BP was only a symptom of an underlying cardiovascular disease (4). If the hypertension was only a secondary event, reduction of BP would not prevent progression of the pathological changes in the heart and arterial system. Prevention of cardiovascular changes after BP reduction provided strong evidence that the changes were the result of the elevated BP and not the reverse, as was formerly believed. Of course, what causes the BP to rise in the first place still remains unknown.

The VA trial is primarily recognized as the first convincing demonstration of the effectiveness of drug treatment in preventing complications associated with moderate and severe hypertension. It provided the first sound evidence that cardiovascular complications such as stroke, heart failure, and renal failure were reduced by drug treatment.

The effectiveness of treatment was directly related to the severity of the hypertension at entry. The greatest reduction of morbid events in treated patients, as compared with control patients, occurred in the group with the most severe hypertension, and the smallest difference occurred in the patients with the mildest elevation of BP. These findings were the opposite of those of the Hypertension Detection and Follow-Up Program (HDFP) (9), which found that the percentage reduction in mortality with treatment was greatest in the mildest forms of hypertension (90 to 94 mm Hg) and decreased progressively with higher levels of pretreatment blood pressure. The reason for this difference between the two trials is not clear.

The most frequent major complications of mild hypertension are those related to coronary heart disease. There were also the most frequent complications in the patients with mild hypertension in the VA trial. Although there were fewer reductions in coronary-related morbidity and mortality with treatment, the differences were not significant (2). On the other hand, so-called ''hypertensive'' complications such as stroke, congestive heart failure, and accelerated hypertension occurred more frequently in patients with moderate to severe hypertension. These complications, unlike the coronary events, were reduced considerably by treatment.

Patients with systolic hypertension were not included in the VA trial. It was recognized that diastolic hypertension was caused by constriction of the arterioles. On the other hand, systolic hypertension was the result of reduced distensibility of the aorta and its major branches caused by atherosclerotic changes associated with aging. The principal risk was not thought to be the elevated systolic BP but rather the underlying atherosclerosis. Indeed, some physicians considered it dangerous to reduce blood pressure when there was possible narrowing of arterial lumen by atherosclerotic plaques. At that time, we did not have the benefit of reliable epidemiological and therapeutic trial data (10) to prove that our concerns were unnecessary.

The patients in the VA trial differed from the general population of hypertensive patients. The untreated patients developed more complications and more accelerated hypertension than in other trials. This was partly because of the manner in which they were selected for the trial. Many of the patients had moderate to severe hypertension on admission. Also, before randomization they were hospitalized for one week and the patients whose diastolic blood pressure fell below 90 mm Hg were excluded. However, these selection procedures did not invalidate the main conclusion of the trial, which was that treatment was effective in preventing the cardiovascular complications of hypertension.

V. CONCLUSION

The VA cooperative study is remembered for changing the management of hypertension. It altered the emphasis from diagnosing and treating secondary forms of hypertension to using drugs to control the BP in the much more prevalent form of hypertension, that is, primary hypertension. The study convinced physicians that such patients could benefit from treatment with antihypertensive drugs. It demonstrated that by controlling the BP, physicians could prevent most of the complications of the disorder as well as its progression to a more severe state.

REFERENCES

1. Veterans Administration Cooperative Study Group on Antihypertensive Agents. Effects of treatment on morbidity in hypertension. Results in patients with diastolic blood pressure averaging 115 through 129 mm Hg. JAMA 1967; 202:1028–1034.
2. Veterans Administration Cooperative Study Group on Antihypertensive Agents. Effects of treatment on morbidity in hypertension. II. Results in patients with diastolic blood pressure averaging 90 through 114 mm Hg. JAMA 1970; 213:1143–1152.
3. Veterans Administration Cooperative Study Group on Antihypertensive Agents. Effects of

treatment on morbidity in hypertension. III. Influence of age, diastolic blood pressure and prior cardiovascular disease. Further analysis of side effects. Circulation 1972; 45:991–998.
4. Goldring W, Chasis H. Antihypertensive drug therapy: an appraisal. Arch Intern Med 1965; 115:523–525.
5. Sokolow M, Perloff D. Five-year survival of consecutive patients with malignant hypertension treated with antihypertensive agents. Am J Cardiol 1960; 6:858–863.
6. Mohler ER, Freis ED. Five-year survival of patients with malignant hypertension treated with antihypertensive agents. Am Heart J 1960; 60:329–335.
7. Collins R, Peto R, MacMahon S, Hebert P, Fiebach NH, Eberlein KA, Godwin J, Qizilbash N, Taylor JO, Hennekens CH. Blood pressure, stroke, and coronary heart disease. Part 2, short-term reductions in blood pressure: overview of randomised drug trials in their epidemiological context. Lancet 1990; 335:827–838.
8. Poblete PF, Kyle MC, Pipberger HV, Freis ED. Effects of treatment on morbidity in hypertension. Veterans Administration Cooperative Study Group on Antihypertensive Agents. Effect on the electrocardiogram. Circulation 1973; 48:481–490.
9. Hypertension Detection and Follow-up Programs. The effect of treatment on mortality in ''mild'' hypertension. Results of the Hypertension Detection and Follow-up Programs. N Engl J Med 1982; 307:976–980.
10. SHEP Cooperative Research Group. Prevention of stroke by antihypertensive treatment in older persons with isolated systolic hypertension: final results of the Systolic Hypertension in the Elderly Program (SHEP). JAMA 1991; 265:3255–3264.

2

The Treatment of Mild Essential Hypertension: The U.S. Public Health Service Hospitals Clinical Trial

W. McFATE SMITH

SRI International, Menlo Park, California

I. BACKGROUND AND RATIONALE

The Public Health Service Hospital intervention trial in mild hypertension (1) was initiated in September 1966. At that time, it was estimated that more than 20 million adults in the United States had definite hypertension defined as 160/95 mm Hg or greater. After using the lower cut-off point of 140/90 mm Hg to define hypertension, the estimate was raised to nearly 50 million persons, the preponderance of whom had so-called "mild hypertension," that is, diastolic blood pressures in the range of 90 to 104 mm Hg.

Data from the Society of Actuaries (2), the Framingham experience (3), and the Pooling Project (4) of the Council on Epidemiology of the American Heart Association had established that excess morbidity and mortality are experienced by both sexes, at all ages, and in direct proportion to the elevation of their blood pressure above diastolic levels of 80 mm Hg. The high prevalence of hypertension noted above, combined with this elevated risk of premature and excess cardiovascular complications, defined a public health problem of enormous proportion.

The treatment of hypertension had been predicated on the assumption that intervention that lowers pressure would prevent the cardiovascular complications. Support for this hypothesis began to accumulate a decade or so earlier, first in the case of the malignant phase of hypertension, and subsequently for severe but benign, or non-"accelerated" primary hypertension. The reports of Hamilton et al. (5), Leishman (6), and Bjork et al. (7), were noteworthy in this regard, and whereas only Hamilton's study was prospective and included concurrent controls, all consistently demonstrated an improved prognosis when pressure was lowered.

By inference, it was logical to expect this should also be the case for less severe and mild hypertension. However, given the natural history of the disease, including the long asymptomatic phase with low incidence of complications, it was expected to be exceedingly difficult to demonstrate. The anticipated difficulties included the need to recruit and provide systematic long-term follow-up of a large representative study population in a well-controlled intervention trial. Moreover, therapists in the Cooperative Study Group of the Public Health Service Hospitals shared a general reluctance to commit individuals with mild hypertension to a lifetime of medication—itself not without hazard, expense, and inconvenience. Accordingly, the Group concluded that there was a need for a well-designed, long-term, prospective intervention study to evaluate the influence of blood pressure control on the complications of mild hypertension.

The first subjects entered the study in September 1966, less than 1 year after the beginning of the Veterans Administration (VA) prospective trial, which had similar objectives (8). The VA trial confirmed the findings of Hamilton for those with diastolic blood pressures in the 115 to 129 mm Hg range, and subsequently extended these observations to their group of subjects in the range of 90 to 114 mm Hg.

II. OBJECTIVES OF THE STUDY

The objective of the trial was to determine whether the lowering of blood pressure with antihypertensive medications would result in reduced incidence of cardiovascular complications, increased survival, or both.

The primary hypothesis for the statistical design was that the survival rate of treated hypertensive patients would be comparable to that of the normotensive population.

The trial was a primary prevention study in the sense that every reasonable effort available at the time was made to exclude individuals who had already sustained demonstrable target organ damage.

III. STUDY DESIGN

The design and time course of the trial is schematized in Figure 1.

A. Selection Criteria (Table 1)

Male and female subjects up to age 55 were qualified for admission to the study if their average diastolic blood pressure (DBP) during a 6-week *home* pressure control period was in the range of 90 to 114 mm Hg. In addition, their ''clinic basal'' (sitting position after resting quietly for 20 minutes without smoking) diastolic pressures were required to equal or exceed 90 mm Hg.

Those thus qualified were admitted to the study if not excluded for the following reasons:

1. Diabetes mellitus, renal insufficiency, or hypercholesterolemia (> 350 g/dl)
2. Abnormal electrocardiogram
3. Radiographic cardiomegaly
4. Grade III or IV retinopathy
5. Clinical history or findings of (a) previous arterial thrombosis or vascular insuf-

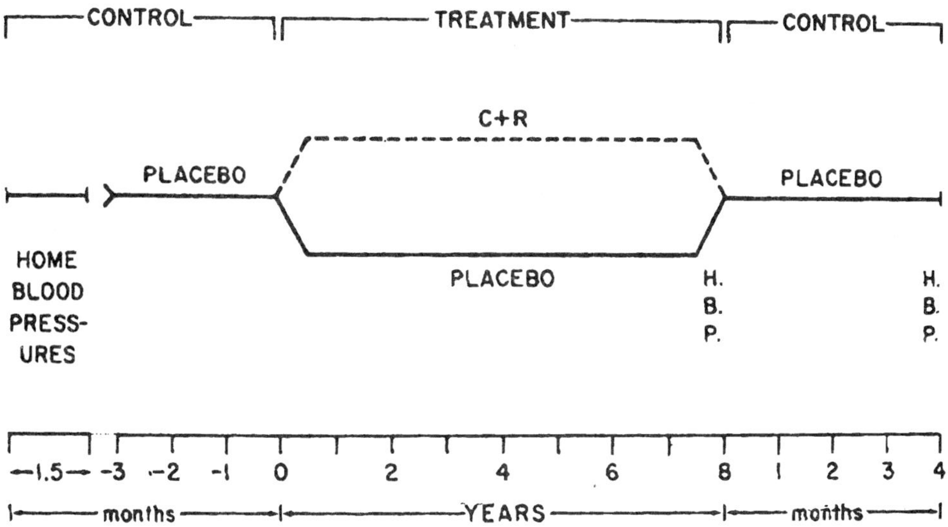

Fig. 1 A schematic diagram of the study design indicating control and treatment (C + R = chlorothiazide and rauwolfia) and the duration of follow-up. Home blood pressures (HBP) were a feature of pre- and post-treatment control periods. *Source*: Ref. 15, published by permission of the American Heart Association.

ficiency, whether coronary, cerebral, or peripheral; (b) congestive heart failure; (c) angina pectoris; (d) valvular heart disease; or (e) secondary or correctable hypertension

6. Known sensitivities to the intervention agents

B. Placebo Trial Period

Qualified subjects were then started on a 3-month trial period of placebo medication, during which time additional baseline blood pressures were obtained. Excluded were those

Table 1 Selection Criteria

Gender	Male and female
Age	55 years and younger
Blood pressure	Home control
	DBP 90 to 114 mm Hg
	Clinic control
	DBP ≥90 mm Hg
Exclusions	Diabetes mellitus
	Renal insufficiency
	Hypercholesterolemia
	Abnormal ECG
	Radiographic cardiomegaly
	Retinopathy grade III or IV
	Clinical history of cardiovascular disease
	Secondary or correctable hypertension

whose diastolic pressures fell to less than 90 mm Hg on two or more of the three visits during the period.

C. Treatment Program

At the conclusion of the trial period, subjects were randomly assigned to either active or placebo treatment. This medication was substituted for the identical placebo of the trial period and administered in double-blind fashion. Active therapy consisted of 500 mg of chlorothiazide plus 100 mg of rauwolfia serpentina combined in a single tablet, taken twice daily, a regimen demonstrated in previous trials to control blood pressure in up to 80% of such cases (9) (Table 2).

D. Follow-Up Procedures

Subjects were followed up bimonthly with determination of blood pressure and heart rate. A pill count was made and adverse effects query carried out.

Semiannually, a limited physical examination, including fundoscopy, was conducted and recorded. Electrocardiogram (ECG), urinalysis, and determination of serum creatinine and potassium were carried out at that time. Annually, an exercise ECG, cardiac series, creatinine clearance, serum cholesterol, and a 2-hour post-load serum glucose were recorded.

Electrocardiograms were interpreted centrally by a single reader who was blinded to treatment assignment. Cardiac series for radiographic cardiac size assessment were interpreted centrally by a cardiovascular radiologist, similarly blinded to treatment, applying the Ungerleider technique of measurement.

E. Morbidity Observations

The statistical endpoints were predefined in terms of specified cardiovascular complications, which were classified into primary, secondary, tertiary, and treatment failure. Endpoints were classified into those morbid events considered direct complications of elevated pressure, per se (hypertensive), and those predominantly associated with vascular sclerosis (atherosclerotic) (Tables 3 and 4). Endpoints were also preclassified as major and minor. Only the major events—death, stroke, and myocardial infarction—were used as endpoints in the sequential analysis.

Treatment failure was defined as ''accelerated hypertension,'' namely, the progressive elevation of DBP to levels exceeding 130 mm Hg on three consecutive visits over a period of not more than one month, or on any single visit if symptomatic, or if associated with the appearance of grade III or IV retinopathy.

Table 2 Drug Regimen

Active	Chlorothiazide 500 mg*
	Rauwolfia serpentina 100 mg*
Control	Identical placebo

* Combined in a single tablet and taken twice daily.

Table 3 Classification of Endpoints

- Primary
  - Cerebral hemorrhage or thrombosis
  - Myocardial infarction
  - Death
    - Cardiovascular disease
    - Sudden
- Secondary
  - Coronary insufficiency
  - Cerebrovascular arterial insufficiency
  - Peripheral arterial insufficiency or occlusion
  - Renal insufficiency
  - Encephalopathy and/or malignant hypertension
  - Congestive heart failure
- Tertiary
  - Cardiac enlargement
  - ECG abnormality
    - LVH/LVI
    - Positive exercise test
    - Arrhythmias and conduction disturbances
- Treatment failure
  - Accelerated hypertension

Abbreviations: *LVH*, left ventricular hypertrophy; *LVI*, left ventricular ischemia.

Table 4 Classification of Complications

- Hypertensive
  - Cerebral hemorrhage
  - Aortic dissection
  - Renal insufficiency
  - Encephalopathy or retinopathy grade III or IV
  - Malignant or accelerated hypertension
  - Cardiac enlargement
  - Left ventricular hypertrophy
- Atherosclerotic
  - Cerebral thrombosis
  - Myocardial infarction
  - Coronary insufficiency
    - Angina pectoris
    - ECG abnormality—ischemia, arrhythmias, and conduction disturbances
  - Claudication syndromes

IV. STATISTICAL DESIGN

The design provided for sequential (truncated binomial boundaries) and for life table analysis, the former to recognize the earliest possible stopping point should results favor either group and to minimize the required sample size. Subjects were randomly assigned to treatment or placebo and then matched by race and sex for two broad age groups (younger than age 46 and ages 46 to 55). This stratified randomization was carried out within each of the six participating clinical centers.

Morbidity data on which to base sample size and duration of follow-up were not available in the literature, so published survival rates were used. These were available both for mild to moderate hypertension (10–13) and for the general male population of the same age groups not dying of cardiovascular diseases (14). Curves were fitted to the survival rates for the two groups (Fig. 2), examination of which reveals that after ten years of follow-up, mild to moderate hypertensive patients had a survival rate of 65%, compared with 85% for the general male population (15).

To demonstrate with a high degree of confidence (α 0.05, β 0.05) that the survival rate of treated hypertensives was comparable to the normotensive population, it was calculated that 328 subjects (164 matched pairs) would be required in the truncated sequential design (16). This assumed that the magnitude of difference to be expected between the treated and nontreated groups would be of the same order of magnitude as illustrated in Figure 2.

Morbidity rates were expected to be somewhat higher than fatality rates, meaning that the desired degree of difference should be seen earlier. The estimate was 7 years,

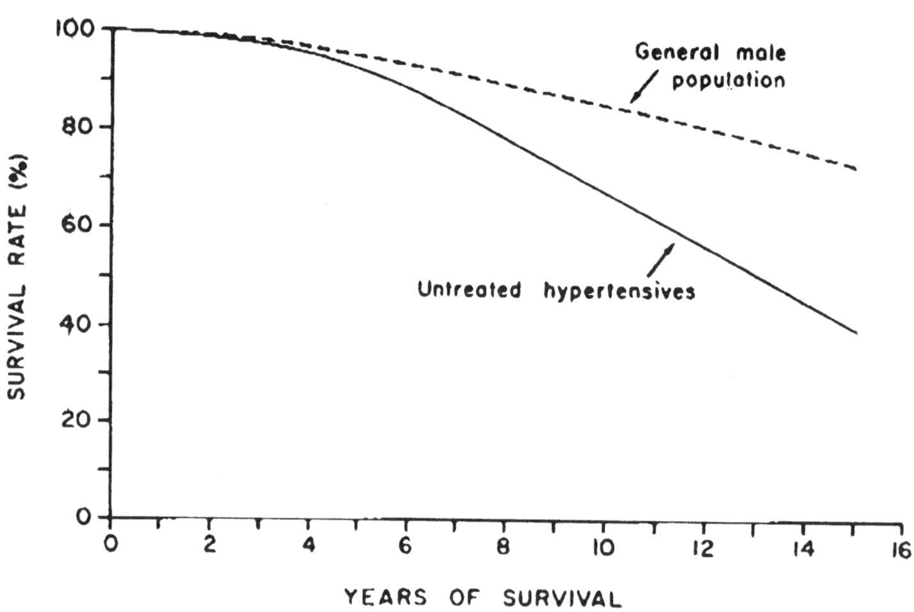

Fig. 2 Survival rates of mild to moderate hypertensive patients and general male population of initial age 45 to 49 years who did not die of cardiovascular diseases. *Source*: Ref. 15, published by permission of the American Heart Association.

and on the basis of anticipated dropouts over that period, a final sample size of 400 to 450 subjects was considered desirable.

V. CHARACTERISTICS OF THE STUDY POPULATION

Of 1600 potential candidates formally screened, 422 were entered into the study, 33 of whom were disqualified early as misadmissions, leaving 389 for follow-up and analysis. Of the nearly 1200 excluded during screening, the most common reason was failure to demonstrate sustained hypertension during the home pressure control period. Subjects averaged 44.4 years of age, with little variation of the distribution by race or gender. Men made up 80% of the total, three-fourths of whom were white. More than half had received no prior therapy for high blood pressure, and of those who had, 90% had responded satisfactorily. The distribution of these and all other pretreatment characteristics into the active and placebo groups by stratified randomization was uniform (Table 5).

A. Blood Pressure (Table 6)

Pretreatment home control blood pressure averaged 148/99 mm Hg, with the highest frequency in the distribution of systolic pressures in the range of 140 to 149 and 90 to 95 for diastolic pressures. It should be noted that 79.1% of the study population were in a group with pretreatment diastolic pressures in the range of 90 to 104 mm Hg.

B. Serum Chemistry

The average pretreatment serum cholesterol was 224 mg/dl, with only 9% of subjects exceeding 275 mg/dl. Uric acid levels were shifted upward in both men and women, with

Table 5 Pretreatment Characteristics

	Active		Placebo	
	Men (148)	Women (45)	Men (163)	Women (33)
Age (years)	44.3	44.3	44.6	43.9
Height (inches)	69.8	64.3	69.9	64.1
Weight (lb)	186.9	151.3	191.6	147.1
Serum cholesterol	228.7 (43.5)*	238.8 (44.7)	226.8 (41.5)	226.5 (39.1)
Serum uric acid	6.9 (1.4)	5.0 (1.3)	6.5 (1.5)	4.6 (1.2)
Serum creatinine	1.1 (0.2)	0.9 (0.3)	1.2 (0.3)	0.9 (0.2)
2-hour glucose	107.1 (19.4)	106.3 (19.0)	109.7 (18.2)	106.0 (18.2)

	Total		Active		Placebo	
	n	%	n	%	n	%
White	280	72.0	138	71.5	142	72.4
Nonwhite	109	28.0	55	28.5	54	27.6
Male	311	80.0	148	76.7	163	83.2
Cigarettes	182	46.7	89	46.1	93	47.4
Hypervoltage	64	16.4	26	13.4	38	19.3
Prior therapy	203	52.2	84	43.5	119	60.7

* ( ) = standard deviation.

Table 6 Control Blood Pressure

Pressure (mm Hg)	Total			Active treatment			Placebo treatment		
	No.		%	No.		%	No.		%
Subjects	389		100.0	193		100.0	196		100.0
Systolic									
< 140	105		27.0	52		26.9	53		27.0
140–159	216		55.5	111		57.5	105		53.6
160–179	60		15.4	29		15.0	31		15.8
180–199	6		1.5	1		0.5	5		2.6
>199	2		0.5	—		—	2		1.0
Average		147.8			146.8			148.7	
SD		13.5			12.4			14.5	
Diastolic									
90–95	152		39.1	77		39.9	75		38.3
96–100	91		23.4	41		21.2	50		25.5
101–105	66		17.0	31		16.1	35		17.8
106–110	41		10.5	23		11.9	18		9.2
111–115	39		10.0	21		10.9	18		9.2
Average		99.3			99.5			99.1	
SD		6.9			7.1			6.9	

Abbreviation: SD, standard deviation.

a mean of 6.2 mg%. The mean value for serum glucose 2 hours after a 100-g oral load was 107 mg%.

C. Electrocardiograms

Left ventricular hypertrophy (defined as hypervoltage) was found in 16.3% of subjects by at least one of three separate criteria. Left axis deviation minus 30 degrees or greater, (not an exclusion factor) was present in 12%.

All of these pretreatment variables distributed uniformly into the two treatment regimens. Furthermore their distributions by age, race, and gender resulted in no clustering whereby subgroups of excess or preferred risk occurred in either treatment group. Thus, it was concluded that on the basis of pretreatment characteristics, each group was potentially equally responsive to the therapeutic agents, and neither was at greater risk from factors other than blood pressure.

VI. RESULTS

Follow-up time in the study ranged from 78 to 108 months, averaging more than seven years. There was no differential dropout rate between the treatment and control groups (33.2% versus 34.7%). This applies to those who simply failed to return (Lost to Follow-up) as well as those who voluntarily ''withdrew'' from assigned therapy but remained under follow-up. The number for whom vital status was unknown was also similar in the two groups (14 versus 12).

A. Blood Pressure Control

Lowering of blood pressure in the active treatment group occurred promptly, was virtually complete in the first 6 months and, for those remaining on therapy, was sustained for the duration of follow-up. Group means for the two regimens at points in time over the entire period of follow-up are illustrated in Fig. 3. The average reduction in systolic pressure varied narrowly around 16 mm Hg, and diastolic was around 10 mm Hg, which was the equivalent of the differential in reduction between the two regimens, as the blood pressure in the placebo group remained essentially unchanged over the duration of the study (Table 7). Women of both races and whites of both sexes had the best response, whereas non-whites had the poorest.

B. Morbid Events

As noted above, the primary endpoints of death, stroke, and myocardial infarction were used in the sequential analysis that determined the earliest possible stopping point. No

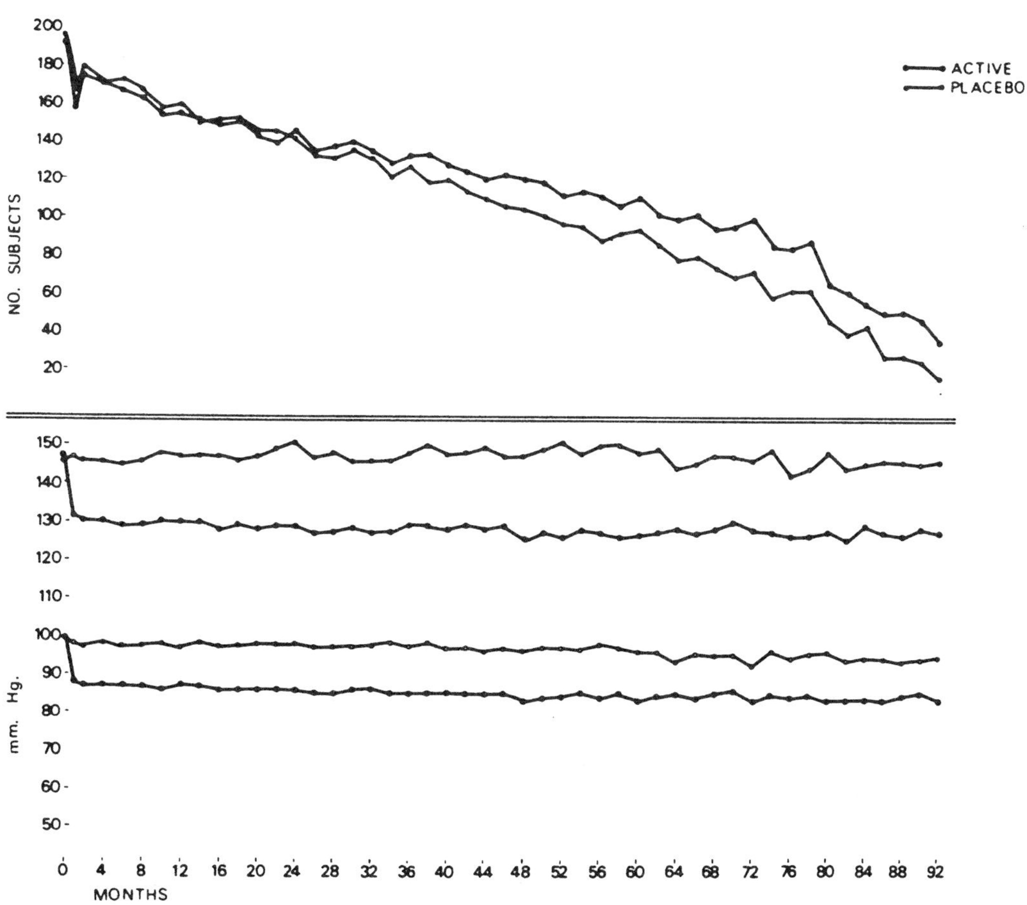

Fig. 3 Average blood pressure and number of subjects by regimen over time.

Table 7 Blood Pressure Change (All Subjects)

	Active			Placebo		
	X	SD	n	X	SD	n
Systolic						
Baseline (placebo control)	147.8	14.5	175	145.9	13.1	178
12 months	131.5	20.0		147.4	18.9	
Difference	−16.5	19.4		+1.5	16.7	
Diastolic						
Baseline	98.8	6.6		99.0	8.3	
12 months	88.4	11.3		98.4	11.9	
Difference	−10.4	11.4		−0.6	11.3	

Abbreviations: n, number of subjects; SD, standard deviation.

stopping point was reached in advance of the planned duration of the study. These major endpoints totaled 17 and were only slightly higher in the controls (9 versus 8) (Table 8). Moreover, the total deaths were fewer than predicted for the placebo group based on published mortality rates. There were six deaths overall, four in the placebo group, two of which occurred subsequent to the subjects having been switched to active therapy. One death in each group was a sudden death, the others subsequent to myocardial infarction. Two strokes occurred in the placebo group. Twelve subjects suffered nonfatal myocardial infarction as their first events, seven while taking active drugs and five taking placebo.

All first morbid events occurring during assigned regimens are shown in Table 9. Such events occurred in 151 of the 389 subjects, the rate in the active treatment group being 31 per 100 (59 of 193). This was about two-thirds that of those receiving placebo, which was 46.9 per 100 (92 of 196). There was no difference in the incidence of ''atherosclerotic'' events, all of the observed difference in endpoints being accounted for by reduction in ''hypertensive'' endpoints in the group receiving active antihypertensive agents. So-called hypertensive endpoints occurred at more than double the rate of atherosclerotic ones in the placebo group, with ECG and x-ray indicators of increased myocardial afterload (minor endpoints) accounting for nearly all the recorded events. Hypervoltage and left ventricular hypertrophy occurred most commonly, together with increased heart size on X-ray. As with myocardial infarction, angina pectoris, abnormal exercise ECGs, and other ECGs, abnormalities ascribable to coronary disease occurred with equal frequency in the treatment groups.

Table 8 Major Morbid Events

	Active	Placebo
Myocardial infarction		
Fatal	1	1
Nonfatal	6	5
Sudden death	1	1
Stroke	0	2
Total	8	9

Table 9 First Morbid Events While on Assigned Regimen

	Active			Placebo		
	n		%	n		%
Total patients on regimen	193			196		
Total patients with morbid events	59		30.6	92		46.9
Hypertensive	28		14.5	64		32.6
CVA		0			2	
Hypervoltage		8	4.1		23	12.2
Left ventricular hypertrophy		9	4.7		21	10.7
Cardiomegaly		11	5.7		15	7.7
Retinopathy		0			3	
Atherosclerotic	31		16.1		28	14.3
Myocardial infarction		5			6	
Death		1			1	
Other CHD		24	12.4		21	10.7
CVD-TIA		0			0	
Arterial insufficiency		1			0	
Treatment failures	0			12		6.1
Asymptomatic		0			7	
Symptomatic		0			5	

Abbreviations: *CVA*, cerebral hemorrhage; *CHD*, coronary heart disease; *CVD*, cerebral thrombosis; *TIA*, transient ischemic attack.

On the other hand, treatment failures without complications, that is, a progressive rise in blood pressure with or without symptoms, occurred exclusively in the group not receiving active antihypertensive agents. If these cases are added to the total of all other events, the event rate in the placebo group becomes 53%, which when compared to 30.6% in the active treatment group, yields an overall effectiveness (difference in percent incidence of complications between control and treatment groups divided by the percent incidence in the control group) of pressure lowering in preventing events of 48%. The effectiveness for "hypertensive" events alone is 56% and, when prevention of treatment failure is included, rises to more than 62%.

By design, the protocol allowed continued double-blind follow-up of subjects without change of regimen after sustaining any endpoint except stroke. Thus, most subjects were at continued risk for additional events. Others were followed up on known medications. During this continued follow-up, an additional 104 events occurred, resulting in a total of 255 events in 166 subjects. The distribution of these events by type and between the treatment groups was essentially the same as for first events on coded therapy. Six additional strokes (five in the placebo group) and four additional deaths occurred (Table 10).

C. Drug Adverse Effects

Based on an incidence of less than 10% of adverse drug reactions or intolerance leading to termination of therapy, it was concluded that the risk attributable to the therapy itself was minimal and acceptable. This conclusion was supported by the absence of a differential dropout rate between the active and placebo-treated groups.

Table 10 All Morbid Events Whether on Assigned or Known Drugs

	Active			Placebo		
	n	Rate/ 100 pts.	%	n	Rate/ 100 pts.	%
Total patients	193			196		
Total events	95	49.2	100.0	160	81.6	100.0
Hypertensive	46	23.8	48.4	104	53.1	65.0
CVA	1*			6	3.1	
Hypervoltage	12	6.2		27	13.8	
Left ventricular hypertrophy	14	7.3		34	17.3	
Cardiomegaly	16	8.3		24	12.2	
Retinopathy	2			9	4.6	
Renal insufficiency	1			2		
Congestive heart failure	0			2		
Atherosclerotic	49	25.4	51.6	56	28.6	35.0
Myocardial infarction	13	6.7		15	7.6	
Death	2			5		
Other CHD	32	16.6		35	17.8	
CVD-TIA	0			0		
Arterial insufficiency	2			1		
Treatment failures	0			24	12.2	
Asymptomatic	0			11		
Symptomatic	0			13		

* $X^2 = 2.265$; $P = 0.13$.

Abbreviations: *CVA*, cerebral hemorrhage; *CHD*, coronary heart disease; *CVD*, cerebral thrombosis; *TIA*, transient ischemic attack.

The overall incidence of adverse effects, based on serial side effects queries during the first one to five years (average follow-up, 33 months), was 42.7% in the active group and 22.3% in the placebo group. The dominant complaint was nasal congestion, with 20.5% in the active group and 11.1% in the placebo controls. No cases of mental depression were recognized. This favorable tolerance of the drug therapy occurred despite diuretic and rauwolfia dosages that were twice those currently recommended.

VII. SIGNIFICANCE OF THE STUDY

In subjects with mild hypertension without discernible target organ damage and with no other predisposing disorders, whose blood pressures were well controlled with antihypertensive agents, there was no reduction in fatal or nonfatal coronary heart disease when compared with placebo-treated controls over a period of nearly 2000 man-years of observation. Indeed, myocardial infarction occurred with equal frequency in the treated and controls whether only first events or all such events were considered.

On the other hand, active therapy was more than 50% effective in preventing the development of ECG evidence of left ventricular hypertrophy and radiographic cardiac enlargement. Although the numbers were too small (1 versus 6) to speak about rates with any confidence, the calculated rate of stroke in the placebo group of 36.4/10,000/year when compared with the 24.8/10,000/year in the National Pooling Project, is at least what might have been expected. Moreover, the difference, although having a 0.13 (X^2 2.26) probability of occurring on a chance basis, cannot be dismissed as unimportant. It should also be emphasized that treatment failure occurred exclusively in the placebo-treated group.

When these results were reported in 1977, their proper interpretation, particularly the failure to favorably impact the incidence of coronary heart disease events, was anything but clear. Was the premise incorrect that blood pressure-related risks for coronary heart disease were preventable? Or was the failure to demonstrate such an effect merely the result of too small a population followed up for too short a time, given its initial low-risk status? It was pointed out that although the control population had a much more favorable survival experience than projected (an observation noted in many subsequent studies), the expected number of major coronary events and strokes had occurred.

The investigators concluded that data from additional well-controlled trials were essential, and new trials should plan for much larger numbers of subjects followed up for longer periods. They cautiously suggested that, in view of the observed low total death rates in the control population in whom deaths due to cardiovascular complications did not exceed that expected in the general population, it was appropriate to consider deferral of drug therapy in such closely followed patients until signs of target organ damage or a progressive rise in blood pressure occurred.

Although it did not provide a definitive or comprehensive answer to the question it was designed to address, the PHS trial served to further define the dilemma, which would be the primary focus of clinical research and remained controversial among investigators in the field of hypertension over the ensuing decade.

World-wide appreciation of this dilemma had arisen somewhat independently and almost simultaneously by 1972 when seven groups in the United States, Australia, and Europe initiated therapeutic trials or feasibility studies in mild hypertension, all driven by the question of "to treat or not to treat?"

The cardiovascular unit of the World Health Organization and the International Society of Hypertension took the lead in establishing a program of information exchange and discussion among the studies, in the hope that certain uniformity of design and methods would strengthen conclusions. Together they convened the initial gathering of lead investigators in Madrid in March 1975. Dr. Ralph Reader, one of the investigators and President of the National Heart Foundation of Australia, served for many years as chairman of the liaison committee responsible for implementing the program, providing periodic reports of progress and interpretation of results. These studies were reported as work in progress at a conference entitled "Mild Hypertension: To Treat Or Not To Treat, sponsored by the New York Academy of Sciences in March 1978 (17).

The contributions of the Veterans Administration Trials, the Hypertension Detection and Follow-Up Program, the Australia Mild Hypertension Study, and the British Medical Research Council Trial, which were major contributors to resolution of the dilemma of mild hypertension, appear in subsequent chapters of this text.

Looked at in retrospect, it is clear that the results of the Public Health Service Hospitals Trial in Mild Hypertension were predictive of both the later definitive demonstrations of the benefits of treating mild hypertension and of the difficulties to be surmounted to do so. Subsequent studies all powerfully confirmed the preventability of the cerebrovascular complications of mild hypertension, as well as the prevention and reversibility of left ventricular hypertrophy, and demonstrated the reduction of total and cardiovascular mortality as well. Perhaps uniquely, and certainly underemphasized in ensuing years, was the clear demonstration in the Public Health Service study, that progression of mild hypertension to levels of higher risk is preventable by antihypertensive therapy that is safe and well tolerated.

Ultimately, and to a lesser degree than for stroke and congestive heart failure, the Hypertension Detection and Follow-Up Program demonstrated a reduction in both fatal and nonfatal myocardial infarction as well as in the incidence of angina pectoris. These findings have subsequently been demonstrated by studies in older populations with mild hypertension or isolated systolic hypertension.

PARTICIPANTS IN THE PHS COOPERATIVE STUDY

Principal Investigators, PHS Hospitals

Baltimore: J. Richard Warbasse, M.D., Richard J. Bouchard, M.D.
Boston: Richard H. Thurm, M.D.
New Orleans: Christfried Urner, M.D.
San Francisco: John A. Vaillancourt, M.D., Jeffrey M. Newman, M.D., M.P.H.
Seattle: Willard P. Johnson, M.D., Robert Wills, M.D.
Staten Island: Anthony N. Damato, M.D.

Coordinating Center (San Francisco): W. McFate Smith, M.D. (Director), Stanley Edlavitch, Ph.D., W. Mark Krushat, M.P.H.

Statistical Unit (Silver Springs, MD): Louis Bromer (Director), Julie Wagner, Lyla Rosloff, Annie Brown, Steven Schwab, Dr. Jerome Cornfield (Consultant)

Advisory Committee: Thomas R. Dawber, M.D., Walter M. Kirkendall, M.D., John R. McDonough, M.D., M.P.H. Mitchell Perry, M.D., Warren Winkelstein, M.D.

REFERENCES

1. Smith WM. U.S. Public Health Service Hospitals Cooperative Study Group: Treatment of mild hypertension. Results of a ten-year intervention trial. Circ Res (suppl I) 1977; 40:98–105.
2. Society of Actuaries. Build and blood pressure study. New York: Society of Actuaries, 1959.
3. Kannel WB, Schwartz MJ, McNamara PM. Blood pressure and risk of coronary heart disease: Framingham studies. Dis Chest 1969; 56:43.
4. Paul O. Risks of mild hypertension: ten-year report. Brit Heart J 1971; 33 (suppl):116.
5. Hamilton M, Thompson EN, Wisniewski TKM. Role of blood pressure control in preventing complications of hypertension. Lancet 1964; 1:235.
6. Leishman AWD. Merits of reducing high blood pressure. Lancet 1963; 1:1284.
7. Bjork S, Sannerstedt R, Falkheden T, Hood B. Effect of active drug treatment in severe hypertensive disease. Acta Med Scand 1961; 169:673.
8. Veterans Administration Cooperative Study Group on Antihypertensive Agents. Effects of treatment on morbidity in hypertension. JAMA 1967; 202:1028–1034.
9. Smith WM, Damato AN, Galluzzi NJ, Garfield CF, Hanowell EG, Stimson WH, Thurm RH, Walsh JJ, Bromer L. Evaluation of antihypertensive therapy-cooperative clinical trial method: I. Double-blind control comparison of chlorothiazide, rauwolfia serpentina, and hydralazine. Ann Intern Med 1964; 61:829.
10. Palmer RS, Loofbourrow D, Doering CR. Prognosis in essential hypertension: eight-year follow-up study of 430 patients on conventional medical treatment. N Engl J Med 1948; 239: 990.
11. Sokolow M, Perloff D. Prognosis of essential hypertension treated conservatively. Circulation 1961; 23:697.

12. Simpson FO, Gilchrist AR. Prognosis in untreated hypertensive vascular disease. Scot Med J 1958; 3:1.
13. Frant R, Groen J. Prognosis of vascular hypertension. Arch Intern Med 1950; 85:727.
14. National Center for Health Statistics. Vital Statistics of the United States, 1964, Vol. II: Mortality, part A. Washington, DC: DHEW, Public Health Service, 1966.
15. Smith WM. United States Public Health Service Cooperative Studies Group. Morbidity and mortality in mild essential hypertension. Circ Res (suppl II) 1972; 30, 31:110–124.
16. Armitage P. Sequential Medical Trials. Springfield, IL: Charles C Thomas, 1960.
17. Mild Hypertension: to treat or not to treat. Perry HM Jr, Smith WM, eds. Vol. 304. Ann NY Acad Sci, 1978.

3

The Hypertension Detection and Follow-Up Program

BARRY R. DAVIS and CHARLES E. FORD

The University of Texas–Houston School of Public Health, Houston, Texas

I. INTRODUCTION

In 1972, the National Heart, Lung, and Blood Institute (NHLBI, then known as the National Heart and Lung Institute) launched two major efforts to address the public health problem of high blood pressure (BP). One, the National High Blood Pressure Education Program, was established to inform the public and health care professionals about the known facts of high BP and its treatment to stimulate more awareness and aggressive treatment of the disease (1). The other effort, the Hypertension Detection and Follow-Up Program (HDFP), was a large-scale clinical study initiated to gain more facts and to resolve several unanswered questions about the treatment of high BP (2, 3). The National High Blood Pressure Education Program is still with us today; the HDFP has receded into the history of hypertension research. This chapter on the HDFP may remind older readers of the major contributions from the HDFP and help their younger colleagues appreciate the role HDFP played in establishing high BP treatment goals and imperatives that are accepted today as standards of care.

Our purpose is not to restate all the HDFP findings with regard to outcomes and subgroups. Numerous publications present these findings in detail (4–17). Rather, our purpose herein is to highlight some of the major findings and to present some new results with regard to combined outcomes and key subgroups. Specifically, we will focus on the overall group, the major subgroup of the lowest entry diastolic blood pressure (DBP) stratum (90 to 104 mm Hg, designated DBP stratum I), and the low risk DBP subgroup—those individuals with an entry DBP of 90 to 94 mm Hg who at entry were untreated and free of major end-organ damage.

II. PRIOR HYPOTHESIS AND WHY THE TRIAL WAS DONE

Since the late 1940s, epidemiologic and actuarial studies had sought to identify risk factors for cardiovascular morbidity and mortality (18–26). By the early 1960s, these studies had identified elevated BP as an important risk factor (26–30), and their findings led to the initiation of a placebo-controlled, randomized clinical trial by the United States Veterans Administration (VA) Cooperative Study Group on Antihypertensive Agents (31). The VA study is the focus of the first chapter of this book, which highlights its importance. The VA Study Group published the results of their trial in 1967, 1970, and 1971 (31–33). They demonstrated a significant benefit in reduction of morbidity and mortality from treating middle-aged, male hypertensive patients with an entry DBP of 115 to 129 mm Hg. Reductions in morbidity and mortality were also achieved in those subjects in the two DBP strata of 90 to 104 mm Hg and 105 to 114 mm Hg. However, in only the latter group were results statistically significant (32). In addition, the reduction in rate of major coronary events in the treated group as compared with the placebo group was not statistically significant. Although the trend was favorable, the sample size provided insufficient power to detect a difference in this lowest DBP stratum. This study among male veterans left unanswered the question of efficacy of antihypertensive treatment of women.

By the early 1970s, several sets of data from United States population surveys had found hypertension to be one of the most prevalent chronic diseases for which treatment was available and had indicated that about 85% of individuals with high BP were undetected, untreated, or inadequately controlled (34–39). The VA study, which had involved highly selected patients, left unanswered several questions:

1. Could hypertensives in an entire community be identified, brought under modern pharmacologic management, and kept under such management?
2. Would intervention of hypertension identified in the population of the community at large reduce the occurrence of associated disease and death?
3. Would therapeutic efficacy exceed toxicity in the mild hypertensive and justify long-term treatment?
4. Would pharmacologic control of elevated BP be effective in young adults and women?
5. Would the occurrence of myocardial infarction and coronary death be decreased by antihypertensive therapy?

Because of these major questions, the NHLBI appointed a special panel in October 1970 to assess the need for additional trials on control of hypertension. This panel recommended, "The first priority need is to determine the effectiveness of antihypertensive therapy in reducing morbidity and mortality from hypertension in the general population. Such studies should include both sexes, all races in a community, and preferably younger (adults) as well as middle age ranges. Such a study would not have a placebo group but could allow randomization of subjects for comparison of optimum drug regimens versus the customary medical care in the community." Acting on these recommendations, the NHLBI began planning for a multicenter, prospective, cooperative study of hypertension detection and therapy in community settings.

The HDFP was a national, multicenter, randomized, 5-year clinical trial of the effectiveness of antihypertensive therapy in reducing all-cause mortality in hypertensive participants screened from the general population. The study was funded under contract by the NHLBI. Participant recruitment for the trial began in February 1973 and was completed in May 1974 (40). Therapeutic intervention ended in June 1979. The 5-year findings of the HDFP were first reported in December 1979 shortly after the close of the trial (4, 5). Post-trial surveys of mortality, BP, and therapeutic status were continued through May 1982, when follow-up of participants terminated (17).

III. OBJECTIVES AND QUESTIONS DESIGNED TO ANSWER IN CONTEXT OF TIME

The primary objective of the HDFP was to determine whether systematic antihypertensive drug treatment of persons with high BP would result in a significant reduction in mortality from all causes over a 5-year period. To accomplish this, a projected total of 10,500 hypertensive participants were to be recruited into the clinical trial. Half the participants were to be randomly assigned to Stepped Care (SC) and half to Referred Care (RC). The SC group was offered antihypertensive therapy in special centers. Therapy was increased stepwise to achieve and maintain reduction of BP to or below set normotensive goals. The RC group was referred for treatment to usual sources of care, with special referral efforts for those with more severe hypertension or pre-existing organ system damage.

The secondary objectives of the HDFP were to determine (a) whether SC treatment would reduce the occurrence of cardiovascular causes of death, fatal and nonfatal stroke, electrocardiographic (ECG) abnormalities, in particular, new evidence of myocardial infarction (MI) and left ventricular hypertrophy (LVH), and other historical evidence of coronary heart disease; (b) possible adverse effects of antihypertensive medication in the SC program; (c) whether hypertensive participants, detected in a community screening program, could be brought under pharmacologic management and kept under such management long-term; and (d) whether pharmacologic control of elevated BP would be as effective in young adults and women, as had been demonstrated in the VA trials for middle-aged, white, and black males.

IV. PROTOCOL SUMMARY

The HDFP was planned as a multicenter clinical trial because of the need for several thousand participants. The study participants were randomized into two groups: SC or RC. A placebo assignment was considered ethically inappropriate in view of the VA Cooperative Study results.

Populations selected for the study were drawn from general population subgroups of the United States and included various age, race, sex, and socioeconomic strata. These populations were community based, and there was as complete a case finding of hypertensives as possible. Only terminally ill and institutionalized persons were excluded, and the selected population included adults from 30 to 69 years of age with an average home screening DBP of 95 mm Hg or above and a confirmed follow-up average DBP of 90 mm Hg or above (Table 1). There were no systolic BP entry criteria and no upper limits of BP.

The study required the periodic observation of all participants to assure their well being, accomplished in such a way as to minimize trial influence on those receiving RC. Data from all centers were pooled for analysis and, thus, had to be gathered uniformly and according to standardized protocols. The data were centrally processed, and there was an overall coordinating center for the operations.

Table 1 HDFP Inclusion and Exclusion Criteria

Inclusion Criteria
1. Men and women aged 30–69 years
2. Average home screening DBP ≥ 95 mm Hg
3. Confirmed follow-up DBP ≥ 90 mm Hg
Exclusion Criteria
1. Terminally ill patients
2. Institutionalized patients

The trial used a method of organization similar to that recommended by a committee of the National Advisory Heart Council (Fig. 1). Clinical centers in 14 communities in the United States were selected by competitive contract review to participate in the study. They were located at Atlanta, Georgia; Baltimore, Maryland; Birmingham, Alabama; Chicago, Illinois; Davis, California; Boston, Massachusetts; East Lansing, Michigan; Evans County, Georgia; Jackson, Mississippi; Los Angeles, California; Minneapolis, Minnesota; New York, New York; and Salt Lake City, Utah (Fig. 2). Also selected were a central laboratory (Chicago) for standardized determinations of participant biochemical values, an ECG center (Minneapolis) for standardized ECG interpretations, and a coordinating center (Houston) for (a) data collection; (b) monitoring and analysis; (c) standardization, staff training, and regulation of study protocol; and (d) overall project coordination. A steering committee composed of the principal investigators from each of the 14 clinical centers, the coordinating center, the biochemical laboratory center, and the ECG center, and an NHLBI staff representative directed the trial, meeting frequently. The coordinating center staff, in consultation with the officers of the steering committee and the NHLBI staff, monitored and supervised the day-to-day problems and progress of the study. A policy advisory board, composed of senior biomedical scientists not participating in the

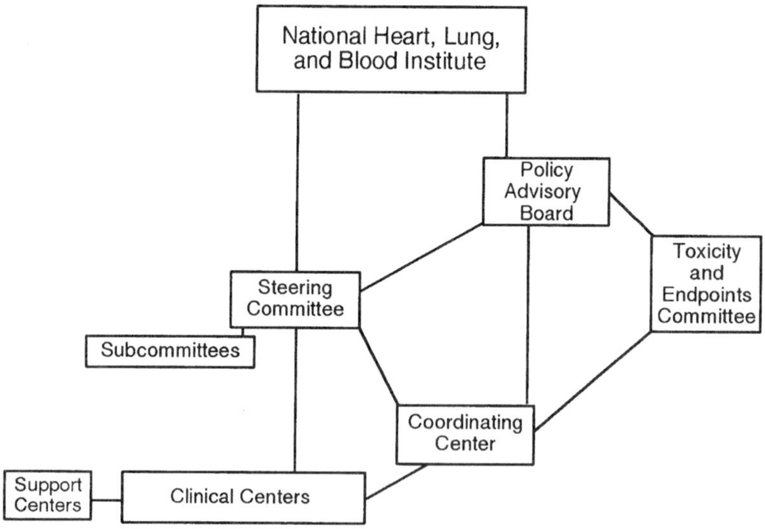

Fig. 1 Hypertension Detection and Follow-Up Program organization chart.

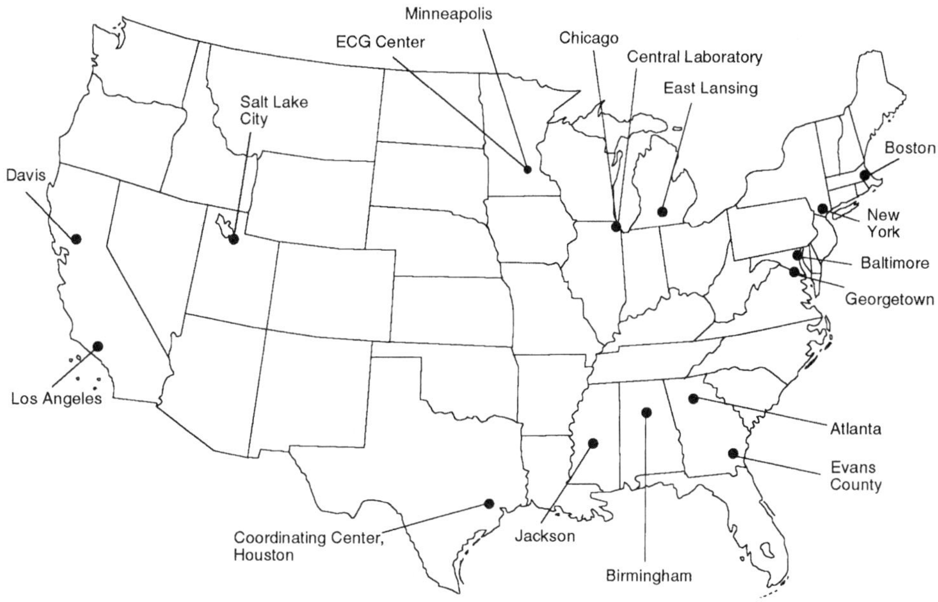

Fig. 2 Hypertension Detection and Follow-Up Program clinical sites and support centers.

program as investigators, acted in an advisory capacity on policy matters throughout the study. A toxicity and endpoints evaluation committee, reporting to the policy advisory board, monitored the trial throughout its course for drug toxicity and for any other unanticipated harm or risk to program participants.

Stepped Care participants were seen several times per year by the HDFP clinical staffs, whereas RC participants were seen only once a year. Therefore, a potential bias in ascertainment of nonfatal clinical outcomes and the determination of cause-specific mortality between the SC and RC groups could not be ruled out. All-cause mortality was selected as the primary endpoint, and every effort was made to ascertain the living status of each participant during the 5-year follow-up period. Because trial intake was staggered over 16 months, some SC participants were followed up for as long as 6.3 years, when trial follow-up was terminated on a common date. However, because comparable survival data were not available for the RC group beyond five years, mortality analysis was restricted to five years. A post-trial surveillance (PTS) study, conducted after the conclusion of the trial, extended the mortality follow-up of all participants to 8.3 years (17).

A. Participant Enumeration, Screening, and Recruitment

Each clinical center defined a population base for enumeration and screening of potential participants (41, 42). Thirteen of the 14 centers identified target populations on the basis of residential areas (census tracts, probability samples of larger areas, or entire housing projects); one center used employment rolls of industries. The purpose of the census enumeration was to prepare a roster of all household members and to identify those between the ages of 30 and 69. Home screening of those ages 30 to 69, which included a health status and health care interview plus BP measurements, then followed in the 13 communities and at the work site in the remaining center. Interviewers were trained to conduct these tasks in a standardized manner. The interview included education and employment status, basic demographic information, information on history of hypertension and its treatment, smoking history, history of heart attack, stroke, and diabetes, information on health beliefs, and status of current health care.

Blood pressures were measured with a standard mercury sphygmomanometer and an appropriate size cuff, with the participant seated and at rest for five minutes. Systolic BP was designated by the first phase Korotkoff sound and DBP was designated as the fifth phase Korotkoff sound (disappearance). To reduce the impact of regression toward the mean, two approaches were used. First, a higher DBP value was chosen for the first screen than for the final entrance criterion for the study. Second, each potential participant had his BP measured three times at each visit so that an average reading could be used to reduce biological variation. If, at the first screen, the average diastolic pressure of the second and third readings was 95 mm Hg or higher, the individual was invited to attend a clinic within a few days, if possible, for a second BP screen. This criterion was used regardless of current antihypertensive treatment status. A major effort was made to screen all enumerated age-eligible persons, and an overall success rate of 89% was obtained (40).

A second-stage screen was obtained in the clinic by taking four BP readings, again in the sitting position. The first and third readings were made with the standard mercury sphygmomanometer, and the second and fourth readings were obtained with the Hawksley ''Random-Zero'' manometer (Hawksley and Sons Limited, Sussex, England), a device that conceals the true zero point on the scale until after the measurement has been taken (43). The device was adopted to minimize observer biases. If the mean fifth phase DBP based on the second and fourth readings was 90 mm Hg or more, the individual was considered hypertensive for the purpose of the trial and randomized to the SC or RC group. A sealed randomization envelope was drawn sequentially and attached to the participant's data form. This sealed envelope contained the assignment of the participant to either the SC or RC group and remained sealed until after baseline examinations were completed.

All hypertensive participants underwent clinical evaluation at the second screen (first baseline clinic visit) as part of the baseline examination. At this visit, health history information, blood and urine analyses, an ECG, and a chest X-ray were obtained. A second baseline clinic visit was scheduled within a week or two, when repeat blood and urine specimens were collected, BP was measured, and a physical examination was administered. The randomization envelope was opened at this time, and the participant and clinic staff were informed of the random allocation.

The process of random allocation of confirmed hypertensive participants between SC and RC was directed and implemented by the coordinating center. Randomization was stratified by center and by three entry DBP strata: 90 to 104 mm Hg, 105 to 114 mm Hg, and 115 mm Hg or higher.

B. Therapeutic Regimen

Stepped Care participants were invited to participate in special HDFP clinics where antihypertensive care, medications, and laboratory tests were provided free of charge. Measures were undertaken to ensure maximum clinic attendance and medication adherence. These included short waiting times, conveniently scheduled appointments, provision of transportation services if needed, and a program physician availability at all times for hypertension-related problems.

Antihypertensive drug treatment was administered according to a standardized protocol. Participants with an entry DBP of 100 mm Hg or more or who were already on antihypertensive medication were assigned a goal pressure of 90 mm Hg or less, whereas those whose entry DBP ranged from 90 to 99 mm Hg were to achieve at least a 10 mm Hg reduction. This "goal blood pressure" was considered a minimum level of BP to be achieved rather than an optimal goal. It was to be achieved by prescribing antihypertensive drugs in a standardized, stepwise fashion. The therapy steps were as described below.

Step 0. No HDFP-prescribed medication.

Step 1. Chlorthalidone (25 to 100 mg/day). Triamterene (50 to 300 mg/day) or spironolactone (25 to 100 mg/day) could be prescribed as supplementary or alternative medication if indicated. If the goal was not reached, maximum durations were 4 weeks per dosage level and 12 weeks total for step 1.

Step 2. Addition of reserpine (0.1 to 0.25 mg/day). If reserpine was contraindicated, methyldopa (500 to 2,000 mg/day) could be substituted. If the goal was not reached, maximum durations were 4 weeks per dosage level and 12 weeks for step 2.

Step 3. Addition of hydralazine (30 to 200 mg/day). If the goal was not reached, maximum durations were 4 weeks per dosage level and 16 weeks maximum for step 3.

Step 4. Addition of guanethidine (10 to 200 mg/day). Reserpine, hydralazine, or both could be deleted at this step.

Step 5. Additional drugs (added only after step 4 failure). Duration was determined by a clinic physician.

Only drugs approved by the Food and Drug Administration were prescribed at steps 1 to 5. During the course of the trial, other newly approved FDA drugs were available for step 5 use, such as propranolol.

Stepped Care participants proceeded through these steps in accordance with their BP response. The aim was to bring each participant's pressure to goal as rapidly and safely as feasible with as little drug as possible. Exceptions to this basic plan were provided on the basis of history (e.g., depression) or specific adverse reactions. Most patients were not advanced beyond 50 mg of chlorthalidone because of a recognition of a lack of additional antihypertensive effect.

C. Follow-Up

Stepped Care participants were seen at intervals determined by their clinic status, but at least every four months and generally every two months. All SC and RC participants were seen at home at years 1, 2, 4, and 5 for a health history and BP measurements and at the clinic at years 2 and 5 for an examination similar to that at entry to the study. At each contact, any RC participant with DBP still 90 mm Hg or higher was advised to visit a physician. If severe hypertension (DBP 115 mm Hg or higher) or major organ system damage was present, special steps were taken to achieve contact with a physician.

An ECG [Minnesota Code (44)], standardized chest X-ray examination for heart size (45), and serum creatinine were obtained at years 0, 2, and 5 on each examined participant as objective measurements of end-organ damage and unbiased assessments of nonfatal secondary endpoints. Automatically timed, three-channel, 12-lead ECGs were obtained using machines that met the recording characteristic standards of the American

Heart Association Committee on Standards for Electrocardiographs. All ECGs were read at an ECG center by trained technicians using a modification of the 1973 Coronary Drug Project (46) revision of the Minnesota Code for Testing ECGs (44). Electrocardiograms were masked as to randomization group.

D. Ascertainment of Endpoints

Mortality. As previously noted, the primary endpoint of the HDFP trial was all-cause mortality. Thus, extensive efforts were made to ascertain the vital status of all participants at regular frequent intervals throughout the study. A special pilot project was carried out early in the trial on methodological approaches to accomplish this task (47). Determination of vital status was based first on surveillance of SC participants in regard to their clinic attendance and in accordance with their schedules of frequent appointments, and for RC participants in relation to planned annual contacts. Any person lost to follow-up was vigorously pursued to encourage continued participation or at least to determine vital status annually. Annual surveillance of death certificates was also carried out by each of the 14 clinics through local and state health departments and state offices of vital statistics. Death certificates were collected for all decedents, along with related autopsy reports and hospital records when available. The vital status of 99.5% of HDFP participants was known at the end of the trial in 1979. In 1982, as part of a posttrial surveillance study, a search for persons whose vital status was still unknown was conducted through the Social Security Administration and the newly established National Death Index (48). It was thus determined that three deaths not previously reported had occurred within the five years of randomization into the trial, one in the SC group and two in the RC group. These three deaths are included in the mortality analyses in this article.

Stroke. The total number of stroke cases ascertained during the 5-year follow-up included fatal and nonfatal strokes occurring in the SC and RC groups. Fatal strokes were identified by a nosologist using only information available from the death certificates. Death certificates assigned Eighth Revision International Classification of Diseases (ICDA) (49) codes 430 to 438 were counted as fatal strokes.

Nonfatal strokes were identified by means of a stroke questionnaire administered during the final clinic evaluation to all SC and RC participants who had survived for five years after randomization (7). The study investigators recognized two possibly serious sources of bias that might interfere with the clinical ascertainment of nonfatal stroke. One source of bias was the fact that physicians from the 14 clinical centers were not equally trained in neurology, and there might be variation in the diagnosis of stroke. A second potential bias existed because of the study design itself. Because SC participants were seen in the clinics far more frequently than RC participants, the chances of detecting either historical or neurological evidence of stroke were enhanced in the SC population. Hence, a stroke questionnaire was developed as an objective method for ascertainment of nonfatal stroke. The administration of this questionnaire by trained interviewers at the end of year 5 reduced the likelihood of these two potential sources of bias. The completed questionnaires were reviewed and evaluated by a board-certified neurologist, blinded as to randomization-assignment of the participants.

Questionnaire findings were classified as positive by the neurologist if the episode of focal neurological deficit was a clearly described event, referable to one of the recognized territories supplied by the major cerebral vessels, with sudden or rapid onset and lasting more than 24 hours. Further division of strokes into subterritories of the vessels or into hemorrhagic versus occlusive types was not feasible based on the questionnaire information.

Fatal coronary heart disease (CHD). Death certificates assigned ICDA 410 to 414 were counted as fatal CHD events.

Nonfatal MI. Unless otherwise specified, the incidence of nonfatal myocardial infarction is defined as either (a) serial ECG changes, (b) history of MI, or (c) Rose Questionnaire MI (50). A detailed report of these findings can be found elsewhere (8).

Electrocardiographic LVH. Electrocardiographic evidence of LVH was based on voltage and repolarization changes seen in limb and chest leads of a standard 12-lead ECG using Minnesota Code (44) criteria. An incident case was required to be free of LVH at baseline (11).

Angina pectoris (AP). Data provided by the Rose Questionnaire at baseline and during subsequent interviews at the end of years two and five were used to estimate 5-year incidence of AP among those participants who had a negative history of AP at baseline (8).

Renal insufficiency. The diagnosis of renal insufficiency was based on serum creatinine change from baseline to year 5. Renal insufficiency was defined as a fifth-year serum creatinine value of 2.0 mg/dl or more and at least 25% greater than the baseline value (12).

Electrocardiographic ischemia. Electrocardiographic evidence of myocardial ischemia was based on criteria used in the Whitehall study (51, 52). An incident case had to be free of such ECG ischemia at baseline.

E. Combined Endpoints

5-year fatal and nonfatal outcomes were used to define three classes of combined endpoints:

1. *Combined total endpoints*: Death, nonfatal stroke, nonfatal MI (including Rose Questionnaire MI), ECG LVH, angina, ECG ischemia, or renal insufficiency
2. *Combined major trial endpoints*: Death, nonfatal stroke, nonfatal MI, ECG LVH, or renal insufficiency
3. *Combined cardiac endpoints*: Fatal CHD, nonfatal MI (ECG criteria or history), or ECG LVH

F. Baseline End-Organ Damage

The definition of end-organ damage at entry included the presence of any of the following at the baseline examination: ECG LVH, a history or ECG evidence of MI, a history or clinical evidence of stroke, a history of intermittent claudication, and a serum creatinine greater than 1.7 mg/dl (>150 μmol/L) (7).

G. Sample Size

A sample size of 10,500 participants was estimated for the HDFP. This number was based on the following assumptions:

1. The primary endpoint would be all-cause mortality.
2. Based on the U.S. Pooling Project and United States population mortality data, 5-year mortality in the RC group would be 96/1000.

3. The expected reduction in mortality for the SC group would be 40% for those adhering to therapy and remaining in the SC program for 5 years.
4. Over the 5 years of follow-up, 50% of the SC group would drop out of the program in the following pattern: 25% in the first year, 10% in the second year, and 5% in each of the last 3 years.
5. After allowing for overall SC dropout plus nonadherence to prescribed therapy, the anticipated net reduction in total mortality rate for the entire SC group was 17.7%.
6. A two-tailed significance level (alpha) of 0.05 and a power of 0.90 would be used.

These assumptions and estimations yielded a sample size of 10,500 hypertensives, aged 30 to 69, 5250 to be randomized to SC and 5250 to RC. Actually, 10,940 participants (5,485 in SC and 5,455 in RC) were enrolled in the program after screening 159,468 individuals.

H. Statistical Methods

Standard life table methods (53) were used to compute the cumulative, all-cause mortality rates for the three intervals of trial and posttrial follow-up reported herein. Specifically, the estimated cumulative proportion dying was computed as one minus the cumulative proportion surviving, using the Cutler-Ederer estimator for the probability of surviving successive 4-month intervals (54). Although it did not take into account exact survival time, the Cutler-Ederer estimator assumes that on average, participants lost or ''withdrawn alive'' survive half the interval in which they withdraw. Participants were considered as ''withdrawn alive'' if they were known to be living on or after the date for which they were last scheduled for contact and if their duration of follow-up was less than that of the life table. Participants whose living status could not be determined after some point in time (within the period covered by the life table) were considered lost to follow-up as of the next successive interval. In the life table analyses of trial mortality, the start of treatment was defined as the date of randomization. For living participants, the respective fifth anniversary of a participant's entry into the trial defined the end of 5-year follow-up. In the 6.7-year life table analysis, the end of trial follow-up was defined as November 30, 1979. In the 8.3-year life table analysis, the date of randomization and the end of the PTS study follow-up were used to demarcate the period of follow-up. The end of PTS study follow-up was defined as the date the participant was last scheduled for contact, that is, home visitation or contact by mail or telephone.

The life table analysis for the full trial period was truncated after 80 months (6.7 years). Only 427 SC and 403 RC participants had any trial follow-up experience beyond 80 months and were withdrawn alive in the next 4-month interval.

Follow-up during the PTS was from 18 to 30 months, but less than one-third of the population was followed up for more than 24 months, and the majority of these participants were withdrawn alive in the 25th and 26th months. To avoid giving too much weight (or too little) to deaths among this declining subset of the PTS study population, the life table was truncated after 100 months (8.3 years; 24 months of PTS study follow-up).

The stroke and combined endpoints analyses were restricted to 5-year trial follow-up because only data on mortality were collected beyond the fifth year of follow-up. A participant who had one or more of the included fatal or nonfatal events during the five years of HDFP follow-up was counted only once as having had a stroke or combined trial endpoint. The time of occurrence for events, other than death, was not generally known. However, all surviving participants had a minimum of five years of follow-up, and 5-year incidence rates, in general, were used in the stroke and combined endpoint analysis.

The 5-year incidence rates of stroke and combined trial endpoints were adjusted by the direct method for distributional differences between the SC and RC cohorts in age, race, and sex using the standard population of the combined SC and RC groups. In comparisons of the two randomized groups (SC and RC), the relative difference in the occurrence of an event was calculated by the formula:

$$\frac{RC - SC}{RC} \times 100 \tag{1}$$

which is the percent reduction in risk. Differences in incidence rates between the SC and RC groups were tested for statistical significance by using standard normal (two-sided) tables. No adjustment for multiple comparisons was done.

The denominators used in the computation of incidence rates are the total cohort at risk at baseline, including those who had incomplete ascertainment of endpoints during the follow-up period. The observed differences in incidence rates between SC and RC, therefore, may be biased, that is, true RC rates may be underestimated to a greater extent than SC rates because of the larger number of RC individuals with incomplete information. If both groups had similar amounts of missing information, the absolute and relative differences between the two treatment groups would be greater.

V. RESULTS

A. Population Screening

Defined populations in 14 communities of varied composition across the United States were enumerated and screened by HDFP from February 1973 through May 1974. From a base population of 442,056 residents of households and employees, the HDFP clinical center staffs identified and enumerated 178,009 men and women aged 30 to 69. Of these, 89% (159, 566) completed the first screen (Fig. 3). Based on the last two of three BP readings, 22,994 (14.5%) had a mean fifth phase DBP of 95 mm Hg or higher and were invited to the HDFP centers for a second screening. Although some individuals declined this invitation to a clinic visit, the majority, 17,499 (76.1%), underwent rescreening. Of these, 11,386 (65.1%) were found to have a mean DBP of 90 mm Hg or above (average of two random zero readings), were designated hypertensive, and were assigned randomization envelopes. However, a systematic violation of the randomization procedure that occurred at one center toward the end of the intake period forced the elimination from analyses of all data on 446 randomized participants. These individuals were all randomized after a specific date, and other than reducing the HDFP sample, they did not affect the validity of the randomization procedure. They continued to have follow-up in the local center, but their data were not pooled with those of the remaining 10,940 properly randomized participants.

The great majority of the 10,940 trial participants (71.5%), as expected (26–30), were in DBP stratum I (90 to 104 mm Hg) (Fig. 3); 18.8% were in stratum II (105 to 114 mm Hg), and 9.7% were in stratum III (115 mm Hg or greater). Stratum III included 140 participants with DBP greater than 129 mm Hg and 124 participants with SBP greater than 219 mm Hg. Another 71 participants with SBP greater than 219 mm Hg were random-

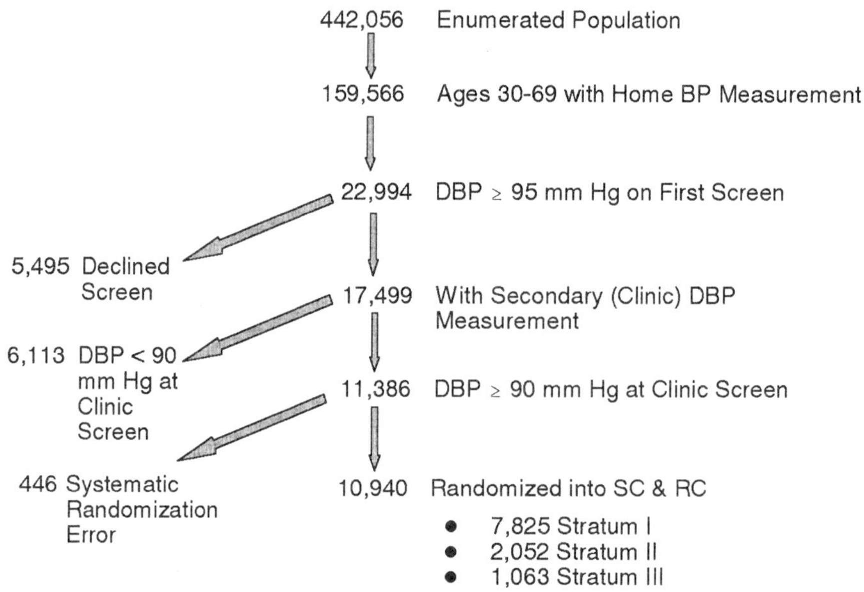

Fig. 3 Number of persons enumerated, screened, and randomized by Hypertension Detection and Follow-Up Program.

ized into strata I and II. Trial participants were followed for 5-year mortality experience, as originally planned.

B. Baseline Comparability of SC and RC Groups

Data on comparability at entry of SC and RC groups overall, for DBP stratum I, and for the low-risk subgroup are shown in Table 2 for a set of variables of potential prognostic import. Overall, differences between the SC and RC for these and other variables were small, indicating the effectiveness of the randomization procedure. This comparability of the RC and SC groups was also true for DBP strata II and III, and for age, race, sex, and other DBP end-organ damage subgroups (55, 56). Compared to overall and DBP stratum I, the low-risk subgroup had a slightly lower mean age, more whites, fewer blacks, fewer participants with a history of diabetes or elevated fasting blood sugar, fewer with Rose Questionnaire angina or MI, fewer with ECG ischemia, and higher levels of education and current employment.

C. Pharmacological Treatment and DBP Response of the SC and RC Groups

The proportion of individuals who were on antihypertensive medication throughout the trial are displayed in Figure 4, overall and for the two highlighted subgroups. For the trial overall and for DBP stratum I, about 25% to 26% of both the RC and SC participants were taking antihypertensive medications at baseline. By the end of the first year, about 80% of the SC group overall and for DBP stratum I were on treatment and remained so throughout the trial. Community treatment of RC participants also began to increase after entry and reached about 65% overall and 60% for DBP stratum I by the trial's end.

Table 2 Baseline Characteristics of Stepped and Referred Care Participants

	All		DBP 90–104		Untreated, free of major EOD at entry DBP 90–94	
Baseline Characteristic	SC	RC	SC	RC	SC	RC
Sample Size	5485	5455	3903	3922	1021	1022
Average age, years	50.8	50.8	50.7	50.7	49.5	49.3
White men, %[a]	34.6	34.2	38.5	37.5	44.4	41.9
Black men, %	19.4	19.9	16.9	17.3	15.6	15.9
White women, %[a]	21.5	21.1	23.4	23.5	23.2	25.0
Black women, %	24.5	24.9	21.2	21.7	16.8	17.2
Systolic BP, mean mm Hg	159.0	158.6	151.9	151.2	145.5	144.5
Diastolic BP, mean mm Hg	101.1	101.2	96.3	96.4	92.0	92.0
Pulse rate, mean beats/min	81.7	82.3	81.2	81.8	81.4	81.7
Serum cholesterol, mmol/L[b]	6.080	6.087	6.054	6.072	6.038	6.015
Body mass index, kg/m^2	28.3	28.5	28.2	28.3	27.7	28.0
Taking antihypertensive medication, %	26.3	25.7	25.5	24.7	0.0	0.0
Cigarette smoker, %	38.6	38.9	36.9	37.5	36.8	39.6
FBS $\geq$ 7.771 mmol/L, %[b]	4.5	4.8	4.6	4.7	3.6	3.0
History of diabetes, %	6.6	7.5	6.7	7.3	4.1	5.2
Rose Questionnaire AP, %	7.5	7.2	6.9	7.0	6.0	3.9
Rose Questionnaire MI, %	5.5	5.5	5.6	5.2	3.5	4.0
ECG ischemia, %	19.3	19.1	16.2	16.2	8.0	9.8
High school graduate, %	50.3	51.3	53.3	54.7	55.1	59.2
Currently employed, %	63.6	64.4	65.3	65.9	69.7	70.7
Major end-organ damage, %	14.9	14.5	13.0	11.9	0.0	0.0
ECG MI, %	1.1	1.0	0.9	0.7		
History of MI, %	5.1	5.2	4.7	4.8		
Stroke, %	2.5	2.5	2.1	2.1		
Major LVH, %[c]	4.8	5.1	3.4	3.6		
Serum creatinine $\geq$ 150.28 μmol/L, %[b]	2.9	2.5	2.4	1.9		
Intermittent claudication, %	1.3	1.3	1.3	1.0		

[a] Includes less than 1% others, e.g., Asians.

[b] Equivalent metric units: FBS, 7.771 mmol/L = 140 mg/dl; serum creatinine, 150.28 μmol/L = 1.7 mg/dl. The metric conversion factor for serum cholesterol is 38.66976 mg/dl per mmol/L.

[c] Based on combined R wave and ST-T segment changes: tall R wave (Minnesota code 3.1) and major ST segment depression (Minnesota code 4.1–4.3) or major T wave inversion (Minnesota code 5.1–5.3).

Abbreviations: *EOD*, end-organ damage; *DBP*, diastolic blood pressure; *SC*, stepped care; *RC*, referred care; *BP*, blood pressure; *FBS*, fasting blood sugar; *AP*, angina pectoris; *ECG*, electrocardiogram; *MI*, myocardial infarction; *LVH*, left ventricular hypertrophy.

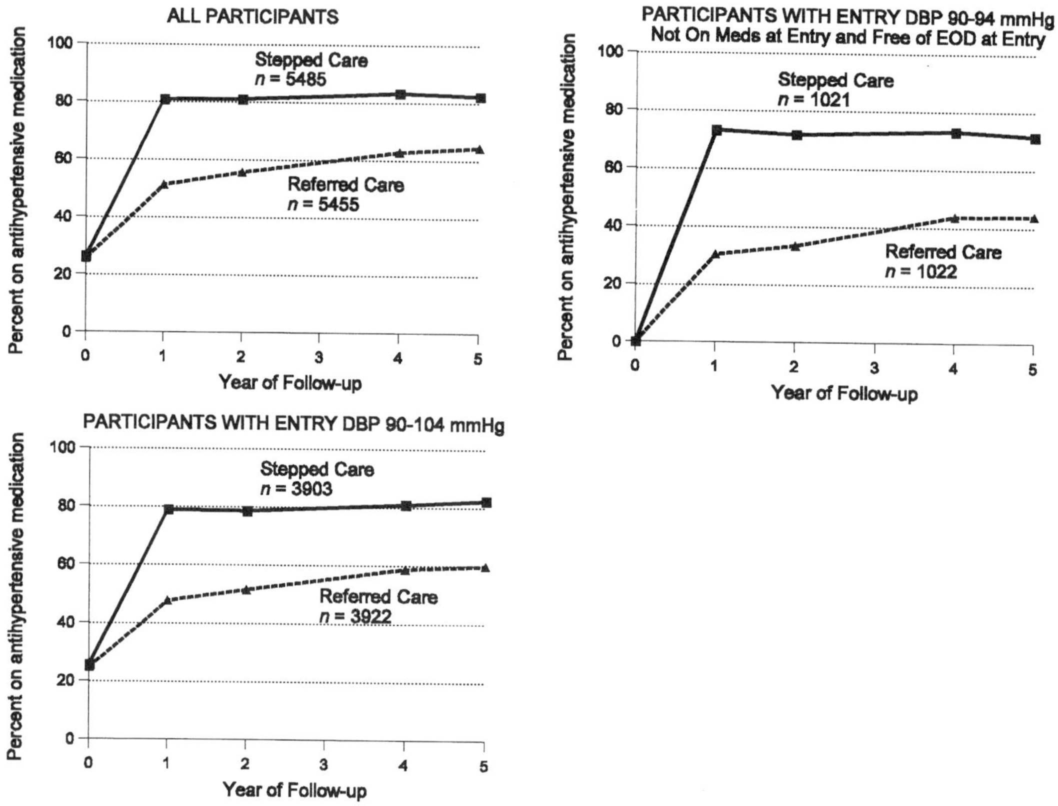

Fig. 4 Percent of participants on antihypertensive medication at entry and at annual home visits.

Within the low-risk subgroup, at baseline no one in the RC or SC group was receiving antihypertensive medication. By the end of the first year, about 73% of the SC group were on treatment and remained so throughout the trial. Community treatment of RC participants also began to increase after entry and reached about 44% by the trial's end.

The DBP and SBP responses of the RC and SC groups are displayed in Figure 5 overall and for the two highlighted subgroups. For the trial overall, the mean baseline SBP/DBP was 159/101 mm Hg in both groups. The greatest decrease in BP occurred in the first year and generally decreased slowly thereafter in both SC and RC groups. In the SC group, BP at year 1 was 133/88 mm Hg and decreased to 130/84 mm Hg by year 5. In the RC group, BP was 145/94 mm Hg at year 1 and 140/89 mm Hg at year 5.

Within stratum I, the mean baseline SBP/DBP was 152/96 mm Hg in both groups. As with the overall results, the greatest decrease in BP occurred in the first year and generally decreased slowly thereafter in both SC and RC groups. In the SC group, BP at year 1 was 131/86 mm Hg and decreased to 129/83 mm Hg by year 5. In the RC group, it was 142/92 mm Hg at year 1 and 138/88 mm Hg at year 5.

Within the low-risk subgroup, the mean baseline SBP/DBP was 146/92 mm Hg in the SC group and 144/92 mm Hg in the RC group. In the SC group, BP at year 1 was 127/84 mm Hg, decreasing to 127/82 mm Hg by year 5. In the RC group, it was 138/90 mm Hg at year 1 and 135/89 mm Hg at year 5.

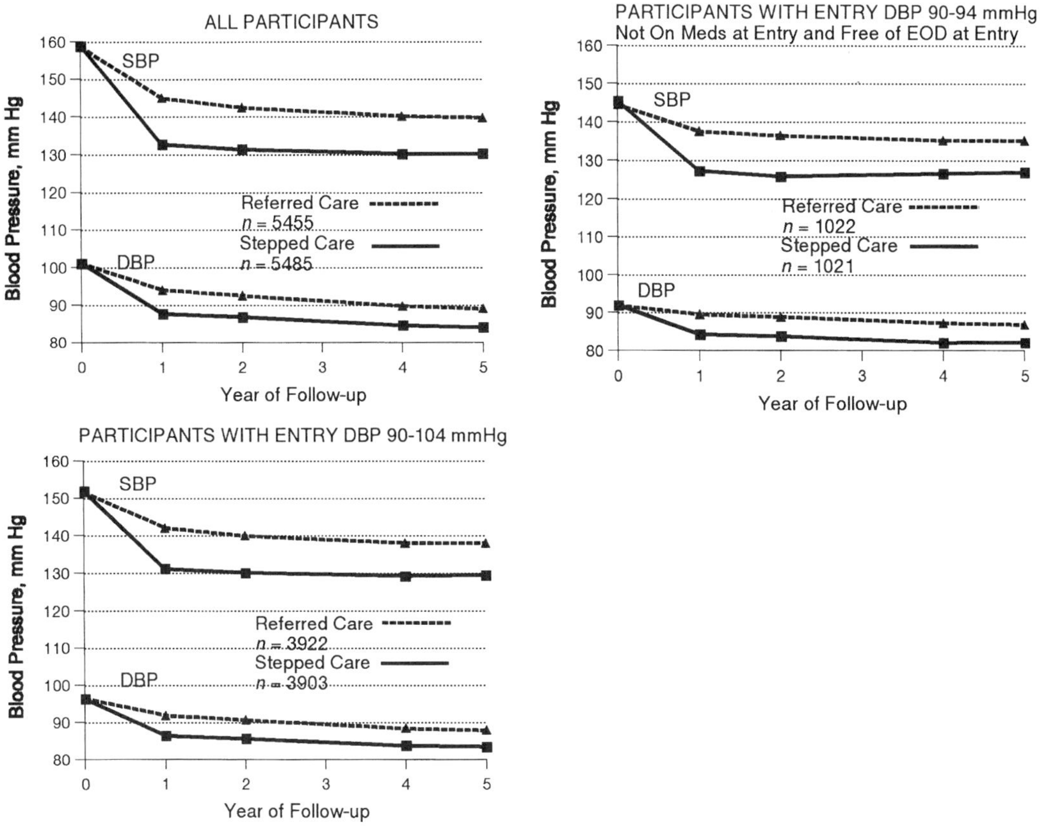

Fig. 5 Mean systolic blood pressure (SBP) and diastolic blood pressure (DBP) for stepped care (SC) and referred care (RC) participants at entry and at annual home visits.

D. Clinic Follow-Up of SC Group

A high percentage of the SC participants remained active in the HDFP over the five years of follow-up, as shown in Figure 6. During the trial, more than 80% of the SC participants continued to receive medication, and more than 80% achieved blood pressure levels within the normotensive range, at or below the HDFP diastolic goal. After 12 months of follow-up, most of these individuals were on a drug regimen that remained constant for the rest of the trial (57). After one year, more than 40% of the SC group were on step 1 monotherapy with a diuretic drug, principally chlorthalidone. At entry, 26% of the SC participants were currently on antihypertensive drugs, which is reflected by the percentages of participants initially on a regimen above step 1. The changing regimen pattern reflects both the shift from non–HDFP-prescribed drugs to HDFP prescriptions and the stepped advance in drug regimen in accordance with individual BP responses.

The HDFP SC participants formed one of the largest groups for which there was detailed surveillance of long-term antihypertensive treatment and drug adverse effects. During the 5-year follow-up, SC participants made 172,569 clinic visits to the 14 HDFP clinical centers. At the end of trial, nearly 80% of SC participants were active in the program. Blood pressure control to defined BP goals was a key objective of HDFP clinic

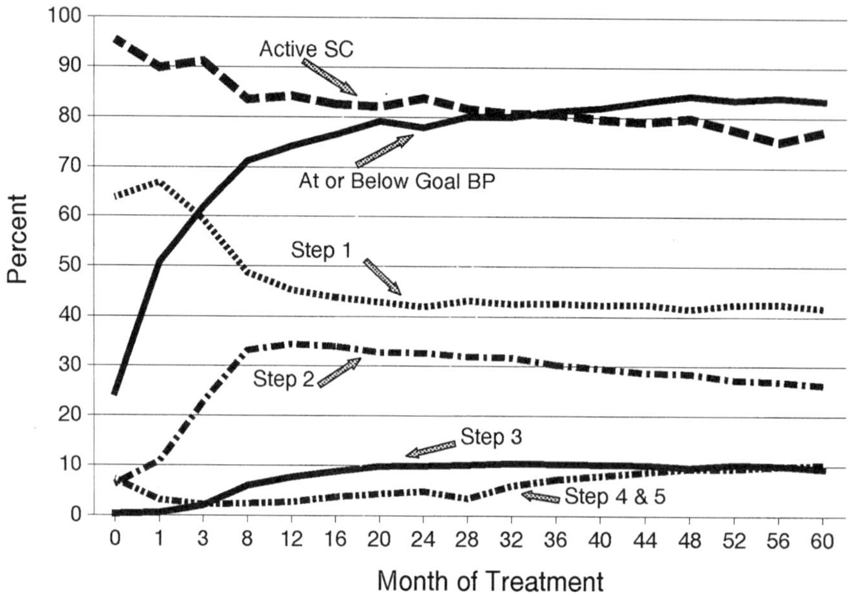

Fig. 6 Percentage of stepped care (SC) (n = 5485) participants with clinic follow-up visits (active SC) by month of follow-up; the percentage of ''active SC'' on specific drug steps and at or below their goal diastolic blood pressure.

staffs, who made every effort to help participants achieve and maintain their respective goal levels. During the course of the trial, about one-third of the active SC participants experienced at least one possible adverse reaction to a medication that prompted the clinical therapist to discontinue the use of one or more drugs; 40% of these individuals had more than one such event (58). The incidence of adverse effects declined over the five years. The occurrence of definite or probable adverse effects during the trial, however, was considerably less frequent (<10%). There were few life-threatening side effects, and no deaths could be directly attributed to drug side effects (58). Only 23 individuals were hospitalized for suspected side effects. In 14 cases, chlorthalidone was implicated as at least a possible cause. Thus, the HDFP confirmed the relative safety of long-term antihypertensive therapy, which was one of the secondary objectives of the program (58).

E. Mortality from All Causes

Numbers of deaths and 5-year death rates for the total SC and RC groups and by entry DBP stratum are given in Table 3. Vital status was ascertained for 99.5% of all participants. All-cause mortality was significantly less for the total SC group compared with the RC group ($P = 0.006$). For every major subgroup listed, a reduction was noted. This was evident particularly for DBP stratum I ($P = 0.007$). These statistically significant differences persisted after multivariate adjustment for the minor differences between SC and RC groups in entry characteristics of potential prognostic import (59). The 5-year mortality was 17.3% less for all SC participants compared with RC participants and 20.2% lower for SC com-

Table 3 All-Cause Mortality

Subgroup	Sample size SC	Sample size RC	Deaths SC	Deaths RC	Life table death rates per 1000 (SE) SC	Life table death rates per 1000 (SE) RC	95% Confidence limits for difference in RC and SC rates	Percent reduction in mortality for SC group	*P* value
Total	5485	5455	350	421	63.9 (3.3)	77.3 (3.6)	(3.80, 23.00)	17.3	0.006
DBP stratum									
90–104 mm Hg	3903	3922	232	292	59.5 (3.8)	74.6 (4.2)	(4.03, 26.17)	20.2	0.007
105–114 mm Hg	1048	1004	70	78	66.9 (7.7)	77.9 (8.5)	(−11.45, 33.45)	14.1	0.337
≥ 115 mm Hg	534	529	48	51	90.0 (12.4)	96.6 (12.8)	(−28.37, 41.57)	6.8	0.711
Sex									
Men	2961	2949	223	266	75.4 (4.9)	90.4 (5.3)	(0.94, 29.06)	16.6	0.036
Women	2524	2506	127	155	50.4 (4.4)	61.9 (4.8)	(−1.22, 24.22)	18.6	0.076
Race									
White	3076	3014	168	181	54.7 (4.1)	60.2 (4.3)	(−6.19, 17.19)	9.1	0.356
Black	2409	2441	182	240	75.6 (5.4)	98.4 (6.0)	(6.95, 38.65)	23.2	0.005
Age									
30–49	2427	2371	81	82	33.4 (3.6)	34.7 (3.8)	(−8.97, 11.57)	3.7	0.804
50–59	1856	1912	116	160	62.5 (5.6)	83.8 (6.3)	(4.70, 37.90)	25.4	0.012
60–69	1202	1172	153	179	127.3 (9.6)	152.8 (10.5)	(−2.42, 53.42)	16.7	0.073
Baseline meds									
On meds	1444	1403	132	144	91.5 (7.6)	102.7 (8.1)	(−10.56, 32.96)	10.9	0.313
Not on meds	4041	4052	218	277	54.0 (3.6)	68.5 (4.0)	(4.06, 24.94)	21.2	0.006
EOD status									
With EOD	817	792	125	148	153.1 (12.6)	187.0 (13.9)	(−2.80, 70.60)	18.1	0.070
Without EOD	4668	4663	225	273	48.3 (3.1)	58.7 (3.4)	(1.27, 19.53)	17.7	0.026
No meds, without EOD									
DBP 90–94 mm Hg	1021	1022	36	54	35.3 (5.8)	52.9 (7.0)	(−0.19, 35.39)	33.3	0.052

Mortality from all causes for stepped care and referred care participants during 5-year follow-up, by diastolic blood pressure at entry, sex, race, age, use of antihypertensive medication (meds) at entry, and presence of major end organ damage at entry.

Abbreviations: *SC*, stepped care; *RC*, referred care; *DBP*, diastolic blood pressure; *Meds*, medication; *EOD*, end-organ damage.

pared to RC participants of DBP stratum I. The relative mortality benefit decreased with increasing DBP strata, reflecting the benefit RC participants in the two upper BP strata received from drug treatment prescribed by their personal physicians (56). The reduction was an impressive 33.3% for the low-risk subgroup, although the mortality difference was not statistically significant ($P = 0.052$).

Figures 7 and 8 present the cumulative mortality curves for the HDFP SC and RC participants at 5, 6.7, and 8.3 years of follow-up. As described in the protocol summary, the original mortality analysis was restricted to a common 5-year follow-up of all participants because comparable survival data were not available on the RC group beyond five years. After the HDFP trial was completed, the PTS study was conducted to collect comparable data on mortality for both the SC and RC participants (17). A second analysis of mortality data on RC and SC participants extended the results to 6.7 years. The SC rates were lower than those for RC in each year of the study and continued to show a significant difference through 6.7 years, at which time the SC rate was 18.2% lower than RC ($P < 0.001$) (17). The PTS study also provided data on mortality through 8.3 years after trial entry and demonstrated a continued separation of the mortality curves and a continued significant 15.0% reduction in mortality in the SC group compared to the RC ($P < 0.001$) three years after the trial concluded (17).

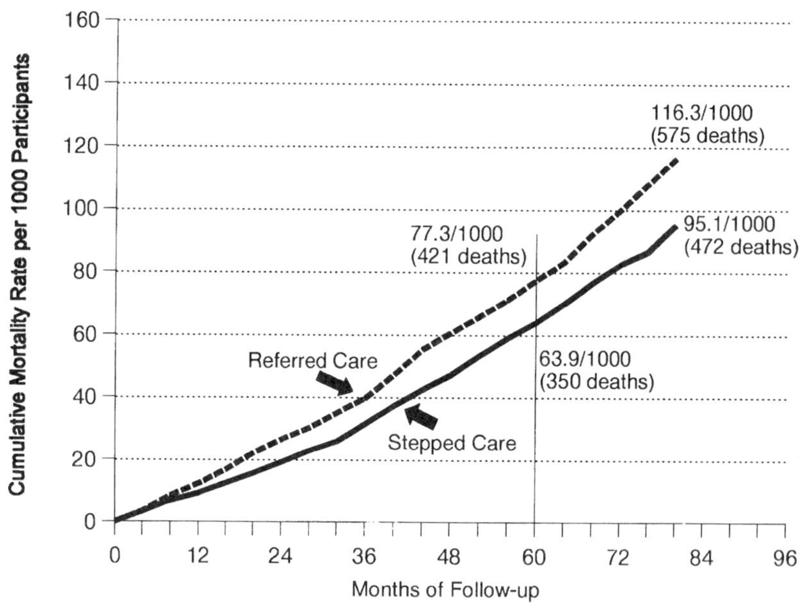

Fig. 7 Hypertension Detection and Follow-Up Program cumulative, life table, all-causes death rates in stepped care (n = 5485) and referred care (n = 5455) participants. All participants were followed up to a common 5-year trial termination date. Deaths beyond 5 years were excluded from the trial's final report (4) because mortality follow-up of referred care participants ended with their year-5 (60-month) visit. Subsequent mortality surveillance identified post-5-year deaths, allowing life table analysis of the trial's full follow-up (17).

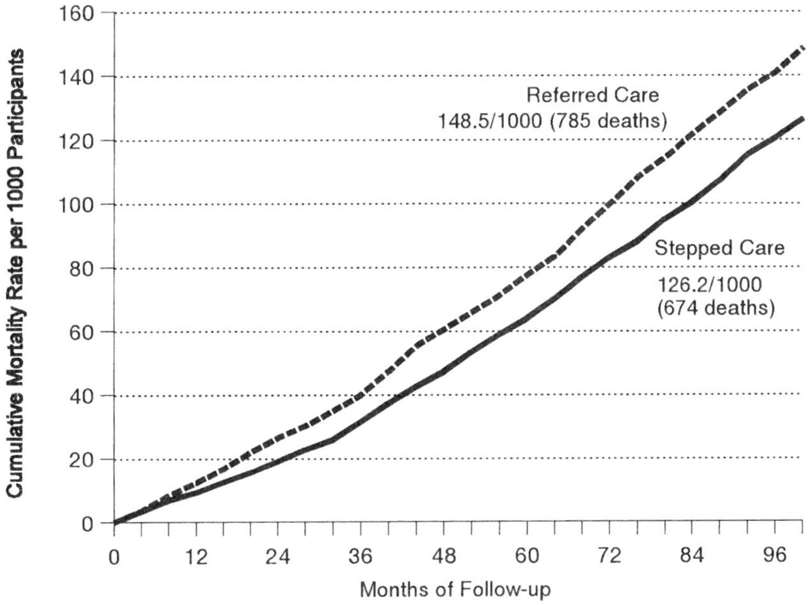

Fig. 8 Hypertension Detection and Follow-Up Program cumulative, life table, all-causes death rates in stepped care (n = 5485) and referred care (n = 5455) participants (1973–1982).

F. Cause-Specific Mortality

Data on cause-specific mortality for the SC and RC groups are presented in Table 4 for all participants, DBP stratum I, and for the low-risk subgroup. As stated in the protocol summary section, the design of the trial precluded assurances of unbiased ascertainment of cause of death. This was an inevitable consequence of the trial's design, including its provision for several visits per year to the center by SC participants, in contrast to no more than one annual exposure of RC participants to the research staff. The findings in Table 4 are solely from the nosologist's ''blind'' single-cause coding of death certificates. No tests of statistical significance are given for the specific causes of death.

Table 4 presents a summary of the data on cause-specific mortality for the total SC compared to the total RC group. Table 5 provides adjusted rates per 1000 participants for selected fatal and nonfatal events. Number of deaths from cerebrovascular diseases was smaller by almost 45% for the SC group. Most frequently, deaths among HDFP participants were attributed to CHD (ICDA codes 410–413): 37% of SC deaths and 35% of RC deaths were assigned to CHD causes (131 SC and 148 RC), as shown in Table 5. There were 26% fewer deaths attributed to acute MI in the SC compared with the RC group (51 and 69, respectively). Deaths from other ischemic heart diseases were similar in both groups. Therefore, for all CHD, the SC group had 15% fewer deaths than the RC group. For the SC group, there were nine deaths certified to hypertension compared with 14 in the RC group. For cardiovascular diseases other than the foregoing, the number of deaths was the same for the SC and the RC groups. For all cardiovascular causes, there were 19% fewer deaths reported for the SC than the RC group—35.7 per 1000 SC versus 43.8 per 1000 RC participants (Table 5).

Table 4 Causes of Death

Cause of death (ICDA codes)[a]	Total SC	Total RC	Stratum I (DBP, 90–104 mm Hg) SC	Stratum I (DBP, 90–104 mm Hg) RC	No medication/ EOD 90–94 mm Hg SC	No medication/ EOD 90–94 mm Hg RC
Total	350	421	232	292	36	54
All cardiovascular diseases	195	240	122	165	17	26
Cerebrovascular diseases (430–438)	29	52	17	31	0	3
Myocardial infarction (410)	51	69	30	56	3	12
Other ischemic heart disease (411–413)	80	79	56	51	9	8
Hypertensive heart disease (402)	5	7	5	5	1	1
Other hypertensive disease (400–401, 403–404)	4	7	2	3	1	0
Other cardiovascular diseases (390–458 exclusive of above)	26	26	12	19	3	2
All noncardiovascular diseases[b]	147	172	105	120	17	27
Renal diseases (580–599)	15	10	7	8	0	0
Diabetes mellitus (250)	5	11	4	5	1	0
Neoplastic diseases (140–239)	61	74	45	57	8	8
Breast cancer (174)	2	5	2	4	0	1
Gastrointestinal diseases (530–537)	12	20	10	15	2	8
Respiratory diseases (460–519)	13	17	9	10	0	3
Infectious diseases (000–136)	6	3	4	2	2	1
Accidents, suicides, and homicides (800–999)	26	25	20	17	3	4
Other diseases	15	15	10	8	3	6
Unknown	8	9	5	7	1	2

Number of deaths by cause, Stepped Care (SC), and Referred Care (RC) participants, Total, DBP Stratum I (DBP, 90–104 mm Hg), and DBP 90–94 who at entry were without EOD and not on antihypertensive medication (low-risk subgroup).

[a] From death certificates. ICDA Codes indicates International Classification of Diseases Adapted Codes, 8th Revision.

[b] In Table 7 of the 1979 Final Report of the HDFP trial findings, the ''All noncardiovascular diseases'' category inadvertently included ''unknown'' causes of death, and the number of DBP stratum I RC deaths attributed to renal diseases was switched with deaths attributed to diabetes mellitus.

Abbreviations: *SC*, stepped care; *RC*, referred care; *DBP*, diastolic blood pressure; *EOD*, end-organ damage; ICDA, International Classification of Diseases, Adapted.

Table 5 Frequency of 5-Year Fatal and Nonfatal Endpoints Among Participants of the HDFP (1973–1979)

Endpoint (Nsc = 5485, Nrc = 5455)	Any event		Adjusted rate per 1000		*P* value for rate diff RC-SC	Combined events[a]	
	SC	RC	SC	RC		SC	RC
Cardiovascular mortality	195	240	35.7	43.8	0.030	195	240
All-cause mortality	350	421	64.2	76.7	0.009	350	421
Fatal stroke	29	52	5.3	9.6	0.008	—	—
Nonfatal stroke	73	107	13.4	19.5	0.013	423	527
All strokes	102	159	18.7	29.1	<0.001	—	—
Fatal CHD	131	148	24.1	26.9	0.346	—	—
Nonfatal myocardial infarction (MI)	194	230	35.6	42.1	0.078	579	721
Prolonged severe chest pain (Rose Questionnaire MI)	320	379	58.4	69.3	0.020	820	1012
Fatal CHD, nonfatal MI, or RQMI	558	669	102.1	122.2	<0.001	—	—
Left ventricular hypertrophy (LVH)	127	183	23.1	33.4	0.001	916	1148
Angina pectoris (AP)	325	449	59.4	82.3	<0.001	1119	1432
AP without fatal CHD or MI	218	322	39.8	59.0	<0.001	—	—
AP with ECG ischemia	64	89	11.6	16.4	0.036	—	—
ECG ischemia	659	673	120.3	123.1	0.653	1565	1796
Without LVH or ECG MI	557	518	101.6	94.9	0.237	—	—
Exclusive of any other event	494	448	90.2	81.9	0.123	—	—
Renal insufficiency	99	101	18.3	18.4	0.969	1628	1853
Any endpoint[b]	1628	1853	297.7	338.7	<0.001	1628	1853
Any major trial endpoint[c]	995	1219	182.2	222.5	<0.001	—	—
Any cardiac endpoint[d]	417	536	76.4	97.7	<0.001	—	—
Any nonfatal endpoint	1344	1507	245.6	275.7	<0.001	—	—

[a] Events are accumulated with each successive row, with only one event per person being counted. Thus, the difference between consecutive rows equals the number of additional events contributed to the total number of combined outcomes.

[b] Total number of combined endpoints.

[c] ''Major trial endpoints'' include death, stroke, nonfatal CHD (ECG MI, history of MI, RQMI), LVH, and renal insufficiency.

[d] ''Cardiac endpoints'' include fatal CHD, MI (ECG or history), and LVH.

Abbreviations: *HDFP*, Hypertension Detection and Follow-Up Program; *SC*, stepped care; *RC*, referred care; *CHD*, coronary heart disease; *MI*, myocardial infarction; *RQMI*, Rose Questionnaire MI; *LVH*, left ventricular hypertrophy; *AP*, angina pectoris; *ECG*, electrocardiogram.

For deaths attributed to renal diseases, 15 occurred in the SC group compared with 10 in the RC group. As to the few deaths certified to diabetes, five were in the SC and 11 in the RC group. There were also fewer deaths in the SC than the RC group attributed to malignant neoplasms, gastrointestinal diseases, and respiratory diseases, whereas the RC group had slightly fewer deaths from infectious diseases. Only seven deaths from breast cancer were recorded: two in the SC and five in the RC group. Numbers of violent deaths (accidents, suicides, and homicides) were almost identical in the two groups. Thus, there were 15% fewer deaths attributed to noncardiovascular causes in the SC than in the RC group. Cause of death could not be ascertained for 17 deaths (8 SC and 9 RC).

For DBP stratum I, there were 45% fewer deaths attributed to cerebrovascular diseases in the SC group compared to the RC group. Similarly, there were 46% fewer deaths due to acute MI in the SC group. Deaths from other ischemic heart diseases were slightly more in the SC group compared with the RC group. Hence, the SC group had 20% fewer CHD deaths than the RC group (86 versus 107). Deaths from hypertensive disease were the same in the two groups, and slightly more deaths in the RC group were attributed to other cardiovascular diseases. Overall, in this DBP stratum, there were 26% fewer deaths from all cardiovascular diseases in the SC group compared with the RC group (122 and 165, respectively). Generally, for the noncardiovascular causes of death, there were fewer deaths (105 and 120, respectively) in the SC than the RC group (13% fewer overall).

For the low-risk subgroup, the overall number of deaths was low in both SC and RC. There were 33% fewer deaths in the SC group compared with the RC. As in the study overall, most frequently, deaths among the low-risk subgroup were attributed to CHD causes: 33% of SC deaths and 37% of RC deaths. Deaths from noncardiovascular causes comprised half of all deaths in the low-risk subgroup. Cancer represented the most frequent noncardiovascular cause of death among the low-risk participants.

G. Mortality Findings Stratified by Other Risk Factors

The HDFP findings demonstrated the predictive value of baseline SPB and pulse pressure (16), serum creatinine (12), ECG abnormalities (9), and of several other baseline risk factors (13) on all-cause mortality. The SC subgroups fared better than did corresponding RC subgroups at all strata of baseline SBP, pulse pressure, body mass index, and serum creatinine. All-cause mortality rates were lower in the SC group than the RC group, both overall and for the 90 to 104 mm Hg stratum, for both cigarette smokers and nonsmokers, and for persons with and without ECG abnormalities, hypercholesterolemia, hyperglycemia, diagnosed diabetes, hyperuricemia, or rapid pulse rate.

H. Fatal and Nonfatal Stroke

Table 6 presents the stroke results from HDFP. There was a total of 159 new fatal and nonfatal strokes ascertained in the RC group and 102 in the SC group during the five years of follow-up. Fatal stroke accounted for 33% of total stroke in RC and 28% of total stroke in SC (Table 5).

A total of 415 RC and 245 SC participants refused to participate in the final interview when the stroke questionnaire was administered (6). For these participants, the ascertainment of the nonfatal stroke endpoint was not achieved (7.6% of the RC group and 4.5% of the SC group). The nonrespondents were treated in the analysis as though they had had no new nonfatal strokes. Thus, the extra number of nonrespondents in RC (415 versus

Table 6 Occurrence of Stroke

Subgroup	Sample size SC	Sample size RC	Strokes SC	Strokes RC	Direct adjusted[a] rates per 1000 (SE) SC	Direct adjusted[a] rates per 1000 (SE) RC	95% Confidence limits for difference in RC and SC rates	Percent[b] reduction in strokes for SC group	*P* value
Total	5485	5455	102	159	18.7 (1.8)	29.1 (2.3)	(4.70, 16.10)	35.7	<0.001
DBP Stratum									
90–104 mm Hg	3903	3922	59	88	15.3 (2.0)	22.4 (2.4)	(1.09, 13.11)	31.7	0.021
105–114 mm Hg	1048	1004	25	36	23.9 (4.7)	36.3 (5.9)	(−2.42, 27.22)	34.2	0.101
≥ 115 mm Hg	534	529	18	35	34.9 (8.0)	63.9 (10.4)	(3.38, 54.62)	45.4	0.026
Sex									
Men	2961	2949	59	90	20.2 (2.6)	30.3 (3.1)	(2.14, 18.06)	33.3	0.013
Women	2524	2506	43	69	17.0 (2.6)	27.6 (3.3)	(2.45, 18.75)	38.4	0.011
Race									
White	3076	3014	46	73	15.0 (2.2)	24.2 (2.8)	(2.27, 16.13)	38.0	0.009
Black	2409	2441	56	86	23.4 (3.1)	35.2 (3.7)	(2.33, 21.27)	33.5	0.015
Age									
30–49	2427	2371	27	35	11.1 (2.1)	14.8 (2.5)	(−2.69, 10.09)	25.0	0.265
50–59	1856	1912	39	62	21.2 (3.4)	32.3 (4.0)	(0.82, 21.38)	34.4	0.034
60–69	1202	1172	36	62	30.1 (4.9)	52.9 (6.5)	(6.76, 38.84)	43.1	0.005
Baseline Meds									
On meds	1444	1403	44	65	30.4 (4.5)	46.2 (5.6)	(1.78, 29.82)	34.2	0.027
Not on meds	4041	4052	58	94	14.4 (1.9)	23.1 (2.3)	(2.82, 14.58)	37.7	0.004
EOD Status									
With EOD	817	792	43	59	53.5 (7.9)	73.5 (9.1)	(−2.80, 70.60)	18.1	0.070
Without EOD	4668	4663	59	100	12.7 (1.6)	21.4 (2.1)	(3.46, 13.94)	40.7	0.001
No Meds, without EOD									
DBP 90–94 mm Hg	1021	1022	4	10	4.2 (2.1)	9.8 (3.1)	(−1.69, 12.89)	57.1	0.132

Fatal and nonfatal stroke for stepped care and referred care participants during 5-year follow-up, by diastolic blood pressure at entry, sex, race, age, use of antihypertensive medication at entry, and presence of major end-organ damage at entry.

[a] Rates were direct adjusted for age, race, and sex distribution differences between the SC and RC groups.

[b] Percent reduction were calculated as 100 × (RC − SC rate)/RC rate.

Abbreviations: *SC*, stepped care; *RC*, referred care; *DBP*, diastolic blood pressure; *Meds*, medication; *EOD*, end-organ damage; SE, standard error.

245) is likely to minimize the actual observed difference in the incidence of stroke between the SC and RC groups.

For every major subgroup listed, a substantial reduction was noted. The overall stroke incidence of 18.7/1000 for SC was significantly lower ($P < 0.001$) than the 29.1/1000 observed among the RC group, a 35.7% reduction in strokes after five years between the SC and RC groups. The reductions were 31.7% for DBP stratum I ($P = 0.021$) and 57.1% for the low-risk subgroup ($P = 0.132$).

There is a direct relationship between the incidence of stroke and the entry level of DBP. In particular, whereas the incidence of stroke among the RC in stratum III was almost triple that in stratum I, the increase in the incidence of stroke by DBP strata among the SC group was less dramatic. Differences in stroke rates between the RC and SC groups are apparent for all three DBP strata: 31.7%, 34.2%, and 45.4%. The largest absolute and relative benefit in terms of fewer strokes in the SC compared to RC was achieved among participants with entry DBP of 115 mm Hg or higher, where the SC rate was nearly half that of RC.

Five-year incidence of fatal and nonfatal stroke by race and sex is also presented in Table 6. Highest incidence were observed in blacks, both men and women (38.5/1000 RC black men, 32.6/1000 RC black women, 30.3/1000 SC black men, and 17.8/1000 SC black women) (6). The stroke rates were lower in the SC group than the RC group in all race and sex categories.

The incidence of stroke increased with age. At all ages, the incidence of fatal and nonfatal stroke was less in the SC than the RC group. Greatest reductions in SC total strokes were observed in those in the oldest age group (60 to 69 years), a 43.1% reduction.

Five-year incidence of total stroke was highest in both SC and RC participants among those who had evidence of long-standing hypertension. Evidence of long-standing hypertension was defined, for the purposes of this article, as being either on a regimen of antihypertensive medication at entry or having evidence of major end-organ damage. End-organ damage was defined as the presence of one or more of the following: LVH by ECG criteria, history of stroke, history of MI, serum creatinine level of 1.7 mg/dl or higher, or a history of intermittent claudication.

When there was no evidence of end-organ damage at entry, or when the participants were not receiving medication at entry, the incidence of stroke was lower than when these two factors were present. Furthermore, participants in the SC group experienced a much lower incidence of stroke than those in the RC group, regardless of whether they were receiving treatment, or had evidence of end-organ damage.

Five-year incidence of fatal and nonfatal stroke for the low-risk group—those with DBP of 90 to 94 mm Hg who were untreated and free of major end-organ damage at entry—is also shown in Table 6. It should be noted that stroke incidence was lowest and relative reduction greatest—57.1%—in this subgroup.

I. Multiple Endpoints

Combined endpoints. The 5-year incidence of combined endpoints, adjusted for age, race, and sex differences between the SC and RC groups, is depicted in Table 5 by type of endpoint. The combined events shown in the fourth column were counted hierarchically, beginning with fatal events and progressing through other events in this order: nonfatal stroke, nonfatal MI, LVH, angina, ECG ischemia, and renal insufficiency. For participants with multiple events, only the first event in the hierarchy was counted. However, the total frequency of each event is given in the first column of the table. There were 1628 SC participants and 1853 RC participants who experienced one or more events. The SC rate for any endpoint event was a significant 12.1% lower than RC ($P < 0.001$)—an absolute difference of 41 events per 1000 participants in five years. For major trial endpoints, the SC rate was 18.1% lower than RC ($P < 0.001$)—an absolute difference of 40 major events per 1000. For cardiac endpoints, the SC rate was 21.8% lower than RC ($P < 0.001$)—an absolute difference of 21 cardiac events per 1000.

Table 7 presents adjusted 5-year event rates for (a) all combined endpoints, (b) major trial endpoints, and (c) cardiac endpoints, overall and by DBP strata. The SC rates were all statistically significantly lower than RC with one exception, a 14.6% lower cardiac event rate for stratum I SC. These differences were large and increased with DBP stratum, both in terms of absolute and relative difference measures. Overall, for total endpoints, major trial endpoints, and cardiac endpoints, the absolute differences were 41.0, 40.3, and 21.3 events per 1000, respectively ($P < 0.001$). The cardiac event rate for stratum III SC was less than half that of RC ($P < 0.001$).

In both SC and RC, the incidence rates of total and major trial endpoints increased with baseline DBP; for cardiac endpoints, this trend was present for RC participants. The rise was much more dramatic for the RC group. For total endpoints, the RC rate ranged from 313.4 per 1000 in stratum I to 428.1 per 1000 in stratum III, a difference of 114.7 events per 1000. In comparison, the SC rates increased by only 63.7 per 1000. For major trial endpoints, the difference between the stratum III and stratum I rates was 106.2 per 1000 for RC participants but only 61.2 per 1000 for SC. For cardiac events, the RC rates increased with DBP by 74.6 per 1000, whereas in the SC group, the stratum III rate was only slightly higher than stratum I.

For any endpoint, the difference was particularly striking among those in the low-risk group, where the SC experienced 47.6 fewer events per 1000 persons than did RC, a 19.3% reduction ($P = 0.009$). For any major endpoint, the difference was still particularly striking: the low-risk SC group experienced 42.6 fewer major events per 1000 persons than did RC, a 29.0% reduction ($P = 0.003$). For any cardiac endpoints, the difference was less striking: the SC experienced 17.2 fewer events per 1000 persons than did RC, a 28.9% reduction ($P = 0.075$).

VI. CONCLUSIONS

The HDFP was a landmark trial. Its implications and influence are still strong in the medical and public health communities (60). The trial demonstrated for the first time that hypertension in the community could be identified by enumeration and screening and that systematic management of hypertension could reduce mortality in people with high BP. Subsequent reports from the HDFP extended this benefit to age, race, and sex subgroups (5), those with uncomplicated mild hypertension (5), and for the outcomes of CHD (8), stroke (6), and LVH (11). In addition, such treatment would, and did, have an enormous public health benefit, as more than 60 million Americans have high BP. The reduction in deaths, strokes, and CHD events, and the economic impact this had, are substantial.

The trial engendered criticism. The HDFP was neither placebo-controlled nor double-blind. The SC participants may have received more intensive medical care because they were seen every 4 months. Perhaps something besides BP reduction could have con-

Table 7 Cardiac Event Occurrences

Subgroup	Sample size SC	Sample size RC	Strokes SC	Strokes RC	Direct Adjusted[a] rates per 1000 (SE) SC	Direct Adjusted[a] rates per 1000 (SE) RC	95% Confidence limits for difference in RC and SC rates	Percent[b] reduction in strokes for SC group	*P* value
Any endpoint									
All	5485	5455	1628	1853	297.7 (6.1)	338.7 (6.3)	(23.83, 58.17)	12.1	<0.001
DBP stratum									
90–104 mm Hg	3903	3922	1104	1233	284.3 (7.1)	313.4 (7.3)	(9.20, 49.00)	9.3	0.004
105–114 mm Hg	1048	1004	339	394	325.1 (14.4)	392.1 (15.3)	(25.93, 108.07)	17.1	0.001
≥ 115 mm Hg	534	529	185	226	348.0 (20.4)	428.1 (21.5)	(21.94, 138.26)	18.7	0.007
No meds, without EOD									
DBP 90–94 mm Hg	1021	1022	202	254	199.6 (12.4)	247.2 (13.3)	(11.87, 83.33)	19.3	0.009
Any major endpoint									
All	5485	5455	995	1219	182.2 (5.1)	222.5 (5.5)	(25.54, 55.06)	18.1	<0.001
DBP stratum									
90–104 mm Hg	3903	3922	659	802	170.0 (5.9)	203.6 (6.3)	(16.69, 50.51)	16.5	<0.001
105–114 mm Hg	1048	1004	213	252	205.1 (12.3)	250.3 (13.5)	(9.50, 80.90)	18.1	0.013
≥ 115 mm Hg	534	529	123	165	231.2 (17.8)	309.8 (19.9)	(26.28, 130.92)	25.4	0.003
No meds, without EOD									
DBP 90–94 mm Hg	1021	1022	106	152	104.5 (9.5)	147.1 (10.9)	(14.14, 71.06)	29.0	0.003
Any cardiac endpoint									
All	5485	5455	417	536	76.4 (3.6)	97.7 (4.0)	(10.85, 31.75)	21.8	<0.001
DBP stratum									
90–104 mm Hg	3903	3922	286	342	73.8 (4.2)	86.7 (4.4)	(1.02, 24.78)	14.9	0.033
105–114 mm Hg	1048	1004	91	109	88.7 (8.7)	107.7 (9.7)	(−6.52, 44.52)	17.6	0.144
≥ 115 mm Hg	534	529	40	85	75.1 (11.4)	161.3 (15.8)	(48.00, 124.40)	53.4	<0.001
No meds, without EOD									
DPB 90–94 mm Hg	1021	1022	43	61	42.3 (6.3)	59.5 (7.3)	(−1.71, 36.11)	28.9	0.075

Adjusted 5-year event rates for any, major, and cardiac events among stepped care and referred care participants of the HDFP (1973–1979), for each diastolic blood pressure stratum and for participants with entry DBP 90–94 mm Hg who were not on antihypertensive medication and were free of major end-organ damage.

[a] The definitions of ''combined endpoints,'' ''major trial endpoints,'' and ''cardiac endpoints'' are given in the Methods Section.

[b] Rates were directly adjusted for distributional differences between the SC and RC cohorts in age, race, and sex.

Abbreviations: *HDFP*, Hypertension Detection and Follow-Up Program; *SC*, stepped care; *RC*, referred care; *DBP*, diastolic blood pressure; *SE*, standard error.

tributed to the apparent benefit. An analysis that examined the major indices of BP treatment showed that a great part of the difference between the two treatment groups could be attributed to antihypertensive therapy (61). Because the primary outcome was total mortality, there could be no ascertainment bias. Finally, the major question looming after HDFP was whether younger persons with mild hypertension and no evidence of end-organ damage should be placed on BP drugs. The answer was yes. In uncomplicated patients with a DBP of 90 to 94 mm Hg, there was substantial benefit from the SC regimen (7). Our analysis of combined endpoints reinforces this dramatically.

The HDFP accomplished many things. It demonstrated that hypertension could be identified in the community (41), brought under pharmacological treatment (42), and effectively treated among younger and older Americans (62), blacks and whites, and men and women (57). It showed that through such treatment, total morality could be reduced in the population and in age, race, and sex subgroups (5). The benefit could be extended to those with mild hypertension (5) and even those with uncomplicated mild hypertension (5). It showed that a large-scale clinical trial could be conducted well and successfully in the community (41).

The HDFP did not accomplish several things. The controversy over an optimal level of DBP control was not resolved. A subsequent analysis of the HDFP data suggested that there might be a ''J-shaped'' relationship for DBP and mortality but not one for SBP (63). Controversy continued to ensue resulting in the Hypertension Optimal Treatment Trial (HOT) (64). That study did not fully answer the J-shaped question, but it did show that treatment of DBP into the 80s mm Hg range demonstrated additional benefit in terms of cardiovascular events. It did not show what treatment might be best for hypertension. This controversy has resulted in several new studies that address clinical outcomes in relation to various treatments, including Antihypertensive and Lipid Lowering Treatment to Prevent Heart Attack Trial (ALLHAT) (65), Controlled ONset Verapamil INvestigation of Cardiovascular Endpoints (CONVINCE) (66), the International Verapamil/Trandolapril Study (INVEST), Second Australian National Blood Pressure Study (ANBP2) (67), African American Study of Kidney Disease and Hypertension (AASK) (68), and others (69).

The HDFP did not address the issue of treating isolated systolic hypertension (ISH), although the data from the screening provided an important look at the cardiovascular risks associated with ISH (70). The Systolic Hypertension in the Elderly Program (SHEP) demonstrated the effectiveness of treating ISH in preventing stroke and CHD (71). Also, the treated SHEP participants had a mean DBP of 68 mm Hg after 5 years, showing that reducing DBP to low levels was not associated with any measurable risk.

The HDFP did not show whether nonpharmacological therapy was useful in treating BP and whether such therapy would be useful in reducing clinical outcomes. Subsequent studies (HPT [72], TONE [73], TOHP [74, 75], TAIM [76]) have shown the effectiveness of nonpharmacological therapy.

What was the influence of this trial on medical practice? It had a major effect on guidelines for hypertension management from the Joint National Committee (77, 78). It heightened awareness of hypertension as a public health problem (78–80). It probably played a major role in resulting in large decreases in stroke mortality, hypertensive renal failure and heart failure in the United States (79). It resulted in the large-scale institution of treatment for patients with mild hypertension, and demonstrated the efficacy of using diuretics in treating hypertension. Although the use of diuretics deceased after the Multiple Risk Factor Intervention Trial (MRFIT) results (81), the success of the SHEP trial, which used chlorthalidone as a first-line drug, revitalized the use of diuretics (71).

The HDFP concluded more than 20 years ago. Since then, its conclusions and implications have been reinforced and expanded by many studies. This trial was and still remains a landmark in the annals of hypertension trials, and of all trials as well.

ACKNOWLEDGMENTS

Many of the HDFP researchers and key advisors are no longer living: Lawrence M. Slotkoff (1930–1983), Arthur S. Littell (1925–1987), B. Frank Polk (1942–1988), Max Halperin (1917–1988), Edward H. Kass (1917–1990), Herbert G. Langford (1922–1991), Walter M. Kirkendall (1917–1991), Richard D. Remington (1931–1992), Aris Apostolides (1937–1993), Nemat O. Borhani (1926–1996), Rose Stamler (1922–1998), Alvin P. Shapiro (1921–1998).

The research on which this publication is based was performed pursuant to contract numbers NO1-HV-124 (83-42), 229 (31, 37-39, 45), 32933, 72915, and 82915 with the National Heart, Lung, and Blood Institute, National Institutes of Health, and U.S. Department of Health, Education, and Welfare.

The HDFP policy advisory board members who monitored the HDFP and advised the National Heart, Lung, and Blood Institute regarding its progress include the following:

Alvin P. Shapiro, M.D., Chairman, University of Pittsburgh School of Medicine, Pittsburgh, PA; Glenn E. Bartsch, Ph.D., School of Public Health, University of Minnesota, Minneapolis; Kenneth G. Berge, M.D., Mayo Clinic, Rochester, MN; Edward S. Cooper, M.D., Hospital of University of Pennsylvania, Philadelphia; Edward D. Frohlich, M.D., Alton Ochsner Medical Foundation, New Orleans, LA; Richard H. Gadsden, Ph.D., Medical University of South Carolina, Charleston; David L. Sackett, M.D., McMaster University Medical Center, Hamilton, Ontario, Canada; Joseph A. Wilber, M.D., Georgia Department of Human Resources, Atlanta; William J. Zukel, M.D., National Heart, Lung, and Blood Institute, Bethesda, MD.

The Toxicity and Endpoints Evaluation Committee members who reviewed data endpoints and toxicity reports at specified intervals include the following:

W. McFate Smith, M.D., M.P.H., Chairman, University of California-USPHS Hospital, San Francisco; Walter M. Kirkendall, M.D., University of Texas Medical School, Houston; Curtis L. Meinert, Ph.D., School of Hygiene and Public Health, Johns Hopkins University, Baltimore, MD; Louis S. Monk, Ph.D., Silver Spring, MD; Richard D. Remington, Ph.D., University of Michigan School of Public Health, Ann Arbor; Alvin P. Shapiro, M.D., University of Pittsburgh School of Medicine, Pittsburgh; Herbert G. Langford, M.D., University of Mississippi Medical Center, Jackson; Jeremiah Stamler, M.D., Northwestern University Medical School, Chicago, IL; Edward H. Kass, M.D., Ph.D., Peter Bent Brigham Hospital Division of Affiliated Hospitals Inc., Boston, MA; Harold W. Schnaper, M.D., University of Alabama in Birmingham; Thomas P. Blaszkowski, Ph.D., PCB, DHVD, NHLBI, Bethesda, MD; Max Halperin, Ph.D., Georgetown University, Bethesda, MD; William J. Zukel, M.D. (Ex Officio), PCB, DHVD, NHLBI, Bethesda, MD.

The HDFP Steering Committee members, the principal investigators in the trial, include the following:

Clinical Centers: Elbert P. Tuttle, Jr., M.D. (Atlanta), George Entwisle, M.D. (Baltimore), Albert Oberman, M.D. (Birmingham, AL), Edward H. Kass, M.D., Ph.D. (Boston), Jeremiah Stamler, M.D. (Vice-Chairman, Chicago), Nemat O. Borhani, M.D. (Davis, CA), John W. Jones, M.D. (East Lansing, MI), Curtis G. Hames, M.D. (Evans County, GA),

Lawrence M. Slotkoff, M.D., Ph.D. (Georgetown, Washington, D.C.), Herbert G. Langford, M.D. (Chairman, Jackson, MS), Morton H. Maxwell, M.D. (Los Angeles), Reuben Berman, M.D. (Minneapolis), M. Donald Blaufox, M.D. Ph.D. (New York), C. Hilmon Castle, M.D. (Salt Lake City).

Coordinating Center: C. Morton Hawkins, Sc.D.; J. David Curb, M.D., M.P.H., Houston

Central Laboratory: Kenneth Schneider, M.D.; Agostino Molteni, M.D., Ph.D., Chicago.

ECG Center: Ronald J. Prineas, M.E., B.S., Ph.D., Minneapolis, MN.

NHLBI Program Office: Gerald H. Payne, M.D., Bethesda, MD.

The 14 clinical centers and four coordination and service centers of the cooperative group, their institutions, coinvestigators, and senior staff were as follows:

Atlanta: Emory University; Neil B. Shulman, M.D., Margaret Chiappini, R.N., Catherine Hampton, R.N.; **Baltimore**: University of Maryland; Aristide Apostolides, D.V.M., Ph.D., J. Richard Hebel, Ph.D.; **Birmingham**: University of Alabama; Harold Schnaper, M.D., James Kitts, P.A., Myra Crawford, M.A., M.F.A.; **Boston**: Peter Bent Brigham Hospital Division of Affiliated Hospitals Inc., Harvard Medical School; James O. Taylor, M.D., B. Frank Polk, M.D., M.Sc.; **Chicago**: Northwestern University; Rose Stamler, M.A., Flora Cass Gosch, M.D.; **Davis**: University of California; Jess F. Kraus, Ph.D., Virginia C. Asbury, B.S., Linda Sigourney, R.N.; **East Lansing**: Michigan State University; Sandra D. Daugherty, M.D., Ph.D.), Robert M. Daugherty, Jr., M.D., Ph.D.; **Evans County, GA**: Evans County Health Department; H. A. Tyroler, M.D., Siegfried Heyden, M.D.; **Georgetown, Washington, D.C.**: Georgetown University; Won Ro Lee, M.D., Charles E. McCauley, M.D.; **Jackson, MS**: University of Mississippi; Myra Tyler, M.D., John D. Abernethy, M.D., Taira Morino, M.D.; **Los Angeles**: Cedars-Sinai and UCLA Medical Centers; Andrew J. Lewin, M.D., Roger Detels, M.D. Joan Ignatius Smith, R.N.; **Minneaplis**: Mount Sinai Hospital and University of Minnesota; Kyuhyun Wang, M.D., Ronald J. Prineas, Ph.D. M.E., B.S., Richard Crow, M.D.; **New York**: Albert Einstein College of Medicine; Sylvia Wassertheil-Smoller, Ph.D., Jeanne Hotchkiss, M.D.; **Salt Lake City**: University of Utah; Joyce Johnson, M.D., Virginia Aldrich, R.N., Irving Ershler, M.D.; **Coordinating Center, Houston**: The University of Texas-Houston; C. Morton Hawkins, Sc.D., Barry R. Davis, M.D., Ph.D., Charles E. Ford, Ph.D., Robert J. Hardy, Ph.D., J. David Curb, M.D., M.P.H., Darwin R. Labarthe, M.D., Ph.D., Arthur Littell, Sc.D., Ph.D., Richard D. Remington, Ph.D., E. O'Brian Smith, Ph.D.; **Central Laboratory, Chicago**: Northwestern Memorial Hospital; Kenneth A. Schneider, M.D., Agostino Molteni, M.D., Ph.D., Edward Fitzsimmons, Ph.D., Frances Gaona, Melanie Palmer; **ECG Center, Minneapolis**: University of Minnesota; Ronald J. Prineas, Ph.D., M.E., B.S., Henry Blackburn, M.D., Deborah Brasseur, Kathy Pickard; and **National Heart, Lung, and Blood Institute, National Institutes of Health, Bethesda, MD**: Gerald H. Payne, M.D., Wallace Williams, Ph.D., James H. Ware, Ph.D., William J. Zukel, M.D.

REFERENCES

1. Roccella EJ, Horan MJ. The National High Blood Pressure Education Program: measuring progress and assessing its impact. Health Psychology 1988; 7(suppl):297–303.
2. Remington RD, on behalf of the HDFP Cooperative Group. The Hypertension Detection and Follow-up Program. INSERM 1973; 21:185–194.
3. Hypertension Detection and Follow-Up Program Cooperative Group. The Hypertension Detection and Follow-Up Program. Prev Med 1976; 5:207–215.
4. Hypertension Detection and Follow-Up Program Cooperative Group. Five-year findings of

the Hypertension Detection and Follow-Up Program: I. Reduction in mortality of persons with high blood pressure, including mild hypertension. JAMA 1979; 242:2562–2571.

5. Hypertension Detection and Follow-Up Program Cooperative Group. Five-year findings of the Hypertension Detection and Follow-Up Program: II. Mortality by race-sex and age. JAMA 1979; 242:2572–2577.
6. Hypertension Detection and Follow-Up Program Cooperative Group. Five-year findings of the HDFP: III. Reduction in stroke incidence among persons with high blood pressure. JAMA 1982; 247:633–638.
7. Hypertension Detection and Follow-Up Program Cooperative Group. The effect of treatment on mortality in ''mild'' hypertension—results of the HDFP. N Engl J Med 1982; 307:976–980.
8. Hypertension Detection and Follow-Up Program Cooperative Group. Effect of stepped care treatment on incidence of myocardial infarction and angina pectoris. Five-year findings of the HDFP. Hypertension 1984; 6(suppl):I-198 through I-206.
9. Hypertension Detection and Follow-Up Program Cooperative Group. The effect of antihypertensive drug treatment on mortality in the presence of resting electrocardiographic abnormalities at baseline: the HDFP experience. Circulation 1984; 70:996–1003.
10. Hypertension Detection and Follow-Up Program Cooperative Group. Five-year findings of the HDFP: mortality by race-sex and blood pressure level. A further analysis. J Community Health 1984; 9:314–327.
11. Hypertension Detection and Follow-Up Program Cooperative Group. Five-year findings of the HDFP: Prevention and reversal of left ventricular hypertrophy with antihypertensive drug therapy. Hypertension 1985; 7:105–112.
12. Shulman NB, Ford CE, Hall WD, Blaufox MD, Simon D, Langford HG, Schneider KA. Prognostic value of serum creatinine and the effect of treatment of hypertension on renal function. Results from the HDFP. Hypertension 1989; 13(Suppl I):I-80–I-93.
13. Hypertension Detection and Follow-Up Program Cooperative Group. Mortality findings for stepped-care and referred-care participants in the HDFP, stratified by other risk factors. Prev Med 1985; 14:312–335.
14. Maxwell MH, Ford CE. Cardiovascular morbidity and mortality in the HDFP patients 50–69 years old at entry. J Cardiovasc Pharmacol 1985; 7(suppl 2):S5–S9.
15. Results and implications of the Hypertension Detection and Follow-up Program. Sonnenblick EH and Lesch M, eds, with MD Blaufox as guest editor. Prog Cardiovasc Dis 1986; 29(suppl 1):1–124.
16. Abernethy J, Borhani NO, Hawkins CM, Crow R, Entwisle G, Jones JW, Maxwell MH, Langford H, Pressel S. Systolic blood pressure as an independent predictor of mortality in the Hypertension Detection and Follow-Up Program. Am J Prev Med 1986; 2:123–132.
17. Hypertension Detection and Follow-Up Program Cooperative Group. Persistence of reduction in blood pressure and mortality of participants in the Hypertension Detection and Follow-Up Program. JAMA 1988; 259:2113–2122.
18. The Framingham Study, Section 30. Kannel WB, Gordon T, eds. DHEW Publications No. (NIH) 74-599. U.S. Government Printing Office, Washington, D.C., 1974.
19. Doyle JT. Risk factors in coronary heart disease. N Y State J Med 1963; 63:1317–1320.
20. Chapman JM, Massey FJ Jr. The interrelationship of serum cholesterol, hypertension, body weight, and risk of coronary disease: results of first ten years' follow-up in the Los Angeles Heart Study. J Chronic Dis 1964; 17:933–949.
21. Epstein FH, Ostrander LD Jr, Johnson BC, Payne MW, Hayner NS, Keller JB, Frances T Jr. Epidemiological studies of cardiovascular disease in a total community, Tecumseh, Michigan. Ann Intern Med 1965; 62:1170–1187.
22. Stamler J, Lindberg HA, Berkson DM, Shaffer A, Miller W, Poindexter A. Prevalence and incidence of coronary heart disease in strata of the labor force of a Chicago industrial corporation. J Chronic Dis 1960; 11:405–420.

23. Tyroler HA, Heyden S, Bartel A, Cassel J, Cornoni JC, Haines CG, Kleinbaum D. Blood pressure and cholesterol as coronary heart disease risk factors. Arch Intern Med 1971; 128: 907–919.
24. Paul O. The risks of mild hypertension: a ten year report. Br Heart J 1971; 33(suppl):116–121.
25. Keys A, Taylor HL, Blackburn H, Brozels J, Anderson JT, Simonson E. Coronary heart disease among Minnesota business and professional men followed fifteen years. Circulation 1963; 28: 381–395.
26. Build and Blood Pressure Study. Vol 1. Chicago: Society of Actuaries, 1959.
27. McGee D, Gordon T. The results of the Framingham study applied to four other US-based epidemiologic studies of cardiovascular disease. In: The Framingham Study: An Epidemiological Investigation of Cardiovascular Disease, publication No. (NIH) 76-1083. Washington, DC: U.S. Dept of Health, Education, and Welfare, Section 31, April, 1976.
28. Pooling Project Research Group. Relationship of blood pressure, serum cholesterol, smoking habit, relative weight and ECG abnormalities to incidence of major coronary events: final report of the Pooling Project. J Chronic Dis 1978; 31:201–306.
29. Shurtleff D. Some characteristics related to the incidence of cardiovascular disease and death: Framingham study, 18-year follow-up. In: The Framingham Study: An Epidemiological Investigation of Cardiovascular Disease, publication No. (NIH) 74-599. Washington, D.C.: US Dept of Health, Education, and Welfare, Section 30, February 1974.
30. Gordon T, Kannel WB. Predisposition to atherosclerosis in the head, heart, and legs: The Framingham Study. JAMA 1972; 221:661–666.
31. Veterans Administration Cooperative Study Group on Antihypertensive Agents. Effects of treatment on morbidity in hypertension: results in patients with diastolic blood pressure averaging 115 through 129 mm Hg. JAMA 1967; 202:1028–1034.
32. Veterans Administration Cooperative Study Group on Hypertensive Agents. Effects of treatment on morbidity in hypertension: II. Results in patients with diastolic blood pressure averaging 90 through 114 mm Hg. JAMA 1970; 213:1143–1152.
33. Veterans Administration Cooperative Study Group on Antihypertensive Agents. Effects of treatment on morbidity in hypertension: III. Influence of age, diastolic pressure, and prior cardiovascular disease; further analysis of side effects. Circulation 1972; 45:991–1004.
34. U.S. Dept of Health, Education, and Welfare. Blood Pressure of Persons 18–74 Years, United States, 1971–72, series 11, No. 150. Washington, D.C.: National Health Survey, National Center for Health Statistics, 1975.
35. Guidelines for the detection, diagnosis, and management of hypertensive populations. In: Wright IS, Fredrickson DT, eds. Cardiovascular Diseases: Guidelines for Prevention and Care, Inter-Society Commission for Heart Disease Resources, Hypertension Study Group. Washington, D.C.: U.S. Government Printing Office, 1974:186–197.
36. Wilber JA. Detection and control of hypertensive disease in Georgia, USA. In: Stamler J, Stamler R, Pullman TN, eds. The Epidemiology of Hypertension. New York: Grune & Stratton Inc, 1967:439–448.
37. U.S. Dept of Health, Education, and Welfare. Blood Pressure of Adults by Age and Sex, United States, 1960–1962, series 11, No. 4. Washington, D.C.: National Health Survey, National Center for Health Statistics, 1964.
38. U.S. Dept of Health, Education, and Welfare. Blood Pressure of Adults by Race and Area, United States, 1960–1962, series 11, No. 5. Washington, D.C.: National Health Survey, National Center for Health Statistics, 1964.
39. Schoenberger JA, Stamler J, Shekelle RB, Shekelle S. Current status of hypertension control in an industrial population. JAMA 1972; 222:559–562.
40. Ford CE, Langford HG, Palmer M. Recruitment in the HDFP. Control Clin Trials 1987; 8: 54S–67S.

41. Hypertension Detection and Follow-Up Program Cooperative Group. Blood pressure studies in 14 communities: A two-stage screen for hypertension. JAMA 1977 237:2395–2391.
42. Hypertension Detection and Follow-Up Program Cooperative Group. Patient participation in a hypertension control program. JAMA 1978; 239:1507–1514.
43. Labarthe DR, Hawkins CM, Remington RD. Evaluation of performance of selected devices for measuring blood pressure. Am J Cardiol 1973; 32:546–553.
44. Prineas RJ, Crow RS, Blackburn H. The Minnesota Code Manual of Electrocardiographic Findings—Standards and Procedures for Measurement and Classification. Littleton, MA: Wright-PSG, 1982.
45. Ungerleider HE, Gubner R. Evaluation of heart size measurements. Am Heart J 1942; 24: 494–510.
46. The Coronary Drug Project Research Group. The Coronary Drug Project: design, methods, and baseline results. Circulation 1973; 47(suppl 1):1–79.
47. Cutter G, Heyden S, Kasteler J, Kraus JF, Lee ES, Shipley T, Stromer M, on behalf of the Hypertension Detection and Follow-Up Program. Mortality surveillance in collaborative trials. Am J Public Health 1980; 70:394–400.
48. Curb JD, Ford CE, Pressel S, Palmer M, Babcock C, Hawkins CM. Ascertainment of vital status through the National Death Index and the Social Security Administration. Am J Epidemiol 1985; 121:754–766.
49. U.S. Department of Health, Education, and Welfare. Eighth Revision International Classification of Diseases, adapted for use in the United States. Public Health Service Publication No. 1693, Washington, D.C., 1968.
50. Rose GA, Blackburn H. Cardiovascular Survey Methods, WHO Monograph Series No. 56. Geneva, World Health Organizations, 1968.
51. Reid DD, Brett GZ, Hamilton PJS, Jarrett RJ, Keen H, Rose G. Cardiorespiratory disease and diabetes among middle-aged male civil servants: a study of screening and intervention. Lancet 1974, 1:469–474.
52. Rose G, Reid DD, Hamilton PJS, McCartney P, Keen H, Jarrett RJ. Myocardial ischemia, risk factors and death from coronary heart disease. Lancet 1977; 1:105–109.
53. Lee ET. Statistical Methods for Survival Analysis. Belmont, CA: Lifetime Learning Publications, Wadsworth, Inc., 1980:88–101.
54. Cutler S, Ederer F. Maximum utilization of the life table method in analyzing survival. J Chron Dis 1958; 8:699–712.
55. Hypertension Detection and Follow-up Program Cooperative Group. Baseline characteristics of the enumerated, screened, and hypertensive participants. Daugherty SA, Entwisle G, Curb JD, Polk BF, Taylor JO, eds. Hypertension 1983; 5(suppl IV):IV–1 through IV–205.
56. Davis BR, Ford CE, Remington RD, Stamler R, Hawkins CM. HDFP design, methods, and baseline characteristics and blood pressure response of the study participants. Prog Cardiovasc Dis 1986; 29:11–28.
57. Hypertension Detection and Follow-up Program Cooperative Group. Therapeutic control of blood pressure after one year in the Hypertension Detection and Follow-Up Program. Prev Med 1979; 8:2–13.
58. JD Curb, NO Borhani, TP Blaszkowski, N Zimbaldi, S Fotiu, W Williams. Long-term surveillance for adverse effects of antihypertensive drugs. JAMA 1985; 253:3263–3268.
59. Langford HG, Stamler J, Wassertheil-Smoller S, Prineas RJ. All-cause mortality in the HDFP: findings for the whole cohort and for persons with less severe hypertension, with and without other traits related to risk of mortality. Prog Cardiovasc Dis 1986; 29:29–54.
60. Ramsay LE. The Hypertension Detection and Follow-Up Program: 17 years on. JAMA 1997; 277:167–170.
61. Hardy RJ, Hawkins CM. The impact of selected indices of antihypertensive therapy on all-cause mortality. Am J Epidemiol 1983; 117:566–574.
62. Curb JD, Borhani NO, Schnaper H, Entwisle G, Kass E, Williams W, Berman R. Detec-

tion and treatment of hypertension in older individuals. Am J Epidemiol 1985; 121:371–376.

63. Cooper SP, Hardy RJ, Labarthe DR, Hawkins CM, Smith EO, Blaufox MD, Cooper C, Entwisle G, Maxwell MH, on behalf of the HDFP Cooperative Group. The relationship between degree of blood pressure reduction and mortality among hypertensives in the HDFP. Am J Epidemiol 1988; 127:387–403.
64. Hansson L, Zanchetti A, Carruthers SG, Dahlof B, Elmfeldt D, Julius S, Menard J, Rahn KH, Wedel H, Westerling S, for the HOT Study Group. Effects of intensive blood-pressure lowering and low-dose aspirin in patients with hypertension: principal results of the Hypertension Optimal Treatment (HOT) randomized trial. Lancet 1998; 351: 1755–1762.
65. Davis BR, Cutler JA, Gordon DJ, Furberg CD, Wright JT Jr, Cushman WC, Grimm RH, LaRosa J, Whelton PK, Perry HM, Alderman MH, Ford CE, Oparil S, Francis C, Proschan M, Pressel S, Black HP, Hawkins CM, for the ALLHAT Research Group. Rationale and design for the Antihypertensive and Lipid Lowering Treatment to Prevent Heart Attack Trial (ALLHAT). Am J Hypertension 1996; 9 (part 1):342–360.
66. Black HP, Elliott WJ, Neaton JD, Grandits G, Grambsch P, Grimm RH Jr, Hansson L, Lacouciere Y, Muller J, Sleight P, Weber MA, White WB, Williams G, Wittes J, Zanchetti A, Fakouhi TD. Rationale and design for the Controlled ONset Verapamil INvestigation of Cardiovascular Endpoints (CONVINCE) Trial. Control Clin Trials 1998; 19:370–390.
67. Wing LM, Reid CM, Ryan P, Beilin LJ, Brown MA, Jennings GL, Johnston CI, McNeil JJ, Marley JE, Morgan TO, Shaw J, Steven ID, West MJ. Second Australian National Blood Pressure Study (ANBP2). Australian comparative outcome trial of ACE inhibitor- and diuretic-based treatment of hypertension in the elderly. Management Committee on behalf of the High Blood Pressure Research Council of Australia. Clin Exp Hypertens 1997; 19:779–791.
68. Agodoa L. African American Study of Kidney Disease and hypertension (AASK)—Clinical trial update. Ethn Dis 1998; 8:249–253.
69. Estacio RO, Jeffers BW, Hiatt WR, Biggerstaff SL, Gifford N, Schrier RW. The effect of nisoldipine as compared with enalapril on cardiovascular outcomes in patients with non-insulin-dependent diabetes and hypertension. N Engl J Med 1998; 338:645–652.
70. Curb JD, Borhani NO, Entwisle G, Tung B, Kass E, Schnaper H, Williams W, Berman R. Isolated systolic hypertension in 14 communities. Am J Epidemiol 1985; 121:362–370.
71. SHEP Cooperative Research Group. Prevention of stroke by antihypertensive drug treatment in older persons with isolated systolic hypertension: final results of the Systolic Hypertension in the Elderly Program (SHEP). JAMA 1991; 265:3255–3264.
72. Meinert CL, Borhani NO, Langford HG. Design, methods, and rationale in the Hypertension Prevention Trial. Hypertension Prevention Trial Research Group. Control Clin Trials 1989; 10(suppl):1S–29S.
73. Whelton PK, Appel LJ, Espeland MA, Applegate WB, Ettinger WH Jr, Kostis JB, Kumanyika S, Lacy CR, Johnson KC, Folmar S, Cutler JA. Sodium reduction and weight loss in the treatment of hypertension in older persons: a randomized controlled trial of nonpharmacologic interventions in the elderly (TONE). JAMA 1998; 279:839–846.
74. The Trials of Hypertension Prevention Collaborative Research Group. The effects of nonpharmacologic interventions on blood pressure of persons with high normal levels. Results of the Trials of Hypertension Prevention, Phase I. JAMA 1992; 267:1213–1220.
75. Hebert PR, Bolt RJ, Borhani NO, Cook NR, Cohen JD, Cutler JA, Hollis JF, Kuller LH, Lasser NL, Oberman A, Miller ST, Morris C, Whelton PK, Hennekens CH. Design of a multicenter trial to evaluate long-term life-style intervention in adults with high-normal blood pressure levels. Trials of Hypertension Prevention (phase II). Trials of Hypertension Prevention (TOHP) Collaborative Research Group. Ann Epidemiol 1995; 5:130–139.
76. Wassertheil-Smoller S, Oberman A, Blaufox MD, Davis B, Langford H. The Trial of Antihypertensive Interventions and Management (TAIM) Study. Final results with regard to blood pressure, cardiovascular risk, and quality of life. Am J Hypertens 1992; 5:37–44.

77. Joint National Committee on Detection, Evaluation, and Treatment of High Blood Pressure. The 1984 Report of the Joint National Committee on Detection, Evaluation and Treatment of High Blood Pressure. Arch Intern Med 1984; 144:1045–1057.
78. Joint National Committee on Detection, Evaluation, and Treatment of High Blood Pressure. The Fifth Report of the Joint National Committee on Detection, Evaluation, and Treatment of High Blood Pressure (JNC V). Arch Intern Med 1993; 153:154–183.
79. Moser M. Historical perspective on the management of hypertension. Am J Med 1986; 80(suppl 5B):1–11.
80. Burt VL, Whelton P, Roccella EJ, Brown C, Cutler JA, Higgins M, Horan MJ, Labarthe D. Prevalence of hypertension in the US adult population: results from the Third National Health and Nutrition Examination Survey, 1988–1991. Hypertension 1995; 25:305–313.
81. Multiple Risk Factor Intervention Trial Research Group. Multiple Risk Factor Intervention Trial: risk factor changes and mortality results. JAMA 1982; 248:1465–1477.

4

The Australian National Blood Pressure Study 1973–1979

RALPH READER

National Heart Foundation of Australia, Canberra, Australia

I. INTRODUCTION

The Australian National Blood Pressure Study (ANBPS) was a randomized, placebo-controlled, single blind, therapeutic trial of antihypertensive drugs in mild, uncomplicated hypertensive subjects conducted in four centers. It was undertaken by the National Heart Foundation of Australia to provide guidelines for its community and professional programs. The Foundation received much encouragement and financial support from government and private research organizations. Screening of 104,171 subjects was carried out between June 1973 and December 1975; 3427 subjects were entered in the trial, which was completed on March 5, 1979 when significantly fewer trial endpoints were found in the actively treated subjects. The primary results were published in 1980 (1), 1981 (2), 1982 (3), and 1984 (4).

II. BACKGROUND

Through the 1950s and 1960s, management of hypertension had been transformed. The groundbreaking paper by Paton and Zaimis in 1948 (5) demonstrated a credible pharmaco-

The author acknowledges, with thanks, permission of editors of the journals to use material from the original papers and to reproduce the following figures and tables: *The Lancet*, Fig. 2, Tables 1, 2, 4, 6–12, 17–20; *Medical Journal of Australia*, Tables 13, 14; *Clinical Science*, Tables 15, 16; and *Circulation*, Figures 3, 4 and Tables 21, 22.

logical basis, and Arnold and Rosenheim in 1949 (6) confirmed that the ganglion blocking agent, pentamethonium iodide, given parenterally, was clinically effective although subject to adverse effects, particularly significant hypotension. There followed a brief period of doubts and reservations about practicality and safety (7). Smirk's two letters to the Lancet (8,9), reporting successful treatment of 80 patients by subcutaneous injections two to three times daily for periods up to nine months and of 130 patients, some given the bromide salt orally, 37 of whom had severe and 9 malignant hypertension, set the scene for one of the most remarkable advances in therapy in medical history.

The fall in blood pressure levels, the relief of congestive cardiac failure, cardiomegaly, and retinal hemorrhages were obvious to the most skeptical observers. The increasing use of antihypertensive drugs, the development of safer alternative preparations, the results of five small therapeutic trials conducted in the 1960s, and the fall in mortality rates from cerebrovascular disease in many countries followed (10). In the 1960s, only patients with severe or symptomatic hypertension were treated by antihypertensive drugs. The conventional wisdom was that patients with milder forms were best simply reassured and observed. Paul D. White, speaking in Australia on national radio in 1958, said ''Much high blood pressure is not serious; it is benign.'' The feasibility of a public health program to identify unrecognized hypertension and treat it was not entertained.

The second report of the United States Veterans Administration (VA) Cooperative Study Group on Antihypertensive Agents (11) reporting significant reduction in hypertensive complications in subjects with diastolic pressures of 90 to 114 mm Hg—''mild hypertension''—led to urgent review of policy. By 1970, prevalence surveys in Australia and overseas were showing that 15% to 20% of adults were hypertensive, and of these, 90% were ''mild,'' a large majority being unaware of their condition; many who were aware were not receiving treatment. The VA study suggested they should be. If so, it was part of the Heart Foundation's charter to campaign vigorously for this. But there were reservations about the applicability for hypertensives identified as mild at mass screenings and of the VA screening criteria that involved a week's hospitalization and then 2 to 4 months of placebo tablets testing compliance with drug therapy.

Accordingly, the Foundation appointed a working group in March 1972 with wide terms of reference to report on ''The need for, feasibility, cost and advantages of a screening program for symptomless hypertension.'' The members were Professor H.M. Whyte, Australian National University (chairman); Professor Austin Doyle, University of Melbourne, who had been assistant to Smirk in his pioneering studies on the methonium antihypertensive drugs (rapporteur); Professor Richard Lovell, University of Melbourne who had led a community survey in Albury (12); Dr. M.G. McCall, University of Western Australia, a principal in the Busselton Community Health Surveys in that state (13); Dr. John McPhie, President, Cardiac Society of Australia and New Zealand, Adelaide; Dr. Peter Leighton, Melbourne, representing The Royal Australian College of General Practice; and myself, Medical Director and CEO, National Heart Foundation. Dr. Ron Prineas, statistician of the University of Melbourne, was recruited.

The group submitted a report in August 1972. The report reviewed and confirmed the observations and reservations referred to above. It recommended a multicenter screening program involving 43,000 subjects, in a three-step screening regimen at 2-week intervals to identify subjects with diastolic blood pressure (DBP) of 95 mm Hg or higher. Those with pressures of 110 mm Hg and higher would be referred to their doctors with documentation. Those with pressures of 95 to 109 mm Hg would be invited to participate in a 5-year therapeutic trial of antihypertensive drug treatment.

The report included draft protocols for screening and for conducting a 5-year therapeutic trial in men and women aged 30 to 69 with mild, uncomplicated hypertension. It proposed that the trial should test the hypothesis that treatment will reduce endpoints by 30% with confidence levels of 95% in a positive result and 90% in a negative result. It estimated that 43,700 subjects should be screened to provide 2400 mild hypertensive subjects after allowing 70% recruitment at first screening, dropout rate of 50% over five years, loss due to spontaneous fall in pressure during prerandomization visits, and loss of 10% due to exclusion factors. Estimates of resources required were based on six centers in four capital cities and two country towns, with salaried staffs appropriate to subject numbers, but including full time director (medical graduate), nurses and secretary, and during the screening phase, additional sessional nurses and cardiologists. Suggested costs were of the order of \$A185,000 including screening in the first year and \$A129,000 in each subsequent year, a total of \$A701,000. At the start of the study in early 1973, \$A1.00 was equivalent to \$US1.415.

The recommendations were debated in the Medical Advisory Committee and by the Board of Directors at its meeting in September 1972. There was general support in principle with reservations that conducting such a research project was not appropriate for the Foundation, whose role was essentially to support the traditional research community by project and training grants. Furthermore the amount of money involved was disproportionate to the annual budget of \$A700,000, two-thirds of which, or \$A466,000, was allocated to the research program. There was anxiety that undertaking the trial would seriously prejudice the traditional grants program that was already overstretched. By good fortune, an unexpected, one-off and uncommitted grant of \$A250,000 had been received from the Federal Government earlier in the year. Approaches were made to four funding bodies to participate in sponsorship; all agreed and continued to do so until clinics closed in 1980.

With the support of those organizations, the Foundation decided, in February 1973, to undertake the management of the trial and to underwrite it. Much preparatory work had been done, including a supplementary report by the working group, the seven members of which formed the nucleus of a management committee of 13. The others were Dr. Gaston Bauer, cardiologist in Sydney; Dr. Ken Edmondson, secretary of the National Health and Medical Research Council; Dr. T.H. Hurley, representing the Royal Australasian College of Physicians; Professor Paul Korner, Director of the Hallstrom Institute of Cardiology, Sydney; Mr. Douglas Oldfield of the Foundation's National Finance Committee; and Professor Michael Rand of the Department of Pharmacology, University of Melbourne.

A protocol for the study based on the recommendations of the working group was drawn up. The preamble referred to the effective pharmacological treatment currently in use for severe hypertension demonstrated by clinical experience and therapeutic trials. It went on, "These observations have clearly indicated that significant benefits may occur from finding unrecognized hypertensives in the community and treating them efficiently. However, they leave unanswered whether treatment is beneficial in mild hypertension (casual DBP less than 110 mm Hg). This project has been designed to provide answers to this question."

III. SCREENING

Screening was carried out in four centers, one in Perth, one in Sydney, and two in Melbourne. The primary factor determining entry of subjects into the trial was blood pressure.

Measurement was usually done by nurses whose training in all centers was conducted by the coordinating center director, Dr. John Abernethy, based in Canberra. Random Zero sphygmomanometers (14), with cuffs 12 × 22 cm, were used throughout the trial, and pressures throughout were recorded as the mean of two readings after sitting for 5 minutes, using disappearance of Korotkoff sounds for DBP. There were two screening visits, S1 and S2, at 2-week intervals in community halls, a ''Heartmobile'' bus, or the clinic headquarters; the mean of the two visits was taken as the ''screening pressure.'' Subjects with pressures within defined mild limits (95 mm Hg ≤ DBP < 110 mm Hg and SBP < 200 mm Hg), who were not excluded for other reasons, were given appointments to attend a laboratory for pathology tests and electrocardiogram (ECG), and to attend a further examination at the study clinic, the C1 visit. Throughout the trial, blood was sent for testing to a single laboratory in Melbourne. If no further exclusion factors were found, the subjects were randomized, with stratification for age and sex, by drawing of envelopes prepared at the coordinating center in Canberra. After randomization, pressure was again measured if DBP was still 95 mm Hg or higher, and subjects were commenced on a randomized tablet regimen. If below threshold, tablets were withheld, but subjects continued in the trial routine; tablets commenced if and when pressure exceeded the threshold. Progression of subjects through the screening process and the C1 clinic visit, with numbers excluded at each stage, are shown in Fig. 1 and the exclusion factors in Table 1.

The first center, under the direction of Austin Doyle, in an outer Melbourne suburb of some 25,000 people, commenced screening on June 8, 1973. Attendance was greatly assisted by members of the local Rotary club; 18,029 had attended when the operation was completed in December 1973. A second center was started in an inner city suburb of Melbourne on August 7, 1973 under the direction of Richard Lovell to coincide with a compulsory X-ray screening for tuberculosis. All in the designated age group in the area were invited by letter to attend the Heartmobile parked alongside the X-ray screening vehicle. The operation was completed on December 5, when 15,900 had attended. A third center started in Perth on September 3, the cohort being groups of office and factory workers and hospital staff. By January 1974, 4164 of the target 6000 had been screened. The fourth center in Sydney, under the direction of Gaston Bauer and Paul Korner, commenced a pilot program for workers of the postal department in November 1973 with plans to start the main effort in the general community in the outer city suburb of Hornsby in April 1974.

Progress was reviewed at six months when screening of 31,000 individuals was completed and 1300 (4.2%) had been randomized (15). To achieve the target of 3200 trial subjects, 50% more than the requirement determined theoretically (16), the management committee estimated that screening of 80,000 subjects would be necessary. This figure was revised upward on several occasions during the screening process, which continued until December 1975 when 3931 subjects had been randomized.

No attempt was made to evaluate the various methods of screening, but it was clear that the Australian community would respond readily if invited. Of the total 104,171 screened, 22,225 (21.3%) were found, at S1, to be hypertensive, that is, above the mild hypertension threshold, or on antihypertensive medication. Of the latter, 7611 (7.3%) of the total screened and 34.2% of all hypertensives knew they had hypertension and were on treatment for it (Fig. 1). Of those on treatment, just over half were normotensive. These figures were roughly similar to findings in two recent surveys in two Australian country towns (12,13).

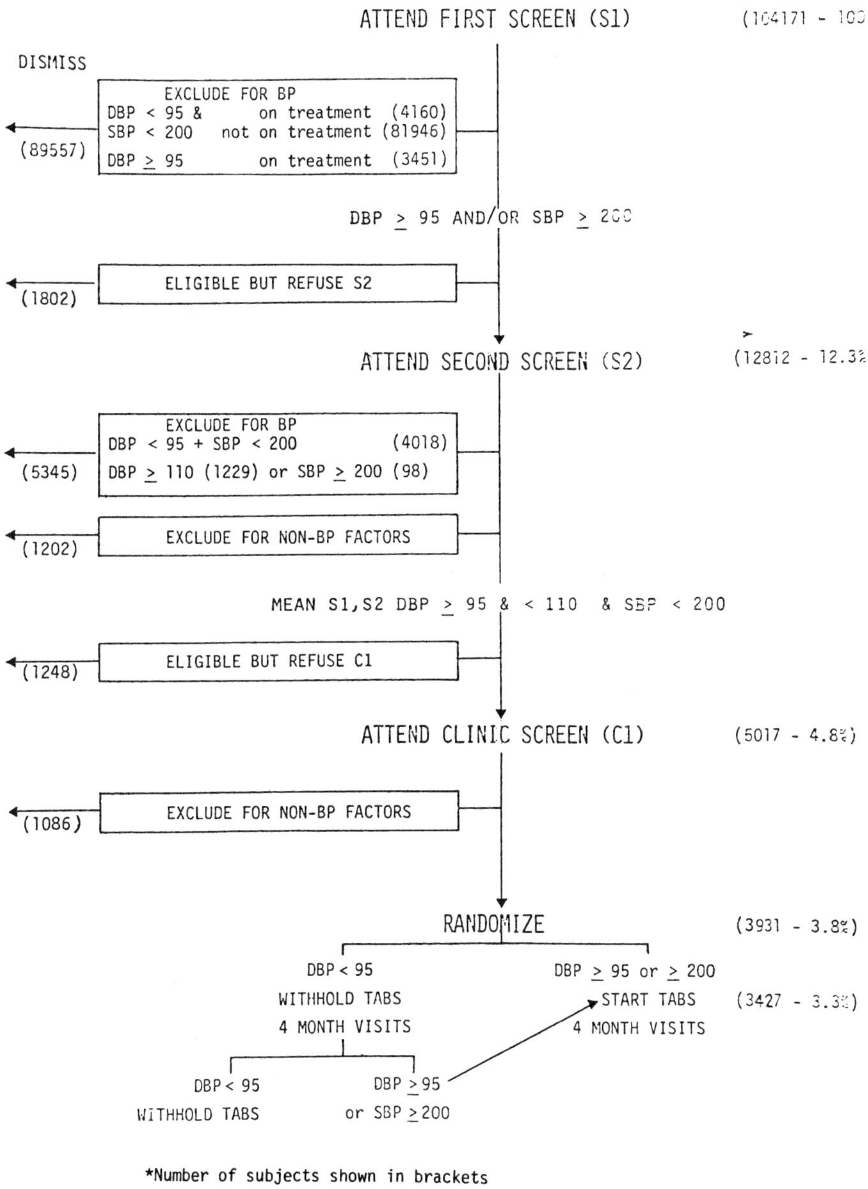

Fig. 1 Recruitment procedure.

Table 1 Exclusion Factors

Visit	Exclusion factors
1st screening	On treatment for hypertension in past 3 months
2nd screening	Angina pectoris by Rose Questionnaire (19)
	History of myocardial infarction in past 3 months
	History of stroke
	Pregnancy
	Taking estrogen and progesterone in combination
	Asthma, diabetes, gout
Clinic	Primary cause of hypertension
	Evidence of cerebrovascular disease, transient cerebral ischemic attacks, acute coronary insufficiency, angina pectoris, plasma creatinine >2 mg/dl*
	Other serious complications of hypertension
	ECG evidence of myocardial ischemia
	Any potentially fatal disease
	Taking tricyclic antidepressants

* >177 μmol/L.

IV. THE TRIAL COHORT

There were 3931 men and women age 30 to 69 years with screening blood pressures (the average of four readings at S1 and S2) within the defined mild limits and who met all other requirements of the trial (Table 1). These were randomized into active and placebo groups on attending the C1 clinic. Of those so randomized, 504 were found to be normotensive at C1 and remained normotensive up to the final censoring date and, according to protocol, were not included in the final cohort.

Thus, there were 3427 trial subjects who had not been taking antihypertensive drugs, had no evidence of hypertensive complications or other condition likely to prejudice their continued participation in the trial, and who started on tablets at C1 or subsequently. All had signed a consent form that included an account of the nature of the trial. All were aware that the tablets to be given might be active or inactive. The numbers and characteristics of the subjects in the active and placebo groups are shown in Table 2.

V. MANAGEMENT AND METHODS

Supervision and management of all subjects were carried out in clinics located at a hospital central to the district in which screening had taken place. Each clinic was staffed by a full-time salaried medical graduate, trained nurses, and a secretary. Pressures were taken, as for screening, with additional readings taken while standing. The mean of the two sitting readings was the index of the subject's progress. The clinic directors were responsible for administering and varying the antihypertensive tablets, or placebo equivalents, throughout the trial. They were aware of each patient's treatment category. All subjects were started on one 500 mg chlorothiazide tablet or the placebo equivalent daily according to their randomized group. If necessary, chlorothiazide was increased to 500 mg twice daily and second- and third-order drugs were given. The schedule for introducing second and lower order drugs is shown in Table 3. Subjects were seen at the clinic at 2-weekly intervals in the initial stage until pressures of the active subjects fell below 95 mm Hg. Thereafter,

Table 2 Comparability of Active and Placebo Groups: Characteristics at Entry

		Active		Placebo	
		No.	Mean (SD)	No.	Mean (SD)
Total subjects		1721		1706	
Age (yr) by 10–yr groups:	30–39	229		223	
	40–49	546		514	
	50–59	653		680	
	60–69	293		289	
	Mean age		50.4 (9.0)		50.5 (8.9)
Sex	Male	1085		1085	
	Female	636		621	
Screening DBP mm Hg	95–99	799		814	
	100–104	589		589	
	105–109	332		303	
	Mean screening DBP mm Hg		100.5 (4.0)		100.4 (3.8)
Screening SBP mm Hg			157.7 (15.0)		157.1 (14.4)
Serum cholesterol mg/dl*	<220	691		742	
	≥220	1030		964	
	Mean mg/dl		231.9 (44.5)		229.8 (44.0)
Smoking	Nonsmokers	1303		1267	
	Smokers	418		439	
Serum uric acid mg/dl†			5.5 (1.4)		5.5 (1.4)
Weight (g)/height^2 (cm)			2.7 (0.4)		2.7 (0.4)
Myocardial infarction before 3 months		6		8	

* 220 mg/dl = 5.69 mmol/l.
† 5.5 mg/dl = 327 μmol/l.
Abbreviations: *SD*, standard deviation; *DBP*, diastolic blood pressure.

subjects were asked to attend at 4-monthly intervals. The object was to maintain DBP of the active treatment patients below 95 mm Hg, but 90 mm Hg was to be regarded as optimal and after two years, the level was lowered to 80 mm Hg. A file for each subject was kept at the clinic and data for each visit was transferred to standardized forms, sent to the Coordinating Center, and entered on computer files.

Efforts were made to match the number and types of tablets and frequency of clinic visits of placebo subjects to those of the active treatment group. At the outset, an estimate was made that 66% of all active subjects would require first-order tablets only throughout the trial, 22% would require second order, and 11% would require third-order tablets. Placebo subjects, therefore, were allocated to tablet regimens in those proportions as part of the randomization procedure at C1. The percentages were 28%, 49%, and 18%, respectively, for the active and 59%, 33%, and 10% for the placebo group.

A special procedure was laid down for any subject of the active or placebo regimens who, at any time through the trial, exceeded 199 mm SBP or 109 mm DBP on three consecutive visits in a 6-week period. These were designated *pressure limits exceeded* and were given active tablets to reduce pressure to optimal levels. They continued in the routine of the trial and continued to be counted in their original randomized group.

Table 3 Recommended Procedure for Altering Active Drug Regimens

Drug	Code	Order of introduction: Austin Hospital	Order of introduction: All other centers	Tablet size	Maximum daily dose
Chlorothiazide	A	1	1	500 mg	1000 mg
Methyldopa	C	3	2	250 mg	2000 mg
Propranolol	F	—	3	40 mg	320 mg
Prindolol	H	2	—	5 mg	30 mg
Clonidine	K	4	4	150 mg	900 mg
Hydralazine	M	5	5	10 mg or 50 mg	200 mg

1. Criteria for introducing a higher order drug into a regimen—DBP
   DBP 90 mg Hg or greater at a follow-up clinic despite maximum doses of drugs in existing regimen.
2. Failure of approved therapy
   a. Providing the DBP remains in the range 95–109 mm Hg and the SBP is less than 200 mm Hg and list of approved drugs had been exhausted, no further action is necessary. The subject continuing with maximum doses of approved drugs.
   b. If the DBP exceeds 109 mg Hg or the SBP exceeds 199 mm Hg at any follow-up visit, the criteria for withdrawal—pressure limits exceeded—would apply, criteria limits exceeded would apply, namely, critical limits exceeded on 3 consecutive occasions in a 6-week period. Providing the list of approved drugs had not been exhausted, there would still be a grace period of at least 4 weeks in which to find an effective regimen.

Drugs approved so far are listed along with information on codes, order of introduction, tablet size, and maximum daily doses.

The management committee was responsible for the overall conduct of the study and for reporting the results. The committee was not aware of the blood pressure or treatment regimen of any subject during the study. It was thus ''blind.'' Much thought was given to ethical considerations, and patient confidentiality and safety were the responsibility of an ethics committee. The terms of reference were: (a) protection of patients' interests; (b) termination of the trial in the event of a positive or negative answer emerging from the ANBPS; (c) surveillance of results from overseas trials. All trial endpoints (Table 4) were reviewed by the ethics committee with full knowledge of the subjects' treatment category. A statement was drawn up detailing possible breaches of confidentiality at the verbal, written, or computer level, and measures taken to avoid them. All personnel of committees and staff were required to sign a document acknowledging confidentiality measures. At one stage, I received a visit, unannounced, from the chairman of the Law Reform Commission of New South Wales asking for details of our ethical standards. He seemed satisfied and we remain friends to this day. He is now a Justice of the High Court of the Commonwealth.

Two other decision-making committees were formed. An ECG committee was based in Sydney. Criteria of myocardial infarction were those defined by the WHO Fifth Working Group for ''Ischaemic Heart Disease Registers,'' Copenhagen, April 26–29, 1971 (17). Precise T-wave changes for chronic ischemia, including those of left bundle branch block, were defined. A trial endpoint review committee was based in Adelaide. Fatal and nonfatal endpoints were defined (Table 4) and diagnostic criteria laid down. Details of a

Table 4 Trial Endpoints

	Endpoints
Fatal	Death from any cause (cause of death specified)
	(a) cardiovascular*
	(b) other
Nonfatal	Thrombotic or hemorrhagic cerebrovascular disease
	Transient cerebral ischemic attacks with observed neurological signs
	Myocardial infarction by WHO category I or II
	Other ischemic heart disease by Rose Questionnaire or defined ECG criteria
	Congestive cardiac failure
	Dissecting aneurysm of the aorta
	Retinal hemorrhages, exudates, or papilledema
	Hypertensive encephalopathy
	Onset of renal failure with plasma creatinine above 2 mg/dl†

* Cardiovascular deaths are limited to those caused by the conditions listed under nonfatal trial endpoints.
† 177 μmol/l.
Abbreviations: *WHO*, World Health Organization; *ECG*, electrocardiogram.

subject with a suspected trial endpoint were referred by the clinic directors to this committee for decision and classification. Both the ECG committee and the trial endpoint review committee were ''blind'' to the subjects' treatment group.

The study was thus a randomized, single-blind, placebo-controlled trial in which the subjects were ''blind'' and the management committee, the trial endpoint review committee, and the ECG review committee were also ''blind.'' The ethics committee and the clinic directors were not, a measure considered necessary for the safety of the subjects and for the efficient management of their blood pressures. It was a comparison of two management regimens for the care of subjects found to have mild hypertension: one to commence antihypertensive drugs on diagnosis, the other to keep the subject under regular surveillance, but to commence antihypertensive drugs should pressure rise above mild limits.

The clinic directors could vary the intervals between visits, if indicated. All subjects were followed up for the duration of the trial, if possible. At each clinic visit, subjects were classified as either:

(A) Failed to attend. This led to: a letter, a second letter, a telephone call at home and at work, a telephone call to the family doctor, and finally, a home visit. The object was to obtain information about a possible trial endpoint, future attendance, or for classification as premature withdrawal and reason for withdrawal. Reasons for withdrawal were defined in detail but under the general headings of ''clinic initiated,'' ''patient initiated,'' or ''local doctor initiated.'' Subjects were withdrawn by the clinic directors if for any reason they did not take tablets or took the wrong tablets for four months. For subjects who were not taking tablets, this period of grace was 8 months. If all these procedures were unproductive, a subject was classified ''premature withdrawal-lost.'' Immediately after the final censoring date, March 5, 1979, two further efforts were made to determine the occurrence of endpoints in this group. A search was made in each state Registrar General's records for death certificates, and secondly, an approach was made to the Federal Electoral Office to find the current address of the missing subjects. The Office could not agree to this but volunteered to identify them in their records and write conveying our

Table 5 Schedule of Biochemistry Tests

	At C1 visit	At 4-monthly visit	At annual visit
Serum uric acid	x		x
Serum potassium	x	x	x
Serum creatinine	x		x
Serum cholesterol	x		x
Urine protein	x		x
Urine glucose	x		x
Urine blood	x		x

request for them to contact the clinics. These measures retrieved some data but in the final count, there were 88 subjects, 42 in the active and 46 in the placebo groups, for whom no data on occurrence of endpoints were available.

(B) Reached a trial endpoint. If the clinic director suspected that an endpoint may have occurred, the case was referred to the trial endpoint review committee, which made the decision.

(C) Classified and managed as pressure limits exceeded.

(D) Continuing. For those continuing, tablet counts and enquiry as to compliance were made and encouragement given, drug intolerance and postural hypotension were investigated and tablet modification implemented, a blood sample for potassium estimation was taken, and a further 4-monthly appointment given. A full clinical, biochemical, and ECG examination was made at the clinic visits nearest to the yearly intervals from the subject's entry into the trial. The schedule for biochemistry tests is shown in Table 5.

VI. STATISTICAL ASPECTS

It was estimated in the protocol that 2428 trial subjects would be required. To allow for imprecision in this estimate, a target of 3640 subjects was set. In all, 3931 persons were randomized, but of these, the 504 referred to above who did not start on tablets were not included in the analysis of the main results. Thus, the trial cohort of the study was 3427.

The trial endpoint rates have been calculated per 1000 person-years of exposure to risk. To calculate whether there were significant differences between subjects of the active and placebo groups, exact significance levels were determined by calculating the relevant binomial probabilities under the hypothesis that the number of trial endpoints was proportional to the exposure to risk. Where appropriate, the significance of the differences was also calculated by the Cox proportional hazards method (18), which uses individual times to failure, or censoring, instead of the total exposure to risk. The two methods gave good agreement; the latter, however, indicated higher levels of significance. In the accompanying results, "not significant" refers to significance at the 5% level.

The outcome of the trial was examined in two ways. In the first, account was taken only of trial endpoints occurring while subjects were continuing their regimen—the *on treatment* analysis. In the second, account was taken of endpoints occurring while subjects were continuing or after they had stopped their treatment regimen—the *intention to treat* analysis. The rationale for these two approaches is considered later.

Data up to the censoring date, March 5, 1979, were entered into the record. On that date, virtually all subjects who had not been withdrawn had forward appointments to the clinics, which remained operative until December 31, 1979 for final examinations and recording of trial endpoints up to censoring date. A standard letter was sent to all local doctors and instructions given to subjects to facilitate an effective transfer. A newsletter was sent to all participants. Four 4-drawer filing cabinets of records, protocols, and minutes of meetings were stored in the archives of the National Heart Foundation in Canberra, including individual patient files. The latter, and much other material, was destroyed ten years later. The two major computer files and several subsidiary data files were stored with Social Science Data Archives of the Australian National University.

VII. TERMINATION OF THE TRIAL

There could be three indications for termination of the trial:

1. Completion of each subject's 5-year period in the study. (The last subject would complete the five-years in November 1980)
2. Because the ethics committee presented an ethical reason
3. Because the results of the trial indicated that significant answers were already available

The latter decision must rest with the management committee but could arise from a recommendation from the ethics committee. However, it must not result from repeated ''looks'' at the results. In fact, the decision was taken by the management committee at its meeting of March 5, 1979, when it looked, for the first time, at results censored at October 26, 1978.

The events leading to the decision were as follows: the ethics committee, at its regular meeting on October 9, 1978, considered data presented by the statistician concerning 201 trial endpoints and average duration of the study for all of the study cohort of 3.5 years. A trend was present that suggested that a result was in sight. The chairman wrote to the management committee to this effect. He emphasized that the trend was of marginal significance at the 5% level and that it did not pose an ethical problem, that the ethics committee proposed to review the situation early in 1979 and recommended that consideration should be given to plans for ensuring an eventual smooth return of subjects to their usual medical care.

No indication was given as to the direction in which the trend tended.

The management committee, at its meeting of October 19, therefore decided that the trial should continue but that a comparison of endpoint rates by the binomial and Cox methods should be undertaken using data as of October 26, 1978. It appointed a subcommittee of Lovell, Reader, and Whyte to meet with the coordinating center staff to consider updated results and recommend either that:

1. The study should continue, in which case the management committee should remain ''blind,'' but the three members of the subcommittee should withdraw from it until a final censoring was effected, or
2. The study should be terminated

The subcommittee received data at censoring date October 26, 1978, by which time a further 38 trial endpoints had been processed. It met twice, on October 30, 1978, and

January 31, 1979, and presented a lengthy report on trends between active and placebo groups by various trial endpoint categories and subsets of patients to the management committee at its meeting of March 5, 1979, thereby committing that group to a decision to terminate the trial.

It did so, setting the final censoring date as the date of the meeting and setting in motion procedures for the scheduled visits over the following months of all subjects, recording their status as of March 5, 1979, tracing lost subjects, returning subjects to their own doctors with appropriate documentation, preparing final analyses, and reporting the results. The decision to stop the trial was thus taken after a single examination of results by the management committee.

VIII. RESULTS

The main results of the trial were published by the management committee in *The Lancet* on June 14, 1980 (1). The paper presented the outcome in the 3427 subjects who were started on a tablet regimen. There were 62 subjects in the active and 46 in the placebo group who, at various stages through the trial and by mistake, were not started on their randomized regimen within four months of becoming eligible. According to protocol, they were included in the trial cohort but withdrawn after the 4- or 8-month period of grace. They accounted for one endpoint in the active and five in the placebo group, all of which occurred after withdrawal.

Comparison of active with placebo subjects in terms of characteristics at entry, length of time in the study, and person-years of exposure are shown in Tables 2 and 6. The attempt to match numbers of visits and tablets taken was only partially successful. In all other respects, the two groups were well matched.

The status of the trial cohort at the final censoring date is shown in Table 7. One third, 1209, were prematurely withdrawn from the regimen and of these, 88 were lost to follow-up, 42 in the active and 46 in the placebo group. The similarity between number

Table 6 Comparability of Active and Placebo Groups: Experience Through Study

	Active	Placebo
Average follow-up (yr):		
Intention to treat	4.06	4.03
On treatment	3.08	3.04
Person-years of exposure to risk:		
Intention to treat	6991	6868
On treatment	5294	5182
Mean number of visits to clinic:		
Intention to treat	16	14
On treatment	14	12
No. of subjects taking antihypertensive drugs or corresponding placebo:*		
One only	492	903
Two only	853	575
More than two	314	182

* Does not include 62 of active group and 46 of placebo group who did not start tablets.

Table 7 Status of the Trial Population at End of Study

	Active		Placebo		Total	
	No.	%	No.	%	No.	%
Continuing on regimen:						
Trial endpoints	91	5.3	127	7.4	218	6.4
No trial endpoints	1047	60.8	953	55.9	2000	58.4
Total	1138	66.1	1080	63.3	2218	64.7
Prematurely stopped regimen:						
Trial endpoints after stopping	47	2.7	41	2.4	88	2.6
No trial endpoints	494	28.7	539	31.6	1033	30.1
Lost to follow-up	42	2.4	46	2.7	88	2.6
Total	583	33.9	626	36.7	1209	35.3
	1721	100	1706	100	3427	100

of trial endpoints after stopping regimen—88—and the 88 subjects lost to follow-up are coincidental.

Comparison of active with placebo subjects who were prematurely withdrawn in terms of entry characteristics, reasons for stopping, trial endpoint rates and person-years of exposure to risk is shown in Table 8, and the numbers and types of endpoint occurring after stopping are shown in Table 9. There was a higher proportion of smokers in the subjects withdrawn (29%) than in those who continued (23%) and a higher proportion of

Table 8 Characteristics of Subjects Prematurely Withdrawn

	Active		Placebo	
	No.	Mean (SD)	No.	Mean (SD)
Total	583	???	626	???
Age (yr)		49.5 (9.6)		49.8 (9.1)
Sex:				
Male	335		362	
Female	248		264	
Screening DBP (mm Hg)		100.2 (3.9)		100.3 (3.8)
Screening SBP (mm Hg)		156.3 (14.7)		157.4 (14.5)
Smoking:				
Smokers	159	???	190	???
Nonsmokers	424		436	
Serum cholesterol (mg/dl)*		229.9 (45.0)		229.6 (44.6)
Reasons for stopping:				
Clinic withdrawal	121		97	
Subject withdrawal	310		288	
Local doctor withdrawal	110	???	195	???
Not known (lost)	42		46	
Trial endpoint rates per 1000 person-years	20.5		16.3	
Person-years of exposure to risk	2288		2518	

* 230 mg/dl = 5.95 mmol/l.

Table 9 Numbers of Trial Endpoints by Diagnostic Category

	A Intention to treat		B On treatment		In premature withdrawals after stopping (A–B)	
	Active	Placebo	Active	Placebo	Active	Placebo
Ischemic heart disease:						
Fatal	5	11	2	8	3	3
Nonfatal						
(a) myocardial infarction	28	22	18	17	10	5
(b) others	65	76	50	63	15	13
Total	98	109	70	88	28	21
Cerebrovascular events:						
Fatal	3	6	2	4	1	2
Nonfatal						
(a) hemorrhage or thrombosis	10	16	7	13	3	3
(b) transient cerebral ischemic attacks	4	9	3	8	1	1
Total	17	31	12	25	5	6
Other fatal:						
Aortic aneurysm	0	1	0	1	0	0
Noncardiovascular						
(a) neoplasm	9	8	1	2	8	6
(b) other	8	9	4	4	4	5
Other nonfatal:						
Retinopathy	2	5	1	4	1	1
Congestive cardiac failure	3	3	2	1	1	2
Renal failure	1	2	1	2	0	0
Total	138	168	91	127	47	41

women (42%) than men (34%). It seemed unlikely that factors associated with premature withdrawal biased the results.

Differences in occurrence of all trial endpoints and all fatal endpoints between the active and placebo groups emerged early and the cumulative occurrence in subjects continuing on their regimen is shown in Figure 2. The differences were analyzed by Cox's method and were significant for all events ($P < 0.01$) and all deaths ($P < 0.05$) in the *on treatment* analysis. The incidence of endpoints and rates per 1000 person-years of exposure for the active and placebo subjects are shown in Table 10. In both modes of analysis, the total endpoints and cardiovascular deaths were significantly lower in the active than in the placebo subjects. Rates for nonfatal endpoints and for total deaths were significantly lower only in the *on treatment* analysis. There were seven fewer endpoints and two fewer deaths per 1000 person-years in actively treated subjects who adhered to their medication. There were fewer endpoints in the active compared with the placebo subjects in men, 67 versus 91 ($P < 0.05$) and women, 24 versus 36 ($P = 0.058$). However, in a multivariate analysis of prognostic factors influencing treatment effect that was reported some years later (4), and described in this chapter, a more powerful model using the Cox proportional hazards method showed the benefit of treatment in women to be

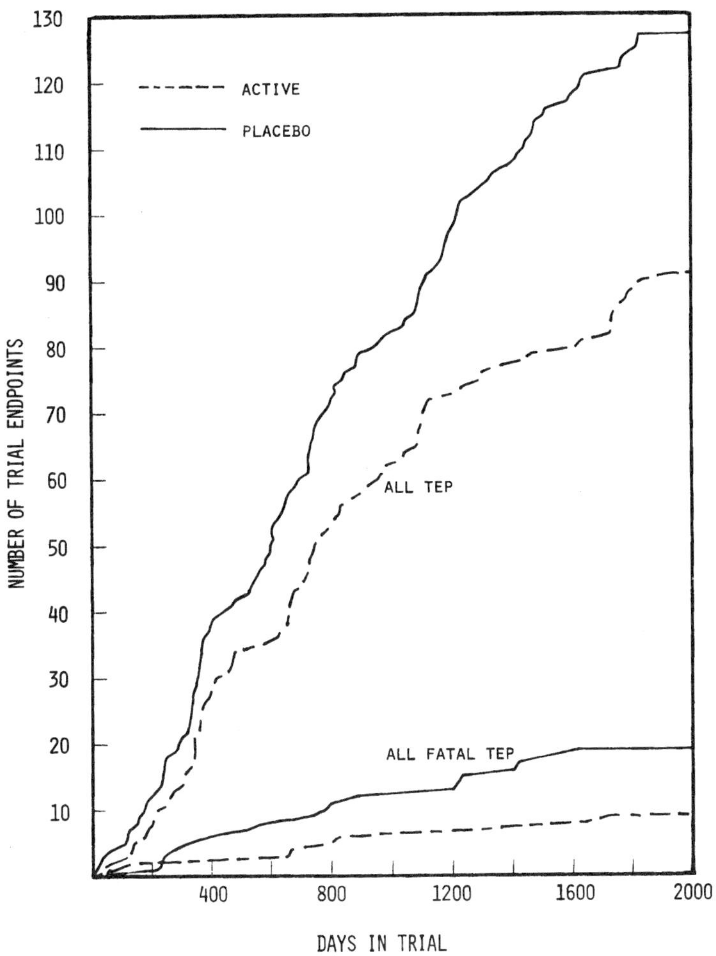

Fig. 2 Cumulative incidence of trial endpoints.

significant, $P = 0.044$. Trial endpoints in subjects younger than age 50 were 22 versus 31 (NS) and older than age 50, 69 versus 96 ($P < 0.025$). The effect of these and other covariates were examined in detail in a later paper (4).

The numbers of trial endpoints in individual diagnostic categories are shown in Table 9. Two-thirds were due to coronary heart disease, mostly nonfatal events that occurred in similar numbers in active and placebo subjects. Less than half as many deaths from coronary heart disease occurred in the active as in the placebo subjects in both *on treatment* and *intention to treat* analyses; the difference was just short of significance ($P = 0.051$) in the former. There were half as many cerebrovascular events in the active compared with the placebo subjects. This was so for both fatal and nonfatal strokes and for transient ischemic attacks with observed neurologic signs. The difference was significant for all cerebrovascular events ($P < 0.025$) and for all nonfatal events ($P < 0.05$).

Table 10 Incidence of Trial Endpoints*

	Intention to treat				On treatment			
	Active n = 1721		Placebo n = 1706		Active n = 1721		Placebo n = 1706	
	No.	Rate	No.	Rate	No.	Rate	No.	Rate
Fatal TEP								
Cardiovascular	8	1.1	18	2.6‡	4	−0.8	13	2.5‡
Noncardiovascular	17	2.4	17	2.5	5	0.9	6	1.2
Total fatal	25	3.6	35	5.1	9	1.7	19	3.7†
Nonfatal TEP	113	16.2	133	19.4	82	15.5	108	20.8‡
All TEP	138	19.7	168	24.5†	91	17.2	127	24.5§

* Rates per 1000 person-years exposure to risk.
† $P < 0.05$;
‡ $P < 0.025$;
§ $P < 0.01$.
Abbreviation: *TEP*, trial endpoint.

Noncardiovascular deaths occurred with similar frequency in the active and placebo groups.

IX. BLOOD PRESSURE LEVELS

The average of all DBP readings for each subject during the trial regimen was taken as an index of response of blood pressure to the regimen. The results are shown in Table 11. In both active and placebo groups, the mean of the average DBPs while on tablets was lower than the screening DBP, and the higher the screening pressure the greater the fall. For each screening DBP class, the fall was greater in the active group, ranging from 9.7 to 16.5 mm Hg, than in the placebo group, ranging from 5.0 to 9.2 mm Hg. Further aspects of blood pressure trends, particularly the fall in pressure in placebo subjects, were considered in a later paper (3).

Table 11 Blood Pressure Levels Throughout the Trial

Screening diastolic pressure (mm Hg)	No. of subjects*		Mean of screening DBP mm Hg		Mean of average DBP mm Hg while on trial regimen		Mean of fall† in DBP mm Hg	
	Active	Placebo	Active	Placebo	Active	Placebo	Active	Placebo
95–99	756	763	96.9	97.0	87.2	92.1	9.7	5.0
100–104	558	563	101.9	101.9	88.8	94.5	13.1	7.4
105–109	320	291	106.7	106.7	90.2	97.5	16.5	9.2
Total	1633	1617	100.5	100.4	88.3	93.9	12.2	6.6

* This table does not include the 176 subjects who did not have any blood pressure readings after entry.
† Difference between screening DBP and average DBP.
Abbreviation: *DBP*, diastolic blood pressure.

Table 12 Trial Endpoint Rates by Average DBP on Trial Regimen and According to Screening DBP Class*

Screening DBP (mm Hg)	95–99				100–104				105–109			
Average DBP (mm Hg)	No. of subjects A	No. of subjects P	Rates† A	Rates† P	No. of subjects A	No. of subjects P	Rates† A	Rates† P	No. of subjects A	No. of subjects P	Rates† A	Rates† P
<90	543	255	12.1	20.5	335	121	17.6	14.7	166	31	12.2	0
90–94	144	244	24.8	15.7	142	174	14.4	17.8	84	64	19.9	12.3
95–99	46	183	69.8	24.6	48	146	38.4	19.3	49	83	58.4	25.4
≥100	23	81	0	46.2	33	122	0	62.2	21	113	131.6	64.6
Total	756	763	15.6	22.3	558	563	17.5	24.5	320	291	20.7	30.5

* This table does not include 176 subjects who did not have any blood pressure readings after starting trial regimen.
† Rates per 1000 person-years.
Abbreviation: *DBP*, diastolic blood pressure.

The relationship of incidence of trial endpoints to average DBP levels is shown in Table 12. The higher endpoint rate in the placebo group as a whole was consistent with the fact that only 25% of placebo subjects had average DBPs below 90 mm Hg compared with 64% of active subjects, and 20% compared to 5% had average pressures above 100 mm Hg. Trial endpoint rates were generally related to average DBP regardless of treatment regimen or screening pressure.

X. DISCUSSION

Subjects of the active and placebo groups were well matched in prognostic characteristics at entry, in management through the trial except for the antihypertensive medication, and in the characteristics at entry of prematurely withdrawn subjects and trial endpoints after withdrawal. Benefit from antihypertensive treatment was shown in both the *on treatment* and *intention to treat* analyses, tending to negate bias caused by inequalities in withdrawal patterns. In fact, bias favoring the placebo group may have resulted in the *intention to treat* analysis from local doctor-initiated withdrawals from the placebo group to start their patients on antihypertensive therapy.

The numbers of endpoints were too small to demonstrate significant differences between active and placebo groups in the various diagnostic categories. Coronary heart disease was responsible for about 70% of endpoints in both regimens and of these, two-thirds were relatively soft, fulfilling the criteria for angina pectoris by Rose Questionnaire (19) or the occurrence of ECG changes defined as ischemic but not fulfilling World Health Organization (WHO) criteria for myocardial infarction (17). In those continuing on treatment, there were 70 coronary events in the active and 88 in the placebo subjects, and two compared with eight of these were fatal. Neither difference was significant, although for the deaths, $P = 0.051$. Considering the natural history of ischemic disease, a possible benefit of treatment of mild hypertension, in its prevention, is likely to take longer to become manifest than for stroke. In this study, the significant reduction in strokes (9 in active, 17 in placebo subjects) that had concerned the ethics committee prohibited prolongation of the trial to allow accumulation of sufficient numbers of ischemic events to demonstrate or refute benefit.

The results were generally in line with those of four other trials of antihypertensive treatment in mild hypertension conducted before or simultaneously with the Australian study. Four, including the ANBPS, were randomized, blind, placebo-controlled studies [U.S. Veterans Affairs 1970 (11), U.S. Public Hospitals Study (USPHS) 1977 (20), ANBPS 1980 (1), the British Medical Research Council (MRC) trial 1985 (21)]. In the fifth study [U.S. HDFP 1979 (22)], the control subjects were managed by "usual care," and neither subjects nor management were blinded. The DBP range varied a little, as did methods and treatments, but the objective of the studies was similar. Considering the *intention to treat* analyses, all five studies showed significant reduction of total trial endpoints and of cerebrovascular events in the active or actively stepped care subjects. Four showed similar reductions in total deaths and cardiovascular deaths; the fifth, the USPHS study, showed two deaths each in active and placebo groups. With respect to fatal coronary heart disease, there was a trend in favor of active treatment in four, but the trend was against in the MRC. For nonfatal coronary heart disease, the HDFP and MRC trials showed a trend in favor, but the other three did not.

A meta-analysis reported in 1986 (23), which included three other randomized, placebo-controlled trials (VA-NHLBI, Oslo, and EWPHE) and a multifactorial intervention study using referred care subjects as controls (MRFIT) showed significant benefits in total mortality (11%), stroke mortality (38%), incidence of nonfatal stroke (43%), and all strokes (39%). For coronary heart disease, there were trends in favor of active treatment for all deaths (8%), nonfatal events (6%), and all events (8%), but none was significant at the 5% level.

The authors of the meta-analysis concluded,

> Collectively the studies indicate a modest but important reduction in mortality in study treatment patients, primarily as a consequence of a substantial reduction of stroke mortality, which accounted for more than 50% of the total reduction in deaths. The risk of non-fatal stroke was also substantially reduced by a similar margin to that of fatal stroke. However, the results of these studies, neither individually nor collectively provide evidence that convinces us of a reduction in mortality from coronary heart disease or clinically diagnosed non-fatal myocardial infarction, although the HDFP reported a significant reduction of myocardial infarction assessed by self report. **Once again it should be stressed that active treatment in control subjects in these trials is likely to have reduced the power to detect a significant effect of study treatments on fatal and non-fatal myocardial infarction**.

The final reservation (the emphasis is mine) raises the question of the relative merits of the *intention to treat* and the *on treatment* analyses of the data. The objective of the trials was to provide guidelines for the control of mild hypertension. Guidelines for whom? Clearly, public health authorities need to know both the benefit, if any, and the scale of benefit from a community-based screening and treatment program. This was a primary objective for the National Heart Foundation of Australia. The *intention to treat* analysis addresses these questions directly, taking account of both the effectiveness of the pharmacological agents and the compliance of the community. The meta-analysis of McMahon and his colleagues based on the *intention to treat* approach shows a "modest but important reduction" in mortality and stroke incidence, in spite of dilution of such benefits by placebo subjects going onto active medication, as the meta-analysis report envisaged they might, which dilution would be further increased if the active subjects ceased antihypertensive medication after withdrawal. Yet the results of the *intention to treat* approach provided evidence in favor of community-based detection and follow-up program.

The *intention to treat* concept had not been widely implemented in the early 1970s when the ANBPS was planned. The committee was indebted to Richard Lovell for proposing it and had no difficulty adopting it. An international anticoagulant review group, of which he was a member, in a meta-analysis of nine controlled trials of anticoagulants in myocardial infarction, wrote in 1970, ''In other words, we have compared mortality experience in terms of the original intention in treatment without regard to changes that might have been made later'' (24). Careful follow-up and recording of data for withdrawn subjects were features of the ANBPS protocol.

Doctors in practice also look to these studies for guidelines. They need to know if antihypertensive medication is effective in preventing complications in mild hypertensive patients, and they will assume that compliance is part of the contract with their patient. Problems of noncompliance are well known, have been highlighted by these studies, and can be reduced by good management. The *on treatment* approach addresses the scale of benefit in patients who continue on their medication. Bias can arise if there are inequalities in levels of risk between active and placebo subjects who are withdrawn, thus distorting the randomization at entry of the two groups. In the Australian study, investigation revealed no evidence of inequality in risk levels in the withdrawn subjects (Table 8), lending support to the *on treatment* analysis.

Thus the *intention to treat* approach in the Australian study, as well as in the meta-analysis, provides evidence in favor of both community based detection and follow-up programs but may well have understated the scale of benefit that may ensue. This benefit may be nearer to that shown in the *on treatment* analysis of the Australian study, with encouragement for doctors in practice to use antihypertensive medication providing they can maintain compliance in their patients.

XI. ELDERLY SUBJECTS

The main study concerned subjects age 30 to 69. As noted earlier, there were fewer endpoints in the active than the placebo subjects; for those younger than 50, 22 versus 31 (NS) and older than 50, 69 versus 96 ($P < 0.025$). At the start of the study, stratification by age had been incorporated in the randomization procedure to test the treatment effect in age-group subsets. The study fulfilled the requirements for a randomized, placebo-controlled, single-blind study in the 582 subjects who were age 60 or older on entry. Because of the special problems perceived at that time for antihypertensive medication in elderly patients, opportunity also was taken to seek evidence of such problems in this subset of subjects older than age 60 and covering ages up to 74 by the final censoring date (2). Active and placebo groups were well matched in characteristics at entry (except for SBP and serum cholesterol levels in women (Table 13) and in length of follow-up (3.93 versus 3.81 years) and person-years of exposure to risk (1152 versus 1100). The proportion of subjects prematurely withdrawn from regimen, 33% from active and 35% from placebo groups, did not differ from the withdrawal rate in the main study, suggesting that the subjects tolerated the therapy and other demands of the trial regimen as well as did their younger counterparts. The occurrence of trial endpoints was higher in the elderly,

Table 13 Comparability of Active and Placebo Group Characteristics at Entry in Elderly Subjects

	Active		Placebo	
	No.	Mean (SD)	No.	Mean (SD)
Total subjects	293		289	
Age 60–64	199		200	
65–69	94		89	
Mean age		63.6 (2.3)		63.5 (2.3)
Sex Male	161		157	
Female	132		132	
Screening DBP				
(mm Hg) 95–99	136		138	
100–104	99		101	
105–109	58		50	
Mean screening DBP		100.7 (4.0)		100.4 (3.9)
Mean screening SBP		166.3 (14.9)		163.9 (14.9)
Cholesterol (mg/dL)				
All subjects <220	103		117	
≥220	190		172	
Mean		236.6 (42.2)		231.1 (45.5)
Men >220	80		75	
Mean		221.6 (38.6)		218.7 (40.5)
Women <220	22		35	
≥220	110		97	
Mean		254.9 (39.2)		246.2 (46.6)
Smoking				
Non-Smokers	241		239	
Smokers	52		50	
Uric acid (mg/dL)		5.5 (1.3)		5.3 (1.4)
Wt (g)/Ht^2 (cm)		2.6 (0.4)		2.6 (0.4)
*Myocardial infarction before 3 months	2		1	

* No TEPs among these three subjects.
Abbreviations: *SD*, standard deviation; *DBP*, diastolic blood pressure; *TEP*, trial endpoint.

14.6% (Table 14), than in the main study, 8.9%, as would be expected. There were fewer endpoints in the active than in the placebo subjects in both *intention to treat* and *on treatment* analyses, the difference being considerably greater in the latter, 30.99 versus 50.82 per 1000 person-years, $P < 0.025$. This was the only comparison that reached significance.

The cumulative difference in incidence of total endpoints analyzed by the Cox method showed a similar pattern to the main study, $P < 0.025$. The mean fall in DBP through the trial was 13.4 mm Hg for the active and 6.7 mm Hg for placebo subjects; the mean difference in average DBP between the regimens was 6.3 mm Hg. Although women had similar DBP to men at entry, they had higher SBP (168.7 versus 164.4 mm Hg,

Table 14 Incidence of Trial Endpoints in Elderly Subjects*

	Intention to treat				On treatment			
	Active no.	Rate	Placebo no.	Rate	Active no.	Rate	Placebo no.	Rate
Fatal TEP								
Cardiovascular	2	1.74	5	4.55	2	2.30	4	4.84
Noncardiovascular	5	4.34	4	3.64	1	1.15	1	1.21
Total fatal	7	6.08	9	8.18	3	3.44	5	6.05
Nonfatal TEP	30	26.05	39	35.46	24	27.55	37	44.77
All TEP	37	32.13	48	43.64	27	30.99	42	50.82†

* Rates per 1000 person-years exposure risk.
† $P < 0.025$.
Abbreviation: *TEP*, trial endpoint.

respectively, in the active and 165.9 versus 162.2 mm Hg in the placebo subjects). These differences may have argued against a benefit from treatment in women. There was also a possible bias against women with a higher serum cholesterol level at entry, 254.9 in active versus 246.2 mg/dl in placebo subjects, which emerged in spite of the randomization process.

XII. DRUG SIDE EFFECTS

In the main study, at each follow-up visit subjects were asked if they had experienced any symptoms. If any were volunteered, questions were directed to determining if these were possibly drug side effects. Although these data were recorded, a formal analysis was not made at the end of the trial. But a study (25) using the 20-symptom Bullpit and Dollery questionnaire was made in the Sydney center of subjects of all ages, two years after they entered the trial. There were 788 subjects of the study cohort, 347 from the active group, 322 from the placebo group, and 119 who had been randomized but not started on tablets because their DBP did not rise to 95 mm Hg throughout the trial after the two screening visits, S1 and S2, and for comparison, a group of 229 subjects, who were randomly selected from the general community and matched for age and sex. The numbers in each group are shown by age and sex in Table 15 and the incidence of ''significant symptoms'' in Table 16. The authors concluded, ''This study demonstrates that there is little justification to attribute symptoms other than sleepiness or a feeling of depression in women to mild hypertension or its drug therapy.'' As stated above, there was no evidence that a preponderance of side effects in the elderly subjects of the main trial led to higher withdrawal rates.

XIII. UNTREATED MILD HYPERTENSION: BLOOD PRESSURE TRENDS AND OCCURRENCE OF HYPERTENSIVE COMPLICATIONS

There were 1943 subjects who were randomized to the placebo group at the C1 visit, including 1706 who started tablets either at the C1 visit or subsequently. The remaining 237 subjects did not start tablets at any time through the study, but in all other respects

Table 15 Age and Sex Distribution and Details of Drug Therapy in Side Effects Study

Treatment category	Age group (years)								Sex distribution	
	30–34	35–39	40–44	45–49	50–54	55–59	60–64	65–69	Male	Female
Active	10	22	37	65	80	59	48	26	221 (64%)	126
Placebo	12	26	36	41	68	55	50	34	219 (68%)	103
No tablets	7	8	16	14	23	21	25	5	80 (67%)	39
Nonstudy	36	42	32	46	26	31	13	3	134 (59%)	95

Drug therapy

One drug	164 (48%)	thiazides 295, propranolol 134,
Two drugs	175 (50%)	methyl-dopa 97, clonidine 12
Three drugs	8	

Table 16 Prevalence of "Significant" Symptoms in Side Effects Study

Treatment category	Sleepiness		Depression		Nocturia		Impotence	Failed ejaculation	Sore gritty eyes		Skin rash	
	M	F	M	F	M	F	M	M	M	F	M	F
Active	17 (38)	29 (36)	8 (17)	25 (31)	41 (90)	49 (61)	19 (39)	9 (17)	22 (48)	21 (26)	13 (28)	14 (17)
Placebo	22 (48)	12 (12)	9 (20)	11 (11)	48 (103)	49 (49)	14 (27)	5 (10)	21 (45)	33 (32)	14 (33)	11 (11)
No tablets	13 (10)	21 (8)	10 (8)	14 (5)	41 (33)	54 (21)	20 (15)	10 (7)	25 (20)	31 (11)	13 (10)	11 (4)
Nonstudy	5 (7)	14 (13)	5 (7)	11 (10)	29 (39)	48 (46)	10 (13)	6 (7)	15 (19)	18 (17)	4 (6)	8 (8)

Values are given as percentages with the number of subjects in parentheses.

continued in the trial regimen so that blood pressure readings were recorded. They provided an opportunity to study the natural history of mild hypertension in subjects who were free of cardiovascular complications, given no antihypertensive medication, and observed for up to five years (3). Analyses of trends of blood pressure and of the incidence of cardiovascular complications (trial endpoints) were made in these subjects, for the total of 1943 subjects observed for periods up to five years, for 1119 who were observed continuously for three years, and for 237 who took no tablets for the period of observation up to five years. The mean systolic and diastolic blood pressures for each of these groups at 4-monthly intervals are shown in Table 17.

The most striking feature of their subsequent course was a sharp fall in pressures in the first four months of follow-up and a continued slight fall for at least four years. The mean pressure of all three sets showed the downward trend. It occurred in both sexes and was not influenced by age, smoking habits, or serum cholesterol level; it occurred in those who lost or gained weight, although it was greater in the former. It occurred at all levels of initial blood pressure and in those whose pressure remained below the mild hypertension level throughout the study and were therefore not given tablets. The phenomenon may have been due to regression to the mean in the early stages, but the continuing fall could not be so explained. It was probably caused by increasing familiarity with the repeated clinic procedures, including use of the sphygmomanometer, the so-called ''white coat effect.'' This phenomenon was noted in other controlled trials in hypertension and was demonstrated by Armitage and Rose in 1966 (26).

Analysis was made of the screening pressures of five subsets of these 1943 subjects, seeking indicators at screening of blood pressure and endpoint status at three years (Table 18): 172 who had exceeded mild limits, 450 who remained in the mild hypertension range, 669 who had fallen below 95 mm Hg DBP, 117 who had experienced a trial endpoint, and 535 who had been prematurely withdrawn. Subjects were classified as within the mild hypertension range at three years if pressures had not exceeded mild limits and if the reading at the 36th month or the mean of three readings through the third year was equal to or greater than 95 mm Hg; a subject was classified as DBP lower than 95 mm Hg at three years if the mean of three readings through the third year and the reading at the 36th month were both less than 95 mm Hg.

The 172 subjects who exceeded mild limits had, on average, higher pressures at S1, S2, and C1. In 148 of them (86%), the mean DBP of the initial three visits was 100 mm Hg or higher and none was less than 95 mm Hg. Not only did these subjects have higher initial pressures but they had, on average, a distinct rise of DBP between the screening visits (S1 and S2) and the third (C1) visit, 26% showing a rise of more than 10 mm Hg. For those remaining in the mild hypertension range at three years, the proportion was 10% and for those with DBP below the mild hypertension range, it was 5%.

During the period of observation, 22 subjects of the placebo cohort suffered a stroke, 6 of which were fatal, and a further 9 subjects suffered transient ischemic attacks. The strokes tended to occur early, 10 in the first year, 7 in the second and third years, and 5 in the fourth and fifth years. The DBP profiles of these subjects, compared with those of matched subjects drawn randomly from placebo subjects who did not suffer a trial endpoint, are shown in Table 19. The former had highest initial pressures and highest average pressures through the trial. Coronary heart disease occurred in 88 subjects. The events were spaced evenly throughout the trial, and the blood pressure profiles did not differ from matched controls.

Table 17 Blood Pressures Over Time in Three Sets of the Control Group*

	Total			Subjects observed for 3 yr			Subjects given no placebo		
Visit	No.	Mean SBP (mm Hg)	Mean DBP (mm Hg)	No.	Mean SBP (mm Hg)	Mean DBP (mm Hg)	No.	Mean SBP (mm Hg)	Mean DBP (mm Hg)
First screening	1943	158.2	102.3	1119	157.4	102.0	237	156.1	101.6
2 wk	1943	155.7	98.5		154.1	98.0	237	149.7	95.5
4 wk	1943	154.6	98.1		152.3	96.9	237	138.7	85.9
4 mo	1677	146.5	93.4		144.6	92.2	185	135.1	83.9
8 ″	1500	146.4	93.3		144.6	92.2	158	134.7	82.7
12 ″	1444	148.0	94.2		146.4	93.6	157	135.2	83.8
16 ″	1339	143.7	91.4		142.9	91.0	148	131.6	82.2
20 ″	1264	145.0	91.9		144.2	91.6	143	133.3	83.1
24 ″	1235	144.9	91.7		144.6	91.6	138	132.9	83.5
28 ″	1155	142.5	90.8		141.9	90.6	134	130.2	81.7
32 ″	1112	142.5	90.1		142.2	90.0	130	129.0	80.7
36 ″	1084	144.3	90.7		144.2	90.7	131	131.3	81.8
40 ″	992	140.2	89.0				112	128.0	80.9
44 ″	818	142.2	89.8				78	131.3	81.8
48 ″	597	142.8	89.6				57	128.0	79.6
52 ″	508	139.9	88.1				49	127.8	79.2
56 ″	412	141.8	89.5				29	129.6	79.2
60 ″	362	144.1	90.0				28	131.5	80.7

* Mean blood pressures for all 1943 control subjects for as long as they continued on their regimen, for 1119 who continued their regimen for at least 3 years, and for 237 borderline subjects whose DBP remained spontaneously below 95 mm Hg and who were not given placebo tablets. At each visit, there were some missing values owing to nonattendance of eligible subjects.

Abbreviations: *SBP*, Systolic blood pressure; *DBP*, diastolic blood pressure.

Table 18 Initial* Blood Pressure Characteristics of 1943 Untreated Control Subjects by Third-Year Status

		Initial blood pressure mm Hg						Distribution by mean DBP of S1, S2, and C1 mm Hg				Distribution by change of DBP from mean of S1 and S2 to C1 visit			
		(S1 + S2)/2		C1		(S1 + S2 + C1)/3						Rise mm Hg		Fall mm Hg	
3rd yr status	No.	SBP	DBP	SBP	DBP	SBP	DBP	<95	95–99	100–104	≥105	>10	≤10	≤10*	>10
Exceeded mild limits	172	164.5	103.4	170.7	108.1	166.6	105.0	0	24	54	94	44	74	41	15
95≤ DBP <110 mm Hg	450	158.3	100.9	156.9	100.0	157.8	100.6	43	161	165	81	47	143	196	64
DBP <95 mm Hg	669	154.1	99.4	149.2	94.7	152.5	97.9	169	307	155	38	32	164	283	190
Trial end-point	117	161.2	100.7	159.1	99.2	160.5	100.2	16	47	32	22	13	30	54	20
Subtotal	1408	157.3	100.5	155.1	98.4	156.6	99.8	228	539	406	235	136	411	574	287
Premature withdrawal	535	156.1	100.1	153.3	97.1	155.2	99.1	107	209	147	72	47	152	197	139
Total	1943	157.0	100.4	154.6	98.1	156.2	99.6	335	748	553	307	183	563	771	426

* Includes no change.

S1 = first screening visit; S2 = second screening visit; C1 = first clinic visit.

Abbreviations: *DBP*, diastolic blood pressure; *SBP*, systolic blood pressure.

Table 19 Mean DBP Throughout the Trial: Comparison of Placebo Subjects Who Experienced a Trial Endpoint with Matched Placebo Controls

	No. at screening	Mean age (yr)	Mean DBP mm Hg through trial								No. at 36 mo	Average* DBP (mm Hg)
			S1	S2	C1	S1 + S2 + C1 3	4 mo	12 mo	24 mo	36 mo		
Neither trial endpoint nor exceeded mild limits	1578	49.7	102.0	98.1	96.9	99.0	92.2	93.3	91.3	90.4	1007	91.1
All trial endpoints	121	55.0	102.3	98.8	98.4	99.8	94.6	95.5	91.8	92.6	31	94.1
Matched controls	121	54.6	101.7	99.2	98.8	99.9	94.0	95.6	94.0	91.4	31	93.3
All IHD	88	54.5	102.4	97.9	96.9	99.1	93.8	95.7	91.6	92.3	24	93.5
Matched controls	88	54.1	101.3	99.1	98.9	99.8	93.2	96.4	94.5	91.8	24	93.1
All CVA	22	57.3	103.3	101.9	102.2	102.5	97.3	95.0	92.7	92.4	5	96.9
Matched controls	22	57.0	101.9	98.8	100.9	100.5	95.6	97.4	94.8	97.8	5	95.6
Exceeded mild limits	198	50.3	104.7	101.5	107.3	104.5	103.4	103.6	99.7	100.7	22	
Matched controls	198	50.4	102.3	97.9	98.4	99.5	91.8	95.3	91.3	89.3	22	

* Mean of the average for each subject of three readings per year throughout the study.

Abbreviations: *DBP*, diastolic blood pressure; *IHD*, ischemic heart disease; *CVA*, cerebrovascular accident.

Table 20 Trial Endpoint Rates by Average DBP Throughout the Study for Active and Placebo Subjects: Entry Characteristics Also Shown

Average DBP	No. of subjects (mean duration yr)		Mean no. of visits per subject		TEP rate per 1000 per year (n)		Entry characteristics									
							% Males		% Smokers		Mean serum cholesterol mg/dl		Mean Davenport index		Mean age (yr)	
mm Hg	A	P	A	P	A	P	A	P	A	P	A	P	A	P	A	P
<85	523 (3.9)	128 (3.3)	11.5	10.5	12.3 (25)	11.8 (5)	57	55	19	25	234	236	2.6	2.6	51.7	51.0
85–89	646 (3.7)	383 (3.3)	11.1	10.5	13.4 (32)	18.8 (24)	69	64	26	21	233	232	2.7	2.6	50.0	49.9
90–94	242 (2.8)	474 (3.5)	8.2	10.4	29.7 (20)	16.2 (27)	66	65	26	25	230	229	2.7	2.7	48.3	50.3
95–99	83 (1.4)	378 (3.5)	4.1	9.9	75.8 (9)	28.7 (38)	67	67	24	25	233	228	2.8	2.7	49.6	50.2
≥100	55 (0.6)	185 (2.4)	1.8	6.4	84.5 (3)	60.4 (27)	64	63	38	26	229	227	2.7	2.7	50.0	51.4

Abbreviations: *TEP*, trial endpoint; *A*, active subjects; *P*, placebo subjects; *DBP*, diastolic blood pressure.

In the initial paper (1) reporting the incidence of trial endpoints in relation to treatment regimens, for each subject, the average of all pressure readings while on their treatment regimen was taken as an index of blood pressure control throughout the study and was found to be related to the incidence of trial endpoints, irrespective of treatment or of screening pressures (Table 12). In a further analysis of data (Table 20) (3), the active and placebo subjects were presented as single groups instead of split into three streams according to classes of screening pressure. There are substantial numbers in each class of average DBP and the mean period of exposure is also substantial in each class, varying from 2.4 to 3.5 years, although allocation was not random. For all subjects with average DBP less than 90 mm Hg and for placebo subjects with average DBP of 90 to 94 mm Hg, endpoint rates in the five classes were similar, varying between 11.8 and 18.8 per 1000 person-years. Above these levels, endpoint rates were much higher, and the higher the average pressure, the higher was the rate in both active and placebo subjects; in each of the classes, the rates for active subjects were higher than for placebo subjects of equivalent average DBP. In fact, the rate for each active DBP class was close to that of the placebo subjects in one class higher. This suggests that for a given average DBP of 90 mm Hg or higher, subjects who have been brought to that level by antihypertensive drugs have a reduced risk of hypertensive complications as a result, but the risk does not fall to that of the subject whose pressure is at the same level naturally.

Dr. John Abernethy, who was director of the coordinating center of the study from 1973 to 1977. He was responsible for introducing the Cox method for statistical analysis of the results and has commented (27) on interpretations of these retrospective data by several authors leading to reservations about the use of antihypertensive drugs in mild hypertension (28–31). Abernethy pointed out the drawbacks of retrospective examination of the results and emphasized that the trial had provided ''unequivocal evidence of the benefit of antihypertensive drug treatment.''

XIV. PROGNOSTIC FACTORS IN TREATMENT

On entry into the trial, characteristics (covariates) that might be associated with prognosis were recorded for each subject, and the similar distribution of these covariates in the active and placebo groups indicated that the randomization procedure was satisfactory. In the fourth and last paper (4) published by the management committee, consideration was given to possible associations between these covariates and treatment. It was pointed out that because the study was not designed to examine such associations and there were relatively small numbers in some covariate sets, such as smokers, the conclusions could not be considered to be definitive.

The apparent relationship of covariates to the incidence of trial endpoints was first examined by comparing rates in the active and placebo groups for high and low levels of each covariate, that is, a univariate, dichotomous analysis of rates. Relationships were examined for age, cut at 50 years, sex, cigarette smoking and non-cigarette smoking, serum cholesterol level cut at 220 mg/dl, body mass index (BMI) (g/cm^2) cut at 2.6, systolic blood pressure (SBP) cut at 160 mm Hg, and DBP cut at 100 mm Hg. The rates of occurrence of endpoints were lower in the active groups than in the corresponding placebo groups for both subdivisions of all covariates, but the differences were by no means uniform, suggesting that interactions between covariates and treatment were operative (Table 21). The most striking results were in relation to serum cholesterol and SBP; for both of these the apparent relative benefit from treatment was greater at lower levels of the covari-

Table 21 TEP Rates in Active and Placebo Groups According to Covariate Level (Univariate Analysis)

	A (rate per 1000 per year)	P (rate per 1000 per year)	Relative difference (P–A as percentage of P)
Age (years)			
<50	9.4	14.0	33
≥50	23.4	32.3	28
Sex			
Male	19.8	27.2	27
Female	12.6	19.6	36
SBP (mm Hg)			
<160	11.0	20.6	47
≥160	25.2	30.1	16
DBP (mm Hg)			
<100	15.5	22.2	30
≥100	18.6	26.4	30
Cholesterol (mg/dl)			
<220	11.0	24.6	55
≥220	21.3	24.4	13
BMI (g/cm^2)			
<2.6	18.1	28.3	36
≥2.6	16.5	21.2	22
Nonsmokers	15.4	21.1	27
Smokers	23.4	35.7	34

Abbreviations: *TEP*, trial endpoint; *A*, active group; *P*, placebo group; *DBP*, diastolic blood pressure; *BMI*, body mass index.

ate. In absolute terms, the apparent benefit from active treatment was greatest in subjects with low cholesterol levels and was greater than the overall average in smokers, those with lower BMI, those with lower SBP, and older subjects.

Because results obtained with this univariate approach may be misleading, multivariate regression analysis was undertaken using the Cox proportional hazards method, and a detailed description of the model by Fazekas and Brewer formed an appendix to the paper. In summary, the analysis was applied in a ''step down'' manner so as to derive a multivariate regression equation that included only those variables that contributed significantly to the prediction of endpoints. The first equation contained 17 variables, which was the limit that available computing services permitted. These variables consisted of the six main covariates, excluding sex, plus a selection from 21 second-order interactions and certain third-order interactions whose inclusion was determined by various preliminary analyses (described in the appendix). The multivariate analyses were done on the males and females separately but were conducted in parallel, so that if a variable was found to be significant in one or the other, it was not eliminated from the joint experience.

A series of equations were then fitted in at each step, the least significant variable was omitted, which provided it was not significant at the 5% level. The step down process terminated when an equation was reached in which all terms were significant and thus contributed significantly to the occurrence of endpoints irrespective of the others. Some results of the analysis are set out below.

Table 22 Observed Number of Trial Endpoints and Rates Per 1000 Per Year by Sex, Smoking, and Treatment in High and Low BMI Groups

	BMI <2.6 g/cm²				BMI ≥2.6 g/cm²			
	Active		Placebo		Active		Placebo	
	TEP no.	Rate	TEP no.	Rate	TEP no.	Rate	TEP no.	Rate
Men								
Nonsmokers	19	18.6	27	23.6	23	15.5	33	24.3
Smokers	13	34.5	18	50.0	12	24.1	13	27.0
Women								
Nonsmokers	9	11.3	14	18.5	12	15.1	10	14.0
Smokers	2	10.8	10	56.6	1	7.2	2	10.8

Abbreviations: *BMI*, body mass index; *TEP*, trial endpoint.

Rates for men in the placebo group were significantly higher than for women, but the difference lessened at low BMI (g/cm^2) and in smokers; thin female smokers had very high rates equal to those found in their male counterparts (Table 22). The only significant relationship of BMI was the adverse effect of its interaction with smoking in both men and women and the benefit of treatment in reducing that effect is demonstrated, for men, in Figure 3, and for both sexes in Table 22.

The treatment effect as analyzed in the main paper (1) showed a 30% lower rate of endpoints for women, 12.6 versus 19.6 per 1000 person-years; the significance level calcu-

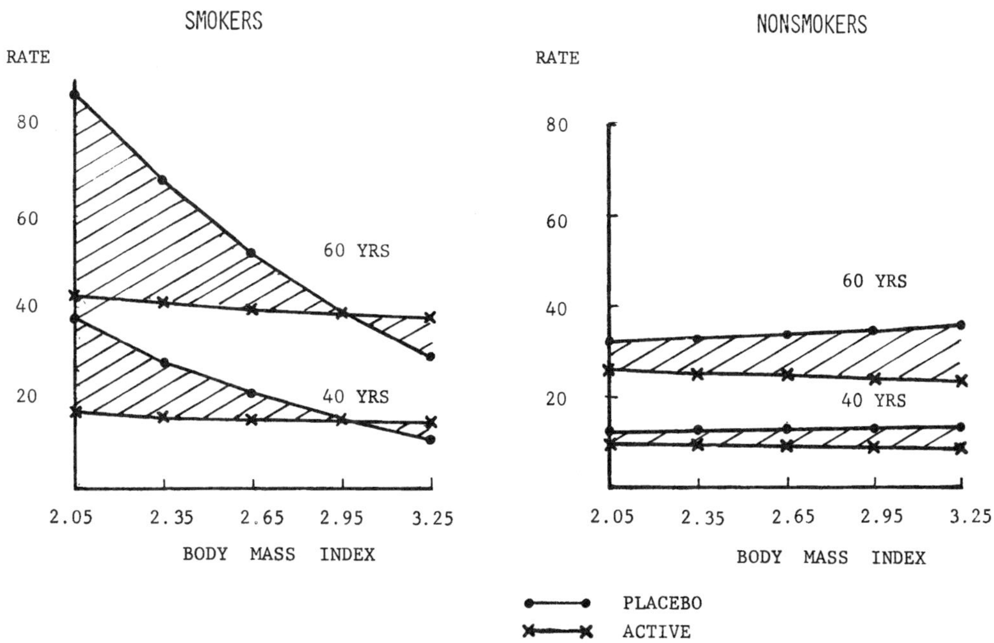

Fig. 3 Trial endpoint rates per 1000 per year by body mass index.

lated by binomial probabilities was $P = 0.058$. However, a later univariate analysis by the Cox method, which uses more information, showed $P = 0.044$ for all trial endpoints, and for all strokes, 1.6 versus 4.9 per 1000 person-years, $P = 0.038$.

The SBP at screening was shown to be significantly related to the incidence of endpoints, but there was no such association for DBP. The incidence of events more than doubled with an increase of SBP from 120 to 195 mm Hg regardless of sex, smoking habits, age, or BMI. However, there was no significant relationship between SBP and treatment effect (Fig. 4).

The multivariate analysis did not confirm the results of the univariate analysis, which suggested that active treatment of mild hypertension was more effective when cholesterol levels were lower. It is worth noting that the interaction between cholesterol level and treatment was among the last to be eliminated in the step down process. Furthermore, a multivariate analysis carried out for both sexes combined with smokers and nonsmokers analyzed in parallel showed a statistically significant inverse relationship between level of cholesterol and benefit from treatment in the nonsmokers. The multivariate analysis also showed a reduction in coronary heart disease events with treatment, reaching significance only in smokers with low BMI.

XV. CONCLUSIONS

The main conclusions from the study were:

1. Mild hypertension is a serious risk factor for cardiovascular disease.
2. Antihypertensive drug treatment is indicated in men and women of all ages, up to at least age 69, with sustained mild hypertension.

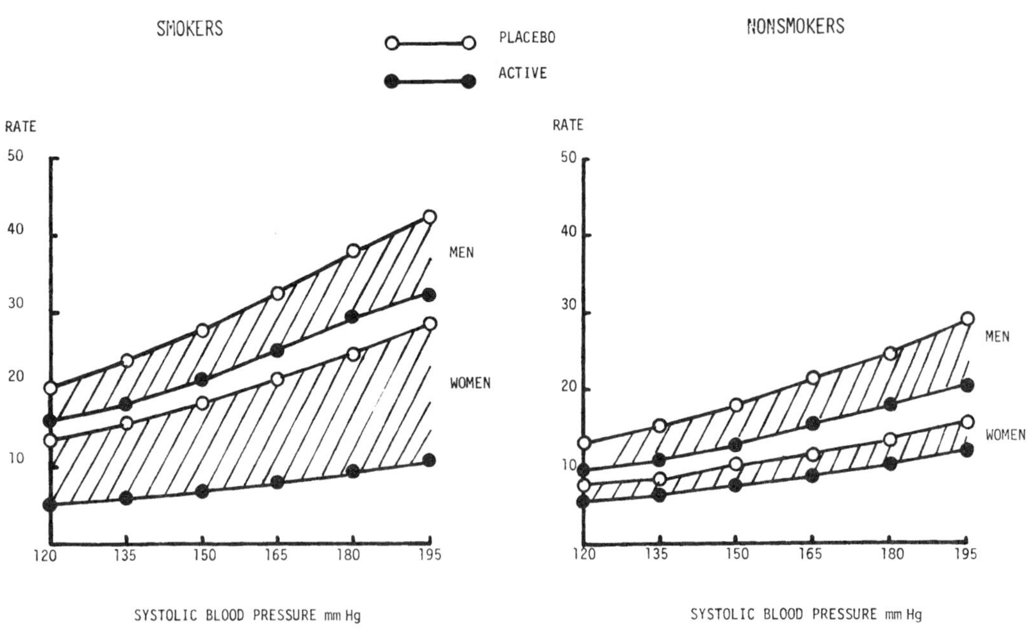

Fig. 4 TEP rates per 1000 per year in men and women by smoking data and SBP at entry.

3. A 4-month observation period is advisable before instituting drug treatment, as a large proportion of subjects with suspected mild hypertension will have normal pressures at that time and will require only periodic review.
4. The major relative benefit of antihypertensive drug treatment is in prevention of cerebrovascular disease, but the study also provided evidence of benefit in coronary heart disease.
5. Systolic blood pressure at screening is a significant predictor of cardiovascular events; diastolic pressure is not; neither is a significant predictor of response to treatment; the average of all of a subject's diastolic pressures while on treatment in the trial was found to correlate well with treatment benefit.
6. The combination of cigarette smoking and mild hypertension involves a high risk of cardiovascular disease in men and women, which is aggravated by low BMI. Antihypertensive medication greatly reduces that risk.
7. Benefit from antihypertensive medication may be significantly reduced in subjects with mild hypertension who have high serum cholesterol levels.

XVI. POSTSCRIPTS

Total direct expenditure on the trial was $A1,640,866. The National Health and Medical Research Council contributed $A457,000, The Life Insurance Medical Research Fund of Australia and New Zealand $A120,000, the Ramaciotti Foundations of New South Wales $A99,500, and the Victorian State Government $A75,000. Other contributions amounted to $A40,405, and the National Heart Foundation's share was $A848,961.

In addition, the Raine Medical Research Foundation of Western Australia bore all costs for the Center in Perth. Accommodation and other administrative resources were provided by the Universities of Melbourne, Sydney, and Western Australia and the Sir Charles Gairdner Hospital, Perth, The Sacred Heart and Box Hill Hospitals, Melbourne, and the Hornsby and District Hospital, Sydney. The Australian National University, Canberra, provided accommodation and subsidized computer services. Active and placebo tablets were provided by the pharmaceutical companies Boehringer Ingelheim, Ciba Geigy, ICI, Sandoz, and Merck Sharp and Dohme. The latter company also provided a fully equipped bus, the "Heartmobile," for screening.

In Australia, mortality rates for both cerebrovascular disease and coronary heart disease have fallen by some 70% since the introduction of antihypertensive medication (32) (Fig. 5). It is probable that control of hypertension has played a significant role in both reductions. The decline in coronary deaths that commenced in 1967 was first reported in 1972 (33). It was not until 1974 (34) that it was noted in the United States. It began some 14 years after cerebrovascular deaths began to decline, possibly because of the different pathogenesis of the two conditions.

Although the premature withdrawal rate of 35% in the Australian study was roughly as predicted, it was too high and did little justice to the committed efforts of study center staffs to retain subjects. The loss of subjects could have been substantially reduced had computer editing and data analysis in the initial stages provided for better consistency checks and management of subject attendances. The flood of incoming data was catered by a succession of quick computer programs, many trying to patch up holes. In April 1978, Mr. Terry Woodings, consultant in computing from the University of Western Australia, spent two weeks at the coordinating center. A comprehensive system based on a "chronological" file of each subject, and a "time point" file containing screening, entry

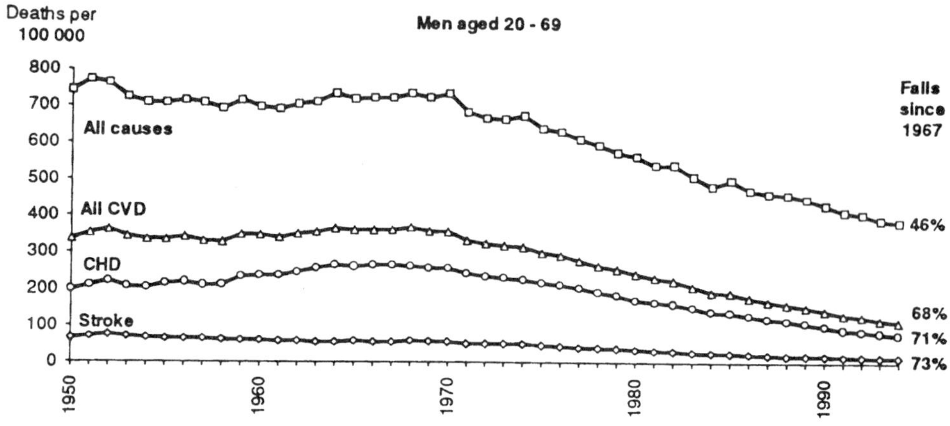

Fig. 5 Age adjusted death rates in Australian men: 1950–1994.

examination, and withdrawal and trial endpoint records in fixed "slots," was set up. These measures facilitated the management of the study and the analysis of results, including the Cox survival analyses, during the final stages. The early tribulations could have been mitigated if a pilot study had been undertaken. It was a great pleasure to find the computer files in such good condition in the data archives of the Australian National University 18 years later, and the assistance of the archives staff in making analyses for this chapter is much appreciated. It is also a pleasure to thank Camilla Fazekas, who was a statistician for the last 2½ years of the trial, for her discussions and assistance in its preparation.

INVESTIGATORS

Management Committee: R. Reader (chairman), G.E. Bauer, A.E. Doyle, B. Edlington, K.W. Edmondson, S. Hunyor, T.H. Hurley, P.I. Korner, P.W. Leighton, R.R.H. Lovell, M.G. McCall, J.M. McPhie, M.J. Rand, H.M. Whyte.
Study director until July 1977: J.D. Abernethy.
Study center directors: J. Baker, M. Bullen, R. Edwards, G. Francis, M. Lamb, M. Stewart.
Statistical consultants: R. Prineas, K.R.W. Brewer.
Statisticians: M.G. Santow, C. Fazekas de St Groth.
Computer programmers: W. Clapton, H. Knight.
Ethics Committee: P.J. Nestel (chairman), K.R.W. Brewer, M. Crawford, P.W. Leighton.
Trial End Point Review Committee: R.J. Craig, J. McPhie, J. Waddy.
ECG Committee: G.E. Bauer, P. Caspari, S. Hunyor.

REFERENCES

1. Management Committee of the Australian National Blood Pressure Study. The Australian therapeutic trial in mild hypertension. Lancet 1980; 1:1261–1267.
2. Management Committee of the Australian National Blood Pressure Study. Treatment of mild hypertension in the elderly. Med J Aust 1981; 2:398–402.

3. Management Committee of the Australian National Blood Pressure Study. Untreated mild hypertension. Lancet 1982; 1:185–191.
4. Management Committee of the Australian National Blood Pressure Study. Prognostic factors in the treatment of mild hypertension. Circulation 1984; 69:668–676.
5. Paton WDM, Zaimis EJ. Clinical potentialities of certain bisquaternary salts causing neuromuscular and ganglionic block (letter). Nature 1948; 162:810.
6. Arnold P, Rosenheim ML. Effect of pentamethonium iodide on normal and hypertensive persons. Lancet 1949; 2:321–323.
7. Turner R. Medical sympathectomy in hypertension. Lancet 1950; 2:353–358.
8. Smirk FH. letter. Lancet 1950; 2:477.
9. Smirk FH. letter. Lancet 1951; 1:347.
10. Reader R. Screening and community control of hypertension. In: Freis ED, ed. The Treatment of Hypertension. England: MTP Press, 1978.
11. Veterans Administration Cooperative Study Group on Antihypertensive Agents. Effects of treatment on morbidity in hypertension: results in patients with diastolic blood pressure averaging 90 through 114 mm Hg. JAMA 1970; 213:1143–1152.
12. Prineas RJ, Stephens WB, Lovell RRH. Blood pressure and its treatment in a community: the Albury blood pressure study. Med J Aust 1973; 1:5–9.
13. McCall MG, Kelsall RG, Rosman DL, Stenhouse NS, Welborn TA. Blood pressure in Busselton, Western Australia. Med J Aust 1973; 2(supp):8–13.
14. Rose GA, Holland WW, Crowley EA. A sphygmomanometer for epidemiologists. Lancet 1964; 2:296–300.
15. Abernethy JD. The Australian National Blood Pressure Study. Med J Aust 1974; 1:821–824.
16. Halperin M, Rogot E, Gurian J, Ederer F. Sample sizes for medical trials with special reference to long term therapy. J Chronic Dis 1968; 21:13–24.
17. World Health Organization Regional Office for Europe. Myocardial infarction and community registers. Copenhagen: WHO, 1976 (Public Health in Europe No. 5).
18. Cox DR. Regression models and life tables. J Royal Statist Soc B 1972; 34:187–220.
19. Rose GA. The diagnosis of ischaemic heart pain and intermittent claudication in field surveys. Bull World Health Organ 1962; 27:645–658.
20. U.S. Public Hospitals Cooperative Study Group; W. McFate Smith. Treatment of mild hypertension: results of a ten-year intervention trial. Circ Res 1977; 40(supp):I-98–I-105.
21. Medical Research Council Working Party. MRC trial of treatment of mild hypertension: principal results. BMJ 1985; 291:97–104.
22. Hypertension Detection and Follow-up Program Cooperative Group. Five-year findings of the Hypertension Detection and Follow-up Program. I. Reduction in mortality of persons with high blood pressure, including mild hypertension. JAMA 1979; 242:2562–2571.
23. MacMahon SW, Cutler JA, Furberg CD, Payne GH. The effects of drug treatment for hypertension on morbidity and mortality from cardiovascular disease: a review of randomized controlled trials. Prog Cardiovasc Dis 1996; 29(supp 1):99–118.
24. An International Anticoagulant Review Group. Collaborative analysis of long term anticoagulant administration after acute myocardial infarction. Lancet 1970; 1:203–209.
25. Bauer GE, Baker J, Hunyor SN, Marshall P. Side effects of antihypertensive treatment: a placebo controlled study. Clin Sci Mol Med 1978; 55(supp):341–344.
26. Armitage P, Rose GA. The variability of measurements of casual blood pressure: a laboratory study. Clin Sci 1966; 30:325–335.
27. Abernethy JD. Comments on Australian therapeutic trial in mild hypertension (letter). Hypertension 1984; 6:774–776.
28. Freis ED. Should mild hypertension be treated? (letter). N Engl J Med 1982; 307:306–309.
29. Alderman MH. Mild hypertension: new light on an old clinical controversy. Am J Med 1980; 69:653–655.
30. Kaplan NM. Whom to treat: the dilemma of mild hypertension (editorial). Am Heart J 1981; 101:867–870.

31. Toth PJ, Horwitz RI. Conflicting clinical trials and the uncertainty of treating mild hypertension. Am J Med 1983; 75:482–488.
32. Heart and stroke facts 1996. Figure 3. National Heart Foundation of Australia, Canberra, Australia.
33. Reader R. Incidence and prevalence of ischaemic heart disease in Australia. Med J Aust 1972; 2(supp):3–6.
34. Walker WJ. Coronary mortality: what is going on? JAMA 1974; 227:1045–1046.

5

The MRC Trial of Treatment in Mild Hypertension

ANTHONY F. LEVER and GORDON T. McINNES

University of Glasgow, Glasgow, Scotland

PATRICK J. BRENNAN

Wolfson Institute of Preventive Medicine, London, England

JOHN ALASDAIR MILLAR

University of Western Australia, Perth, Western Australia

LAWRENCE E. RAMSAY

Royal Hallamshire Hospital, The University of Sheffield, Sheffield, England

I. INTRODUCTION

Recently Doll (1) described 1948 as a ''watershed year'' in the history of clinical trials. It was the year of publication of the Medical Research Council trial of antituberculous drugs (2). New techniques of randomization (3) had made possible, and short supplies of streptomycin had made ethically acceptable, the first published randomized double-blind, placebo-controlled trial (2). The trial succeeded because of its design. The natural history of tuberculosis, with its long and variable course, was such that a new drug could only be assessed this way.

Meanwhile, assessment of antihypertensive drugs had just begun. Malignant-phase hypertension was examined first. The methods were simpler but just as effective as those in the tuberculosis trial: the natural history of malignant hypertension, with its short and uniform course, allowed it to be assessed by a simple comparison of mortality before and after introduction of antihypertensive drugs. Before introduction of these drugs in the late 1940s, less than 20% of patients survived one year and almost none survived three years

(4–6). During the 1950s, 5-year survival was between 15% and 25% (7–9). As drugs improved, so did survival (10, 11); by the 1960s, 5-year survival was between 25% (12) and 40% (13); by the 1970s, it was almost 50% (14); by the 1980s and early 1990s, it was more than 70% in two studies (13, 14) and close to 90% in a third (15). On this evidence alone, malignant hypertension is accepted as a life-threatening condition needing treatment from the day of diagnosis. A randomized, placebo-controlled trial has never been done and would have been unacceptable at any stage on ethical grounds.

At the opposite end of the blood pressure scale is mild hypertension, the subject of this study. Unlike malignant hypertension, its importance lies in the very large number of affected patients who are at only slightly increased risk. This and the natural history of a long and varied course make necessary a randomized, placebo-controlled trial in testing treatment with antihypertensive drugs.

The MRC first considered such a trial in 1970. Up to that time, there had been three placebo-controlled trials of antihypertensive drugs in more severe forms of nonmalignant hypertension: two randomized (16, 17) and one in which patients were assigned in alternating fashion to placebo and active treatment (18). Each trial reported a significant reduction of cardiovascular events in those randomized to active treatment.

During 1970, and after much discussion (19), an MRC working party (Appendix 1) was given the task of organizing a pilot study of mild hypertension (phase V diastolic 90 to 109 mm Hg). If successful, this could be extended to a full-scale trial. Between 1973 and 1977, 1800 patients were recruited, randomized, and treated in a study comparing two forms of active treatment with placebo. As described below the pilot succeeded (20) and expansion to a full-scale trial began in 1977. It was based on 18,000 patients followed up for 5½ years. It ended in 1985 and the principal results were published later that year (21).

II. PLANNING THE TRIAL

A. Trial Design

The trial was to be prospective, multicenter, randomized, placebo-controlled and single blind. It would test separately two active treatment regimens, with 50% of patients being randomized in equal number to bendrofluazide or a placebo tablet resembling bendrofluazide and 50% to propranolol or a tablet resembling propranolol (Table 1). Where blood pressure control was inadequate in actively treated patients, methyldopa was added (except

Table 1 Treatment Regimens

% Randomized	Primary regimen	Supplementary treatment	Active Treatment Needed
25%	Bendrofluazide	Methyldopa	—
25%	Placebo resembling bendrofluazide		Bendrofluazide
25%	Propranolol	Guanethidine early stages of trial; methyldopa later	—
25%	Placebo resembling propranolol		Propranolol

Table 2 Screening of Mild Hypertensives

Invited to screening	First screening visit	Second screening visit	Entry visit
695,000	515,000 Not on antihypertensive treatment DBP 90-109 (trial limits) or SBP >200 mmHg	54,000 BP within trial limits DBP 90–109 SBP < 200 mm Hg	33,000 Randomized 17,354

Abbreviations: *DBP*, diastolic blood pressure; *SBP*, systolic blood pressure; *BP*, blood pressure.

in the early stages of the trial when guanethidine was added to patients taking propranolol) (19, 21).

The trial was multicenter because 500,000 subjects needed screening in a large number of general practices throughout the U.K. It was single blind (patients blinded to treatment) because doctors and nurses managing patients, measuring blood pressure, and taking blood samples, would come to know which treatment patients were taking, particularly where patients attend the same clinic and saw the same doctors and nurses for more than five years. However, the sphygmomanometers used (22, 23) did blind observers to the value of their measurements at the time they were made, and assessment of trial events was by an independent arbitrator blind to treatment of patients (21).

B. One or Two Active Treatment Regimens?

Up to 1972 placebo-controlled trials of antihypertensive drugs had tested one active drug regimen (16–18). In early discussions, the working party had considered testing two active treatments separately. Doing so might distinguish effects of a drug attributable to blood pressure lowering from effects attributable to other mechanisms—to a cardioprotective action of a beta-blocker, for example. After much discussion (19), it was decided to test the two regimens described in Table 1 separately.

C. Statistical Power and Numbers Needed

An estimate of participants needed was based on numbers needed in a 5-year trial with a 95% chance of demonstrating a 40% reduction in fatal and nonfatal strokes taken together or in deaths attributable to hypertension (ICD 400–404). Significance was to be at the 1% level with two-tail testing (19, 21). Data on risk from epidemiological studies (24) and from the Registrar General's statistics (25) suggested that 18,000 mild hypertensives in the age range of 35 to 64 years would provide this power, with half randomized to placebo and half to active treatment. The power for separate comparisons of propranolol and bendrofluazide with placebo would be less than this.

In the event, 500,000 men and women aged 35 to 64 were screened, 17,354 mild hypertensives (phase V diastolic pressure 90 to 109 mm Hg) were identified and randomized) (Table 2). Together they provided 85,572 patient-years of observation.

III. PILOT STUDY

A. Objectives and Plan

The purpose of the pilot study was to assess on a small scale methods to be used and findings anticipated in a full scale study. Particularly relevant were methods of screening, responses to treatment, and the frequency and severity of drug side effects. Was screening best based on hospital clinics, on population surveys, or on general practice? Initially, the working party favored the first, perhaps because several of its members were hospital physicians, but events soon proved this the least effective (19). Recruitment and management in general practice, particularly where practices were small, proved highly effective, so much so that it was the only method used in the main trial (19).

Another objective was to assess the willingness of patients to be screened for a condition with few, if any, symptoms and to be followed up in a trial testing drugs known to have side effects but not known to reduce risk in mild hypertension.

B. Findings

More than 90% of eligible patients, a total of 1849, entered the pilot trial. After one year, 87% had taken at least 75% of tablets prescribed. Changes of serum potassium and urate in those taking bendrofluazide and of pulse rate in those taking propranolol suggested good compliance (20).

1. Psychological Assessment

A self-administered questionnaire devised by the Institute of Psychiatry (26) was completed by a group of patients before and after screening and, where these patients were eligible for the trial, before and after entry. Controls for the second group were subjects screened but not eligible for the trial. Subjects with positive questionnaire results underwent a psychological assessment.

The results were interesting and reassuring: the incidence of psychological disturbance was no greater in those entering the trial than in those not entering. Indeed, among subjects with neurotic symptoms at the outset, those entering the trial had a significantly greater "cure rate" for these symptoms than had nonentrants (26, 27). Thus, screening had no apparent harmful psychological effect and entering the trial might even have had psychological benefits.

2. Changes of Blood Pressure

Blood pressure fell after entry in placebo and actively treated groups. Compared with placebo controls, the fall in those receiving active treatment was greater by 13 to 17 mm Hg systolic and 6 to 8 mm Hg diastolic (20). The fall in placebo controls was greater than expected and was to be seen later in the main trial (21). It was not a consequence of taking placebo tablets because, in a substudy (19, 20), changes of blood pressure were identical in patients taking either a placebo tablet or no tablet at all.

Findings in the pilot trial were generally satisfactory. A great deal had been learned about methods of screening and managing patients in a large trial. The full-scale trial appeared feasible and justified on scientific and ethical grounds (20). Costs based on expenses up to that time were put at £23.50 per randomized patient per year. With follow-up of 90,000 patient-years, the total at 1977 prices became £2.1M (19): £7.5M at 1999 prices. This prediction was to prove accurate at the trial's end and on the basis of the estimate, the MRC authorized expansion to a full-scale study involving 18,000 patients.

IV. TRIAL ORGANIZATION

An experiment that entailed screening 500,000 subjects in different parts of the U.K., randomizing 18,000 to a trial and assessing each subject every 6 months for 5 years,

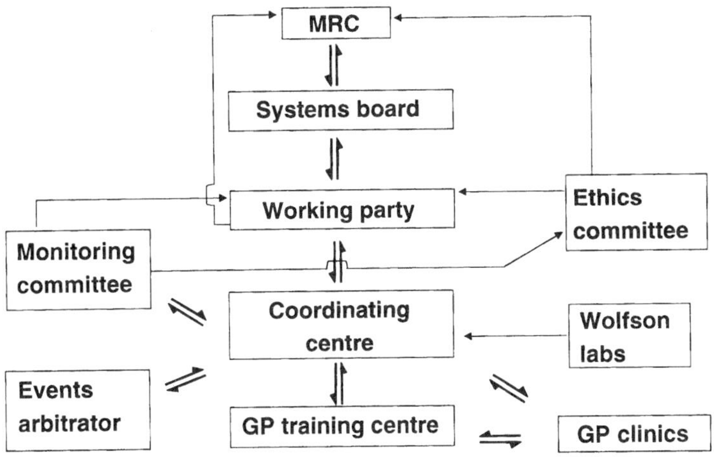

Fig. 1 Organization of MRC Mild Hypertension trial. Interrelation of the parts. (Modified from Ref. 19.)

needed careful coordination. Figure 1 illustrates the interrelation between different parts of the trial. Organization was from a coordinating center at Northwick Park, London. Doctors from the center visited general practitioners interested in joining the trial. Once they had decided to participate, a practice nurse was recruited and the nurse and the doctor attended a trial training center at Stratford-upon-Avon. Here, a senior nurse and a doctor trained the visitors in techniques of blood pressure measurement, blood sampling, and centrifugation. The training center also became a meeting place for general practice physicians and nurses whose high morale and efficiency were regarded by those running the trial as the principal factor in its successful administration (19, 28).

The working party was responsible for planning and, through the coordinating center, for organization of the trial (Fig. 1). Fatal and nonfatal events were classified by an arbitrator blind to treatment (19, 21). Information provided by the center included electrocardiograms (ECGs) and records from general practitioners, hospitals, and the Registrar General. Data on events and the arbitrator's classification of these were sent, via the center, to the monitoring committee (Appendix II). Their responsibilities were to determine during the trial whether event rates were sufficient to provide the statistical power needed for analysis and to ensure that event rates in actively treated patients were not such as to raise ethical questions about continued treatment. Should the second occur, the ethical committee (Appendix III) and the working party would be informed. As discussed later, an ethical problem did arise in patients taking bendrofluazide.

In all patients, blood samples were taken at entry and at intervals during the trial. Twelve tests were done using the Technicon SMA 12 analyzer. Those of greatest interest to the trial were potassium, sodium, urate, urea, cholesterol, and glucose. Objectives here were to exclude from the trial patients whose hypertension was secondary in nature and manifest by biochemical abnormality, to monitor drug-induced biochemical changes, and to collect data for later analysis. Important in the biochemical work was its centralization at the Wolfson Research Laboratories, Birmingham, allowing one set of standards and methods in a single laboratory to ensure consistency. Special packs were designed to mail blood samples to Birmingham. These methods worked well and tests of quality control were satisfactory.

V. SCREENING, RECRUITMENT, AND RANDOMIZATION

A. First and Second Screening Visits

All 695,000 subjects, aged 35 to 64, were invited to attend a screening at one of 176 general practices; approximately 515,000 (Table 2) came. Examinations were in practice clinics or, where accommodation was insufficient, in one of six mobile screening caravans. During their busiest period (1979–1980), up to 14,000 patients were screened each month in these caravans (19).

At the first screening visit, blood pressure was measured twice by a trained nurse using either the Hawksley Random Zero sphygmomanometer (22) or, less often, the London School of Hygiene sphygmomanometer (23). In cases in which the mean of these measurements was between 90 and 109 mm Hg diastolic (trial limits), or when systolic pressure was greater than 200 mm Hg (above trial limits) the patient was referred to a second screening visit usually a week later. If, at this visit, diastolic pressure was below 90 mm Hg, patients were reassured, thanked for attending, and discharged. If pressure was within trial limits (diastolic blood pressure 90 to 109, systolic less than 200 mm Hg), the patient was referred for a third visit, the entry examination.

B. Entry Examination

On this occasion, blood pressure was measured twice by a doctor. If the mean of these measurements was close to the upper or lower limits, the patient was asked to attend on a fourth occasion for further measurements (19). The decision on whether the patient entered the trial was then based on the mean of four measurements by a doctor on two separate occasions. At the entry examination, a detailed history was taken by the nurse or doctor.

Reasons for exclusion from the trial during screening were known hypertension on treatment (23,413 patients excluded); asthma (1611); gout (933); diabetes (679); psychiatric disorders (138), or other serious illness that might compromise attendance (1004). Peak rates of recruitment and randomization were about 500 monthly. In all, 17,354 patients were randomized to one of the four regimens (two of active treatment, two of placebo). Randomization was in stratified blocks of eight in each sex, 10-year age group, and general practice clinic (21).

C. The Screened Population

The following analysis was based on 156 of 176 general practice clinics (19). Screening in these was based on a population of 556,000 men and women, all invited to attend the first screening visit; 411,000 (73.9%) came. Of these, 53,700 (13.1%) had acceptable blood pressure and were invited to attend a second screening visit; 51,521 came to the second screening and of these, 32,987 (8%) were referred to the entry visit. At the entry visit, 17,354 were randomized (the last number is based on all 176 practices).

VI. THE RANDOMIZED PATIENTS

As expected with such large numbers, randomization produced closely similar mean values in bendrofluazide, propranolol, and placebo groups for variables such as age, body weight, blood pressure, serum electrolytes, urea, and cholesterol (Table 3), smoking habit, and frequency of ECG changes (19, 21). However, trial patients were not a random sample

Table 3 Randomization of Patients

	Bendrofluazide		Propranolol		Placebo	
	Entry	3 Years	Entry	3 Years	Entry	3 Years
Serum K mmol/l	4.11	3.72***	4.11	4.22***	4.13	4.17
Serum Na mmol/l	141.6	140.9***	141.6	141.5	141.7	141.6
Serum uric acid μmol/l	386.3	432.0***	373.7	393.5***	372.6	380.8
Serum urea mmol/l	5.43	5.98***	5.44	5.76*	5.40	5.63
Serum cholesterol mmol/l	6.26	6.36***	6.23	6.31**	6.24	6.25
Serum glucose mmol/l	5.48	5.69*	5.48	5.50*	5.46	5.58

Biochemical changes in men in samples taken at entry and at third annual visit in bendrofluazide, propranolol, and placebo groups. Significance testing: $*P < 0.05$; $**P < 0.01$; $***P < 0.001$ is the difference between entry and third annual visit.

of hypertensives in the U.K. Screening was concentrated in areas likely to yield most patients and rural general practices, particularly those in the English Midlands, were overrepresented; inner city areas were underrepresented. As a result, social classes I, II, and III were probably overrepresented. In this classification, social classes I to VI relate inversely to socioeconomic status. Exclusion of conditions that might worsen with treatment, that is, diabetes, gout, and asthma, could also have contributed to lower all-cause mortality in the trial population.

VII. FALL OF BLOOD PRESSURE IN PLACEBO GROUP

The fall of blood pressure in placebo group patients of the pilot study was seen also in the full-scale trial (Fig. 2) (29). It was not unique to this trial: similar falls occurred in the Australian Therapeutic trial of mild hypertension (30) and in the MRC trial of older adults (31). The fall here was most marked in the first two weeks, continuing for up to 3 months (Fig. 2). At least three processes contributed.

A. Decrease of a Pressor Response at Entry

Blood pressure in placebo group patients was higher at the entry visit than at all other times (Fig. 2, lower panel). Suggesting strongly that this was the peak of a pressor response was the highly significant correlation in individuals between the rise of pressure at entry and the fall of pressure after entry (29). Respectively, these are the differences of pressure between the second screening visit and entry and the differences of pressure between entry and the first visit after randomization. Several workers have suggested that it was a response to the stressful conditions at entry and possibly ''a white coat'' pressor effect (19, 29, 32, 33), and there is much to support the idea: the measurement at the entry visit was the first by a doctor; earlier measurements during screening were by nurses; on all other occasions, when doctors made measurements, at annual visits, pressure was higher than at intermediate visits when measurements were by nurses (Fig. 2, lower panel). Also the increase between the second screening visit and entry was greater in women (10/4 mm Hg) than in men (5/3 mm Hg) (29, 34). White coat responses are known to be more pronounced in these circumstances (35, 36), particularly when doctors making the measurement are male and patients are female (37, 38). Interestingly, an analysis by Millar

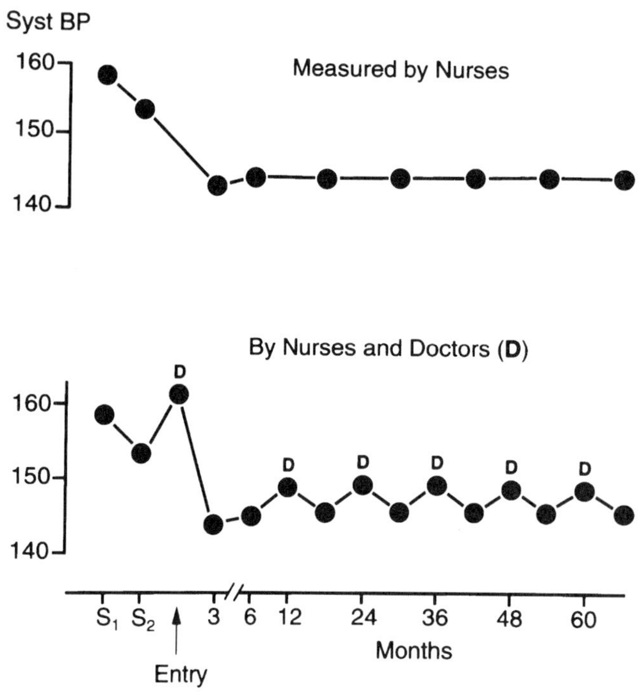

Fig. 2 Placebo Group MRC Trial. **Upper panel**. Measurement of systolic blood pressure (Syst BP) made by nurses at two screening visits (S_1 and S_2) and during 5-year follow-up. **Lower panel**. Measurements by nurses, as in upper panel, but with additional measurements made by doctors (marked **D**), the latter give higher values than the former, particularly at the entry examination. (From Ref. 29, used with permission.)

and colleagues (29) suggests that the increase of pressure at entry did not confer an increased risk of stroke commensurate with that seen with the same increase of pressure measured at other times. In support of this, multiple regression analysis showed that blood pressure measured at screening visits predicted stroke, but that blood pressure measured at the entry visit did not (29).

These observations suggest that a variable pressor response occurred at entry, that it was probably a ''white coat'' response, and that it did not confer additional risk. Whatever the explanation, the decrease from its peak value will have contributed to the fall of blood pressure after entry.

B. Seasonal Effect on Blood Pressure

Blood pressure is known to be higher in winter than in summer, a phenomenon seen in placebo-treated patients of the MRC trial (19, 39). This seasonal effect was not randomly distributed among trial patients, however. Because a greater proportion entered the trial during winter months (19, 39) and because blood pressure falls between winter and summer, predominance of winter recruits in the trial will have contributed to the fall of blood pressure in the placebo group patients during the first six months. This effect on the change in the first two weeks would have been small.

C. Regression to the Mean

A third contribution to the fall of pressure was made by regression to the mean. In this process, subjects from the upper part of a distribution of blood pressure show a decrease of pressure during serial measurements, subjects from the lower part an increase (40, 41). Millar and colleagues (29) have examined the mechanisms involved in the MRC trial placebo group. Patients were classified in quintiles of systolic pressure measured at the third annual visit (Fig. 3, right panel). The distribution of quintile means was broader at this time than at visits before or after the classification (Fig. 3). During follow-up, those in the upper quintiles showed a decrease of pressure, those in the lower quintiles an increase (Fig. 3). That these changes result from the classification was shown by their absence at the third visit when the classification was made at entry (Fig. 3, left panel).

The principal mechanism producing dispersal of quintile means at classification was the selection for upper quintiles of individuals whose blood pressure was higher at the time than their personal mean value (taken here as the mean value of pressure for the five annual visits). Selection for lower quintiles was of individuals whose pressure was lower than their personal mean. That this did contribute to dispersal of quintile means at classification was shown by the greater deviation of individuals from their personal mean at the time of classification. Eighty-one percent of patients in the top quintile had pressure higher than personal mean, and this contributed a 7.7 mm Hg upward shift to the average value for that quintile. In the bottom quintile, systolic pressure was below personal mean in 72% of patients, and this contributed 6.8 mm Hg to the downward shift of average value for the quintile (Fig. 4).

How might such a process contribute to the fall of blood pressure in the placebo group after entry? We suggest the following: (a) That screening subjects for a hypertension trial involves selection of those with blood pressure in the upper part of the distribution for the screened population. Only 2.5% of those screened were selected and, overall, only

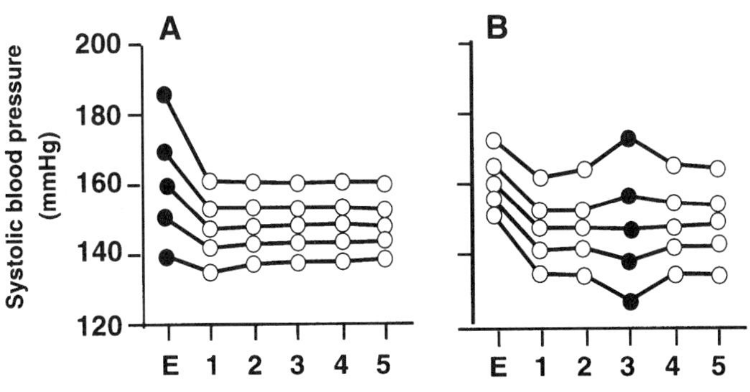

Fig. 3 Systolic blood pressure in patients of MRC trial placebo group at entry, E (solid circle), and at annual visits thereafter. In **left panel**, **(A)** patients were classified in quintiles of systolic pressure at entry. Quintile mean values maintain their position after the first annual visit. In **right panel (B)**, a quintile classification by systolic pressure was made at the third annual visit. The changes seen before and after this classification were of these quintile groups. (From Ref. 29, used with permission.)

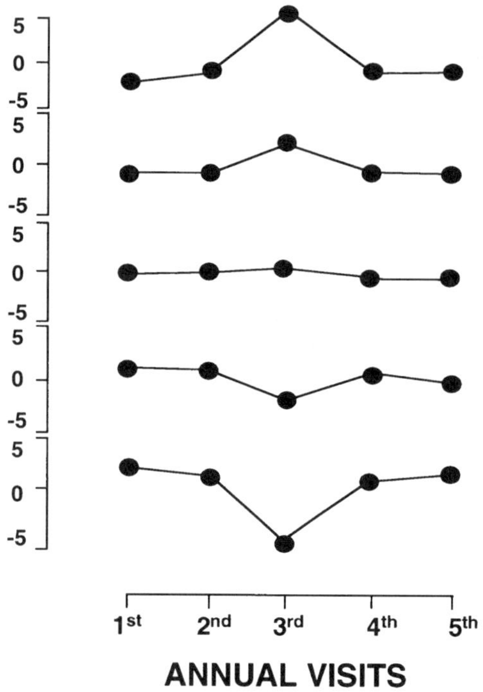

Fig. 4 Deviation of systolic blood pressure for individual patients from their personal mean value at the third annual visit, the time of quintile classification in Fig. 3b. Upward deviation from personal mean value was seen in upper quintiles, downward deviation in lower quintiles. (From Ref. 29, used with permission.)

8% of the screened population had hypertension. (b) That the selective process of screening is similar to that of making the quintile classification at the third annual visit (Fig. 3b). (c) In this event, a number of patients qualifying for a trial during screening and at an entry visit would be those showing, by chance, a higher blood pressure than their personal mean. (d) The fall of pressure in such patients after entry would then be regression of blood pressure to their personal mean. This does not imply that regression is the principal contributor to the fall of blood pressure after entry. The size of the contribution from any one of the three processes described here is difficult to assess in the presence of two others.

D. Diastolic Pressure Fell Below 90 mm Hg in Some Placebo Group Patients

Between one-third and one-half of placebo-group patients had a fall of diastolic pressure during follow-up to less than 90 mm Hg, the lower limit acceptable for admission to the trial. Does this imply, as some suggest (32,42), that these patients had ''normal'' blood pressure and, for this reason, the trial was not strictly one of mild hypertension?

The issue is not so clear. Often, the fall of pressure to ''normal'' did not persist. In only 18% of the 7141 patients having measurements at the first three follow-up visits was diastolic pressure below 90 mm Hg on each occasion. It was more common in these patients for pressure to fall below limits at one visit and to rise above limits at the next. How are such patients to be classified? Probably not as normal subjects.

E. Large Variability of Blood Pressure Among Individuals

Figure 5 illustrates the marked variability of blood pressure underlying these observations. Plotted are changes of quintile position for systolic blood pressure between the first and fifth annual visit in placebo-group patients. More than 50% of these patients changed position. Some starting in the top quintile reached the bottom quintile 5 years later; others in the bottom quintile reached the top quintile. Thus, the appearance of stability of blood

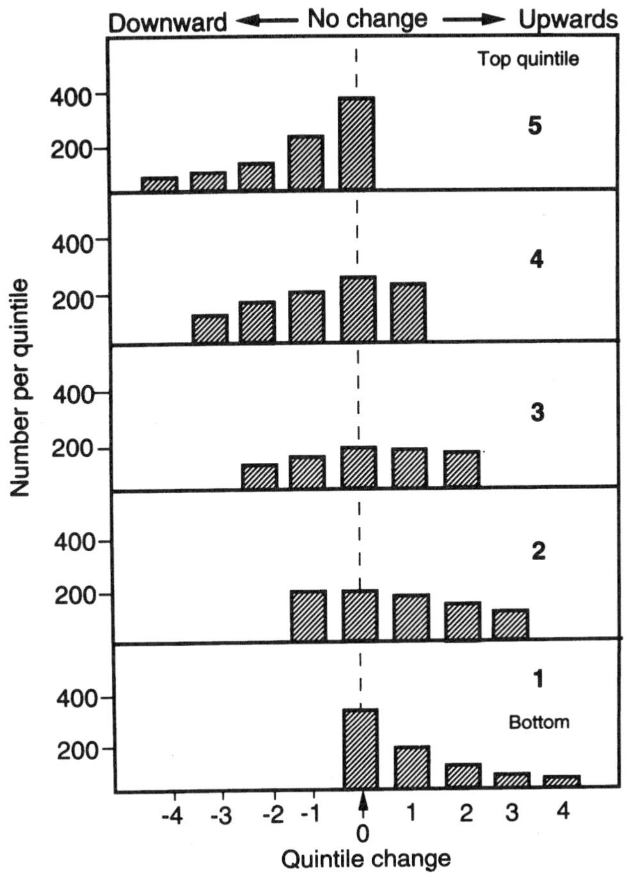

Fig. 5 Changes of systolic blood pressure between the first and the fifth annual visit in placebo group patients. The five panels show changes from quintiles classified at the first annual visit. The top panel shows those with highest pressure at the first visit; the bottom panel those with lowest. By the fifth year, a majority of those in the top quintile had moved downward, some by as much as four quintile positions. For those in the bottom quintile, a similar number had moved upward, some by as much as four quintiles. (From Ref. 29.)

pressure during follow-up (Fig. 3, left panel) does not necessarily represent stability of blood pressure among individuals; more likely, it reflects an exact balance among individuals of large upward and downward movement (Fig. 5).

Many patients in the bottom quintile of systolic pressure at the first annual visit (Fig. 5) will have had a diastolic pressure below 90 mm Hg. Although the direction of change differed, the magnitude of change of pressure for individuals in this quintile thereafter was little different from that of patients in the top quintile. Thus, patients in the bottom quintile showed no more tendency to remain low than did patients in the top quintile to remain high. None of these observations accords with the view that placebo-group patients in whom diastolic blood pressure drops below 90 mm Hg are normal subjects qualitatively distinguishable from mild hypertensives. At a more practical level, such variability makes particularly difficult selection for a trial of placebo-group patients whose blood pressure is certain at all times to remain within limits set for the trial. Simpson and colleagues (32) suggest that more frequent measurements should be made before randomization, particularly where these are made in a quiet environment giving more "basal" conditions. Almost certainly, this would reduce the number of randomized patients whose blood pressure falls below trial limits. However, it would also increase the time spent in screening and its cost. More important, it would make the circumstances in which patients are tested in a trial less like those used routinely by general practitioners in screening for and then treating mild hypertension. The methods used in the MRC trial—three or four visits with a pair of measurements at each—resembled closely those used routinely for screening in general practice.

F. Is Mild Hypertension a Disease Entity?

> The tendency has always been strong to believe that whatever receives a name must be an entity or being having an independent existence of its own; and if no real entity answering to the name could be found man did not for that reason suppose that one existed, but imagined that it was something peculiarly abstruse and mysterious, too high to be an object of sense.
>
> —J. S. Mill

This remarkable statement, attributable to John Stuart Mill, the 19th-century philosopher (43), is certainly relevant to other aspects of hypertension research: low renin hypertension, for example, is regarded by some as a diagnostic nonentity (44). For reasons already discussed, it may be relevant here also. However, even if hypertension is not a disease entity separable from normal blood pressure, "mild hypertension" could still be a perfectly adequate term to describe patients whose blood pressure remains within a specified range on a specified number of occasions. Such patients are known to be at risk and are now known to benefit from treatment. It is the granting of entity status, with its implication of a clear dividing line, that creates the problem, one in which some patients fail to live up to expectation. It is better that mild hypertension makes no claim to entity status and that its management is purely pragmatic.

G. Change with Time in the Relation of Blood Pressure and Risk

Prediction of outcome from levels of blood pressure in a placebo group is usually based on measurements at entry to a trial. For predictions based on blood pressure measured 3 months after entry, the curve of risk and blood pressure in the MRC trial (29) was steeper (because of the fall of pressure during the 3 months). Predictions from this second curve are more precise because of its steepness than are those made from measurements at entry. Contributing to imprecision of entry measurements is the possible ''white coat'' response, particularly if, as seems likely, that response confers no additional risk (29). An analysis by Collins and MacMahon (45) shows that measurements of blood pressure at entry to a trial are more susceptible to regression dilution bias and are thus less reliable than measurements made later in a trial.

VIII. RISE OF PRESSURE AND ACTIVE TREATMENT OF PATIENTS IN THE PLACEBO GROUP

Before September 1980, the upper limit for systolic pressure in the trial was 210 mm Hg or a diastolic pressure of 115 mm Hg or more. After 1980, and because recent work had suggested benefit from treatment at these levels (46, 47), the limits were lowered to less than 200 mm Hg for systolic and to less than 110 mm Hg for diastolic (19).

Over its 5½ year course, 18% of male and 13% of female patients were withdrawn from placebo treatment and actively treated because their blood pressure had exceeded these limits. Withdrawn patients are important because they are at highest risk and are most likely to benefit from active treatment.

A. Intention-to-Treat Analysis

In an intention-to-treat analysis, placebo group patients needing active treatment are assessed as though they remained in the placebo group. If that active treatment reduced risk, their presence as beneficiaries in the placebo group will falsely lower event rates for that group, thereby falsely lowering absolute benefit (event rate in placebo group minus event rate in treated group) (48, 49). That withdrawn placebo group patients did benefit in the MRC trial is strongly suggested by their *lower* cardiovascular event rate compared with age- and sex-matched placebo group patients whose pressure did not exceed the limit and who were not actively treated (19).

B. On-Treatment Analysis

On-treatment analysis was more often used in the past. It too is flawed, although for a different reason (48, 49): withdrawal of high-risk placebo-group patients with blood pressure exceeding trial limits will, *by their absence* from the placebo group in an on-treatment analysis, falsely lower average event rates for the placebo group.

Thus, both methods falsely underestimate benefit by falsely lowering event rate in the placebo group: intention-to-treat analysis by including in the placebo group beneficiaries of active treatment; on-treatment analysis by excluding from the placebo group and from its analysis those most likely to have had an event (48). The underestimate of benefit from reduction of strokes may have been as high as 35% in the MRC trial (50).

A common and perhaps justified criticism of the MRC trial was that average blood pressure for entrance to the trial was set too low. Judged by blood pressure in the placebo group one year after entry, the average value was 149/92 mm Hg. This is in the lower half of the acceptable range (90 to 109 mm Hg diastolic). To some extent, this was unavoidable. Because screening was concentrated on patients whose blood pressure was in the upper part of a bell-shaped distribution, those with pressure between 90 and 99 mm Hg would be more common and likely to be recruited in greater numbers. Average pressure would be lowered for this reason.

Also, the problem created by placebo-group patients whose blood pressure fell below limits was more than balanced at the upper end of the blood pressure range by placebo-group patients whose blood pressure exceeded trial limits. Thus, aiming for a higher average pressure in a trial might decrease the number of placebo-group patients whose blood pressure fell below the limits, but it would also increase the number withdrawn from the trial because blood pressure exceeded these limits.

IX. WITHDRAWAL FROM TREATMENT AND LOSSES TO FOLLOW-UP

Withdrawals and losses of patients to follow-up are important because they can seriously compromise interpretation of a trial's findings.

A. Uniform Nomenclature Needed on "Withdrawal" and "Losses"

Different trials often report different rates of withdrawal; criticism then focuses on those with highest rates. Differences of nomenclature contribute to this variation. A comparison of "losses to follow-up" in three trials (51) showed rates of 25% for the MRC trial of treatment in elderly hypertensives (31); 15% for the European trial (52), and zero for the Swedish Trial in Old Patients (STOP) (53). The definition of "loss" was broad in the MRC trial, narrow in the European trial, narrower still in STOP. When MRC losses were recalculated using the European definition, loss decreased from 25% to 11.7% (51). When definitions are clear, differences between trials decrease: as a result of drug side effects, 3.7% of patients were withdrawn yearly from randomized treatment in the MRC elderly trial; 3.1% from placebo and active treatment groups of STOP; and 2.9% from the active treatment group of Systolic Hypertension in the Elderly Program (SHEP) (54) (see analysis in 48).

Before further comparisons are made of "loss" in hypertension trials, international agreement is needed on terminology.

Table 4 Withdrawals from Randomized Treatment

	5.1/2 year cumulative %			
	Bend	Prop	Plac	All
Group I: Withdrawal from randomized treatment but follow-up continued				
A. Drug side effects	17	19	4	11
B. BP above trial limit	1	3	14	8
C. Others	7	7	12	10
Group I total:	25	28	30	28
Group II: Withdrawn from randomized treatment, follow-up not continued				
A. Terminal event	5	5	6	5
B. Moved house	3	4	3	3
C. Avoidable lapses	14	15	14	14
Group II total (not incl. subgroup A)	18	19	18	18

Abbreviation: *BP*, blood pressure.

Table 5 Side Effects and Withdrawal from Randomized Treatment

	Rates of withdrawal					
	Bendrofluazide		Propranolol		Placebo	
Side effects	Male	Female	Male	Female	Male	Female
Impaired glucose tolerance	7.7*	5.9*	3.4	2.1	3.3	2.0
Gout	12.8*	1.5*	1.5*	—	0.9	—
Impotence	12.6*	—	6.3*	—	1.3	—
Raynaud's phenomenon	—	0.3	5.1*	4.5*	0.2	0.3
Dyspnea	0.1	0.3	7.1*	7.1*	0.4	0.2
Lethargy	3.6*	1.7*	5.3*	8.3*	0.5	0.3
Nausea, dizziness, headache	4.2*	7.4*	4.1*	9.4*	1.4	1.8

* Significant difference from rate in controls. Rates of withdrawal/1,000 patient-years of follow-up.
Source: Ref. 19.

B. MRC Mild Hypertension Trial

Withdrawals and losses to follow-up in this trial are shown in Table 4. In group 1 of this table, patients were withdrawn from randomized treatment but follow-up continued. An important contribution here was made by drug side effects. Rates for the seven most common are given separately in Table 5. Most were known side effects of these drugs but nonspecific symptoms, such as lethargy, nausea, dizziness, and headache, all more common in actively treated than in placebo-treated patients, also contributed (Table 5). Single blindedness in the study may have influenced these assessments.

Withdrawal of patients because blood pressure exceeded upper limits for the trial, the second category in this group, was, as expected, much more common in placebo-treated patients (Table 4). The third category in group 1, "Others," was of patients in whom clinical features needing a change of treatment developed, such as cardiac failure, angina, and silent myocardial infarction (19).

The second principal group in Table 4 is of patients who were withdrawn but not followed up thereafter. Subgroups here include: (a) Those suffering a terminal event, one that would have contributed to the analysis of outcome. Most reports on clinical trials do not include these patients as withdrawn or lost to follow-up. They are listed here. (b) This is a subgroup of patients who moved to an area not containing a general practice contributing to the trial. (c) This is a larger subgroup, including failure to attend appointments and failure to take tablets. These lapses of follow-up could be described as "dropouts."

Total withdrawals in group 1 in which follow-up continued after withdrawal was 28%. The total for group 2, not including those having a terminal event, was 18%. A figure of at most 18% was, in the view of trial organizers, a credit to the efficiency of general practitioners and nurses running the trial (19).

X. DECREASE OF BLOOD PRESSURE IN ACTIVELY TREATED PATIENTS

The target for active treatment was a diastolic pressure of 90 mm Hg or below. When this was not reached, supplementary treatment was to be added.

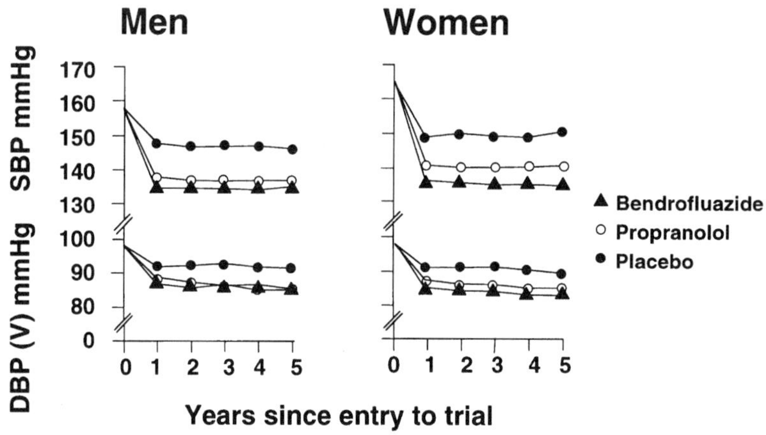

Fig. 6 Changes of blood pressure in male and female patients of MRC Mild Hypertension trial: placebo group (solid circles); bendrofluazide (triangles); propranolol group (open circles). (From Ref. 21, with permission.)

Within 2 weeks of the onset of treatment, blood pressure had fallen, the fall being present in both groups but more significant with active treatment (Fig. 6). The percentage below target was greatest with bendrofluazide (66% to 70% at annual visits in men; 71% to 79% in women). This difference of response to treatment was greater in older subjects of both sexes (19). However, supplementary treatment was needed more often in those randomized to bendrofluazide, and this difference was clearest in younger patients (19).

Overall, blood pressure control was better in those randomized to bendrofluazide than in those randomized to propranolol. However, a higher proportion in this group needed a supplementary drug to achieve this control.

Compared with placebo, lower systolic and diastolic pressures were seen with both forms of active treatment at all times (Fig. 6) and in all age groups (19). The smallest difference of systolic pressure (7.2 mm Hg) was in young men of the propranolol group; the largest (16.4 mm Hg) was in older women taking bendrofluazide (19).

XI. STUDIES DURING THE COURSE OF THE TRIAL

A. Sequential Analysis

During the first year of follow-up, fatal coronary events and sudden deaths were more common (not significantly so) in men taking bendrofluazide as compared with men taking placebo (19). In men taking propranolol, there was no increase. Coronary events were more common in men taking bendrofluazide than in men taking propranolol. On sequential analysis, this crossed the 10% significance line twice, once also crossing the 5% line (19). At about this time, the monitoring committee became aware that ECG changes of ischemia and ectopic arrhythmias were more common in men taking thiazides (19, 55). The ethical committee and the working party were alerted. The view of the working party was that the trial should continue unchanged, partly because the findings with thiazide were of borderline significance, but mainly because a decision to abandon thiazides, a widely used class of drug, must be based on irrefutable evidence (19). There are other good reasons for not stopping large controlled trials prematurely (56).

The decision to continue was fortunate. By the end of the trial, the excess of coronary events in men taking thiazide was smaller and far from significant. A few years later, the working party of a new MRC trial testing antihypertensive treatment in elderly hypertensive patients (31) chose thiazide as part of a diuretic-based regimen for comparison with beta blocker and placebo. On this occasion, the diuretic regimen proved superior to both in prevention of cardiovascular events. Had thiazide treatment been abandoned in the first MRC trial, it would probably not have been tested in the second.

During these analyses, propranolol had served as a second control group for assessment of possible adverse effects of thiazide. These roles were reversed in a later analysis when bendrofluazide served as a second control group for what seemed an adverse interaction between cigarette smoking and propranolol (discussed below). These uses of one class of drug as a control for another were unforeseen dividends of testing the two classes separately.

B. Biochemical Changes

The expected decrease of serum potassium and increases of blood sugar and serum urate occurred in patients taking bendrofluazide (19, 57). Table 3 shows these and other minor changes in men. The pattern of findings was similar in women (19). In a substudy comparing 10 mg and 5 mg daily of bendrofluazide, these changes were more marked with the higher dose; blood pressure changes were no different (19). Biochemical changes with propranolol were increases of serum potassium and of uric acid (19, 57).

XII. FORM OF FIRST REPORT

The working party had considered two forms for their first report (19). A minority favored a full paper based on the principal findings with subgroup analyses and discussion of recommendations on treatment. A majority favored a simpler paper with a full description of principal findings, but with few subgroup analyses and no recommendations on treatment; the findings, they felt, should stand on their own. The problem with subgroup analysis is its vulnerability to chance findings and bias (58, 59). However, without subgroup analysis, the analyst must assume homogeneity of risk and benefit in those receiving treatment. Recommendations can then be of two options only; to treat all mild hypertensive patients or none (49, 60, 61).

The working party chose the simpler form of report. Its conclusion, reflecting the "all or none" basis for recommendations, was that if 850 mild hypertensive patients were treated for one year, one stroke would be saved. It was a bleak conclusion, one that was not very helpful in making a decision on whether an individual patient needed treatment.

Fortunately, it was not the working party's last word on the matter: subgroup analyses were done. One, using logistic regression analysis, compared risk of stroke in two groups of men characterized by the presence or absence at entry of risk factors other than blood pressure (19, 62); factors included advanced age, increased cholesterol and body mass index, an ischemic ECG, and cigarette smoking. In the high-risk group, sharing all these factors, treatment of only 20 men for one year with bendrofluazide was needed to save one stroke. To save one stroke in the low-risk group without any of these risk factors 1250 men would need treatment for one year (62). Although the number eligible in such groups is small, this was clear evidence that an "all or none" policy of treatment for mild hypertension is untenable. Options now were to treat some, but not others.

Reflecting this are recent guidelines on treatment from the World Health Organization (WHO), International Society of Hypertension (ISH) (63), and the British Hypertension Society (64). These guidelines are to treat hypertensive patients with blood pressure consistently in the mild hypertensive range, but only those with additional risk factors (as in the regression analysis above). Patients with lower pressure and without these risks should be followed up, untreated, but with an option of treatment if serial blood pressure measurements show an increase or if other risk factors appear. Increasing age can raise risk above this threshold for intervention even if other risk factors remain stable.

XIII. PRINCIPAL FINDINGS

Antihypertensive drug treatment produced a large reduction of stroke events in men and women, with little or no reduction of coronary events or all-cause mortality (Fig. 7, Table 6). These were the patterns seen in the Australian (30) and European Working Party on Hypertension in the Elderly (EWPHE) (52) trials but, with smaller numbers, their confidence intervals were wider (Fig. 7). Behind these changes lie some interesting observations on the relation between cardiovascular causes of death and cigarette smoking.

A. Cigarette Smoking Alters in Two Ways Cardiovascular Risk and Benefits from Treatment

The relevant findings on the influence of smoking are in Table 7. Four conclusions can be drawn. (a) In patients randomized to placebo, cigarette smoking increases risk from stroke and coronary disease. These well-recognized effects were particularly significant

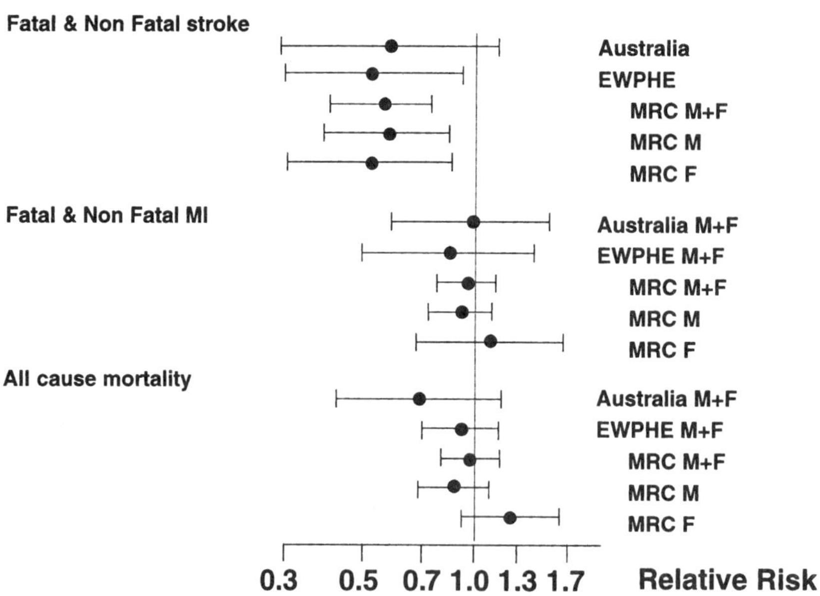

Fig. 7 Relative risk (ratio of rate in treated group and rate in placebo group) for stroke, coronary events, and all-cause mortality in men and women of MRC trial (mean ± 95% CI). Comparison is with Australian trial (30) and the European trial of high blood pressure in elderly patients, EWPHE (52).

Table 6 Principal Results

	Bendrofluazide			Propranolol			Both active treatments		
	Men	Women	Both	Men	Women	Both	Men	Women	Both
Stroke events	↓***	↓**	↓***	—	—	—	↓**	↓***	↓***
Coronary events	—	—	—	—	—	—	—	—	—
All cardiovascular events	—	—	↓*	—	—	↓*	—	—	↓**

Arrows indicate significant reduction compared with placebo group. Effects of cigarette smoking are given in Table 3. $*p < 0.05$; $**p < 0.01$; $***p < 0.001$.
Source: Ref. 19.

in women (Table 7). (b) In nonsmokers, both forms of active treatment reduced stroke to a similar extent (Table 7). (c) Among smokers, only those randomized to bendrofluazide showed benefit from reduction of stroke. (d) Propranolol reduced stroke in nonsmokers but, importantly, not in smokers. Part of this failure may have resulted from a smaller reduction of blood pressure by propranolol in smokers (65) and part from a significant adverse interaction on outcome between smoking and propranolol (19, 21). The nature and size of this interaction is unclear. One possibility discussed by Miall and Greenberg (19) is that cigarette smoking increases catecholamines that, in the presence of nonspecific beta blockade, may raise blood pressure or increase event rates by an alpha-adrenergic action.

The findings for coronary events (Table 7) were as follows: (a) In smokers, coronary events were more common than in nonsmokers in all treatment groups and in both sexes—also a well-recognized observation. (b) As with stroke, relative risks (smokers/nonsmokers) were greater in women than in men. (c) Among smokers, coronary events were not significantly reduced in men or women by propranolol or by bendrofluazide (Table 7). (d) In male nonsmokers, there was a small, just-significant reduction of coronary events

Table 7 Influence of Smoking

	Stroke events			Coronary events		
	Bendro.	Prop.	Plac.	Bendro.	Prop.	Plac.
Men						
Smokers	0.9**xx	5.2	4.3	12.7	13.8	12.6
Nonsmokers	1.1*	1.1*	2.4	7.4	5.0*	7.5
Women						
Smokers	1.1	3.4	3.9	5.1	4.5	3.5
Nonsmokers	0.5	0.9	1.5	0.8	0.8	1.0
Men and Women						
Smokers	1.0***xxx	4.3	4.0	9.3	9.5	8.5
Nonsmokers	0.8**	1.0*	1.9	4.1	2.9*	4.3

xxx, xx Dif. bendrofluazide v. propranolol. $P < 0.001, 0.01$.
***, **, * Dif. active treatment v. placebo, respectively 0.01 and 0.05.
Events are age-adjusted rates/1,000 patients years.
Source: Refs 19, 62.

in those taking propranolol. When all cardiovascular events are taken together, this reduction was more significant in men ($P < 0.01$) (19). Thus, propranolol may reduce cardiovascular events but only in nonsmokers.

B. Reduction of Stroke

The reduction of stroke or of other cardiovascular events can be expressed in three ways:

(1) As a relative risk: $\frac{\text{event rate in treated patients}}{\text{event rate in placebo group}}$

(2) As a proportionate reduction of risk (proportionate benefit) expressed as a percentage: $100 - \frac{\text{event rate in treated group}}{\text{event rate in placebo group}} \times 100\%$

(3) As an absolute reduction of risk (absolute benefit)

event rate in placebo group minus event rate in treated group. Logistic regression analysis makes possible an extension of this method, an example being the comparison described earlier of two groups of men with the same blood pressure, one having a series of risk factors measured at entry, and the other not having them (62).

These methods make clear that stroke is significantly reduced in actively treated patients, men and women separately (Fig. 7); in patients receiving bendrofluazide (Table 7), and in nonsmokers receiving propranolol (Table 7). Significant reductions were also seen in bendrofluazide-treated patients with diastolic pressure at entry above and below 100 mm Hg (19). For propranolol, the reduction was significant only in those with higher diastolic pressure at the outset (19).

C. Constant Proportionate Benefit from Reduction of Stroke but with Wide Variation of Absolute Benefit

It is interesting that proportionate benefit from reduction of stroke in hypertension using antihypertensive drugs is relatively constant across a wide range of severity. Figure 8 is from an earlier analysis (49) showing this for seven placebo-controlled trials, including the trial reviewed here. The index of severity in each, the rate of stroke events in its placebo group, varies widely. A mathematical consequence of this variation in the presence of constant proportionate benefit is that absolute benefit from reduction of stroke is steeply graded. Thus, patients in trials at the upper end of the range of risk appear, in proportionate terms, to benefit no more than those at the lower end of the range. In absolute terms, however, benefit in these patients is much greater.

We have applied this principle to an analysis of subgroups of patients within the MRC Mild Hypertension trial. Subgroups, all previously published (19, 62), were selected by age, sex, level of blood pressure at entry, smoking habit, and treatment. The pattern of findings (Fig. 9) is similar to that seen in the comparison of trials (Fig. 8). Again, proportionate benefit among subgroups is relatively constant across a wide range of risk in the placebo group. Because of this, absolute benefit is graded across the same wide range. Also shown in this figure are two points from the logistic regression analysis described previously; point A is of men at very low risk, point B is of men at very high risk.

The slope seen in the lower panel of Figure 9 is not a correlation: some patients appear in more than one analysis and one term—stroke rate in the placebo group—is

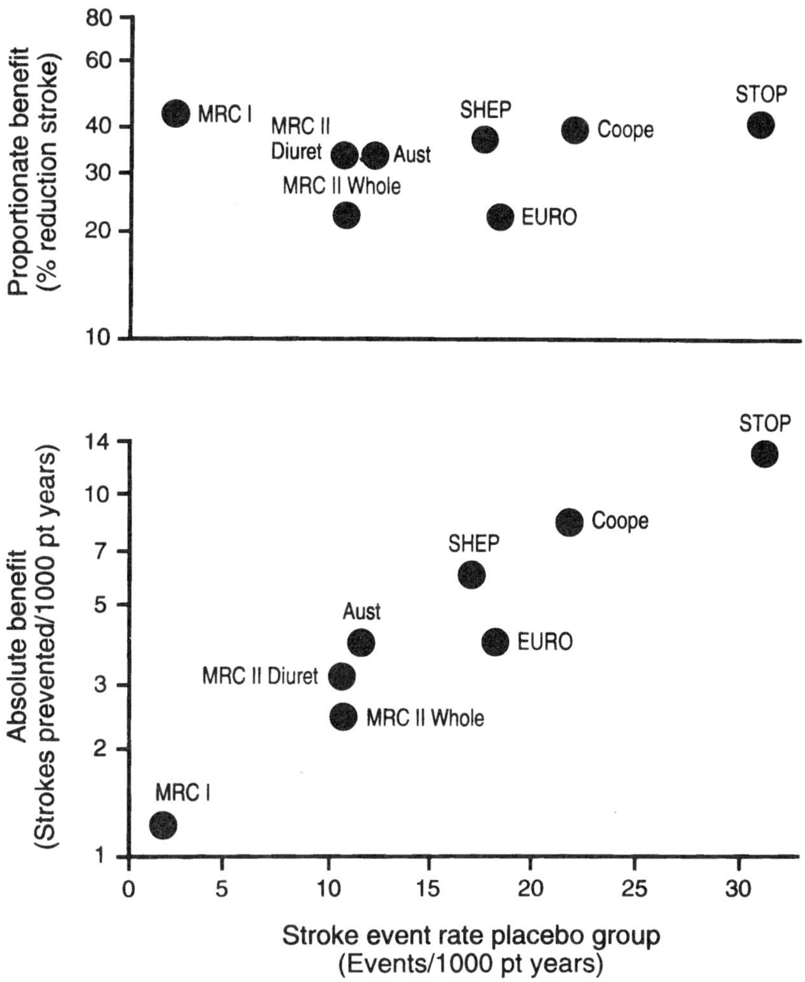

Fig. 8 Comparison of absolute and proportionate benefit (see text) in seven trials. The analyses show over a wide range of risk in the placebo groups of these trials a relatively constant proportionate benefit but with steeply graded absolute benefit. (From Ref. 49, with permission.)

common to both axes of the graph. The purpose of the analysis was not this. It was to test the hypothesis that, although proportionate benefit remains relatively constant across a wide range of risk in treated patients, absolute benefit will vary markedly within subgroups of a trial. The implication is that, whereas comparisons of relative risk and of proportionate benefit are important in assessing outcome of trials (Fig. 7), absolute benefit is more discriminating and thus more useful as a basis for recommendations on treatment. Policy guidelines (63, 64) make this point in their recommendations on management of mild hypertension. Indeed, the WHO/ISH proposal (63) bases its recommendations on a stratification of risk that is the equivalent of increasing absolute benefit by concentrating treatment on patients in the upper right hand part of the distribution in Figure 9. The

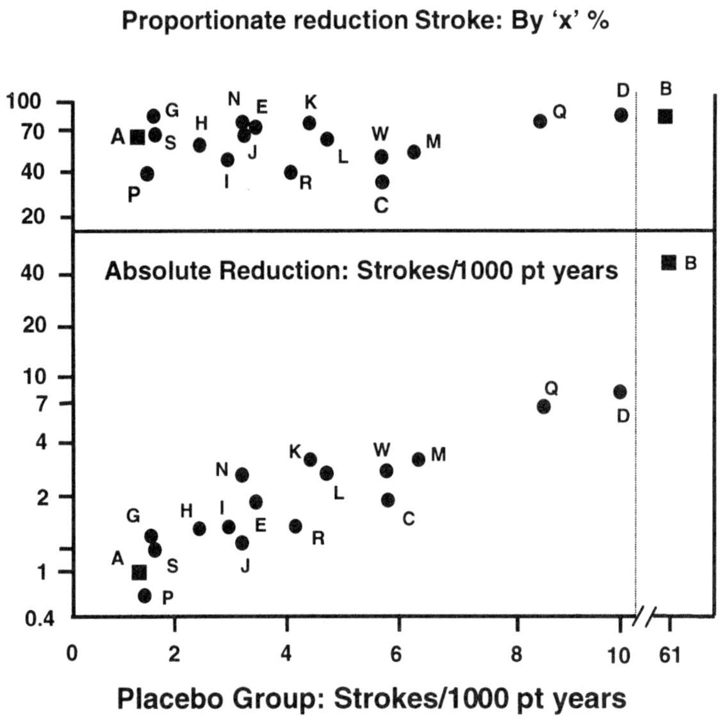

Fig. 9 Upper panel. Proportionate benefit from reduction of stroke in subgroups of MRC trial (see below). **Lower panel**. Absolute benefit in the same subgroups. A = low risk group from regression analysis; B = high risk group; C = men aged 55–64 nonsmokers (NS), SBP > 160 (Ref. MRC 1988); D = men aged 55–64 smokers, SBP > 160; E = women aged 55–64 NS, SBP > 160; G = Ref. 19, Table 9.2, M + F DBP < 95; H · · · G, DBP 95–99; J as G, DBP 100–104; K as G, DBP 105+; L-Table 9.4, men aged 55–64, DBP < 100; M as L, DBP 100+; N Table 9.5, women aged 55–64, DBP 100+; P as N, DBP < 100; Q-Table 10.5, men aged 55–64, smokers; R as Q, NS; S-Table 10.6 women NS; W-Table 10.5, men 55–64 NS; T-Ref. 62, women 55–64, prop NS.

patterns seen in Figure 9 are not peculiar to the MRC trial. Ramsay and colleagues (66) found similar patterns from subgroup analyses of this sort using data from other trials.

D. Influence of Treatment on Coronary Events and All-Cause Mortality

Overall, active treatment had no significant effect on coronary events (Fig. 7). However, comparison of thiazides and propranolol did show several differences: (a) Sudden deaths, that is deaths occurring within one hour of the onset of symptoms and assumed to be coronary events, were significantly more common in men of the thiazide group (rate 2.7/1000 patient-years) than in men of the propranolol group (1.1). For men given placebo, the rate was 1.9. The difference between the two forms of active treatment was significant ($P < 0.01$) (19). An early trend in this direction was a reason for discussion during the trial of a need on ethical grounds to stop testing thiazides. (b) Does propranolol have a cardioprotective effect? Coronary events overall were fewer in men taking propranolol (rate 7.6) than in men taking placebo (9.0), an insignificant difference. As noted earlier and in Table 3, the coronary event rate in nonsmoking men taking propranolol (5.0) was significantly lower than in controls (7.5). It was insignificantly lower than in nonsmoking men of the thiazide group (7.4). Taking both sexes together, the cardiovascular event rate was significantly lower in the propranolol group among nonsmokers (19).

The lack of overall benefit for coronary events with the two forms of active treatment (Fig. 7) may in part reflect a balance between the small adverse effect of thiazide and the small protective effect of propranolol among nonsmokers.

E. Influence of Treatment on Incidence of New ECG Abnormalities

Electrocardiograms were recorded on all patients at entry and at the five annual visits. Each trace was Minnesota-coded independently by two readers; a third arbitrated when discrepancies arose. The findings are expressed as incidence rates for new ECG changes developing during the trial (19).

(1). *Transmural ischemic changes* (Minnesota code $1_{1\text{–}3}$): Compared with placebo controls, propranolol reduced significantly ($P < 0.05$) the incidence of transmural infarction: 19.8 and 16.8 cases/1000 patient-years, respectively. Thiazide marginally increased these changes: 22.7 cases/1000 patient-years compared with placebo ($P < 0.05$). The difference between propranolol and thiazide-treated groups was highly significant ($P < 0.001$) (19). Although this pattern of new ECG changes resembles the pattern for coronary events occurring during the trial in nonsmokers (Table 7), the pattern of ECG changes did not differ in smokers and nonsmokers. This was surprising given the findings for coronary events in smokers (Table 7). An explanation considered by Miall and Greenberg (19) was that smoking increased coronary events by a mechanism less dependent on coronary atheroma, possibly one involving activation of fibrinogen (67).

(2). *Left ventricular hypertrophy* (Minnesota code 3_1); any drug lowering blood pressure would be expected to reduce the incidence of left ventricular hypertrophy developing during treatment, and this was seen in patients of bendrofluazide and propranolol groups. Interestingly, the reduction with bendrofluazide, 44%, was greater than that with propranolol, 20%. Some of this difference may be explained by the greater reduction of blood pressure with bendrofluazide (Fig. 6). However, when this was allowed for in multiple regression analysis, a smaller but still significant difference favoring thiazide persisted (19).

F. All-Cause Mortality

All-cause mortality was little different in controls and actively treated patients (respectively, 5.9 and 5.8 deaths/1000 patient-years). Behind this lay an interesting balance of opposite effects: in men a 13% reduction, in women a 25% increase (Fig. 7), a just-significant difference between sexes ($P = 0.05$) using the more stringent system of P value testing with Yates correction (19). In nonsmoking women, rates were 4.4, 3.6, and 2.3 for bendrofluazide, propranolol, and placebo groups, respectively. The increase in women of the bendrofluazide group, by 91%, was significant ($P < 0.01$). This most likely is a chance finding, a by-product perhaps of multiple subgroup analyses.

However, there is another possibility, one we have discussed previously (61): that within a group of patients receiving an antihypertensive drug, there is a balance between its recognized favorable effect on outcome—a reduction of stroke for example—and a much smaller adverse effect, one causing a small but constant absolute increase of mortality at all levels of risk. When overall risk is low, the balance favors the adverse effect because absolute benefit from reduction of stroke is now also small. Because women, particularly younger women, are those standing to gain least from the reduction of stroke, it would be in such a group that a small absolute increase of risk could be first manifest. Whether this is the explanation for the 91% higher mortality in nonsmoking women on thiazide is far from sure. The possibility cannot be dismissed. Whatever the explanation, the increase of this size in all-cause mortality certainly weakens the case for prescribing thiazides in such women.

G. Active Treatment Prevents Mild Hypertension Becoming Moderate/Severe Hypertension

As can be seen in Table 4, in 14% of patients taking placebo, blood pressure rose to exceed trial limits. These patients had developed moderate/severe hypertension. On ethical grounds they were withdrawn and actively treated. Active treatment from the outset almost completely prevented this rise of pressure. In only 1% of patients taking diuretic and in only 3% of those taking propranolol did blood pressure rise to exceed trial limits. This preventative effect of active treatment is an important positive outcome from treatment of mild hypertension.*

XIV. COURSE OF BLOOD PRESSURE ON STOPPING ANTIHYPERTENSIVE TREATMENT

An interesting substudy was done of the timing and completeness of the return of blood pressure to control values after stopping treatment (68). One thousand four hundred eighteen men and 1347 women taking bendrofluazide, propranolol, or placebo at the end of the 5-year study were randomized to stopping their original treatment or continuing with that treatment. Continuing treatment had no effect on blood pressure in actively treated groups, as did stopping or continuing treatment in the placebo group. Stopping bendrofluazide (gradually withdrawn over 1 week) led to a near-complete return of blood pressure to placebo values 1 month later and complete return 3 months later. Stopping propranolol (withdrawn more gradually in 50% of patients over 1 month) led to near-complete return of pressure at 3 months, to complete return at 12 months (68).

These changes are a mirror image of those occurring after starting treatment in the MRC trial in which a rapid decline of pressure occurred in early weeks with active treatment, a slow decline followed for up to 6 months. Thereafter, blood pressure remained stable (Fig. 2). Clearly, the processes governing these changes are slow acting, much slower than rates at which propranolol produces beta blockade or diuretics produce a balanced state, with equal input and output of salt and water. The ability of quick-acting agents, often given in low doses, to promote slow-developing but ultimately large pressor responses is an interesting but unexplained finding in hypertension research. Slow-developing and slow-regressing structural vascular change might be important here (69).

* We thank Sir James Black for emphasizing this point in correspondence he had with one of us over the form taken by the first report on the MRC trial (21).

XV. ECONOMICS AND OTHER RESEARCH BASED ON MRC TRIAL PATIENTS

Actual expenditure at the end of the trial, just over £2.0M during 5 years at 1977 prices, was close to the cost predicted at the outset (19). By any standards then and now, it was a large and expensive trial. Even so, on medical and economic grounds it was important to determine whether a condition affecting up to 10% of the adult population is best managed by treating all, some, or none of the affected patients. Recommendations of the WHO/ISH Committee (63) and all other guidelines are partly based on findings in the MRC trial. We agree with the WHO/ISH system of stratifying risk at the outset (63): risk relating partly to the level of blood pressure, but also to risk less clearly related to blood pressure—age, the presence of ischemic heart disease, diabetes, high cholesterol, and others. Where overall risks are high, treatment should begin; where risks are low, patients should be followed up in the clinic, possibly with ''lifestyle changes'' only. These changes include reduction of body weight, increase of exercise and, most important of all, cessation of smoking. More lives could have been saved in the MRC trial had smokers stopped smoking than were saved as a result of active treatment (61). The economic implications of this are large but complex politically.

To evaluate outcome in treated and untreated patients was an objective of the MRC trial; its expense was certainly commensurate with the cost of drugs prescribed in the trial. More relevant is the cost of treating hypertension generally. A recent health survey for England (70) suggests that just under 20% of adults are hypertensive and that half of these are receiving antihypertensive drugs. The cost of prescriptions in these patients, approximately 3 million and most having mild hypertension, will greatly exceed the cost of testing these drugs in the MRC Mild Hypertension trial.

It is common for large clinical trials to provide opportunities for types of research not otherwise possible because of high costs. For example, screening was the most expensive element in the MRC trial (19) and, after the trial's end, major opportunities were taken for studies in screened subjects. Screening of a representative subsample of the population of Paisley was the basis of a subsequent cohort study of 15,000 subjects followed up for more than 25 years. Studies based on this cohort since have embraced epidemiology, cardiology, respiratory medicine, genetics, cancer, and sociology. Three references (71–73) describe recent studies and list some of the earlier work. Studies at Ladywell in Edinburgh were of subjects screened in the MRC trial and of their offspring. These have examined phenotypic and environmental factors influencing blood pressure. Two recent papers (74, 75) give examples and information on earlier studies. As in other large trials, the placebo group of the MRC trial has been used in numerous studies; one by Millar and colleagues (29) is represented in this chapter by data from Figures 2–5.

It is relevant to the cost of the MRC trial that these studies are represented in more than 50 publications and that all were dividends, mostly unforeseen, from the original £2.0M invested by the MRC.

XVI. CONCLUSIONS

The MRC trial succeeded in its primary objective of testing separately two widely used antihypertensive drugs. Good organization on a large scale and the enthusiasm and skill of general practice physicians and their nursing colleagues played a major part (19, 28). Benefit from reduction of stroke with active treatment was highly significant but because risks were small, absolute benefits were also small. The importance of mild hypertension lies in the large number of patients at risk. Strokes prevented by treating this large number would be considerable and worthwhile.

The decision to test separately two classes of drug in the trial was probably wise. Differences of outcome comparing these drugs were considerable and most were unrelated to differences of blood pressure. The use of two active treatments lent further support to the view that there is more to treatment of hypertension than the lowering of blood pressure.

The decision to report simply the principal findings without subgroup analyses and with little discussion of recommendations on treatment was understandable but almost certainly unwise. The prospect of treating 850 patients to save one stroke has haunted discussion of the trial, despite clear evidence from papers published since (19, 62) using subgroup analysis that absolute benefit within the trial varied markedly. The analysis in Figure 9 of this chapter adds to this showing a wide range of absolute benefit among subgroups of MRC trial patients.

An interesting but probably less important matter was the identity of patients whose blood pressure on three occasions during screening and at entry was within trial limits, but on one or more occasions after randomization fell below trial limits. Are these intruders from below with normal blood pressure, or are they no more than mild hypertensives defined in pragmatic fashion by six measurements of blood pressure on three visits? We favor the second theory. The problem with questions such as these is that mild hypertension has only a weak claim for status as an entity, much weaker than that of malignant-phase hypertension with its characteristic retinopathy and predictable course in the untreated state.

APPENDIX I

Members of the Working Party

Professor Sir Stanley Peart (Chairman)
Mrs. G.R. Barnes (until 1983)
Mr. P.M.G. Broughton
Professor A.L. Cochrane (until 1977)
Professor C.T. Dollery
Dr. K.G. Green (until 1983)
Dr. J.E. Harrison (until 1977)
Professor W.W. Holland (until 1977)
Dr. M.F. Hudson
Dr. D.M. Humphreys (until 1978)
Dr. A.F. Lever
Dr. T.W. Meade
Dr. W.E. Miall (Secretary until 1983)
Professor G.A. Rose
The late Dr. B.C. Smith (until 1980)
Dr. P. Wilding (until 1977)
Dr. G. Greenberg (Secretary)

APPENDIX II

Members of the Monitoring Committee

Professor G.A. Rose (Chairman)
Dr. M.W. Adler (until 1978)
Mr. P.J. Brennan
Dr. E.C. Coles (until 1978)
Dr. G. Greenberg
Dr. M. Hamilton
Dr. J.A. Heady
Dr. T.W. Meade
Dr. W.E. Miall
Dr. E.B. Raftery (until 1978)
Dr. S.G. Thompson (until 1984)
Professor H.D. Tunstall Pedoe

APPENDIX III

Members of the Ethical Committee

Professor Sir Richard Doll (Chairman)
Dr. J. Fry
Dr. M. Hamilton (until 1980)
Dr. J.A. Heady (until 1980)
Professor Sir Raymond Hoffenberg
Professor J.H. Ledingham
Dr. P.J. Taylor

REFERENCES

1. Doll R. Controlled trials: the 1948 watershed. Br Med J 1998; 317:1217–1220.
2. Medical Research Council. Streptomycin in Tuberculosis Trials Committee. Streptomycin treatment for pulmonary tuberculosis. Br Med J 1948; ii:769–782.
3. Yoshioka A. Use of randomisation in the Medical Research Council's clinical trial of streptomycin in pulmonary tuberculosis in the 1940s. Br Med J 1998; 317:1220–1223.
4. Pickering GW. The cerebrospinal fluid in arterial hypertension. Clin Sci 1934; 1:397–413.
5. Keith NM, Wagener HP, Barker NW. Some different types of essential hypertension: their course and prognosis. Am J Med Sci 1939; 197:332–343.
6. Kincaid-Smith P, McMichael J, Murphy EA. The clinical course and pathology of hypertension with papilloedema (malignant hypertension). Q J Med 1958; 27:117–153.
7. Sokolow M, Perloff D. Five-year survival of consecutive patients with malignant hypertension treated with antihpertensive agents. Am J Cardiol 1960; 6:858–863.
8. Mohler ER, Freis ED. Five-year survival of patients with malignant hypertension treated with antihypertensive agents. Am Heart J 1960; 60:329–335.
9. Harrington M, Kincaid-Smith P, McMichael J. Results of treatment in malignant hypertension. Br Med J 1959; 2:969–980.
10. Pickering GW, Cranston WI, Pears MA. The Treatment of Hypertension. Springfield, IL: Charles C Thomas, 1961:29.
11. Isles CG. Malignant hypertension and hypertensive encephalopathy. In: Swales JD ed. Textbook of Hypertension. Oxford: Blackwell Scientific Publications, 1994; 1233–1248.

12. Breckenridge A, Dollery CT, Parry EHO. Prognosis of treated hypertension: changes in life expectancy and causes of death between 1952 and 1967. Q J Med 1970; 39:411–429.
13. Lip GYH, Beevers M, Beevers DG. Complications and survival of 315 patients with malignant-phase hypertension. J Hypertens 1995; 13:915–924.
14. Isles CG, Link G, Boulton Jones M, Cameron H, Lever AF, Murray G. Factors influencing outcome in malignant hypertension. J Hypertens 1985; 3(suppl 3):S405–S407.
15. Webster J, Petrie JC, Jeffers TA, Lovell HG. Accelerated hypertension—patterns of mortality and clinical factors affecting outcome in treated patients. Q J Med 1993; 86:485–493.
16. Veterans Administration Co-operative Study Group. Effects of treatment on morbidity in hypertension. Results in patients with diastolic blood pressures averaging 115 through 129 mmHg. JAMA 1967; 202:1028–1034.
17. Wolf FW, Lindeman RD. Effects of treatment in hypertension: results of a controlled study. J Chronic Dis 1966; 19:227–240.
18. Hamilton M, Thompson EN, Wisnewski TKM. The role of blood pressure control in preventing complications of hypertension. Lancet 1964; i:235–238.
19. Miall WE, Greenberg G. Mild Hypertension: Is There Pressure to Treat? Cambridge: Cambridge University Press, 1987.
20. MRC Working Party on Mild to Moderate Hypertension. Randomised controlled trial of treatment for mild hypertension: design and pilot trial. BMJ 1977; ii:1437–1440.
21. Medical Research Council Working Party. MRC trial of treatment of mild hypertension: principal results. BMJ 1985; 291:97–104.
22. Wright BM, Dore CF. A random-zero sphygmomanometer. Lancet 1970; i:337–338.
23. Rose GA, Holland WW, Crowley EA. A sphygmomanometer for epidemiologists. Lancet 1964; i:296–300.
24. Miall WE, Chinn S. Screening for hypertension: some epidemiological observations. BMJ 1974; iii:595–600.
25. Registrar General. Statistical Review of England and Wales 1970. London: HMSO, 1971.
26. Mann AH. The psychological effects of a screening programme and a clinical trial upon the participants. Psychol Med 1977; 7:431–438.
27. Mann A. In: Hypertension: Psychological Aspects and Diagnostic Impact in a Clinical Trial. Psychological Medicine Monograph 5. Cambridge: Cambridge University Press, 1984.
28. Peart WS. The pharmaceutical industry: research and responsibility. Lancet 1980; ii:465–466.
29. Millar JA, Isles CG, Lever AF. Blood pressure, white coat response and cardiovascular risk in placebo group patients of the MRC Mild Hypertension trial. J Hypertens 1995; 13:175–183.
30. Australian National Blood Pressure Study Management Committee. The Australian Therapeutic Trial in Mild Hypertension. Lancet 1980; i:1261–1267.
31. MRC Working Party. Medical Research Council trial of treatment of hypertension in older adults: principal results. BMJ 1992; 304:405–413.
32. Simpson FO. Fallacies in the interpretation of the large-scale trials of treatment of mild to moderate hypertension. J Cardiovasc Pharmacol 1990; 16(suppl 7): S92–S95.
33. Waal-Manning HJ, Paulin JM, Simpson FO. MRC trial of treatment of mild hypertension (letter). BMJ 1985; 291:972.
34. Millar JA, Lever AF. Effect of sex-related changes in blood pressure at entry to the MRC trial on prediction of cardiovascular risk. Clin Exper Pharmacol Physiol 1994; 21:167–169.
35. Mancia G, Parati G, Grassi G, Caseder R, Zanchetti A. Alerting reaction and rise in blood pressure during measurement by physician and nurse. Hypertension 1987; 9:209–215.
36. Pickering TG. White coat hypertension. In: JH Laragh, BM Brenner, eds. Hypertension, Pathophysiology, Diagnosis and Management. 2nd ed. New York: Raven Press, 1994; 1913–1928.
37. McCubbin JA, Wilson JF, Bruehl S, Brady M, Clark BA, Kort E. Gender effects on blood pressure obtained during an on campus screening. Psychosomatic Med 1991; 53:90–100.
38. Pickering TG, Devereux RB, Gerin W, James GD, Pieper C, Schlussel YR, Schoall PL. The

role of behavioural factors in white coat and sustained hypertension. J Hypertens 1990; 8(suppl 7): S141–S147.
39. Brennan PJ, Greenberg G, Miall WE, Thompson SG. Seasonal variation in arterial blood pressure. BMJ 1982; 285:919–923.
40. Oldham PD. A note on the analysis of repeated measurements of the same subjects. J Chronic Dis 1962; 15:969–977.
41. Svardsudd K, Blomquist N. A new method for investigating the relation between change and initial value in longitudinal blood pressure data I. Description and application of the method. Scand J Soc Med 1978; 6:85–95.
42. Robertson JIS, Hansson L. How well is hypertension treated? Summary of the proceedings of a workshop held at North Cape, Norway (14th–16th June 1986). J Hypertens 1986; 4(suppl 6):S638–S641.
43. Ogden CK, Richards IA. The Meaning of Meaning. 10th ed. London: Routledge & Keegan Paul, 1949.
44. Mason P, Beevers DG, Beretta-Piccoli C, Brown JJ, Cumming AMM, Davies DL, Fraser R, Lever AF, Morton JJ, Padfield PL, Young J. In: MP Sambhi, ed. Fundamental Fault in Hypertension. Mill's Disease Amongst Medical Specialists in Hypertension. Boston: Martinus Nijhoff, 1984:105–116.
45. Collins R, MacMahon S. Blood pressure, antihypertensive drug treatment and risks of stroke and coronary heart disease. Br Med Bull 1994; 50:272–298.
46. Anonymous. The pressure to treat. Lancet 1980; i:1283–1284.
47. Anonymous. Millions of mild hypertensives. BMJ 1980; 281:1024–1025.
48. Lever AF, Brennan PJ. MRC trial of treatment in elderly hypertensives. High Blood Pressure 1992; 1:132–137.
49. Lever AF, Ramsay LE. Treatment of hypertension in the elderly. J Hypertens 1995; 13:571–579.
50. Millar JA, Lever AF. Adjustment of the apparent benefits of treatment on stroke risk in the MRC Mild Hypertension trial using data from the placebo group. J Hum Hypertens 1995; 9: 409–512.
51. Lever AF, Brennan PJ. MRC trial of treatment in elderly hypertensives. Clin Exper Hypertens 1993; 15:941–952.
52. Amery A, Birkenhager W, Brixko P, Bulpitt C, Clement D, Deruyttere M, De Schaepdryver A, Dollery C, Fagard R, Forette F, Forte J, Hamdy R, Henry JF, Joosens JV, Leonetti G, Lund-Johansen P, O'Malley K, Petrie J, Strasser T, Tuomilehto J, Williams B. Mortality and morbidity results from the European Working Party on high blood pressure in the elderly trial. Lancet 1985; i:1349–1354.
53. Dahlof D, Lindeholm LH, Hansson L, Schersten B, Ekbom T, Wester PO. Morbidity and mortality in the Swedish trial in old patients with hypertension (STOP-Hypertension). Lancet 1991; 338:1281–1284.
54. SHEP Cooperative Research Group. Prevention of stroke by antihypertensive drug treatment in older persons with isolated systolic hypertension. Final results of the Systolic Hypertension in the Elderly Program. JAMA 1991; 265:3255–3264.
55. Medical Research Council Working Party on Mild to Moderate Hypertension. Ventricular extrasystoles during thiazide treatment: sub-study of MRC Mild Hypertension Trial. BMJ 1983; 287:1249–1253.
56. Editorial. On stopping a clinical trial before its time. Lancet 1993; 342:1311–1312.
57. Medical Research Council Working Party on Mild to Moderate Hypertension. Adverse reactions to bendrofluazide and propranolol for treatment of mild hypertension. Lancet 1981; ii: 539–543.
58. Pocock SJ, Hughes MD, Lee RJ. Statistical problems in the reporting of clinical trials. N Engl J Med 1987; 317:426–432.
59. Bulpitt CJ. Subgroup analysis. Lancet 1988; ii:31–34.

60. Schwartz D, Flamant R, Lellouch J (transl by MJR Healy). Clinical Trials. London: Academic Press, 1980.
61. Isles CG, Brown JJ, Lever AF, Murray GD. In: FR Buhler, JH Laragh, ed. Handbook of Hypertension: The management of Hypertension. Vol 13. What Clinical Trials Have Taught Us. Amsterdam: Elsevier Science, 1990: 18–31.
62. Medical Research Council Working Party. Stroke and coronary disease in mild hypertension: risk factors and the value of treatment. BMJ 1988; 296:1565–1570.
63. Guidelines Sub-Committee 1999. WHO/ISH guidelines for management of hypertension. J Hypertens 1999; 17:151–183.
64. Sever P, Beevers DG, Bulpitt C, Lever AF, Ramsay LE, Reid JL, Swales J. Management guidelines in essential hypertension: report of the second Working Party of the British Hypertension Society. BMJ 1993; 306:983–987.
65. Greenberg G, Thompson SG, Brennan PJ. The relationship between smoking and the response to antihypertensive treatment in mild hypertension in the Medical Research Council's Trial of Treatment. Int J Epidemiol 1987; 16:25–30.
66. Ramsay LE, Wallis EJ, Yeo WW, Jackson PR. The rationale for differing national recommendations for the treatment of hypertension. Am J Hypertension 1998; 11:79S–88S.
67. Meade TW, Mellows S, Brozovic M, Miller GJ, Chakrabarti RR, North WRS, Haines AP, Stirling Y, Imeson JD, Thompson SG. Haemostatic function and ischaemic heart disease: principal results of Northwick Park Heart Study. Lancet 1986; 2:533–537.
68. Medical Research Council Working Party on Mild Hypertension. Course of blood pressure in mild hypertensives after withdrawal of long-term antihypertensive treatment. BMJ 1986; 293:988–992.
69. Lever AF, Harrap SB. Essential hypertension: a disorder of growth with origins in childhood? J Hypertens 1992; 10:101–120.
70. Colhoun HM, Dong W, Poulter NR. Blood pressure screening, management and control in England: results from the Health Survey for England. J Hypertens 1994; 16:747–752.
71. Hole DJ, Watt GCM, Davey-Smith G, Hart CL, Gillis CR, Hawthorne VM. Impaired lung function is the strongest clinical indicator of mortality risk in men and women. Findings from the Renfrew/Paisley study. BMJ 1996; 313:711–715.
72. Lever AF, Hole DJ, Gillis CR, McCallum IR, McInnes GT, MacKinnon PL, Meredith PA, Murray LS, Reid JL, Robertson JWK. Do inhibitors of angiotensin-l-converting enzyme protect against risk of cancer? Lancet 1998; 352:179–184.
73. Isles CG, Hole DJ, Hawthorne VM, Lever AF. Relation between coronary risk and coronary mortality in women of the Renfrew/Paisley survey: comparison with men. Lancet 1992; 399: 702–706.
74. Watt GMC, Harrap SB, Foy CJW, Holton DW, Edwards HV, Davidson HR, Connor JM, Lever AF, Fraser R. Abnormalities of glucocorticoid metabolism and the renin-angiotensin system: a four-corners approach to identification of genetic determinants of blood pressure. J Hypertens 1992; 10:473–482.
75. Harrap SB, Fraser R, Inglis GC, Lever AF, Beastall GH, Dominiczak MH, Foy CJW, Watt GCM. Abnormal epinephrine release in young adults with high personal and high parental blood pressures. Circulation 1997; 96:556–561.

6

Beta-Blockers Versus Diuretics in Hypertensive Men: The HAPPHY Trial

LARS WILHELMSEN

Göteborg University, Göteborg, Sweden

I. INTRODUCTION

When the Heart Attack Primary Prevention in Hypertensives (HAPPHY) Trial was designed in 1975 to 1976, a few randomized antihypertensive trials with placebo groups had been published and had shown positive effects, primarily on stroke incidence and mortality. The effects on coronary heart disease (CHD), morbidity and mortality, were less apparent (1, 2). At that time, thiazide diuretics and beta-blockers were becoming used as first-line drugs in hypertension in many countries, and studies in Sweden indicated that these two modalities were used by about 50% each. Some available results indicated beneficial effects of beta-blocker treatment after myocardial infarction (MI) (3–5). Since then, several large trials have confirmed that beta-blockers reduced the risk of death and reinfarction by more than 20% in overviews including more than 20,000 patients (6).

II. OBJECTIVES OF THE TRIAL

The main objective of the HAPPHY Trial was to determine whether antihypertensive treatment with beta-blockers differed from thiazide diuretic treatment with respect to the incidence of nonfatal MI, mortality from CHD, and total mortality in men with mild to moderate hypertension. The design and results were published in 1987 (7). A prerequisite for the main objective was that an equal blood pressure reduction was achieved in both treatment groups. In addition to the main objectives, the occurrence of side effects and reported symptoms in each treatment group were assessed.

Two other trials designed to examine the incidence of major endpoints in hypertensive patients on a beta-blocker based regimen compared with placebo, a non–

Table 1a Classification of Risk Groups

Systolic blood pressure	Cholesterol	Nonsmoker	Ex-smoker	Smokes g/day*	
	≥ 8.7	H	H	H	H
≥ 190 mm Hg	7.0–8.6	M	H	H	H
	< 7.0	L	M	H	H
	≥ 8.7	M	H	H	H
< 190 mm Hg	7.0–8.6	M	M	H	H
	< 7.0	L	L	M	H

* For calculation of tobacco consumption in grams the following values are used: 1 cigarette = 1 g; 1 cheroot = 2 g; 1 cigar = 5 g. A packet of pipe tobacco normally contains 50 g. The consumption per week is divided by 7 to obtain the daily consumption.
H, high-risk group; M, medium-risk group; L, low-risk group.

Table 1b Randomization Groups

Age	40–49	50–59	60–64
H, High-risk group	3	6	9
M, Medium-risk group	2	5	8
L, Low-risk group	1	4	7

From Ref. 11, with permission.

beta-blocker regimen including thiazide diuretics, or both were also initiated in 1977 (8, 9).

III. DESIGN

For the study to have the highest power possible, we tried to include patients with a high expected endpoint incidence. Therefore, only men with their higher CHD endpoint incidence compared to women were included. We also used a stratification scheme in nine groups according to the predicted CHD risk based on serum cholesterol, smoking habits, and systolic blood pressure (SBP) (10), as well as age group (40–49, 50–59, and 60–69 years). The stratification procedure is presented in Table 1 (11).

The incentive to launch the trial came from researchers not related to any pharmaceutical company. However, financial support and help in recruiting collaborators and patients were given by the ASTRA as well as the ICI (later Zeneca) companies.

Individual centers chose to use either atenolol or metoprolol, and bendrofluazide or hydrochlorothiazide. Thus, there was no randomization between centers choosing different alternatives. Therefore, it would not be possible to compare the two beta-blockers or the two diuretics. The effects of beta-blockers and diuretics, respectively, were predicted to be similar on the endpoints studied (class effects).

Assumptions made about distribution of high- and low-risk patients in participating centers gave a predicted CHD endpoint (fatal plus nonfatal) rate of 20/1000 patient-years. To demonstrate a (somewhat optimistic) 30% lower incidence of nonfatal plus fatal CHD in the beta-blocker group compared with the diuretic group, a two-tailed test with acceptable statistic certainty (alpha = 0.05, beta = 0.90) called for accumulation of 20,000

Table 2 Inclusion Criteria

- Men aged 40–64 years free of clinical coronary heart disease.
- Patients with treated hypertension may be included if antihypertensive treatment had been withdrawn for at least 4 weeks.
- Mean value of four diastolic blood pressures (phase V) ≥100 mm Hg measured at two occasions, 14 days apart. Screening blood pressures must not be used for this calculation.
- Patients may be recruited via population screening, hospital clinics, or practices.

patients-years allowing for a 10% noncompliance rate. At a meeting with the steering committee in April 1984, it was expected that this number of patient-years should be reached during the autumn of 1985, and the formal closing date was set at December 31, 1985.

At the closure of the main trial, the ASTRA company decided that it would be of interest to continue follow-up of patients randomized on metoprolol versus diuretics, and 66 of these 70 centers decided to do so. That study is presented in another contribution (Chapter 7) in this volume.

A. Patients and Procedures

Men aged 40 to 64 years with a diastolic blood pressure (DBP) between 100 and 130 mm Hg (mean of four readings on two different occasions) were recruited to the trial. The first two readings were taken at an interval of 15 minutes and the remaining two were taken at the same interval at least 14 days later. The pressure was measured with the patient in the sitting position with a device that allowed blind registration (Hawksley Random Zero Sphygmomanometer).

Between 1976 and 1984, 6569 patients from 184 centers in 15 countries were recruited to the trial. Patients were randomized to treatment with either diuretic (3272 patients) or a beta-blocker (3297 patients). More than 99% of the patients were Caucasians (5548 from Europe and 1021 from the United States). Most of the men in the trial were recruited from population screening examinations or from physicians' offices. Patients already receiving antihypertensive treatment could be recruited to the study, providing they fulfilled the inclusion criteria after a treatment-free interval of four weeks. Thirty-five percent of all patients included had been undergoing antihypertensive treatment before randomization. Inclusion criteria are listed in Table 2 and exclusion criteria are listed in Table 3.

Table 3 Exclusion Criteria

A history of:
Myocardial infarction
Angina pectoris
Stroke
Malignant or secondary hypertension
Cancer or other malignancy
Liver cirrhosis
Alcoholism
Other serious disease

At their initial visit, all men eligible for the study were questioned about previous diseases, cardiovascular symptoms, and smoking habits. Patient well-being, initially and during the trial, was assessed using a standardized symptom questionnaire. Patients were first asked whether the treatment had resulted in any side effects since their last visit, and then were questioned more specifically regarding 23 specified symptoms.

B. Treatment

Drugs and doses are given in Table 4. Doses were chosen in an attempt to achieve equipotent antihypertensive effects. If the initial drug did not give a satisfactory blood pressure reduction, adjuvant drugs were added until the therapeutic goal was reached, that is, a sitting DBP less than 95 mm Hg. If the goal blood pressure was not attained with the drugs and doses shown in the schedule, other drugs, free of choice, were added. Any dose increase and the need for additional antihypertensive medication were assessed at scheduled visits 2 months after entry and every 6 months thereafter, or at closer intervals if deemed necessary by the physician. Reduction of the dose was undertaken if hypotensive symptoms or other side effects developed. The two basic drugs (beta-blockers and thiazide diuretics) were not to be crossed over or given together. However, for ethical reasons and at the discretion of the physician in charge, a patient with a nonfatal MI in the diuretic group could be treated with a beta-blocker, and a patient with cardiac failure randomized to beta-blocker was allowed diuretic treatment.

Until 1981, a second dose step amounting to twice the original dose was used in both the diuretic and the beta-blocker groups. However, because of concern regarding an increased risk of side effects with high doses and, as the blood pressure dose-response curve for both beta-blockers and diuretics was relatively flat, it was decided to terminate the use of the second dose step in all patients in 1981.

At the check-up that was performed every 6 months, it was found that compliance to these changes were followed very rapidly. An important reason for this good compliance

Table 4 Treatment Schedule

Diuretics	Daily dose (mg)	Beta-blockers	Daily dose (mg)
Initial treatment			
Bendroflumethiazide*	5	Atenolol	100
or		or	
Hydrochlorothiazide	50	Metoprolol[†]	200
Additional treatment step			
(1) Hydralazine	75		
(2) Hydralazine	150		
(3) 2 + spironolactone	75		
(4) 2 + spironolactone	150		
(5) 4 + optional drug			

Until 1981, a second dose step was used for both diuretics and beta-blockers. These doses were twice those shown in the table. Propranolol (160 mg daily) was given to 46 patients in one center. In centers where beta-blockers were given twice daily, the diuretic was also given twice daily.

* K^+ supplementation was optional; built-in amiloride and triamterene were also allowed.

[†] Metoprolol was given either as ordinary tablets, 100 mg twice daily, or as extended release tablets (Durules®, 200 mg daily.

was most probably the generally accepted tradition by the medical community to use those lower doses.

C. Follow-Up

Data were collected at entry, after 2, 6, 9, and 12 months, and every 6 months thereafter. At each visit, blood pressure and heart rate were recorded. Data on serum potassium, serum uric acid, serum creatinine, serum cholesterol, urine tests for albumin and glucose, electrocardiogram, and weight were obtained annually. All patients were followed up to the end of the study even if they reached a nonfatal endpoint before hand. If a patient was withdrawn from randomized treatment, the reason was stated in the follow-up form. We used an intention-to-treat analysis, so these patients were still included in the study. However, in the very early phase, there were some patients for whom only an initial record form but no other information was achieved, and these patients (fewer than 10) were excluded from the trial according to a decision by the steering committee during the first year of the trial.

D. Assessment of Endpoints

During the whole trial, death (cause specific), nonfatal MI, and stroke were recorded on follow-up record forms. The trial was closed at midnight, December 31, 1985. All endpoints occurring between entry to the trial and this endpoint were included in the analysis. A special form reporting the status of every patient at this closing time (with or without an endpoint) was completed and signed by the investigator during early spring of 1986. Sixty-four patients (1%) could not be traced for this assessment. These patients, who were equally distributed between the two treatment groups, were included in the analysis by using the endpoint information recorded on earlier follow-up visit forms.

All the relevant information required to validate the diagnoses of endpoints was collected from patient files, death certificates, coroner's reports, and autopsy records and assessed by the independent (blinded) endpoint committee.

For the diagnosis of MI to be confirmed, at least two of three criteria (typical chest pain, ECG changes, and elevation of serum transaminases) had to be fulfilled. In addition, an event that fulfilled only one of these criteria was diagnosed as a possible MI. The diagnosis of fatal acute MI was also confirmed if given as the main cause of death or by the presence of recent myocardial necrosis at a postmortem examination. Sudden cardiac death was defined as death not resulting from extra coronary causes occurring within 24 hours of the onset of symptoms.

Stroke was defined as unequivocal signs of focal or global neurological deficit of sudden onset with a duration of at least 24 hours, judged clinically to be of vascular origin. Fatal stroke was recorded when stated as the main cause of death on a death certificate.

Diabetes mellitus was defined as fasting blood sugar higher than 6.8 mmol/L and at least two positive dip tests for glucosuria. Heart failure and gout were recorded when clinically diagnosed.

The trial was open to both physicians and patients, but the assessment of endpoints was done blindly, with care taken to record every possible endpoint even if it had been missed during the running of the trial. This methodology since has been used by others and has been given the name Prospective Randomized Open-Label Blinded End-Points (PROBE) design.

E. Trial Committees

All major decisions during the trial were taken by an international steering committee. The working party, consisting of the Göteborg-based members of the steering committee, managed the day-to-day running of the trial. An independent safety committee reviewed the incidence of endpoints for safety when half the required number of patient-years was achieved and did not recommend to stop the trial from a safety point of view. An independent endpoint committee reviewed the diagnoses of the endpoints without knowing to which treatment patients had been randomized. An independent data auditor made personal visits to a number of randomly selected centers to review data quality and checked all the available information at the coordinating center in Göteborg.

Names of committee members and participating centers are listed at the end of this chapter.

F. Statistical Methods

The analyses were made on an "intention-to-treat" basis. Comparisons of rates between groups were carried out using Fisher's exact test. The life table method according to Kaplan-Meier (12) was applied to take into account the time from randomization to the endpoint. When analyzing mortality, patients who experienced a nonfatal event during the trial were followed up until death or until the closure of the trial, that is, they were not censored at the time of the nonfatal event. The Cox regression analysis (13) was used to adjust for differences in baseline variables between the two treatment groups. Two-tailed tests were used and P values less than 0.05 were considered as significant when testing the main hypothesis. Some subgroup analyses were performed. As stated above, the two beta-blockers used were considered to have comparable effects on the endpoints. The two beta-blockers were not randomly allocated and it was considered inappropriate to perform statistical testing between the two beta-blocker groups.

IV. RESULTS

At the time of closing the trial, 24,665 patient-years had been achieved. Baseline characteristics were well balanced in the two treatment groups with two exceptions: body weight and serum uric acid levels were higher in the beta-blocker group than in the diuretic group (Table 5). The estimated CHD risk based on the combination of age, serum cholesterol, SBP, and smoking habits did not differ between the treatment groups. An average of 37.1 months total follow-up time was collected on follow-up visit forms, whereas the mean follow-up to the closure of the trial was 45.1 months.

A. Antihypertensive Drug Treatment

Of the patients randomized to diuretics and beta-blockers, 83.4% and 85.9%, respectively, were on the scheduled treatment. About 4% in both the diuretic and the beta-blocker group were taking the opposite drug, and approximately 3% were taking drugs other than those stipulated in the protocol. Of those randomized to diuretics and beta-blockers, 6.0% and 5.5%, respectively, were not taking any antihypertensive drug treatment. In the diuretic group, 61.9% were receiving monotherapy compared with 68.0% in the beta-blocker group ($P < 0.001$). Of the patients randomized to diuretics and beta-blockers, 22.5% and 17.7%, respectively, were prescribed the second dose step until it was omitted in 1981. Of patients

Table 5 Patient Data at Entry and Treatment Years at Risk

	Diuretics		Beta-blockers		P-values for difference
Patient number	3,272		3,297		
Patient years at risk	3,272		3,297		
Until December 31, 1985	12,238		12,427		
Until last visit	10,012		10,279		
On randomized drug until last visit	8,922		9,291		
Smoking habits (%)					
Current smoker	34		35		
Ex-smoker	22		20		>0.40
Nonsmoker	44		45		
Major Q-wave	1.7		2.3		
Mean values and s.d.					
Age (years)	52.3	7.1	52.2	6.9	>0.40
Blood pressure (mm Hg)					
Systolic	166	19	166	19	>0.40
Diastolic	107	7	107	7	>0.40
Heart rate (beats/min)	77	12	77	12	>0.40
Body weight	83.0	13.0	83.7	13.0	0.051
Body mass index (kg/m^2)	27.1	3.7	27.3	3.8	0.078
S-cholesterol (mmol/L)	6.25	1.23	6.25	1.45	>0.40
S-creatinine (μmol/L)	93.5	16.1	93.7	16.4	>0.40
S-potassium (mmol/L)	4.27	0.43	4.29	0.44	0.200
S-urate (μmol/L)	356	80	360	79	0.046
Proportion (%) of patients in					
High-risk groups	27.4		27.0		
Medium-risk groups	25.3		26.0		>0.40
Low-risk groups	47.3		46.8		
Multiple risk score	0.1252		0.1253		>0.40

* Minnesota code 1: 1–2.

randomized to diuretics and beta-blockers, 24.2% and 21.0%, respectively, were given hydralazine as the second drug, and 5.2% in both groups had spironolactone as the third drug treatment. The crude withdrawal rate, calculated as the number of withdrawn patients divided by the total number of patients, was 8.9% and 7.9% in the diuretic and beta-blocker groups, respectively (nonsignificant [NS]), corresponding to an annual withdrawal rate of 2.4% per year for the diuretic-treated group and 2.1% for the beta-blocker-treated group. About the same number of patients in the two groups were receiving treatment during follow-up—90.4% of the total follow-up time in the beta-blocker group compared to 89.1% in the diuretic group.

B. Effects on Blood Pressure and Other Variables During Follow-Up

There was a major and similar reduction in blood pressure during the first year from 166/107 to 141/90–91 in the two treatment groups, and until the last visit only a further decrease of 1 mm Hg systolic and 2 mm Hg diastolic. Heart rate decreased more in the beta-blocker group, whereas body weight increased slightly in that group but remained unchanged in the diuretic group. Prevalence of smoking decreased to 28% in both treatment groups during the trial. There was a slight decrease in serum total cholesterol (6.25 vs. 6.13 mmol/L, $P = 0.018$) in the beta-blocker group but not in the diuretic group. Serum potassium was unchanged in the beta-blocker group but decreased in the diuretic group (4.29 to 3.98 mmol/L, $P = 0.001$). Serum urate increased in both treatment groups, but significantly more so in the diuretic group (356 to 396 μmol/L, $P = 0.001$).

C. Mortality and Morbidity

As seen in Table 6, there was no significant difference in the incidence of fatal and nonfatal CHD events between the two groups, but the incidence was slightly higher in the beta-blocker group. Stroke mortality and the incidence of nonfatal stroke tended to be lower in the beta-blocker group than in the diuretic group, but not significantly so. Cox regression analyses were performed on the relationship between randomized treatment and endpoints, adjusting for differences in entry characteristics, but the results did not differ from those of the comparisons of the crude endpoint rates. None of the patients withdrawn from diuretic treatment (n = 292) experienced a CHD event. Among the patients withdrawn from beta-blocker treatment (n = 261), eight experienced a CHD event. Four of the patients withdrawn from diuretics, but none of those withdrawn from beta-blockers, experienced a stroke. Four patients in the diuretic withdrawal group and six patients in the beta-blocker withdrawal group died.

D. Side Effects and Reported Symptoms

The percentage of patients withdrawn because of side effects was 2.4% and 2.0% in the diuretic and beta-blocker groups, respectively. More patients on beta-blockers than on diuretics reported symptoms related to treatment: 19.1% and 16.0% ($P < 0.001$), respectively. Most of the symptoms according to the standardized questionnaire were less common after the start of treatment than initially. Symptoms that were more common in the beta-blocker group were breathlessness, decreased physical capacity, cold hands and feet, slow heart rate, diarrhea, unusual tiredness, and nightmares. Irregular heart rhythm and dry mouth were more common in patients taking diuretics.

E. Incidence of CHD in Relation to Predicted CHD Risk at Entry

There was a clear increase in CHD incidence with increasing predicted risk, but there was no difference in any of the quartiles of predicted risk between diuretic and beta-blocker groups. The risk increased from 4% in the first quartile to 6%, 10%, and 17% in the second, third, and fourth quartiles, respectively.

Total mortality was twice as high among smokers compared with nonsmokers; rate per 1,000 patient-years was 13.96 and 12.08 in the diuretic and beta-blocker groups, respectively. For nonfatal and fatal CHD, there was a slightly higher incidence in the beta-blocker group: 16.26 versus 14.68 per 1,000 patient-years, respectively. The stroke rate was 4.81 and 3.95 per 1,000 patient-years in the diuretic and beta-blocker groups, respectively. No difference was shown between smokers and nonsmokers regarding the effects of beta-blockers versus diuretics, and there was no significant difference regarding new heart failure, incidence of diabetes, or gout.

Table 6 Total and Cause-Specific Mortality, Nonfatal Myocardial Infarction, and Nonfatal Stroke

	Diuretics (n = 3272)		Beta-Blockers (n = 3297)			
	n	Rate/1000 patient-years	n	Rate/1000 patient-years	Odds ratio diuretics/beta-blocker	Confidence interval (95%)
CHD events						
Fatal CHD	50	4.09	54	4.35	0.93	(0.64–1.37)
Nonfatal MI	75	6.13	84	6.76	0.90	(0.66–1.23)
Fatal and/or nonfatal CHD*	116	9.48	132	10.62	0.88	(0.68–1.14)
Stroke events						
Fatal stroke	10	0.82	3	0.24	3.37	(0.96–9.53)
Nonfatal stroke	32	2.61	29	2.33	1.11	(0.68–1.83)
Fatal and/or nonfatal stroke*	41	3.35	32	2.58	1.29	(0.82–2.04)
Deaths						
Fatal CHD	50	4.09	54	4.35	0.93	(0.64–1.37)
Fatal stroke	10	0.82	3	0.24	3.37	(0.96–9.53)
Other deaths	41	3.35	39	3.14	1.06	(0.69–1.64)
All deaths	101	8.25	96	7.73	1.06	(0.80–1.41)
Patients with an endpoint†	192	15.69	197	15.85	0.98	(0.80–1.20)
Total number of endpoints†	224		225		1.00	(0.83–1.21)

All differences $P > 0.20$ except for the difference in stroke mortality. $P = 0.09$.

* Patients who had suffered both a nonfatal and a fatal endpoint were only counted once.

† Death, nonfatal myocardial infarction, nonfatal stroke.

Abbreviations: *CHD*, coronary heart disease; *MI*, myocardial infarction.

V. DISCUSSION

A. Design Considerations

This study was not blinded for physicians or patients. The trial was planned for a duration of 5 years or more. It was believed to be difficult to keep patients and doctors blinded to the type of treatment during that long period, especially as additions of several drugs could be expected. The reduction and heart rate produced by beta-blockade and the occurrence of hypokalemia associated with thiazide diuretic treatment would rather easily break the code. The management of patients would also mirror the clinical situation much better if physicians were able to tailor the therapy to control blood pressure as well as possible.

To counterbalance the problems of the nonblinding, maximum efforts were undertaken to avoid bias when assessing the major endpoints of the trial. An independent endpoint committee, which was not aware of the patients' treatment, scrutinized all endpoints. Withdrawals caused by side effects might, however, be biased given the prejudices of participating physicians.

Another way of preventing bias was the use of a special closing-out form that was signed for every patient, with or without endpoints, just after the close of the trial. A few, previously unknown endpoints were in fact detected by this procedure.

The special 23 question assessment of side effects could well be biased. Beta-blockers were associated with more subjective side effects, whereas diuretics showed lower levels of serum potassium and higher levels of serum urate than beta-blockers during follow-up. Patients' knowledge about subjective side effects of beta-blockers might have influenced their tendencies to respond, but we have no way of assessing this.

A placebo group was not included because of the knowledge at start of the trial that some mortality and morbidity endpoints were reduced by antihypertensive treatment, and the knowledge that some large trials were underway. The Hypertension Detection and Follow-Up Program (14) showed that effective step care treatment decreased mortality compared with usual care. The Australian National Blood Pressure Trial (15) showed a significant effect on diuretic-based treatment on total mortality. The overview of randomized drug trials in hypertension later showed clear benefits on stroke and also significant benefits on CHD, even though these benefits were smaller than expected from epidemiological studies (16).

The general consensus has been that moderately to severely increased blood pressure levels have to be treated. However, we have recently demonstrated in a large random population sample that patients with hypertension, even those who were brought down to completely normal blood pressures, still had an increased risk for both stroke and CHD during 20 years of follow-up (17). Interestingly, the risk among the hypertensives was not increased during the first 6 to 8 years, corresponding to the duration of the previously mentioned positive intervention trials. Thus, there is still a need for finding better treatment modalities among hypertensive patients, and it might be that treatment has to be tailored to the specific metabolic or other abnormalities that are related to the blood pressure increase. One such group of abnormalities that has received different names is the so-called insulin-resistance syndrome (18). In a population study, we found these disturbances in 6% of hypertensives and 3% among nonhypertensives (19). Interestingly, at age 50, people with these metabolic disturbances also had bigger heart volumes, which indicate a multifaceted disease with definitely worse long-term prognosis. Most treatments used in hypertensive patients until today have not affected these apparently basic, and probably genetically determined, abnormalities.

B. Beta-Blockers Versus Diuretics

The findings of the present trial are consistent with the main results of the International Prospective Primary Prevention Study in Hypertension (IPPPSH) and Medical Research Council (MRC) trials (8, 9). The very positive results of beta-blockers used both in the acute phase of MI and long-term follow-up could not be found in these three trials that did not include patients with clinical CHD.

There are several possible explanations for this lack of effect among hypertensives.

1. Not even in the highest risk stratum in this study did we find any significant difference between beta-blockers and diuretics with respect to CHD incidence or mortality. In one of the very first trials of beta-blockade in MI in which stratification was used, we found mortality only in the high-risk groups during 2 years of follow-up, and the effect of beta-blockade was only seen in these groups (20). These high-risk groups had a considerably higher mortality during follow-up than was seen even in the highest risk quartile of the present hypertensive patients. Similarly, in a much larger trial of patients with acute MI, it was found that the benefit of beta-blockade versus placebo was only seen among the highest risk groups (21). Thus, the first reason for the lack of difference between beta-blockers and diuretics in the present study might be that there were too few patients high risk enough to enable demonstration of any difference between diuretics and beta-blockers during follow-up.
2. Another explanation might be that beta-blockers exert their cardioprotective effect only in an ischemic myocardium as, for example, when an MI has occurred. There are similar conditions in other situations. Ventricular ectopic beats do not seem to have the same poor prognostic importance in healthy people as they have in patients with ischemic heart disease.
3. Adverse side effects on metabolic variables such as potassium, uric acid, and lipids might be other explanations for lack of effect. However, hypokalemia developed significantly more frequently in the diuretic group, and sudden cardiac death or fatal MI did not occur more frequently in the diuretic group than in the beta-blocker group. Beta-blockers have sometimes been associated with adverse effects on lipid levels, especially triglycerides. The latter were not routinely measured in the present trial. However, serum total cholesterol decreased significantly in the beta-blocker group compared with the diuretic group, where it remained unchanged during the trial. In summary, it does not seem that metabolic adverse effects were responsible for the lack of effects in the trial.
4. Body weight did not increase in the diuretic groups but increased by 1.1 kg in the beta-blocker group, which is a known effect of beta-blockade. An increase in body weight would not have materially reduced the possible effects of beta-blockade on hard endpoints during this limited period of the trial. The same effect on body weight has been seen in beta-blocker groups in secondary prevention.

Subgroup analyses of the MRC and IPPPSH trials (8, 9) have suggested that smokers benefit less from beta-blocker treatment than nonsmokers. We found no evidence of such a difference in this trial. As in many earlier and later trials, this discrepancy indicates the dangers in putting emphasis on post hoc subgroup analyses. These findings might well be the result of chance. In the two other trials, however, nonselective beta-blockers were used, and there is a slight possibility that the catecholamine-induced pressor response to smoking may be greater in subjects receiving a nonselective rather than beta_1-selective beta-blocker (22).

ACKNOWLEDGMENTS

The author acknowledges members of the various trial committees and participating centers, as listed at the end of this chapter.

HAPPHY COLLABORATIVE GROUP

Steering Committee: Berglund G, Elmfeldt D (Department of Medicine, Göteborg University); Fitzsimons T (Macclesfield, United Kingdom); Holzgreve H (Medizinische Universitätsklinik, München); Hosie J (general practitioner, Glasgow); Hörnkvist P-E (Göteborg); Tuomilehto J (Department of Epidemiology, National Public Health Institute, Helsinki); Wedel H (Department of Epidemiology and Biostatistics, Nordic School of Public Health, Göteborg); Wikstrand J, Wilhelmsen L (Chairman, Department of Medicine, Göteborg University).

Working Party: Berglund G (Secretary); Elmfeldt D, Hörnkvist P-E, Pennert K, Wedel H, Wikstrand J, Wilhelmsen L (Chairman).

Safety Committee: Jesdinsky HJ (Institut fur Medizinische Statistik und Biomathematik, Dusseldorf); Leren P (Medical Out-Patients Clinic, Ullevål Sykehus, Oslo); Odén A (Kungälv); Pyörälä K (Department of Medicine, University of Kuopio).

Endpoint Audit Committee: Persson S (Department of Cardiology, University of Lund); Kallio V (Folkpensionsanstalten för Rehabiliteringsforskning, Åbo); Johansson BW (Department of Cardiology, Allmänna sjukhuset, Malmö).

Data Auditor: Nissinen A (Department of Epidemiology, National Public Health Institute, Helsinki).

HAPPHY Investigators

Belgium: Libotte J (Kortessem), Marlier R (Gent), Orye R (Hasselt), Rorive G, Taziaux P (Liege).

Canada: Balram C, Chockalingham A, Fodor JG, Handa PS (Saint John), Hardacre GD (Toronto), Lebel M (Quebec), Robitaille NM (Quebec), Shearer R (Ontario), Wollam RC (Ontario).

Czechoslovakia: Boudik F (Prague), Bultas J (Prague), Cifkova R (Prague), Hejl Z (Prague), Valkova L (Prague).

Denmark: Jastrup B (Odder).

Finland: Honkavaara M (Outokumpu), Koponen H (Janakkala), Kuusisto P (Ilomantsi), Mustaniemi H (Joensuu), Mönkkönen M (Hammaslahti), Mörttinen A (Polvijärvi), Pohjola M (Juuka), Tuomilehto J (Helsinki), Vinni S (Eno), Vänskä O (Joensuu).

France: Barabe P (Marseille), Duret JC (Bordeaux), Hardel PJ (Dijon), Hout D, (Cherbourg), Lacoste J (Lille), Lantrade P (Brest), Ollivier JP (Paris), Seigneuric A (Versailles).

Germany: von Eiff AW (Bonn), Friedrich G (Bonn), Holzgreve H (Munich), Mideke M (Munich), Schulte W (Bonn).

Greece: Karatzas NB (Athens).

Great Britain: Adams-Strump BG (Glasgow), Anderton JL (Edinburgh), Barkataki N (Durham), Beevers DG (Birmingham), Bird S (Leeds), Cahill A (Cheadle), Campbell LM (Glasgow), Caswell S (Stockport), Causer M (Lichfield), Cochran G (London), Daengsvang PADC (Liverpool), George M (Durham), Gostick NK (Rugby), Goves JR (Cardiff), Grundy PF (Cardiff), Hackett GI (Holmes Chapel), Harding KG (Cardiff), Harvard Davis R (Cardiff), Henry PJ (Sherwood), Hosie J (Glasgow), Hosie G (Glasgow), Korlipara K (Bolton), McLauchlan JH (Glasgow), Mayhew SR (Huntingdon), Milson JE (Stockport), Muir

AL (Edinburgh), Newson-Smith G (Slough), Owen S (Bexley), Petrie JC (Aberdeen), Presley AP (Gloucester), Renton R (Slough), Roberts JJK (Edinburgh), Saul PA (Bolton), Sharp H (Glastonbury), Simmons RLL (Bexley), Sudhakar C (South Croydon), Taylor S (Leeds), Wathen CG (Edinburgh), Wayne DJ (Gorleston), Welch RB (Leeds).

Holland: Berge BS ten (Groningen), Bloem THJJM (Tilburg), Jansen LJ (Hertogenbosch), May JF (Groningen), Nube MJ (Alkmaar), Westerman RF (Amsterdam).

Iceland: Regnarsson J (Reykjavik), Snorrason S (Reykjavik).

Italy: Ambrosioni E (Bologna), Corea L (Perugia), Daglio M (Pavia), de Divitis O (Napoli), Fogari R (Pavia), Marchetta F (Bologna), Pirelli A (Bari), Pettene A (Pavia), Poletti L (Pavia), Tettamanti F (Pavia).

Norway: Andersen L (Oslo), Bratland S (Dokka), Brattegard T (Oslo), Dahl Å (Fyllingsdalen), Falkum E (Oslo), Haraldson A (Kopervik), Helgeland A (Oslo), Humerfeldt S (Bergen), Lyche-Saether (Börgenhaugen), Piatkowski W (Oslo), Rolfstad J (Rakkestad).

Sweden: Atmer B (Vallentuna), Bengtsson LE (Hässleholm), Bergner C-G, (Norrköping), Bergstad B (Gävle), Brounéus B (Ludvika), Bruhn A (Helsingborg), Dahlman A (Borlänge), Egelius NM (Linköping), Ekblad G (Lidköping), Eliasson K (Stockholm), Ellborg Å (Varberg), Elmfeldt D (Göteborg), Engström K (Linköping), Ernerot H (Göteborg), Fagerberg SE (Örebro), Fries L (Hällefors), Frisell JE (Ludvika), Gumaelius K (Grimsås), Gunnarson K (Örnsköldsvik), Hagströmer R (Stockholm), Hassler L (Luleå), Hellman P (Falun), Hjalmers S (Båstad), Hulsten K (Tibro), Hylander B (Stockholm), Häggmark A (Skärholmen), Johansen B (Åmål), Jonsson H (Dingle), Jonsson J (Varberg), Jönsson S (Mölndal), Kjellberg J (Lidköping), Kylin B (Sandviken), Larsson ST (Mölndal), Lindfors H (Falun), Lindgren LG (Norsborg), Linné G (Örkelljunga), Lins LE (Stockholm), Luptovics J (Tingsryd), Magnusson PO (Tidaholm), Marcus K (Göteborg), Nilsson L (Malmö), Norrby A (Göteborg), Ohlsson E (Jönköping), Persson LG (Habo), Schultz PO (Nässjö), Sjöstrand Å (Tranås), Stobéus NA (Motala), Strömvall T (Luleå), Sundman L (Gävle), Svensson M (Skene), Tilling B (Åtvidaberg), Tovi T (Skärholmen), Weiner L (Karlskoga), Wikman G (Skene).

USA: Balfour DC (San Diego, CA), Black PL (San Diego, CA), Blevins DD (Salem, VA), Brandman C (Greenbrae, CA), Brehm JG (Dubuque, IA), Brown SG (Menomonie, WI), Buchanan JL. (Corvallis, OR), Bullard HV (Wilson, NC), Fogel MA (Champaign, IL), Fournet J (Lafayette, LA), Frost J (Rhinelander, WI), Glode JE (Longmont, CO), Hainer JW (Everett, WA), Hancock CW (Sheboygan, WI), Hilty RW (Boulder, CO), Holmburg CE (Menomonee Falls, WI), Hughes SO (Winona, MN), Kern JW (Portland, OR), Krabill LD (Wilson, NC), Kretschmar PO (Vancouver, WA), Lewis JE (Sunnyvale, CA), Mocklin KE (Lake Charles, LA), Nasr H (Palm Springs, CA), O'Brien JT (Arlington, VA), Prabhu R (San Diego, CA), Prather ND (Shreveport, LA), Rao R (Janesville, WI), Rodrigues-Viera V (Vero Beach, FL), Rietbrock MJ (Oconomowoc, WI), Santilli RJ (Milwaukee, WI), Sharp RW (Rustin, LA), Sood SJ (Modesto, CA), Stafford JM (St Joseph, MI), Stamler J (Chicago, IL), Sugar DM (Evansville, IN), Sullivan EM (LaHabra, CA), Thompson MT (Redondo Beach, SA), Vig SD (Tucson, AZ), Welch C (Milwaukee, WI), Wong JWH (Visalia, CA), Wyskoarko NP (Covina, CA).

REFERENCES

1. Veterans Administration Cooperative Study Group on Antihypertensive Agents. Effects of treatment on morbidity in hypertension. I. Results in patients with diastolic blood pressure averaging 115 through 129 mmHg. JAMA 1967; 202:1028–1034.
2. Veterans Administration Cooperative Study Group on Antihypertensive Agents. Effects of

treatment on morbidity in hypertension. II. Results in patients with diastolic blood pressure averaging 90 through 114 mmHg. JAMA 1970; 213:1143–1152.
3. Wilhelmsson C, Vedin JA, Wilhelmsen L, Tibblin G. Reduction of sudden deaths after myocardial infarction by treatment with alprenolol. Lancet 1974; ii:1157–1159.
4. Ahlmark G, Saetre H, Korsgren M. Reduction of sudden deaths after myocardial infarction. Lancet 1974; 11:1563.
5. A Multicentre International Study. Improvement in prognosis of myocardial infarction by long-term beta-adrenoceptor blockade using practolol. BMJ 1975; 3:735–740.
6. Yusuf S, Peto R, Lewis J, Collins R, Sleight P. Beta-blockade during and after myocardial infarction: an overview of the randomized trials. Prog Cardiovasc Dis 1985; 27:335–371.
7. Wilhelmsen L, Berglund G, Elmfeldt D, Fitzsimons T, Holzgreve H, Hosie J, Hörnkvist P-E, Pennert K, Tuomilehto J, Wedel H, on behalf of the Heart Attack Primary Prevention in Hypertension Trial Research Group. Beta-blockers versus diuretics in hypertensive men: main results from the HAPPHY Trial. J Hypertens 1987; 5:561–572.
8. Medical Research Council Working Party. MRC Trial of Treatment of Mild Hypertension: principal results. BMJ 1985; 291:97–104.
9. IPPPSH Collaborative Group. Cardiovascular risk and risk factors in a randomized trial of treatment based on the beta-blocker oxprenolol: the International Prospective Primary Prevention Study in Hypertension (IPPPSH). J Hypertens 1985; 3:379–392.
10. Wilhelmsen L, Wedel H, Tibblin G. Multivariate analysis of risk factors for coronary heart disease. Circulation 1973; 48:950–958.
11. Wilhelmsen L, Berglund G, Elmfeldt D, Wedel H. Beta-blockers versus saluretics in hypertension. Prev Med 1981; 10:38–49.
12. Kaplan EL, Meier P. Non-parametric estimations from incomplete observations. J Am Stat Assoc 1958; 53:457–481.
13. Cox DR. Regression models and life-tables (with discussion). J R Stat Soc Ser B 1972; 34: 182–202.
14. Hypertension Detection and Follow-up Program Cooperative Group. Five year findings of the hypertension detection and follow-up program. I. Reduction in mortality of persons with high blood pressure, including mild hypertension. JAMA 1979; 242:2562–2571.
15. Australian National Blood Pressure Study Management Committee. The Australian therapeutic trial in mild hypertension. Lancet 1982; 1:1261–1267.
16. Collins R, Peto R, MacMahon S, Hebert P, Fiebach NH, Eberlein KA, Godwin J, Qizilbash N, Taylor JO, Hennekens CH. Blood pressure, stroke, and coronary heart disease. Part 2. Short-term reductions in blood pressure: overview of randomized drug trials in the epidemiological context. Lancet 1990; 335:827–838.
17. Andersson OK, Almgren T, Persson B, Samuelsson O, Hedner T, Wilhelmsen L. Survival in treated hypertension: follow-up study after two decades. BMJ 1998; 317:167–171.
18. Reaven GM. Role of insulin resistance in human disease. Diabetes 1988; 37:1595–1607.
19. Eriksson H, Welin L, Wilhelmsen L, Larsson B, Ohlson L-O, Svärdsudd K, Tibblin G. Metabolic disturbances in hypertension: results from the population study of "Men born in 1913". J Intern Med 1992; 232:389–395.
20. Wilhelmsson C, Vedin JA, Wilhelmsen L, Tibblin G, Werkö L. Reduction of sudden deaths after myocardial infarction by treatment with alprenolol. Lancet 1974; II:1157–1159.
21. The MIAMI Trial Research Group. Metoprolol in acute myocardial infarction (MIAMI). A randomized placebo-controlled trial. Eur Heart J 1985; 6:199–226.
22. Greenburg G, Thompson SG. The effect of smoking on blood pressure in mild hypertensives, and on their response to antihypertensive treatment. J Hypertens 1984; 2:553.

7

Metoprolol Versus Thiazide Diuretics in Hypertension: Results from the MAPHY Study in Perspective

JOHN WIKSTRAND

Sahlgrenska University Hospital, Göteborg University, Göteborg, and AstraZeneca, Mölndal, Sweden

MARTIN KENDALL

Birmingham Medical School, Edgbaston, Birmingham, England

GÖRAN BERGLUND

Malmö General Hospital, Lund University, Lund, Sweden

I. PRIMARY PREVENTION OF SUDDEN DEATH

The goal of treating patients with hypertension is to prevent morbidity and mortality associated with high blood pressure and to control blood pressure by the least intrusive means possible (1). Sudden death is the major challenge as it is the most common cause of death in patients with hypertension (2). Primary preventive trials have not yet produced data indicating that any of the agents—diuretics, angiotensin-converting enzyme (ACE) inhibitors, AII-blockers, calcium antagonists, or alpha-blockers—can affect the risk of sudden death (1–7). Evidence from randomized clinical trials with beta-blockers, however, indicate an important role for these agents in the primary prevention of sudden death (2–4). One of these studies was the Metoprolol Atherosclerosis in Hypertensives (MAPHY) study comparing metoprolol and diuretics (8–12).

A. Study Design: The MAPHY Study

1. *The Original Study: Beta-Blockade Versus Saluretics in Hypertension*

Plans were drawn up in 1975 in Göteborg, Sweden, for a study comparing beta-blockade with thiazide diuretic treatment in hypertensive patients. This study, entitled ''Beta-Blockers Versus Saluretics in Hypertension,'' (13) is the parent trial for both the MAPHY study (8–12) and the Heart Attack Primary Prevention in Hypertensives (HAPPHY) study (14). For reasons of statistical power, it was decided to only include patients at increased risk for coronary events: male patients with untreated diastolic blood pressure at or above 100 mm Hg (13).

Inclusion criteria were as follows:

- Male sex.
- Age 40 to 64 years at randomization.
- Untreated diastolic blood pressure 100 to 130 mm Hg.
  Comment: Blood pressure recordings were taken after 5 minutes' rest twice at 15-minute intervals. Blood pressure was measured blindly (Hawksley random-zero sphygmomanometer or London School of Hygiene Blind Manometer) in the right arm with the patient in a sitting position (mean of four readings on two different occasions at least 2 weeks apart).
- Informed consent.

Exclusion criteria were as follows:

- Because this was a primary preventive study, a history of myocardial infarction, angina pectoris, or stroke was an exclusion criterion.
- Malignant or secondary hypertension.
- Malignant disease, liver cirrhosis, alcoholism, or other serious disease.
- Relative or absolute contraindications to beta-blockers or thiazide diuretics.
- Patients with other nonhypertensive conditions requiring treatment with a beta-blocker or a diuretic.

Recruitment was aimed at 20,000 patient-years with a statistical power of $\alpha = 0.05$ and $\beta = 0.90$ for the detection of a hypothesized 30% difference in coronary events. When the study was initiated, data existed to show that in hypertensive men with diastolic blood pressure above 100 mm Hg, thiazide diuretics reduced the risk for stroke (15). For ethical reasons, therefore, a placebo group could not be included. The original protocol from 1976 stipulated that patients should be randomly assigned to treatment with a thiazide diuretic (hydrochlorothiazide or bendroflumethiazide) or one of the three beta-blockers, metoprolol, propranolol, or alprenolol. A fixed therapeutic schedule should be used to reach the treatment goal of diastolic blood pressure less than 95 mm Hg in all patients randomized (8, 13). Propranolol was used in only one center with a total of 88 patients (11, 16, 17). None of the centers chose to use alprenolol. The first patient was randomized at the center in Sahlgrenska Hospital, Göteborg, Sweden, March 15, 1976, a center that chose metoprolol as the beta-blocker. Thus, the study following the original protocol essentially compared metoprolol and thiazide diuretics.

2. *The HAPPHY Study: Pooling of Metoprolol, Propranolol, and Atenolol Data*

In 1978, more than 2 years after the first patient was randomly assigned according to the original protocol, atenolol had become available in many countries, and the original protocol was modified to allow for centers that could randomly assign patients to either atenolol or diuretics (Fig. 1) (11). The metoprolol, propranolol, and atenolol parts were run in parallel and kept completely separate regarding randomization and follow-up, because the original protocol stipulated that only one beta-blocker could be used within each center (13, 16, 17). The reason for adding a new beta-blocker was to increase recruitment, and

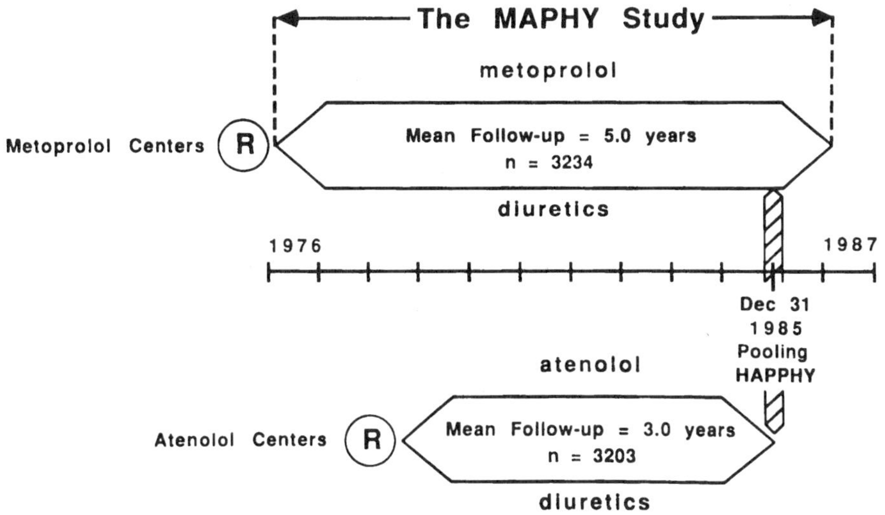

Fig. 1 Schematic design of the study *Beta-Blockers Versus Saluretics in Hypertension*. which was the parent trial for both the MAPHY study (8–11) and the HAPPHY study (14). For reasons of simplicity, the single propranolol center has not been illustrated. R = randomization. (From Ref. 11, by permission.)

the design was not planned for a comparison of different beta-blockers. After 1981, this joint study was called HAPPHY. Results from 6569 men covering 20,000 patient-years with the pooled data, known as the HAPPHY study, were initially analyzed and published in 1987 (14). Because atenolol was introduced to the HAPPHY study 2 years after metoprolol, the mean follow-up time was considerably shorter in the atenolol part as compared with the metoprolol part (Fig. 1).

3. The MAPHY Study

In October 1985, it was decided to close the HAPPHY study on December 31 because the pooled data had accumulated 20,000 patient years. The pooled data did not show any difference between patients randomized to beta-blockade or diuretics (14). An immediate decision (October 1985) was taken to continue follow-up at metoprolol centers according to the original study protocol from 1976. No information was available whatsoever for anyone involved about endpoints in the different beta-blocker arms of HAPPHY when the decision to continue follow-up at metoprolol centers was made in October 1985 (9). Such information did not become available until 1989 (16, 17). The background for the decision to continue follow-up at the metoprolol centers was as follows: in 1985, the results of the Medical Research Council (MRC) study and the International Prospective Primary Prevention Study in Hypertension (IPPPSH), performed in both men and women, were published (18, 19). The results in the two sexes combined suggested that beta-blocker therapy was not effective in terms of reducing coronary events. However, at that time, and as summarized in the original mortality report from MAPHY (8), evidence was accumulating to suggest that certain beta-blockers had various actions that indicated the potential for antiatherosclerotic and cardioprotective effects. In addition, the long-term postinfarct studies with timolol, propranolol, and metoprolol had produced positive results (2).

Furthermore, there was some evidence in data published in 1985 from MRC and IPPPSH that in men, relative risk was lower with beta-blockade as compared with a mainly thiazide diuretic-based schedule (20). However, 60% of those on beta-blockade in IPPPSH also received a diuretic, making it hard to compare drug effects in a valid way. Accordingly, it could be considered that the MRC and IPPPSH had failed to yield positive results for a number of reasons, one of which was that women with a low absolute risk for coronary events had been included and had diluted the results, and because the number of events in the men was not large enough to allow for a powerful statistical analysis. With this in mind and knowing the animal and postinfarct data, it was decided that follow-up should continue at the metoprolol/thiazide diuretic centers. Four U.S. centers with 59 randomized patients were unable to participate in this follow-up (8). The vital status of these patients was checked, and as of February 28, 1987 (the closing date for MAPHY, see below), 58 were alive, and one was unavailable for follow-up (this patient was randomized to diuretics). The aim of this follow-up was to obtain additional data regarding the possible cardioprotective benefits of metoprolol. At the meeting of the MAPHY study steering committee in March 1987, data were presented on the number of patients with combined use of beta-blockade and thiazide diuretics in the two randomization groups. The data showed an increasing use of beta-blockade in the diuretic group as the follow-up period lengthened (20.4% taking beta-blockers in the diuretic group in the fourth quartile follow-up, more than 6.15 years) (8). It was decided to close the study by February 28, 1987. At this point, several hundred patients were reported as unavailable for follow-up.

B. Follow-Up and Administrative Routines

The MAPHY Study followed the original protocol of ''Beta-Blockade Versus Saluretics in Hypertension'' as defined in 1976, although the aim of having data on 20,000 years was not achieved. Every patient entered on the randomization list was included in the follow-up, regardless of treatment status. The start of treatment was defined as the date of randomization. For living patients, the end of the study was defined as the day of the last follow-up interview. The latest follow-up date for any patient was February 28, 1987.

All information on whether patients were alive, dead, or unavailable for follow-up was gathered by using specially designed questionnaires. A specially designed questionnaire was also sent to all investigators who reported that patients had died during the follow-up, asking for detailed information on death certificates, hospital files, and necropsies. A major operation was run during 5 months to trace patients initially reported as unavailable for follow-up. At the close of the study, 3085 patients were reported to be alive and 148 dead. One patient was unavailable for follow-up (randomized to diuretic). Of the 3085 patients alive, 3039 were seen by the investigators, 27 were contacted personally by telephone, three were reported alive by relatives, and 16 were reported alive by an up-to-date population register (8).

In the 148 patients who died, death certificates were available for 115 patients; hospital-based files, but no death certificate, were available for 17; signed letters from investigators defining identity and the circumstances of death were available for nine, and other information, such as police reports and non–hospital-based medical files, was available for seven patients. The autopsy rate was 51%.

C. Main Endpoints and Classification of Endpoints

The main endpoints were total mortality, sudden cardiac death, the pooled incidence of fatal and nonfatal coronary events (sudden death and acute and silent myocardial infarction, time to first event; for definition see below), and stroke. A classification of all reported fatal and nonfatal symptomatic events was made by the Independent End-Point Committee. Agreement between two independent members defined the final classification. This classification, the Minnesota coding of electrocardiograms (ECGs) (see below) and data quality, were audited by the Independent Data Audit Committee. All cases were judged without any knowledge of actual treatment or of the treatment to which the patients had originally been randomly assigned.

D. Classification of Cause-Specific Mortality

The cause of death was defined by using all available information, such as hospital records, physicians' reports, police reports, death certificates, and necropsy reports. If the death occurred within 28 days of the onset of an event, that event was classified as the fatal event; otherwise the event was classified as nonfatal, and a subsequent event, if fatal, was coded as the cause of death (8). A decision regarding the cause of death was made by the Independent End-Point Committee on each of the 148 deaths. Sudden cardiovascular death was defined as death occurring within 24 hours of onset of symptoms without obvious extracardiovascular cause of death. Sudden cardiovascular deaths were further subdivided into deaths occurring within 1 hour, and deaths occurring after more than 1 hour but less than 24 hours after the onset of symptoms (10). Patients found dead with no obvious extracardiovascular cause of death have been coded as sudden deaths, even if the time between onset of symptoms and time of death is unknown. In all these patients, however, circumstances indicated that death occurred suddenly.

E. Classification of Nonfatal Endpoints

1. Nonfatal Myocardial Infarctions

a. Acute Myocardial Infarction

For a diagnosis of an acute myocardial infarction to be confirmed, at least two of the following three criteria were to be fulfilled: central chest pain of more than 15 minutes' duration, transient elevation of enzymes indicating myocardial necrosis, or typical ECG changes. If myocardial infarction was suspected but only one criterion was fulfilled, the condition was reported as a possible myocardial infarction.

b. Silent Myocardial Infarction

A 12-lead resting ECG was recorded at randomization, repeated on a yearly basis, and sent to the administrative center at the Sahlgrenska University Hospital, Göteborg University, for Minnesota coding. Altogether 16,987 ECGs were each coded by two independent technicians: 8575 from patients randomly assigned to metoprolol and 8412 from patients randomly assigned to diuretics (11). The occurrence of a new major Q/QS item (Minnesota code 1 : 1 or 1 : 2) without other clinical signs of myocardial infarction was defined as a definite silent myocardial infarction. Similarly, a new minor Q/QS item (code 1 : 3) was defined as a possible silent myocardial infarction.

2. Nonfatal Stroke

For a diagnosis of nonfatal stroke to be recorded, unequivocal signs of focal or global neurological deficit with sudden onset, with a duration longer than 24 hours and were thought to be vascular in origin, were to be present.

Table 1 Clinical Characteristics of Patients at Entry and at Last Follow-Up Visit (n = 3234)*

Characteristics	Entry: Patients randomized to metoprolol (n = 1609)	Entry: Patients randomized to diuretics (n = 1625)	Last follow-up: Patients randomized to metoprolol (n = 1609)	Last follow-up: Patients randomized to diuretics (n = 1625)
Systolic blood pressure, mm Hg	166.9 ± 17	166.8 ± 17	142.4 ± 17	142.7 ± 16
Diastolic blood pressure, mm Hg	107.6 ± 6	107.5 ± 6	88.7 ± 8	89.5 ± 8†
Heart rate, beats/min	78.2 ± 11	77.3 ± 10	64.1 ± 10	74.1 ± 11‡
Age, years	52.6 ± 7	52.6 ± 6	57.7 ± 7	57.6 ± 7
Body weight, kg	83.2 ± 12	82.7 ± 12	84.7 ± 12	82.6 ± 12‡
Body mass index, kg/m^2	27.3 ± 3.5	27.1 ± 3.5	27.6 ± 3.7	26.9 ± 3.5‡
Serum cholesterol, mmol/L (mg/dL)	6.32 ± 1.2 (244 ± 46)	6.29 ± 1.2 (243 ± 46)	6.15 ± 1.2 (237 ± 46)	6.32 ± 1.2 (244 ± 46)§
Serum creatinine, mol/L (mg/dL)	93.1 ± 17 (1.05 ± 0.19)	93.1 ± 16 (1.05 ± 0.18)	97.7 ± 19 (1.10 ± 0.21)	96.8 ± 16 (1.09 ± 0.18)
Serum potassium, mmol/L (mEq/L)	4.28 ± 0.4	4.27 ± 0.4	4.28 ± 0.4	3.97 ± 0.4‡
Serum urate, mol/L (mg/dL)	349 ± 76 (5.9 ± 1.3)	347 ± 80 (5.8 ± 1.3)	364 ± 75 (6.1 ± 1.3)	384 ± 82 (6.4 ± 1.4)‡
Serum potassium <3.6 mmol/L (mEq/L), %	5.2	6.3	1.7	13.0‡
Serum urate >450 mol/L (>7.5 mg/dL), %	9.2	9.0	11.9	18.2‡
Glucosuria, %	1.5	0.4	2.3	1.6
Albuminuria, %	4.7	3.9	3.0	2.7
Smokers, %	34	33	23	25

* Values are mean ± SD.
† P = .012, between-group comparison at last follow-up visit.
‡ P < .001 between-group comparison at last follow-up visit.

F. Statistical Methods

All data were analyzed at the Computing Center of Göteborg University using the SAS program. With the Gehan-Wilcoxon nonparametric test for survival analysis, the null hypothesis was tested, that is, that there was no difference between the two treatments (intention-to-treat) in event rates (8–11).

For quantitative variables regarded as normally distributed, that is, blood pressure and heart rate, parametric tests were used (Student's *t*-test). Differences in proportions were tested by Fisher's exact test. *P* values below 0.05 (two-sided) were considered significant for all variables.

G. Comments to Study Design

The MAPHY study was an international, multicenter, stratified, randomized, open, controlled study of primary prevention in parallel groups preceded, for previously treated patients, by a 4- to 8-week run-in period without treatment. The vast majority of patient-years came from previously untreated patients, found partly by screening procedures. The open study design has the advantage that it mirrors everyday clinical practice. The stratification and randomization procedures, together with the results of baseline characteristics, the blind recording of blood pressure, the blind evaluation of hard endpoints, and the completeness of follow-up make it unlikely that there is any significant bias stemming from the study design (Prospective, Randomized, Open, Blind End-point Evaluation [PROBE] design). Critical comment has been made regarding the follow-up made after the closing date of HAPPHY. However, data are very similar in MAPHY if instead analyzed with the same closing date as HAPPHY (December 31, 1985).

Before randomization, patients were stratified according to risk of coronary heart disease into nine risk groups depending on age (40 to 49, 50 to 59, or older than 60 years), first systolic blood pressure recorded ($<$190 or $\geq$190 mm Hg), cholesterol level ($<$7.0, 7.0 to 8.6, or $\geq$8.7 mmol/L [$<$270, 270 to 330, or $\geq$330 mg/dL]), and smoking habits (never smoked, ex-smoker, 1 to 14 g/day, or $\geq$ 15 g/day [one cigarette = 1 g]) (8, 13). An ex-smoker was defined as a smoker who had stopped at least one month previously.

After stratification, patients were randomized to treatment with 200 mg/day of metoprolol or a thiazide diuretic (50 mg/day of hydrochlorothiazide or 5 mg/day of bendorflumethiazide). These dosages were doubled, or additional drugs (hydralazine, spironolactone, or others, but not beta-blockers or thiazide diuretics) were given, if necessary, to reach the treatment goal of diastolic blood pressure lower than 95 mm Hg in both randomization groups. To modernize the therapy, the maximum daily doses of the baseline drugs were reduced to 200 mg/day of metoprolol or 50 mg/day of hydrochlorothiazide (5 mg/day of bendroflumethiazide) in 1981.

According to protocol criteria stated in an addendum to the protocol from 1982, a patient in the diuretic group could receive beta-blockade if the physician considered this to be indicated for clinical reasons (that is, in some patients suffering a nonfatal myocardial infarction during the study).

H. Summary of Clinical Characteristics at Randomization and During Follow-Up

Before treatment started, risk factors for coronary events were very similar in the two treatment groups (Table 1). There was a highly significant reduction in systolic and dia-

Table 2 Blood Pressure and Heart Rate at Randomization and at the Last Follow-Up Visit in the Two Treatment Groups in the MAPHY Study by Smoking Status at Randomization (8, 9)

	Metoprolol mean		Diuretic mean	
	SBP/DBP (mm Hg)	HR (bpm)	SBP/DBP (mm Hg)	HR (bpm)
Smokers				
At randomization	168/108	80	169/108	79
At last visit	143/89	66	144/90	76
Nonsmokers				
At randomization	166/107	77	166/107	77
At last visit	142/89	63	142/90	73

Abbreviations: SBP, systolic blood pressure; *DBP*, diastolic blood pressure; *HR*, heart rate; *bpm*, beats per minute.

stolic blood pressure to similar levels in the two treatment groups. Heart rate was 10 beats/min lower with metoprolol compared with diuretics. Comparable control of blood pressure was achieved in subgroups of nonsmokers and smokers (Table 2) (8, 9). Reduction in serum cholesterol in the metoprolol group (3%) was significant, with no change in the diuretic group. At the last visit, serum cholesterol was significantly lower in the metoprolol group than in the diuretic group ($P < 0.001$; Table 1) (8).

I. Summary of Mortality and Morbidity Results

The results showed that total mortality was lower in patients randomized to metoprolol than in those randomized to thiazide diuretics ($P = 0.028$; Fig. 2) (8). The explanation for the reduced risk for total mortality was a reduced risk for sudden cardiovascular deaths ($P = 0.017$; Fig. 2) (10).

The morbidity results support the conclusions from the mortality data (11). Altogether, 255 patients suffered a definite coronary event—sudden death or a fatal or definite nonfatal acute or silent (unrecognized) myocardial infarction during the course of the trial. The incidence of coronary events was significantly lower during follow-up in patients randomized to metoprolol than in patients randomized to diuretics: 111 versus 144 cases, respectively ($P = 0.001$, time to first event; Fig. 3). There was no difference in stroke rates between the two treatment groups (Fig. 3), although stroke was fatal in more patients in the diuretic group compared with the metoprolol group (9 versus 2 deaths, $P = 0.043$) (8, 11).

Post hoc subgroup analyses showed that total mortality and coronary heart disease mortality were significantly lower in smokers taking metoprolol than in smokers on diuretics ($P = 0.012$ and $P = 0.021$, respectively; Fig. 4) (9). Furthermore, analyses also showed that the incidence of all first definite coronary events (fatal plus nonfatal, time to first event) was significantly lower in nonsmoking patients taking metoprolol than in nonsmoking patients taking diuretics ($P = 0.0008$; Fig. 4) (11).

An analysis of cost effectiveness of hypertensive treatment based on the results from the MAPHY study showed that metoprolol was more cost effective than thiazide diuretics due to the more favorable effect on coronary events (12).

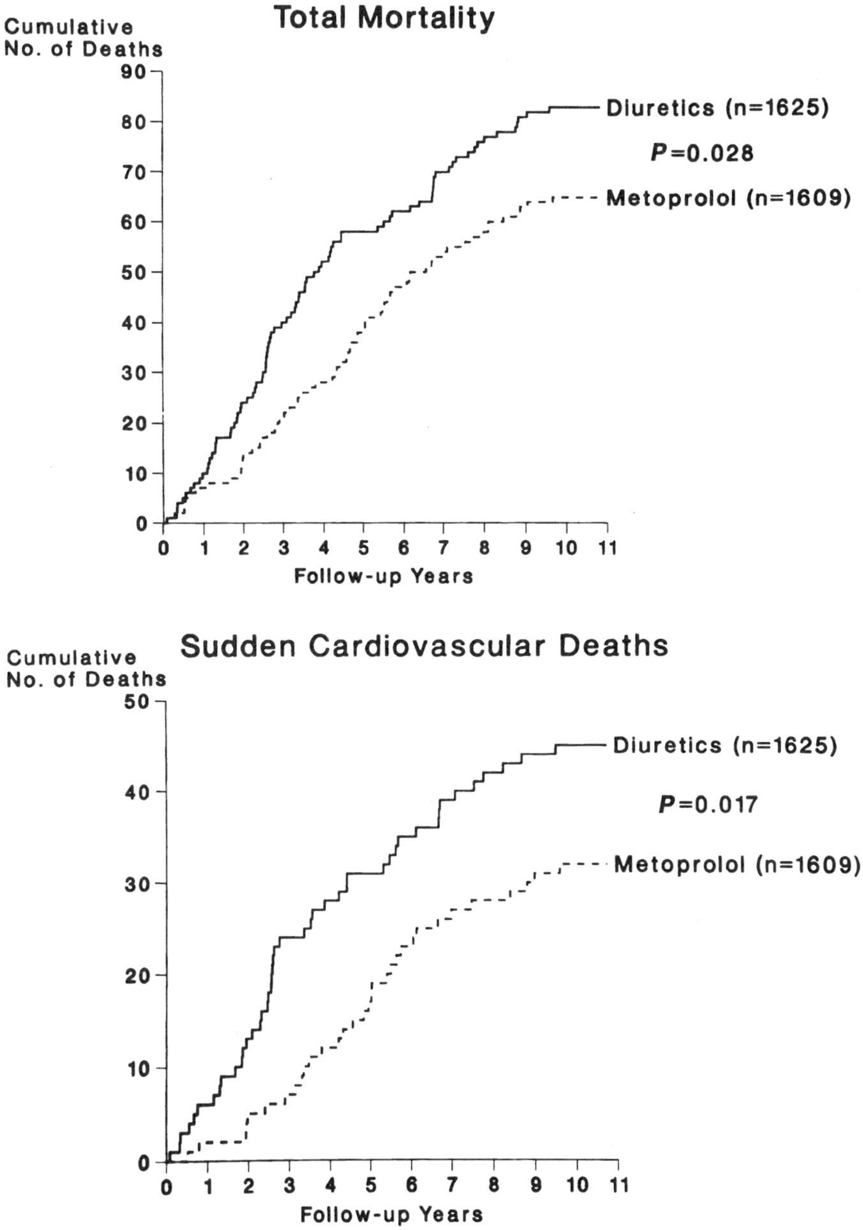

Fig. 2 Cumulative numbers for all-cause mortality (**upper panel**), and sudden cardiovascular deaths (**lower panel**) in the MAPHY study. The *P* values refer to the difference in the survival experience between the two randomization groups during the entire study period. (From Ref. 8 [**upper panel**] and Ref. 10 [**lower panel**], by permission.)

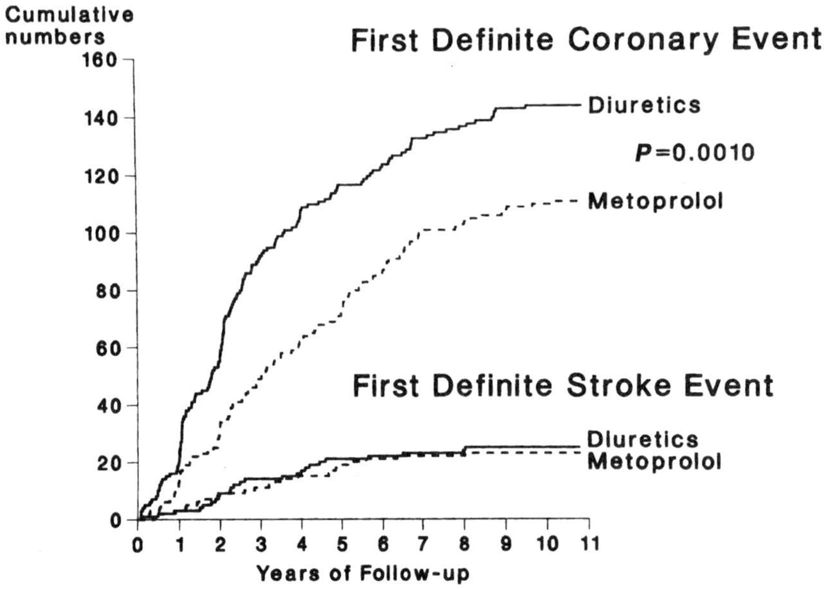

Fig. 3 Cumulative numbers for all first definite coronary events and stroke events in the two randomization groups in the MAPHY study. The *P* value refers to difference in risk between the two randomization groups during entire study period. (From Ref. 11, by permission.)

II. COMMENTS ON SUPPORTING EVIDENCE FOR A CARDIOPROTECTIVE EFFECT OF BETA-BLOCKERS IN HYPERTENSION

The high mortality from coronary heart disease in men with hypertension can be substantially reduced only if the treatment can reduce the risk for sudden death (2, 21). For statistical and biological reasons, any preventive effect on sudden death and myocardial infarction is hard to demonstrate in women in the primary preventive trials performed because of the low incidence of coronary events in middle-aged, white women (13, 20, 22–24). Therefore, in this summary, special attention will be focused on the effect in men.

There are no data from primary preventive studies to indicate that hydrophilic beta-blockers reduce the risk of sudden death (Table 3) (2, 4, 17, 25), nor are any positive data available from long-term secondary preventive postinfarction studies with hydrophilic beta-blockers on this important mode of death (2, 22, 26). A theoretical explanation for the possible lack of impact of hydrophilic beta-blockers on ventricular fibrillation and sudden death is discussed in a later section.

Pooled data from randomized primary preventive trials in men with hypertension in which lipophilic beta-blockers have been used—MRC: propranolol (18, 25, 27, 28); IPPPSH: oxprenolol (19); and MAPHY: metoprolol (8–11), representing 11,000 patients and the experience from more than 51,000 patient years of follow-up, show a statistically significant 20% lower total mortality, a 35% reduction in sudden death, and a 22% lower incidence of definite coronary events (time to first event), as compared with a non–beta-

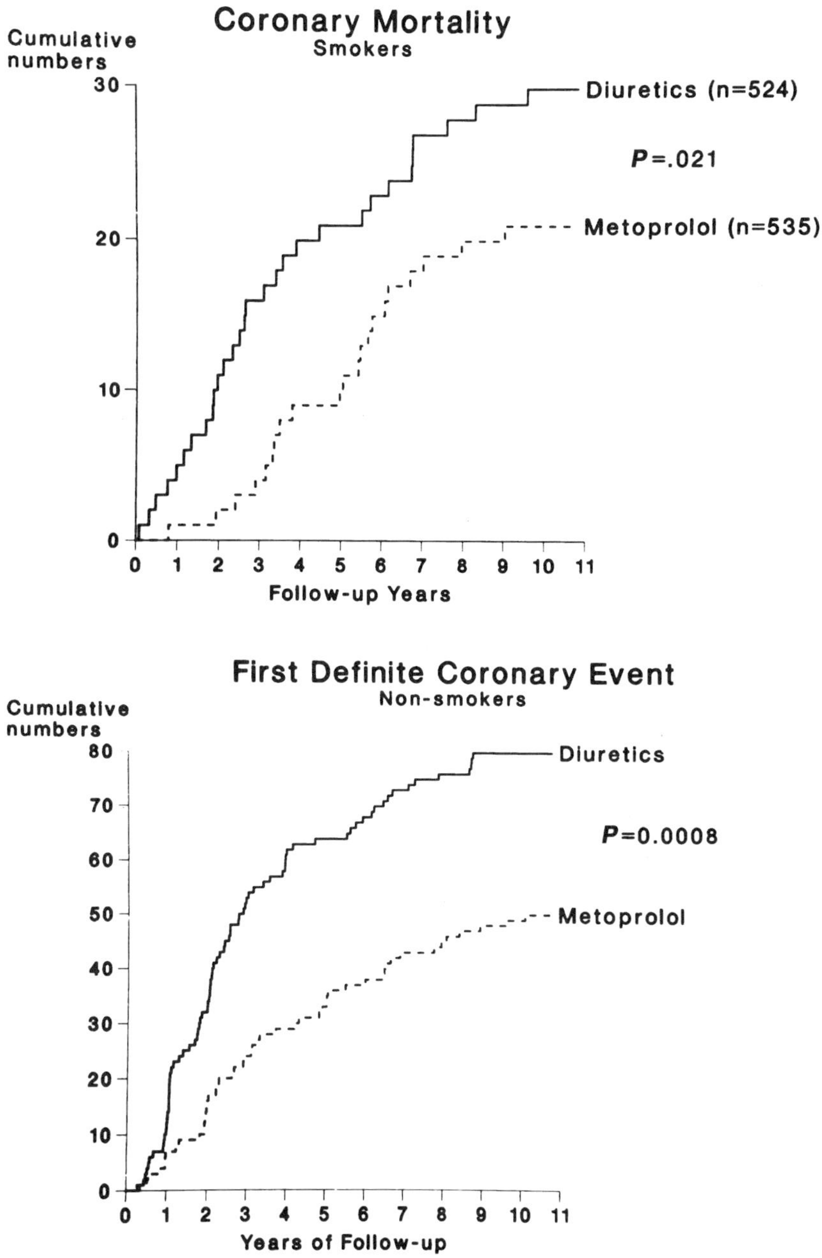

Fig. 4 Cumulative numbers of coronary mortality in smokers (**upper panel**) and of coronary events (sudden death + fatal and nonfatal acute and silent myocardial infarctions) (**lower panel**) in the MAPHY study. The *P* values refer to the difference in risk between the randomization groups during the entire study period. (From Ref. 9 [**upper panel**] and Ref. 11 [**lower panel**], by permission.)

Table 3 Total Mortality in the Atenolol Arm of the HAPPHY Study (17) and in the MRC Older Adults Study (25)

	Number of deaths	
	Atenolol	Diuretics
HAPPHY, atenolol arm	33	26
MRC older adults	167	134
Total	200	160

blocker, mainly a diuretic-based schedule (Table 4). Pooled data from MRC, IPPPSH, and MAPHY show that baseline characteristics and the reduction in blood pressure achieved are very similar in patients treated with beta-blockers and thiazide diuretics (8, 20). Therefore, the difference in relative risk is caused by mechanisms other than blood pressure control.

In addition, secondary preventive studies with relatively lipophilic beta-blockers including propranolol, timolol, and metoprolol have shown very convincingly a reduction in sudden death as compared with placebo (29, 30). Around 30% of patients in these studies have been hypertensive and the effect in the subgroup of hypertensives has been impressive (31–33). Two large-scale survival studies using lipophilic beta-blockers in patients with heart failure have also demonstrated a highly significant reduction in sudden death (34, 35).

A. Comments on the Effects in Smokers and Nonsmokers

In smokers, no effect was observed on coronary events (fatal plus nonfatal) with beta-blockade in MRC and IPPPSH using nonselective beta-blockers (propranolol and oxprenolol, respectively) (18, 19). In the MAPHY study, using metoprolol, a cardioselective beta-blocker, total and coronary mortality was significantly lower in smoking men on beta-blockade than in those taking diuretics (Fig. 4) (9). The importance of the cardioselectivity of metoprolol for the reduced relative risk in smokers has been discussed elsewhere (8, 9, 11). The favorable results in smokers in MAPHY are also supported by results from animal experiments that have shown protection against smoke-induced endothelial injury with metoprolol in guinea pigs (36). The risk for coronary events was significantly lower in nonsmoking patients randomized to metoprolol than in nonsmoking patients randomized to diuretics in the MAPHY study (Fig. 4) (11). Post hoc subgroup analysis from the MRC study also showed that the risk for coronary events (fatal plus nonfatal) was significantly lower in nonsmoking men taking propranolol than in nonsmoking men taking placebo (18, 27, 29).

The IPPPSH also showed a significantly lower risk for coronary events (fatal plus nonfatal) in nonsmoking males randomized to beta-blockade (oxprenolol) compared with the men randomized to a non–beta-blocker, mainly a thiazide diuretic-based treatment schedule (19). Thus, results in nonsmoking men are consistent in three randomized clinical trials with relatively lipophilic beta-blockers (23).

Table 4 Meta-Analysis Regarding Total Mortality, Sudden Death, and the Pooled Incidence of Nonfatal and Fatal Coronary Events from Men in MRC (18, 27, 28), IPPPSH (19), and MAPHY (8, 9, 19, 11) Studies Using Relatively Lipophilic Beta-Blockers

	Beta-blockade	Non-Beta-blockade*	*P* value†	Percentage reduction with Beta-blockade	95% Confidence interval
Number randomized	5499	5452			
Patient years‡	25941	25491			
Total mortality	202	247	0.024	20%	1 to 32%
Sudden death§	68	105	0.0042	36%	13 to 54%
CHD (nonfatal plus fatal)	262	330	0.003	22%	6 to 33%

* Mainly diuretic.
† The optimal test for comparison of two Poisson distributions.
‡ For total mortality.
§ Data from MRC are given for men and women combined, as data are not available for subgroups of men and women in the MRC study (from Ref. 28).
Abbreviation: *CHD*, coronary heart disease.

III. IS THERE NO "CLASS EFFECT"?

Is it possible that different beta-blockers could have different efficacy in preventing ventricular fibrillation and sudden death because there is no class effect (2–4, 6)?

An important difference between lipophilic and hydrophilic beta-blockers is that lipophilic beta-blockers pass the blood-brain barrier and produce the same drug concentration in the brain as in the heart, which hydrophilic beta-blockers do not. The question arises as to whether there is any important $beta_1$-mechanism in the brain that effects ventricular fibrillation threshold and the risk of sudden death? Data indicate that activity in the frontocortico-brain-stem pathway, in combination with myocardial ischemia, triggers a state of increased vulnerability of the heart to the initiation of ventricular fibrillation and sudden death in susceptible subjects (37–41). One of nature's illustrations of emotional stress triggering sudden death is the Northridge earthquake (41). Animal data also indicate that psychosocial stress in combination with myocardial ischemia triggers the initiation of ventricular fibrillation and sudden death (37–39, 42). A reasonable strategy for the prevention of sudden death would be to interrupt the linkage between the trigger and the event (37, 38, 41). The proposed mode of action for the preventive effect of lipophilic beta-blockers on ventricular fibrillation and sudden death is as follows (2, 38, 39):

1. $Beta_1$-blockade in the brain maintaining electrical stability of the heart through prevention of vagal withdrawal during stressful situations
2. $Beta_1$-blockade in the heart through prevention of increased cardiovascular sympathetic tone during stressful situations (anti-ischemic effect and prevention of increases in heart rate, blood pressure, and contractility)

IV. CONCLUSION

In conclusion, the results from the MAPHY study showed improved survival and a decreased risk of sudden cardiovascular death with metoprolol compared with diuretics in men with diastolic blood pressure above 100 mm Hg at randomization. Results from men in the MRC and IPPPSH studies provide additional evidence that beta-blockers reduce the risk of sudden death. The survival benefit may be attributed to $beta_1$-blockade, and positive data are only available from trials in which lipophilic beta-blockers have been studied. Furthermore, experimental data indicate that beta-blockers that pass the blood-brain barrier make an important contribution to a decrease in the risk of ventricular fibrillation and sudden death. Among the lipophilic drugs, the choice of a $beta_1$-selective blocker is suggested because such an agent may more effectively reduce the risk in those who cannot quit smoking. The MAPHY study, an open study, was not designed to detect differences in unwanted subjective symptoms between the two regimens. However, another study, the Metoprolol in Elderly Hypertensive Patients (MEPH) study, a randomized double-blind study in 600 patients, was specifically designed to tackle this question (43), and results showed that metoprolol was very well tolerated (43, 44). Interestingly, an efficacy tolerance index analyzed in the study showed a statistically significant difference between the beta-blocker and the thiazide diuretic regimen in favor of metoprolol. In the MAPHY study, a similar rate of noncardiovascular deaths was seen in the two randomization groups (23 noncardiovascular deaths on metoprolol and 26 on diuretics), indicating that the metoprolol regimen is safe (8). Cardioselectivity and tolerability may be further enhanced by using a long-acting preparation like metoprolol CR/XL (45–49).

The sixth report of the Joint National Committee (JNC VI) stated that the optimal formulation of an antihypertensive agent should provide 24 hours efficacy with a once-daily dose with at least 50% of the peak effect remaining at the end of 24 hours (1). Long-acting formulations that provide 24 hours efficacy are preferred over short-acting drugs for many reasons, one being protection against risk for sudden death, heart attack, and stroke caused by the abrupt increase of blood pressure or other triggers in early morning hours or after arising from overnight sleep (1, 49). The MAPHY study included high-risk hypertensive patients: men with diastolic blood pressure higher than 100 mm Hg before randomization. In this category of patients, combination treatment is needed in the majority of cases. Metoprolol may be combined with any other antihypertensive drugs such as diuretics, calcium antagonists, ACE inhibitors, AII-blockers, or alpha-blockers. In addition to the choice of antihypertensive drug, primary prevention and risk reduction also require the detection and appropriate management of other cardiovascular risk factors (1, 50).

INVESTIGATORS

Independent Data Audit Committee: Aram Chobanian, M.D., Cardiovascular Institute, Boston University School of Medicine, Boston, MA; Göran Berglund, M.D, Ph.D., Department of Medicine, Malmö Hospital, Lund University, Malmö, Sweden.

Steering Committee: Gunnar Olsson, M.D., Ph.D., Department of Medicine, Danderyd Hospital, Karolinska Institute, Stockholm, Sweden; Jaakko Tuomilehto, M.D., Ph.D., Department of Epidemiology, National Public Health Institute, Helsinki, Finland; Ingrid Warnold, Ph.D. (nonvoting secretary), Medical Department, Hässle Cardiovascular Research Laboratories, Mölndal, Sweden; John Wikstrand, M.D., Ph.D., Wallenberg Laboratory for Cardiovascular Research, Sahlgrenska University Hospital, Göteborg, and Senior Medical Advisor, AstraZeneca, Mölndal, Sweden.

Advisory Committee: Hamish J. Barber, M.D., Department of General Practice, University of Glasgow, Scotland; Keith Eliasson, M.D., Ph.D., Department of Internal Medicine, Karolinska Hospital, Karolinska Institute, Stockholm, Sweden; Birthe Jastrup, M.D., Medical Clinic, Odder Sygehus, Odder, Denmark; Nicholas B. Karatzas, M.D., Hypertension Research Clinic, First Department of Propedeutic Medicine, Laikon Hospital, University of Athens, Athens, Greece; John Leer, M.D., Legecenteret i Florvåg, Florvåg, Norway; Fausto Marchetta, M.D., Ospedale S Orsola, Bologna, Italy; Johann Ragnarsson, M.D., Medical Department, Reykjavik City Hospital, Reykjavik, Iceland; Michelle Robitaille, M.D., Institut de Cardiologie, Quebec, Canada; Liba Valkova, M.D., Department of General Practice, National Institute of Health, Prague, Czechoslovakia; Harry Wesseling, M.D., Ph.D., Department of Pharmacology and Clinical Pharmacology, University of Groningen, The Netherlands.

The Independent End Point Committee: Cause-specific mortality: Robert Bergstrand, M.D., Ph.D. and Lars Wilhelmsen, M.D., Ph.D., Department of Internal Medicine, Eastern Hospital, Göteborg University, Göteborg, Sweden. Nonfatal end points: John Kjekshus, M.D., Ph.D., Department of Internal Medicine, Baerum Hospital, Oslo University, Oslo, Norway and Lars Rydén, M.D., Ph.D., Department of Cardiology, Karolinska Hospital, Karolinska Institute, Stockholm, Sweden.

Statistical Consultant: Andes Odén, Ph.D., Department of Mathematics, Göteborg University, Göteborg, Sweden.

Data System Manager: Jonny Lindqvist, Computing Centre, Göteborg University, Göteborg, Sweden.

Investigators: *Canada* (8.5% of patient-years): J. George Fodor, M.D., Ph.D., S. Paul Handa, M.D., Gordon D. Hardacre, M.D., N. Michelle Robitaille, M.D., M.P.H., Robin S. Shearer, M.D., Robin C. Woollam, M.D.; *Czechoslovakia* (3.5% of patient-years): Frantisek Boudik, M.D., Zdenek Hejl, M.D., Zbynek Pisa, M.D., Jiri Valek, M.D., Liba Valkova, M.D.; *Denmark* (0.4% of patient-years): Birthe Jastrup, M.D.; *Finland* (21.2% of patient-years): Matti Honkavaara, M.D., Pasi Kuusisto, M.D., Martti Mönkkönen, M.D., Arto Mönttinen, M.D., Matti Pohjola, M.D., Jaakko Tuomilehto, M.D., Ph.D., Seija Vinni, M.D., Olavi Vänskä, M.D.; *Greece* (0.6% of patient-years): Nicholas B. Karatzas, M.D.; *The Netherlands* (2.2% of patient-years): Bart S. ten Berge, M.D., Theo H.J.J.M. Bloem, M.D., Johan Frans May, M.D., Menso J. Nubé, M.D., Jo L.J. Jansen, M.D.; *Iceland* (5.9% of patient-years): Thordur Hardarson, M.D., Johann R. Ragnarsson, M.D., Snorri Snorrason, M.D.: *Italy* (2.7% of patient-years): Ettori Ambrosioni, M.D., Roberto Fogari, M.D., Fausto Marchetta, M.D., Anna Pirrelli, M.D.; *Norway* (1.9% of patient-years): Svein Z. Bratland, M.D., Åge Dahl, M.D., Arne Haraldson, M.D., John Leer, M.D.; *Sweden* (43.8% of patient-years): Bernd Atmer, M.D.; Agneta Brouneus, M.D., Birger Brouneus, M.D., Arne Bruhn, M.D., Jan Candefjord, M.D., Gunnar Ekblad, M.D.; Keith Eliasson, M.D., Ph.D., Åke Ellborg, M.D., Dag Elmfeldt, M.D., Ph.D., Sven-Erik Fagerberg, M.D., Ph.D., Lars Fries, M.D., Johan Erik Frisell, M.D., Karl Gumaelius, M.D., Christer Gunnarsson, M.D., Raoul Hagströmer, M.D., Leo Hassler, M.D., Staffan Hjalmers, M.D., Kjell Hultsten, M.D., Brita Hylander, M.D., Anders Häggmark, M.D., Bertil Johansen, M.D., Jörgen Jonsson, M.D., Jan Kjellberg, M.D., Lars-Göran Lindgren, M.D., Gösta Linné, M.D., Janos Luptovics, M.D., Per-Olof Magnusson, M.D., Lennart Nilsson, M.D., Lars-Göran Persson, M.D., Åke Sjöstrand, M.D., Ted Strömvall, M.D., Tunc Tovi, M.D., Halina Wajntraub, M.D.; *United Kingdom* (9.4% of patient-years): Barry J. Adams-Strump, M.D., Steven Bird, M.D., L. Malcolm Campbell, M.D., Allan R. Cuthill, M.D., John R. Goves, M.D., Peter F. Grundy, M.D., Keith G. Harding, M.D., Robert Harvard Davis, M.D., John H. McLauchlan, M.D., Chris J.L. Morgan, M.D., Alexander L. Muir, M.D., Trevor G. Pinker, M.D., Sudhi Sudhakar, M.D., Stanley H. Taylor, M.D., Chris G. Wathen, M.D..

REFERENCES

1. The Sixth Report of the Joint National Committee on Prevention, Detection, Evaluation, and Treatment of High Blood Pressure (JNC VI). National Institutes of Health, November 1997.
2. Wikstrand J, Kendall M. The role of beta receptor blockade in preventing sudden death. Eur Heart J 1992; 13(suppl D):111–120.
3. Kendall MJ, Lynch KP, Hjalmarson Å Kjekshus J. Beta-blockers and sudden cardiac death. Ann Intern Med 1995; 123:358–367.
4. Soriano JB, Hoes AW, Meems L, Grobbee DE. Increased survival with beta-blockers: importance of ancillary properties. Prog Cardiovasc Dis 1997; XXXIX:445–456.
5. Kaplan NM. Beta blockade in the primary prevention of hypertensive cardiovascular events with focus on sudden death. Am J Cardiol 1997; 80:20J–22J.
6. Staessen JA, Wang JG, Birkenhäger WH, Fagard R. Treatment with beta-blockers for the primary prevention of the cardiovascular complications of hypertension. Eur Heart J 1999; 20:11–25.
7. Wikstrand J. Reducing the risk for coronary heart disease and stroke in hypertensives-comments on mechanisms for coronary protection and quality of life. J Clin Pharm 1992; 17:9–29.
8. Wikstrand J, Warnold I, Olsson G, Tuomilehto J, Elmfeldt D, Berglund G, on behalf of the Advisory Committee. Primary prevention with metoprolol in patients with hypertension. Mortality results from the MAPHY Study. JAMA 1988; 259:1976–1982.

9. Tuomilehto J, Wikstrand J, Olsson G, Elmfeldt D, Warnold I, Barber H, Eliasson K, Jastrup B, Karatzas N, Leer. J. Decreased coronary heart disease in hypertensive smokers. Mortality results from the MAPHY Study. Hypertension 1989; 13:773–780.
10. Olsson G, Tuomilehto J, Berglund G, Elmfeldt D, Warnold I, Barber H, Eliasson K, Jastrup B, Karatzas N, Leer J, Leer J. Primary prevention of sudden cardiovascular death in hypertensive patients: mortality results from the MAPHY study. Am J Hypertens 1991; 4:151–158.
11. Wikstrand J, Warnold I, Tuomilehto J, Olsson G, Elmfeldt D, Berglund G, on behalf of the Advisory Committee. Metoprolol versus thiazide diuretics in hypertension. Morbidity results from the MAPHY study. Hypertension 1991; 17:579–588.
12. Johannesson M, Wikstrand J, Jönsson B, Berglund G, Tuomilehto J. Cost-effectiveness of antihypertensive treatment. Metoprolol versus thiazide diuretics. Pharmacoeconomics 1993; 3:36–44.
13. Wilhelmsen L, Berglund G, Elmfeldt D, Wedel H. β-Blockers versus saluretics in hypertension. Comparison of total mortality, myocardial infarction, and sudden death: study design and early results on blood pressure reduction. Prev Med 1981; 10:38–49.
14. Wilhelmsen L, Berglund G, Elmfeldt D, Fitzsimons T, Holzgreve H, Hosie J, Hörnkvist P-E, Pennert K, Tuomilehto J, Wedel H. Beta-blockers versus diuretics in hypertensive men: main results from the HAPPHY trial. J Hypertens 1987; 5:561–572.
15. Veterans Administration Cooperative Study Group on Antihypertensive Agents. Effect of treatment on morbidity in hypertension. II. Results in patients with diastolic blood pressure averaging 90 through 114 mm Hg. JAMA 1970; 213(7):1143–1152.
16. Olsson G, Tuomilehto J, Wikstrand J, for the MAPHY Steering Committee. MAPHY and the two arms of HAPPHY. In reply to letter to the editor. JAMA 1989; 262:3272–3273.
17. The Steering Committee of the HAPPHY Trial (Berglund G, Elmfeldt D, Fitzsimons T, Holzgreve H, Hosie J, Hörnkvist P E, Tuomilehto J, Wedel H, Wikstrand J, Wilhelmsen L). MAPHY and the two arms of HAPPHY. In reply to letter to the editor. JAMA 1989; 262:3273–3274.
18. Medical Research Council Working Party. MRC trial of treatment of mild hypertension: principal results. BMJ 1985; 291:97–104.
19. The IPPPSH Collaborative Group. Cardiovascular risk and risk factors in a randomized trial of treatment based on the beta-blocker oxprenolol: the International Prospective Primary Prevention Study in Hypertension (IPPPSH). J Hypertens 1985; 3:379–392.
20. Wikstrand J. Betablockers and cardioprotection—Is there any good news from the recent trials? (Editorial.) J Clin Pharm Ther 1987; 12:347–350.
21. Kannel WB, Thomas HE Jr. Sudden coronary death: the Framingham study. In: Greenberg HM, Dwyer EM Jr. (eds) Sudden Coronary Death. Vol 382. New York: New York Academy of Sciences 1982:3–20.
22. MacMahon SW, Cutler JA, Furberg CD, Payne GH: The effects of drug treatment for hypertension on morbidity and mortality from cardiovascular disease: a review of randomized controlled trials. Prog Cardiovasc Dis 1986; 29(suppl 1):99–118.
23. Wikstrand J. Reducing the risk for coronary events and stroke in hypertensive patients: comments on present evidence. Clin Cardiol 1991; 14 (suppl III):25–35.
24. Wikstrand J, Berglund G, Tuomilehto J. Beta-blockade in the primary prevention of coronary heart disease in hypertensive patients. Review of present evidence. Circulation 1991; 84(suppl VI):VI-93–VI-100.
25. Medical Research Council Working Party. Medical Research Council trial of treatment of hypertension in older adults: principal results. BMJ 1992; 304:405–412.
26. Yusuf S, Peto R, Lewis J, Collins R, Sleight P. Beta blockade during and after myocardial infarction: an overview of the randomized trials. Prog Cardiovasc Dis 1985; 27:335–371.
27. Medical Research Council Working Party on Mild Hypertension. Coronary heart disease in the Medical Research Council trial of treatment of mild hypertension. Br Heart J 1988; 59: 364–378.
28. Green KG. British MRC trial of treatment for mild hypertension—A more favorable interpretation. Am J Hypertens 1991; 4:723–724.
29. Olsson G, Wikstrand J, Warnold I, Manger Cats V, McBoyle D, Herlitz J, Hjalmarson A,

Sonneblick EH. Metoprolol induced reduction in postinfarction mortality: Pooled results from five double-blind randomized trials. Eur Heart J 1992; 13:28–32.

30. Teo KK, Yusuf S, Furberg CD. Effects of prophylactic antiarrhythmic drug therapy in acute myocardial infarction. An overview of results from randomized controlled trials. JAMA 1993; 270:1589–1595.
31. Pedersen T. A multicenter study on timolol in secondary prevention after myocardial infarction. Acta Med Scand 1983; (suppl 674):1–129.
32. Olsson G, Rehnqvist N. Reduction of non-fatal reinfarctions in patients with a history of hypertension by chronic postinfarction treatment with metoprolol. Acta Med Scand 1986; 220:33–38.
33. Herlitz J, Hjalmarson Å. Effect of metoprolol on mortality and morbidity among hypertensives with suspected acute myocardial infarction. CV World Report 1990; 3:40–43.
34. CIBIS-II Investigators and Committees. Lancet 1999; 353:9–13.
35. The MERIT-HF Study Group. Effect of metoprolol CR/XL in chronic heart failure: metoprolol CR/XL Randomised Intervention Trial in Congestive Heart Failure (MERIT-HF). Lancet 1999; 353:2001–2007.
36. Bondjers G, Hansson G, Olsson G, Pettersson K. Smoking, catecholamines and their effects on endothelial cell integrity. In: Diana JN, ed. Tobacco Smoking and Atherosclerosis. Pathogenesis and Cellular Mechanisms. New York: Plenum Press, 1990. Adv Exp Med Biol 273, pp 51–59.
37. Skinner JE. Regulation of cardiac vulnerability by the cerebral defense system. J Am Coll Cardiol 1985; 5:88B–94B.
38. Parker GW, Michael LH, Hartley CJ, Skinner JE, Entman JE. Central β-adrenergic mechanisms may modulate ischemic ventricular fibrillation in pigs. Circ Res 1990; 66:259–270.
39. Åblad B, Bjurö T, Björkman J-A, Edström T, Olsson G. Role of central nervous beta-adrenoceptors in the prevention of ventricular fibrillation through augmentation of cardiac vagal tone. JACC 1991; 17(2):165A.
40. Meisel SR, Kutz I, Dayan KI, Pauzner H, Chetboun I, Arbel Y, David D. Effect of Iraqi missile war on incidence of acute myocardial infarction and sudden death in Israeli civilians. Lancet 1991; 338:660–661.
41. Leor J, Poole WK, Kloner RA. Sudden cardiac death triggered by an earthquake. N Engl J Med 1996;334:413–419.
42. Dellsperger KC, Martins JB, Clothier JL, Marcus ML. Incidence of sudden cardiac death associated with coronary artery occlusion in dogs with hypertension and left ventricular hypertrophy is reduced by chronic β-adrenergic blockade. Circulation 1990; 82:941–950.
43. Wikstrand J, Westergren G, Berglund G, Bracchetti D, van Couter A, Feldstein C, Siu Ming K, Kuramoto K, Landahl S, Meaney E, Pedersen EB, Rahn KH, Shaw J, Smith A, Waal-Manning H. Antihypertensive treatment with metoprolol or hydrochlorothiazide in patients aged 60–75 years. JAMA 1986; 255:1304–1310.
44. Wikstrand J. New concepts in the treatment of the elderly hypertensive. Am Heart J 1988; 116(suppl): 296–300.
45. Kendall MJ. Introduction. Eur J Clin Pharmacol 1988; 33(suppl):S1.
46. Sandberg A, Ragnarsson G, Jonsson UE, Sjögren J. Design of a new multiple-unit controlled-release formulation of metoprolol—metoprolol CR. Eur J Clin Pharmacol 1988; 33(suppl):S3–S7.
47. Blomqvist I, Westergren G, Sandberg A, Jonsson EU, Lundborg P. Pharmacokinetics and pharmacodynamics of controlled-release metoprolol: a comparison with atenolol. Eur J Clin Pharmacol 1988; 33(suppl):S19–S24.
48. Dimenäs E, Dahlöf CG, Heibel B, Moore RG, Olofsson BK, Westergren GE, Lücker PW. Subjective symptoms and pharmacokinetics/dynamics of metoprolol CR in elderly subjects—A comparison with atenolol. Eur J Clin Pharmacol 1990; 30:S92–S9.
49. Agewall S, Kendall M. Treatment with beta-blockers. The value of an even plasma concentration over 24 hours. J Clin Pharm Ther 1997; 22:171–179.
50. Fagerberg B, Wikstrand J, Berglund G, Samuelsson O, Agewall S, for the Risk Factor Intervention Study Group. Mortality rates in treated hypertensive men with additional risk factors are high but can be reduced. A randomized intervention study. Am J Hypertens 1998; 11:14–22.

8

The European Working Party on High Blood Pressure in the Elderly (EWPHE) Trial

ROBERT H. FAGARD, JAN A. STAESSEN, and LUTGARDE THIJS

University of Leuven, Leuven, Belgium

CHRISTOPHER J. BULPITT

Imperial College School of Medicine, London, England

I. INTRODUCTION

It has long been recognized that hypertension is a major risk factor for stroke and coronary heart disease in the elderly (1, 2). However, such an association does not necessarily imply that morbidity and mortality are reduced when blood pressure is lowered by antihypertensive drugs. In 1972, the European Working Party on High Blood Pressure in the Elderly (EWPHE) initiated a double-blind multicenter trial to assess the effects of antihypertensive drug therapy in patients who were at least 60 years old (3, 4). The trial was brought to an end in 1984 when the Steering Committee reported that some preset trial endpoints had been reached (5). The present chapter reviews the objectives, protocol, and results of the main trial, as well as the results of various analyses on subsidiary research questions based on the EWPHE data.

II. OBJECTIVES

The primary objective of the trial was to either detect a 40% reduction of cerebrovascular mortality and morbidity at the 5% level of significance or exclude a 40% reduction of cerebrovascular mortality and morbidity with a 90% power (3). Secondary objectives included the collection of data about effects of antihypertensive therapy on biochemical variables, left ventricular size, and general well-being in elderly patients.

III. METHODS

A. Protocol

The study was double-blind and randomized with one control group and one treatment group in each of eight stratified groups of patients (3, 5). After a preliminary selection, apparently suitable patients were placed on one capsule daily of a placebo for at least one month, during which they were seen at least three times. If at the end of the single-blind

Table 1 Criteria for Randomization

Inclusion criteria

1. Age 60 years or older at randomization
2. Blood pressure in sitting position on placebo during the run-in period
   - systolic: not less than 160 mm Hg and not more than 239 mm Hg
   - diastolic: not less than 90 mm Hg and not more than 119 mm Hg

   For selection of the subjects, the sitting blood pressure was measured three times on three different visits; the last reading of each visit was recorded and these three readings were averaged to yield the final figure
3. Willingness of patients to cooperate—informed consent, either oral or written, was obtained—and high likelihood of regular follow-up

Exclusion criteria

1. Certain causes of blood pressure elevation
   - specific causes of systolic blood pressure elevation, such as hyperthyroidism
   - conditions correctable by surgery, such as coarctation of the aorta, Cushing's and Conn's syndrome, renovascular hypertension, pheochromocytoma
2. Certain complications of hypertension

   Presence of
   - vascular retinopathy grade III (hemorrhages or exudates) or grade IV (papilloedema);
   - congestive heart failure, not corrected without diuretics or antihypertensive drugs (low salt diet and cardiac glycosides, however, were allowed)
   - enlarging or dissecting aneurysm
   - severe renal failure (serum creatinine of 2.5 mg/dl or more)

   History of
   - repeated severe nasal bleeding, not controlled by local measures
   - certified cerebral or subarachnoid hemorrhages
   - hypertensive encephalopathy
3. Certain other diseases
   - acute hepatitis or active cirrhosis
   - severe diseases not related to hypertension (e.g., carcinoma, insulin-dependent diabetes)
   - a physical infirmity prohibiting a sitting position
   - orthostatic hypotension, severe enough to prohibit antihypertensive drug therapy
   - clinical gout: repeated attacks or a single attack caused by thiazides, or serum uric acid of 10 mg/dl or more on repeated examinations, despite uricosuric therapy
   - conditions not related to hypertension that necessitate the continued administration of diuretics, beta-blocking agents or Rauwolfia derivatives
4. Lack of collaboration

   Patients found, by means of the pill count during the run-in period, not to have complied with prescribed drug intake (a maximum deviation of 10% less or 5% more than prescribed was acceptable) run-in period, the patient remained within the selection criteria (Table 1), the patient was randomized after stratification for center, age, gender, and cardiovascular complications. The latter included cerebrovascular accidents, cardiac events, and mild renal insufficiency. The schedule of drug therapy in the double-blind part of the trial is summarized in Table 2. All patients began treatment with one capsule of a diuretic (a combination of 25 mg of hydrochlorothiazide and 50 mg of triamterene) or matching placebo. The dose could be increased after an interval of not less than 2 weeks to a maximum of two capsules per day. When sitting blood pressure remained at 160/90 mm Hg or above after at least one month, alpha-methyldopa (500-mg tablets) or matching placebo were added. This treatment was started at a daily dose of 1/2 tablet in the evening and was increased when necessary by 1/2 tablet at intervals of not less than 2 weeks, to a maximum of 4 tablets, or 2000 mg per day. Thereafter the patients had to be seen at least every 3 months. The fatal events and nonfatal cardiovascular and renal events that withdrew individual patients from the trial are listed in Table 3, as well as the cardiovascular events that were considered as nonterminating. Other reasons for withdrawing from the trial were completion of the study period, being lost to follow-up, and interruption of all study treatment for more than 3 months. Patients who left the double-blind part of the study were followed up on whatever treatment was necessary, but only the date and cause of death were recorded.

B. Sample Size Calculations

At the onset of the trial, it was calculated that either 600 men or 1400 women would have to be followed up for 5 years to detect a 50% reduction in cerebrovascular events, a positive answer being significant at the 5% level with the power of the trial being 90% (3). As the gender mix became apparent, the numbers were recalculated so that 850 patients should be followed up for 8 years to detect a 40% reduction in cerebrovascular events.

Table 2 Schedule of Drug Therapy

	Time of drug intake		
	Morning	Noon	Evening
First-line treatment: diuretic*			
1 capsule	1	—	—
2 capsules	2	—	—
Additional treatment: alpha-methyldopa†			
½ tablet	—	—	½
1 tablet	½	—	½
1½ tablet	½	—	1
2 tablets	1	—	1
2½ tablets	1	½	1
3 tablets	1	1	1
3½ tablet	1	1	1½
4 tablets	1	1	2

* 1 capsule contains 25 mg of hydrochlorothiazide and 50 mg of triamterene.
† 1 tablet contains 500 mg of alpha-methyldopa.

Table 3 Events Leading to Withdrawal of a Patient from the Double-Blind Part of the Trial

1. *Terminating fatal events*
   - All causes
   - Cardiovascular
     - cerebrovascular
     - cardiac
     - other cardiovascular
   - Renal
   - Noncardiovascular, nonrenal
2. *Terminating nonfatal cardiovascular and renal events*
   - Nonfatal, morbid cardiovascular terminating events
     - cerebral hemorrhage
     - papilloedema, retinal hemorrhage or exudates
     - severe congestive heart failure
     - dissecting aneurysm
     - hypertensive encephalopathy
   - Nonfatal, nonmorbid cardiovascular terminating events
     - severe increase in blood pressure ($\geq$250/130 mm Hg, or $\geq$40/$\geq$20 mm Hg increase on $\geq$3 visits)
     - therapy required with diuretic, beta-blocker, calcium-antagonist
     - severe left ventricular hypertrophy or dilatation ($\geq$30% increase in ECG voltages and $\geq$20% increase of cardiothoracic ratio on chest X-ray)
   - Renal
     - severe increase in serum creatinine ($\geq$ 4.0 mg/dl, or $\geq$100% increase at two successive measurements)
3. *Nonterminating cardiovascular events*
   - Cerebrovascular
     - cerebral thrombosis
     - cerebral embolism
     - transient ischemic attack
   - Cardiac
     - myocardial infarction
     - moderate congestive heart failure
     - arrhythmias
     - heart block
   - Other vascular events

C. Statistical Methods

Both analyses on randomized treatment in the double-blind part of the trial (per-protocol or on-treatment analysis) and an overall intention-to-treat analysis were performed, the latter being confined to mortality. The life table approach was used to compare the outcome in the actively treated and placebo groups; tests of significance were performed with the log-rank statistic.

IV. RESULTS OF THE MAIN TRIAL

An interim analysis provided highly significant results, and the main trial findings were published in 1985 (5).

Table 4 Blood Pressure Measured in the Sitting Position During the Double-Blind Part of the Trial

	Blood pressure (mm Hg)		
	Placebo	Active	P
Randomization	$\frac{182 \pm 16}{101 \pm 7}$ (424)	$\frac{183 \pm 17}{101 \pm 7}$ (416)	$\frac{0.65}{0.98}$
After 1 yr	$\frac{172 \pm 23}{95 \pm 12}$ (287)	$\frac{151 \pm 17}{88 \pm 9}$ (300)	<0.001
3 yr	$\frac{172 \pm 25}{94 \pm 11}$ (171)	$\frac{149 \pm 16}{85 \pm 9}$ (187)	<0.001
5 yr	$\frac{171 \pm 25}{95 \pm 9}$ (93)	$\frac{150 \pm 20}{85 \pm 9}$ (108)	<0.001
7 yr	$\frac{167 \pm 22}{90 \pm 9}$ (27)	$\frac{148 \pm 18}{85 \pm 10}$ (39)	<0.001

Number of patients is shown in brackets.

A. Patient Characteristics

The 840 patients were randomized to placebo (n = 424) or active treatment (n = 416). The placebo and active treatment groups were similar in sex ratio (70.5% and 69.0% were women, respectively), sitting blood pressure (182/101 and 183/101 mm Hg), and percentage with cardiovascular complications (36% and 35%) on admission to the trial. During the double-blind part of the trial, blood pressure was lower ($P < 0.001$) in the actively treated patients than in those receiving placebo (Table 4); for example, after 3 years of follow-up, blood pressure averaged 172/94 mm Hg in the placebo group and 149/85 mm Hg in the active treatment group. At the end of the double-blind part of the trial, the diuretic was taken by 96% of those on active treatment, and methyldopa by 35%; these percentages were, respectively, 98% and 63% for the patients in the placebo group.

Table 5 Mortality in the Intention-to-Treat Analysis

	Rate per 1,000 patient-years (number of deaths)		Difference (active minus placebo)	
Causes of death	Placebo	Active	% Rate (95% CL)	P
All causes	76 (149)	69 (135)	−9 (−28 to +15)	0.41
Cardiovascular	47 (93)	34 (67)	−27 (−46 to −1)	0.04
cerebrovascular	16 (31)	11 (21)	−32 (−61 to +19)	0.16
cardiac	24 (47)	15 (29)	−38 (−61 to −1)	0.04
other	8 (15)	9 (17)	NC	NC
Renal	NC (1)	2 (4)	NC	NC
Noncardiovascular nonrenal	28 (54)	31 (61)	+14 (−21 to +64)	0.48
Unknown	NC (1)	2(3)	NC	NC

Abbreviation: CL, confidence level; *NC*, not calculated.

Table 6 Events on Randomized Treatment

	Rate per 1,000 patient-years (number of events)		Difference (active minus placebo)	
	Placebo	Active	% rate (95% CL)	P
	1. Terminating fatal events			
All causes	70 (89)	52 (73)	−26 (−45 to +1)	0.08
Cardiovascular	48 (61)	30 (42)	−38 (−58 to −8)	0.02
cerebrovascular	15 (19)	9 (12)	−43 (−72 to +18)	0.15
cardiac	23 (29)	12 (17)	−47 (−71 to −3)	0.05
myocardial infarction	13 (16)	5 (7)	−60 (−84 to −4)	0.04
others	10 (13)	7 (10)	−30 (−69 to +59)	0.44
pulmonary embolism	6 (7)	6 (8)	NC	NC
others	5 (6)	4 (5)	NC	NC
Renal	0 (0)	1 (1)	NC	NC
Noncardiovascular nonrenal	22 (28)	21 (30)	−3 (−42 to +62)	0.96
	2. Terminating nonfatal cardiovascular and renal events			
Morbid cardiovascular				
cerebral hemorrhage	2 (3)	3 (4)	NC	NC
papilloedema/retinal	4 (5)	0 (0)	NC	NC
severe heart failure	13 (17)	5 (7)	−63 (−85 to −10)	0.01
Nonmorbid cardiovascular				
severe BP increase	15 (19)	1 (2)	−90 (−98 to −59)	<0.001
therapy required	10 (8)	6 (10)	NC	NC
LV hypertrophy/dilatation	1 (1)	0 (0)	NC	NC
Severe creatinine increase	1 (1)	3 (4)	NC	NC
	3. Nonterminating cardiovascular events			
Cerebrovascular	20 (24)	9 (13)	−52 (−76 to −7)	0.03
thrombosis	10 (12)	4 (5)	−62 (−87 to +7)	0.05
embolism	2 (2)	2 (2)	NC	NC
TIA	12 (15)	6 (8)	−53 (−80 to +11)	0.08
Cardiac	31 (37)	32 (42)	+3 (−34 to +61)	0.98
myocardial infarction	9 (12)	14 (19)	NC	NC
moderate heart failure	5 (6)	9 (12)	NC	NC
arrhythmias	7 (8)	12 (16)	NC	NC
heart block	12 (15)	10 (14)	−16 (−60 to +73)	0.57
Other vascular	4 (5)	4 (5)	NC	NC

Abbreviations: CL, confidence limits; *NC*, not calculated; *TIA*, transient ischemic attacks.

B. Mortality in the Intention-to-Treat Analysis

The duration of follow-up in the intention-to-treat analysis averaged 4.6 years in the placebo and 4.7 years in the active treatment group; the patient-years of observation were, respectively, 1963 and 1950 years. The results on mortality are given in Table 5. In the placebo group, the total death rate was 76 per 1,000 patient-years, including 47 deaths per 1,000 patient-years from cardiovascular causes. The small reduction in mortality rate from all causes was not significant (−9%; $P = 0.41$), but the reductions in all cardiovascular mortality (−27%; $P = 0.04$) and in cardiac mortality (−38%; $P = 0.04$) were both significant.

C. Fatal and Nonfatal Events in the Double-Blind Part of the Trial

The duration of follow-up in the double-blind part of the trial averaged 3.0 years in the placebo group and 3.4 years in the actively treated group. The results of the on-treatment analysis are summarized in Table 6. The total and cardiovascular death rates amounted to 70 and 48 per 1,000 patient-years, respectively, in the placebo group. Whereas the reduction in all-cause mortality did not reach statistical significance (−26%; $P = 0.08$), the total cardiovascular mortality rate was significantly reduced (−38%; $P = 0.02$). The incidence of terminating nonfatal morbid cardiovascular events was reduced from 20 to 8 per 1,000 patient years (−60%; $P = 0.006$), mainly related to the reduction of severe congestive heart failure from 13 to 5 events per 1,000 patient years (−63%; $P = 0.01$); few other events occurred in this category, which included cerebral hemorrhage and eyeground complications. Terminating events, that is, fatal and nonfatal morbid events combined, were reduced in the active treatment group, both cardiac (−54%; $P = 0.002$) and cerebrovascular (−46%; $P = 0.06$). Terminating nonfatal nonmorbid cardiovascular events, that is, less hard data or premorbid events such as a rise in blood pressure, were reduced by 70% ($P < 0.001$).

Nonterminating cardiovascular events, that is, events that did not necessitate withdrawal from the trial, were reduced by 25% ($P = 0.12$) in the actively treated group. This was due mainly to a reduction of cerebrovascular events (−52%; $P = 0.03$), whereas the nonterminating cardiac event rate was unchanged.

The total cardiovascular event rate, including cardiovascular deaths, terminating nonfatal morbid cardiovascular events, and nonterminating cardiovascular events was reduced by 36% ($P = 0.0015$) in the actively treated group.

It can be calculated that, in 1000 hypertensive subjects older than age 60, 1 year of active treatment would prevent six fatal and 11 nonfatal cerebrovascular events, 11 fatal cardiac events and eight cases of severe congestive heart failure (6).

V. SECONDARY ANALYSES

A. Efficacy of Antihypertensive Drug Treatment According to Age, Gender, Blood Pressure, and Previous Cardiovascular Disease

The relation between outcome and randomization group, age, gender, cardiovascular complications at entry, and baseline systolic and diastolic blood pressure was determined by means of the Cox proportional hazard regression model (7).

1. *Cardiovascular Mortality*

In the intention-to-treat analysis cardiovascular mortality was higher in men than in women, higher in patients with than in those without cardiovascular complications at entry, increased with advancing age and with increasing systolic blood pressure at presentation; it was not related to diastolic blood pressure. The effect of treatment was significant in the Cox regression model even after age, gender, the presence of cardiovascular complications, and systolic and diastolic pressure at randomization were taken into account ($P = 0.01$). There were no statistically significant interactions ($P > 0.8$) between the effect of treatment and, respectively, gender, systolic blood pressure, or the presence of cardiovascular complications at entry. However, a negative age-treatment interaction was demonstrated ($P = 0.048$), related to a decrease in treatment effect with advancing age, especially in patients older than age 80.

The per-protocol analysis yielded similar results on cardiovascular mortality as the intention-to-treat analysis, but the treatment-age interaction was not significant ($P = 0.20$).

2. *Cardiovascular Study Terminating Events*

The incidence of study-terminating cardiovascular events, that is, fatal events and nonfatal morbid study-terminating events (Table 3) was higher in men and in patients with previous cardiovascular complications, increased with age and with increasing systolic blood pressure at randomization, but was not related to diastolic blood pressure. The effect of treatment on these events remained significant after adjustment for age, gender, presence of cardiovascular complications, and blood pressure. No significant interactions were present but interactions between treatment and age ($P = 0.18$) were not excluded with confidence.

B. Effect of Diuretic Treatment on Cardiovascular Events

A post hoc analysis examined the effect of the diuretic treatment on cardiovascular events, both when given alone and in conjunction with methyldopa by calculating the relative hazard rate for cardiovascular mortality and morbidity (8, 9).

In the patients treated with diuretics, the relative hazard rate for cardiovascular mortality was 0.67 in the first step of the Cox model when treatment with diuretics alone was compared with the total placebo group. This suggests that in patients receiving diuretic treatment only (57% of the active treatment group), cardiovascular mortality was reduced by 33%. After cumulative introduction of other variables into the Cox model, including age, gender, systolic blood pressure, and cardiovascular complications at randomization, the relative hazard rate was still 0.66 (95% confidence level [CL]: 0.44–0.97; $P < 0.05$). It should be realized, however, that those taking only a diuretic were a very selected group. Compared with the total placebo group, the influence of combined treatment with active methyldopa and diuretics was not significant ($P = 0.14$), but the estimated hazard rate was 0.84 and the 95% CL (0.56–1.25) overlapped that for diuretics alone (0.44–0.97).

The relative hazard rate associated with diuretic treatment, independent of other variables, was 0.48 (95% CL: 0.30–0.76; $P < 0.01$) for study-terminating cardiovascular events, that is, cardiovascular mortality and nonfatal morbid cardiovascular events. The relative hazard rate was 0.62 (0.40–0.95; $P < 0.05$) for patients receiving both active diuretic and methyldopa.

C. Influence of Antihypertensive Drug Treatment on Electrocardiographic Left Ventricular Mass

Standard 12-lead electrocardiograms (ECG) were obtained at randomization and at each yearly visit thereafter (10). The height of the R wave in aVL (RaVL) and in V5 (RV5) and the depth of the S wave in V1 (SV1) was measured. At baseline RaVL averaged 7 ± 4 (SD) mm, SV1 10 ± 5 mm and RV5 15 ± 7 mm. At randomization, RaVL was positively correlated with age and body mass index (BMI) and was lower in men than in women ($P < 0.001$). The sum of SV1 + RV5 was inversely related to age, and was higher in men than in women. After controlling for these covariates, RaVL was positively related to systolic ($r = 0.10$; $P < 0.01$) and diastolic blood pressure ($r = 0.09$; $P < 0.05$) and SV1 + RV5 to systolic pressure only ($r = 0.15$; $P < 0.001$). On follow-up, the ECG amplitudes showed divergent trends in the two treatment groups. After 1 year, they had decreased in the patients on active treatment and increased in the patients on placebo:

RaVL, −0.25 versus +0.46 mm ($P < 0.01$); SV1 + RV5, −1.6 versus +1.2 mm ($P < 0.001$). After 4 years these values were: RaVL, −0.3 versus +0.8 mm ($P < 0.01$); SV1 + RV5, −1.2 versus +3.2 mm ($P < 0.001$). Significant relationships were found between changes in ECG voltages and changes in blood pressure.

D. Risks and Benefits in the EWPHE Trial

Adverse effects were assessed in the double-blind period of the trial by calculating investigator reports of diseases and prescription of concomitant therapy, the incidence of abnormal biochemical results, and a self-administered symptom questionnaire completed by the patients (6). Questions on the following symptoms were included: faintness, sleepiness, hours of sleep, weakness in the limbs, a showed walking pace, headache, blurred vision, depression, diarrhea, nocturia, dry mouth, nasal stuffiness, nausea, poor mental concentration, and vivid dreams.

No unexpected adverse treatment effects were observed. Both the active and placebo treatment groups had similar rates for malignant neoplasms (lower than 20 per 1,000 person years), fractures (12 per 1,000 person years) and diseases of the stomach and gall bladder (less than 7 per 1,000 person years). Anemia, parkinsonism, disorders of the pancreas, and liver disease had an incidence of lower than 5 per 1,000 person years. A significant excess incidence rate was found in the active treatment group compared with placebo for:

1. Impaired renal function, that is, a serum creatinine greater than 2.0 mg/dl ($P < 0.001$)
2. Mild hypokalemia, that is, a serum potassium less than 3.5 mmol/L ($P < 0.001$)
3. Reports of gout ($P < 0.05$)
4. An elevated serum uric acid, that is, greater than 8.7 mg/dl in men or >7.7 mg/dl in women ($P < 0.001$).

More patients reported a dry mouth, blocked nose, and diarrhea in the active treatment group compared with placebo ($P < 0.05$). Dry mouth and diarrhea were associated with methyldopa rather than the diuretic. Finally, clinical reports of headache were significantly fewer in the actively treated group ($P < 0.01$).

Elevated blood sugar and prescriptions for hypoglycemic drugs tended to be more frequent in the actively treated group (6). The effect of diuretic treatment on glucose tolerance was analyzed in more detail in a subset of the patients who had entered the study by December 1983 (11). Five hundred and forty-two had a fasting blood sugar recorded initially and one or more years later. Patients receiving oral hypoglycemic drugs or insulin were excluded from the analyses. Blood sugar level was available at entry and after 1 year in 507 patients, at entry and after 2 years in 371 patients, and at entry and after 3 years in 270 patients. Blood glucose estimations were also made 1 and 2 hours after taking 50 g of glucose in 386 patients (71%). In the placebo group, small increases of 4 and 0.6 mg/dl in fasting blood sugar were observed during the second and third year in the trial. These rises followed a fall of 1.4 mg/dl in the first year. In contrast, for actively treated patients receiving a diuretic, the average fasting blood sugar rose by about 3 mg/dl for every year in the trial. The differences between the two groups in fasting blood sugar were statistically significant after 1 ($P < 0.05$), 2 ($P < 0.05$), and 3 ($P < 0.01$) years. The average blood sugar 60 minutes after the glucose load fell 6 mg/dl during the first year in the placebo group but returned almost to baseline after 3 years. In contrast, in the actively treated group, the average 60-minutes glucose increased after 2 years when it was, on average, 10 mg/dl above that of the placebo group ($P = 0.06$). The average 120 minutes glucose increased by 2 to 3 mg/dl/yr in the placebo group and about 4 mg/dl/yr in the actively treated group. These increases did not differ significantly from one another. In the actively treated group the average fasting blood sugar increased by 3 mg/dl/yr in both men and women and in both the age groups 60 to 69 and 70 to 79 years.

Another analysis assessed the influence of the antihypertensive regimen on serum cholesterol (12). During a period of up to 3 years, the average fall in cholesterol was 5.9 mg/dl/yr in the placebo group and 5.0 mg/dl/yr in the actively treated group. Thus, the changes in serum cholesterol were similar whether the patients received active or placebo medication. In particular, there was no evidence for an increase in cholesterol or for a smaller decrease during diuretic therapy.

E. Relation Between Mortality and Treated Blood Pressure

Mortality was related to the blood pressure during randomized treatment (per-protocol analysis) (13). Treated blood pressure was defined as the blood pressure at nine months of follow-up. In the two treatment groups, patients were subdivided into thirds by the 33rd and 66th centiles of their treated systolic and diastolic pressures. Mortality in the thirds of treated pressure was compared after adjustment for age and gender.

The analyses were of 339 patients randomized to placebo and 352 patients randomized to active treatment and followed up for at least 9 months. The two groups were similar at randomization in sex ratio, mean age, systolic and diastolic blood pressures, and proportion of patients with cardiovascular complications. From the visit at nine months until the end of the double-blind study, 65 patients in the placebo group and 56 in the group taking active treatment died. In patients taking placebo, total, cardiovascular, and noncardiovascular mortality tended to increase from the lower to the upper third of treated systolic pressure. In patients taking active treatment, fewer died in the middle than in the highest and lowest thirds ($P < 0.05$). A U-shaped relation was apparent between treated systolic pressure and total mortality, and a similar trend was observed for cardiovascular and for noncardiovascular mortality (Fig. 1).

When the thirds of diastolic pressure were considered, mortality from all causes was lower ($P < 0.05$) in the middle than in the two other thirds in the placebo group. Cardiovascular and noncardiovascular mortality showed a similar U-shaped tendency. In patients taking active treatment, both total ($P < 0.004$) and noncardiovascular ($P < 0.007$) mortality were higher in the lowest than the highest third of blood pressure, and a similar trend was seen for cardiovascular mortality (Fig. 2).

The increased mortality in the lowest thirds of diastolic pressure was not associated with an increased proportion of patients with cardiovascular complications at randomization or with an excessive fall in diastolic pressure. However, patients in the lowest thirds of treated pressure showed greater decreases in body weight and hemoglobin concentration than those in the middle and upper thirds of pressure. Presumably, the fall in pressure was caused by other factors (associated with increased mortality) and, as this was also observed in the placebo group, not to active antihypertensive treatment.

F. Prognostic Factors in Elderly Hypertensive Patients

In addition to age, gender, blood pressure, and cardiovascular complications at baseline, the EWPHE investigators also assessed the prognostic significance of BMI (14), serum cholesterol (15), uric acid (16), and ECG voltages (10).

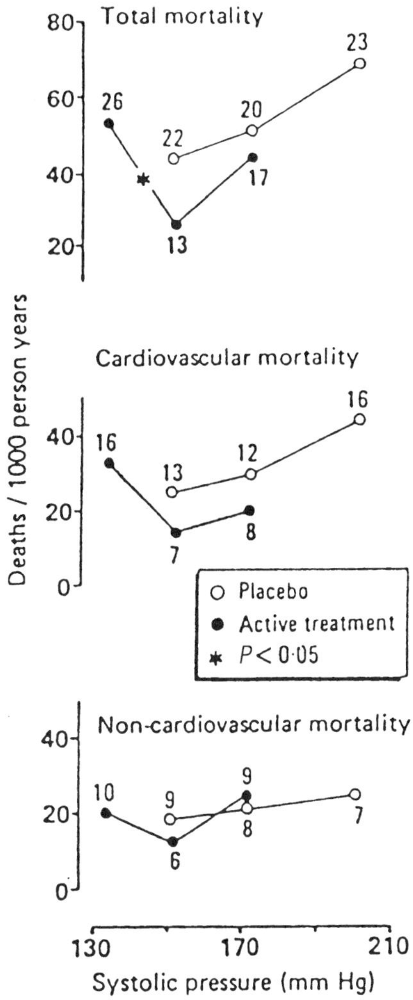

Fig. 1 Total, cardiovascular, and noncardiovascular mortalities adjusted for age and gender in thirds of treated systolic pressure in patients randomized to placebo or active treatment. Figures are numbers of deaths in each third. (From Ref. 13, used with permission.)

The initial mean BMI was 26.7 kg/m^2 in women and 25.7 kg/m^2 in men. During the trial, total mortality and cardiovascular and noncardiovascular terminating events were highest in the patients belonging to the leanest BMI quintile. The association between BMI and cardiovascular endpoints was U-shaped, whereas noncardiovascular mortality decreased with increasing BMI. The U-shaped relation was confirmed with Cox's proportional hazards model, controlling for age, gender, systolic blood pressure, hemoglobin, serum cholesterol, blood glucose, and cardiovascular complications at entry. The BMI level with the lowest risk was 28 to 29 kg/m^2 for total mortality and cardiovascular terminating events, 26 to 27 kg/m^2 for cardiovascular mortality, and 31 to 32 kg/m^2 for noncardiovascular mortality. Body mass index did not modify the favorable effects of drug treatment. There was no evidence that obesity would protect elderly hypertensive men or women from cardiovascular complications (14).

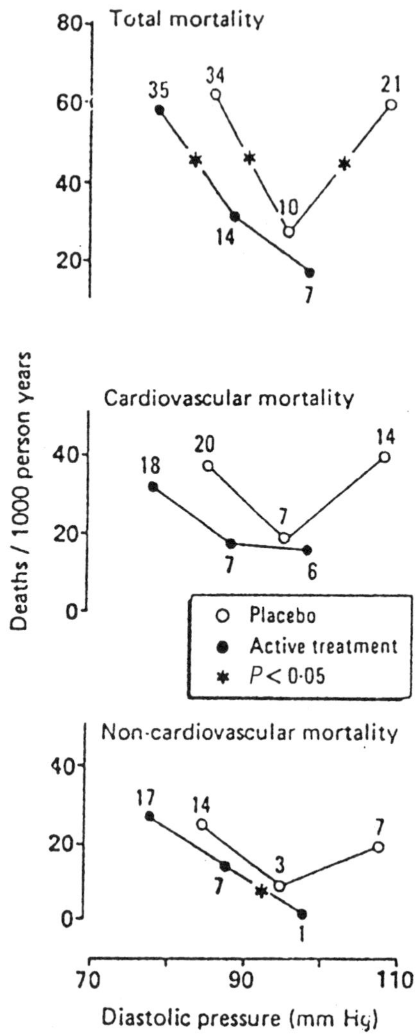

Fig. 2 Total, cardiovascular, and noncardiovascular mortalities adjusted for age and gender in thirds of treated diastolic pressure in patients randomized to placebo or active treatment. Figures are numbers of deaths in each third. (From Ref. 13, used with permission.)

Serum cholesterol averaged 246 mg/dl at baseline. Cox's proportional hazards model showed that pretreatment serum total cholesterol levels were independently and inversely correlated with the incidence of total mortality ($P = 0.03$), noncardiovascular mortality ($P = 0.02$), and cancer mortality ($P = 0.04$) during treatment. All factors being equal, an increase in total serum cholesterol of 89 mg/dl was associated with a one-year prolongation of survival. After adjustment for gender, age, pretreatment cardiovascular complications, and systolic pressure, the correlations between serum cholesterol and cardiovascular and cardiac mortality were not significant (15).

Pretreatment serum uric acid levels averaged 5.4 mg/dl, were significantly higher in men than women and had positive correlation with serum creatinine. After adjustment for serum creatinine, positive correlations of serum uric acid with body weight and fasting blood glucose in women and with serum cholesterol in men were significant. Total, cardiovascular, and noncardiovascular mortality were unrelated to initial serum uric acid levels (16).

Finally, in Cox's regression model, the amplitude of RaVL was significantly related to total mortality and to cardiovascular mortality in the data from the double-blind part of the trial; the overall results were similar in the intention-to-treat analysis. However,these correlations disappeared after adjustment for age. No significant correlation was found between SV1 + RV5 and total mortality or cardiovascular mortality (10).

VI. DISCUSSION

In 1971, when the EWPHE trial was originally planned, trials undertaken by the Veterans Administration (17, 18) and by Hamilton et al. (19) had provided evidence of efficacy of antihypertensive treatment in moderate to severe hypertension, but most of the patients included in these trials were younger than age 60. On the other hand, epidemiological evidence showed that hypertension was common in the elderly, that it was an important risk factor for cardiovascular disease in this age group, and that cardiovascular event rates in the elderly were high (1,2). Therefore, the EWPHE designed a double-blind, placebo-controlled randomized trial of antihypertensive treatment in patients ages 60 and above (3). The overall intention-to-treat analysis, combining the double-blind part of the trial and all subsequent follow-up, revealed a nonsignificant change in total mortality (−9%) but a significant 27% reduction in cardiovascular mortality rate. The latter was the result of a reduction in cardiac mortality (−38%) and a nonsignificant decrease in cerebrovascular mortality (−32%). In the double-blind part of the trial, total mortality rate was not significantly reduced (−26%), whereas cardiovascular mortality was reduced in the actively treated group (−38%) owing to a reduction in cardiac death (−47%) and a nonsignificant decrease in cerebrovascular mortality (−43%). Cardiovascular study-terminating events were significantly reduced by active treatment by 45%, and cardiovascular terminating plus nonterminating events by 36%. Active treatment reduced the incidence of severe congestive heart failure but not of mild congestive heart failure. In the patients randomized to active treatment, there were 29 fewer cardiovascular events and 18 fewer cardiovascular deaths per 1000 patient years during the double-blind part of the trial (5). In addition, the trial provided evidence of a favorable effect of antihypertensive treatment on left ventricular mass (10).

Cox proportional hazard analysis showed that cardiovascular mortality and the cardiovascular study-terminating events were significantly and independently related to treatment, age, gender, cardiovascular complications at randomization, and systolic but not diastolic blood pressure. The relative benefits of treatment observed in the trial seemed to be independent of gender, baseline blood pressure, and the presence or absence of cardiovascular complications at entry. There was some evidence that the treatment effect decreased with advancing age. Little or no benefit from treatment could be demonstrated in patients older than age 80, the great majority of whom were women. However, only 155 patients older than age 80 were included in the trial. As the proportional reductions were similar in most of the subgroups, the absolute reduction in events was greatest among those at highest risk, that is, men, and patients with cardiovascular complications at entry. However, the benefit of treatment was not established in patients older than age 80 (7).

The first-line treatment in the EWPHE-trial was a diuretic. To avoid possibly harmful decreases in serum and whole body potassium, the designers of the trial used hydrochlorothiazide, a thiazide diuretic, combined with triamterene, a potassium-sparing agent. Nevertheless, metabolic disturbances were expected, such as glucose intolerance, decrease in serum magnesium, and increases in serum uric acid, cholesterol, and triglycerides. Furthermore, part of the beneficial effect of treatment on outcome in the EWPHE trial might have been the result of the concurrent use of methyldopa for better blood pressure control. Therefore, a post hoc analysis examined the effect of the diuretic treatment on cardiovascular events, both when given alone and in conjunction with methyldopa, which was added in 35% of the patients. Using the Cox proportional hazard model, compared with placebo, a 34% reduction in cardiovascular mortality in the per-protocol analysis was demonstrated in the diuretic group; the 16% decrease in the group treated with diuretics and methyldopa was not significant. Cardiovascular study-terminating events were reduced by 52% in those on the diuretic only, and the effect of treatment was also significant in the combined group (−38%) (8, 9). It must be recognized, however, that the decision to add methyldopa to the diuretic was taken because the blood pressure was difficult to control with a diuretic alone. Thus, the group given combined therapy may well have differed from the monotherapy group in other ways that were not adjusted for in the Cox model. It is important, therefore, to be cautious about the interpretation of the data. The trialists prudently concluded that the reduction of cardiovascular events in the EWPHE-trial cannot be explained solely by the addition of methyldopa.

With regard to metabolic disturbances, only small changes were observed under treatment with a thiazide diuretic combined with a potassium-retaining agent; the difference in serum potassium between the active treatment group and the placebo group was, however, significant and averaged about 0.2 mmol/L. Serum creatinine and uric acid remained unchanged in the placebo group but increased in the active treatment group. The between-group differences averaged 0.17 mg/dl for serum creatinine and 1.2 mg/dl for uric acid (6, 9). Overall there was an increase in fasting blood sugar of 5 mg/dl in the active treatment group, which occurred mainly in the first year. The hyperglycemic effect of the diuretic appeared to be at least partly related to potassium loss, as, in both groups, impairment of glucose tolerance was most significant in those in whom serum potassium decreased (11). The serum cholesterol level was similar in both groups during the run-in period and its changes over time did not differ between the two groups (12).

Fletcher et al. (6) made an overall assessment of adverse effects by calculating the incidence of abnormal biochemical results, investigator reports of diseases, and prescriptions of concomitant therapy and the results of the self-administered symptom questionnaire. The authors concluded that the adverse effects did not outweigh the benefits of treatment in preventing stroke events, cardiac deaths, and heart failure.

The major strength of the EWPHE trial is that it was the first trial to show that treatment of elderly patients with systolic-diastolic hypertension would benefit from antihypertensive treatment. This finding was later confirmed by other trials in the elderly (20) and was readily incorporated in guidelines for the management of hypertension. Furthermore, the patients in the EWPHE trial were drawn from a wide variety of sources—community, general medical, and geriatric services in different European countries—so that the findings should have wider application than data generated from a single country or from a single source of patients. The investigators not only looked at hard endpoints, but also at symptomatic well-being. Finally, the EWPHE database was used to get a better insight into the risk factors in elderly hypertensives and to help understand the so-called J-curve phenomenon.

On the other hand, several weaknesses have to be considered. The number of randomized patients was relatively small and the number of patients who stopped the trial prematurely amounted to 36% of all randomized patients. Furthermore, the patients who left the double-blind part of the trial were only followed up for mortality and not for nonfatal events, which limited the intention-to-treat analysis to fatal events only. Nevertheless, as an American colleague would say, this was a ground-breaking, ''pivotal'' study.

ACKNOWLEDGMENT

The authors gratefully acknowledge the secretarial assistance of N. Ausseloos.

EUROPEAN WORKING PARTY ON HIGH BLOOD PRESSURE IN THE ELDERLY

Coordinators: A. Amery (Leuven) and A. De Schaepdryver (Ghent)

Steering Committee: A. Amery, A. De Schaepdryver, C. Dollery, J.V. Joossens, and T. Strasser.

Advisors: E. Freis, F. Gross, M. Healy, S. Hoobler, P. Milliez, and J. Willems.

Statistical analysis was supervised by R. Grauwels; technical assistance was provided by K. Byttebier, N. De Pue, R. Deruyck, M. Stinissen, V. Mariën, and Y. Toremans.

Collaborating centers: University Hospital Haukeland, Bergen, Norway (P. Lund-Johansen, O.J. Ohm, P. Omvik); North Karelia Project, Helsinki, Finland (A. Alasoini, A. Koistinen, A. Nissinen, P. Puska, J. Tuomilehto, R. Varis); Zuiderziekenhuis, Rotterdam, The Netherlands (W. Birkenhäger, P. de Leeuw, P. Willemse); Victoria Geriatric Unit, Glasgow, Scotland (K. Beard, J.L. C. Dall, J.P.R. MacFarlane, B.O. Williams); Aberdeen Royal Infirmary, Aberdeen, Scotland (J.C. Petrie, J. Webster); Royal College of Surgeons, Dublin, Ireland (M. Laher, P. McCormack, F. Meagher, E. O'Brien, W. O'Callaghan, K. O'Malley); Hammersmith Hospital, London, England (C.J. Bulpitt, P. Lewis, M. Murphy); St. John's Hospital, London, England (R.C. Hamdy, N.H. Perera); St. Charles' Hospital, London, England (X. Chellappah, J. Morris, A.I. Suchett-Kaye); University Hospital, Köln, West Germany (H. Feltkamp, A. Konrads, U. Laaser, K. Meurer); University Hospital Gasthuisberg, Leuven, Belgium (R. Fagard, J. Hellemans, W. Pelemans); University Hospital, Ghent, Belgium (M. Bogaert, D. Clement); Geriatric Hospital Le Valdor, Liège, Belgium (P. Brixko, A. Ernould, A. Mutsers); University Hospital St. Luc, Brussels, Belgium (J.F. De Plaen, Ch. van Ypersele); Medisch Centrum voor Huisartsen, Leuven, Belgium (M. Deruyttere); Hôpital Charles Foix, Ivry, France (P. Berthaux, F. Forette, J.F. Henry); Centro di Fisiologia Clinica e Ipertensione, Milan, Italy (G. Leonetti, X. Tammaro, L. Terzoli, A. Zanchetti); University Hospital Santa Maria, Lisbon, Portugal (F. de Padua, J. Forte, J.M. Pereira-Miguel).

The trial was carried out in consultation with WHO and supported by the Belgian National Research Foundation (NFWO) and the Belgian Hypertension Committee through grants from Merck, Sharp, and Dohme and Smith, Kline, and French. Yearly meetings of the EWPHE investigators were also sponsored by the European Economic Community, ICI, and Astra; Boehringer Pharma, Belgium, collaborated in performing the quality control.

REFERENCES

1. Kannel WB, Dawber TR, Sorlie P, Wolfe PA. Component of blood pressure and risk of atherothrombotic brain infarction: the Framingham Study. Stroke 1976; 7:327–331.
2. Amery A, Hansson L, Andrén L, Gudbransson T, Sivertsson R, Svensson A. Hypertension in the elderly. Acta Med Scand 1981; 210:221–229.
3. European Working Party on High Blood Pressure in the Elderly (EWPHE). An international trial of antihypertensive therapy in elderly patients. Objectives, protocol and organization. Arch Int Pharmacodyn Ther 1985; 275:300–334.
4. Amery A, Berthaux P, Birkenhäger W, Bulpitt C, Clement D, De Schaepdryver A, Dollery C, Ernould H, Fagard R, Forette F, Hellemans J, Kho T, Lund-Johansen P, Meurice J, Pierquin L. Antihypertensive therapy in elderly patients. Pilot trial of the European Working Party on High Blood Pressure in the Elderly. Gerontology 1977; 23:426–437.
5. Amery A, Birkenhäger W, Brixko P, Bulpitt C, Clement D, Deruyttere M, De Schaepdryver A, Dollery C, Fagard R, Forette F, Forte J, Hamdy R, Henry JF, Joossens JV, Leonetti G, Lund-Johansen P, O'Malley K, Petrie J, Strasser T, Tuomilehto J, Williams B. Mortality and morbidity results from the European Working Party on High Blood Pressure in the Elderly trial. Lancet 1985; 1:1349–1354.
6. Fletcher A, Amery A, Birkenhäger W, Bulpitt C, Clement D, de Leeuw P, Deruyttere ML, de Schaepdryver A, Dollery C, Fagard R, Forette F, Forte J, Henry JF, Koistinen A, Leonetti G, Lund-Johansen P, Nissinen A, O'Brien E, O'Malley K, Pelemans W, Petrie J, Staessen J, Terzoli L, Thijs L, Tuomilehto J, Webster J, Williams B. Risks and benefits in the trial of the European Working Party on High Blood Pressure in the Elderly. J Hypertens 1991; 9: 225–230.
7. Amery A, Birkenhäger W, Brixko P, Bulpitt C, Clement D, Deruyttere M, De Schaepdryver A, Dollery C, Fagard R, Forette F, Forte J, Hamdy R, Henry JF, Joossens JV, Leonetti G, Lund-Johansen P, O'Malley K, Petrie JC, Strasser T, Tuomilehto J, Williams B. Efficacy of antihypertensive drug treatment according to age, sex, blood pressure, and previous cardiovascular disease in patients over the age of 60. Lancet 1986; 2:589–592.
8. Amery A, Birkenhäger W, Bulpitt C, Clement D, de Leeuw P, Deruyttere ML, De Schaepdryver A, Dollery C, Fagard R, Fletcher A, Forette F, Henry JF, Koistinen A, Leonetti G, Nissinen A, O'Brien E, O'Malley K, Pelemans W, Petrie JC, Terzoli L, Tuomilehto J, Williams B. Diuretics—a risk in the long-term treatment of hypertensive patients? J Hypertens 1988; 6:925–930.
9. Fagard R, Staessen J, Amery A. Experience with diuretics in the study conducted by the European Working Party on High Blood Pressure in the Elderly (EWPHE). Prog Pharmacol Clin Pharmacol 1992; 9:463–472.
10. Van Hoof R, Staessen J, Fagard R, Thijs L, Amery A, on behalf of the EWPHE. The effect of antihypertensive treatment on electrocardiogram voltages in the EWPHE trial. J Cardiovasc Pharmacol 1991; 17(suppl 2):S101–S104.
11. Amery A, Birkenhäger W, Brixko P, Bulpitt C, Clement D, Deruyttere M, De Schaepdryver A, Fagard R, Forette F, Forte J, Hamdy R, Leonetti G, O'Malley K, Murphy M, Petrie J, Tuomilehto J, Webster J, Williams B. Glucose intolerance during diuretic therapy in elderly hypertensive patients. A second report from the European Working Party on High Blood Pressure in the Elderly (EWPHE). Postgrad Med J 1986; 62:919–924.
12. Amery A, Birkenhäger W, Bulpitt C, Clement D, Deruyttere M, De Schaepdryver A, Dollery C, Fagard R, Forette F, Forte J, Hamdy R, Leonetti G, Lund-Johansen P, MacFarlane JPR, Mutsers A, O'Malley K, Tuomilehto J. Influence of anti-hypertensive therapy on serum cholesterol in elderly hypertensive patients. Acta Cardiol 1982; 37:235–244.
13. Staessen J, Bulpitt C, Clement D, de Leeuw P, Fagard R, Fletcher A, Forette F, Leonetti G, Nissinen A, O'Malley K, Tuomilehto J, Webster J, Williams BO. Relation between mortality

and treated blood pressure in elderly patients with hypertension: report of the European Working Party on High Blood Pressure in the Elderly. BMJ 1989; 298:1552–1556.

14. Tuomilehto J, for the European Working Party on High Blood Pressure in the Elderly (EWPHE). Body mass index and prognosis in elderly hypertensive patients: a report from the European Working Party on High Blood Pressure in the Elderly trial. Am J Med 1991; 90(suppl 3A):34S–41S.
15. Fagard R, for the European Working Party on High Blood Pressure in the Elderly (EWPHE). Serum cholesterol levels and survival in elderly hypertensive patients: analysis of data from the European Working Party on High Blood Pressure in the Elderly trial. Am J Med 1991; 90(suppl 3A):62S–63S.
16. Staessen J, for the European Working Party on High Blood Pressure in the Elderly (EWPHE). The determinants and prognostic significance of serum uric acid in elderly patients of the European Working Party on High Blood Pressure in the Elderly trial. Am J Med 1991; 90(suppl 3A):50S–54S.
17. Veterans Administration Co-Operative Study Group on Anti-Hypertensive Agents. Effects of treatment on morbidity in hypertension. Results in patients with diastolic blood pressure averaging 115 through 129 mm Hg. J Am Med Assoc 1967; 202:1028–1034.
18. Veterans Administration Co-Operative Study Group on Anti-Hypertensive Agents. Effects of treatment on morbidity in hypertension. II. Results in patients with diastolic blood pressure averaging 90 through 114 mm Hg. J Am Med Assoc 1970; 213:1143–1152.
19. Hamilton M, Thompson EN, Wisniewski TKM. The role of blood pressure control in preventing complications of hypertension. Lancet 1964; I:235–238.
20. Thijs L, Fagard R, Lijnen P, Staessen J, Van Hoof R, Amery A. A meta-analysis of outcome trials in elderly hypertensives. J Hypertens 1992; 10:1103–1109.

9

The Swedish Trial in Old Patients with Hypertension (STOP-Hypertension)

LARS H. LINDHOLM

Umeå University Hospital, Umeå, Sweden

TORD EKBOM

Lund University, Malmö, Sweden

LENNART HANSSON

University of Uppsala, Uppsala, Sweden

I. INTRODUCTION

It is generally accepted that high blood pressure is a major risk factor for cardiovascular morbidity and mortality in middle-aged subjects (1–5). Does this also hold true for the elderly? In some studies, the answer is yes (6–11); in other studies, there is an inverse relation (12–15), yet others have been more indecisive and unable to show any relation between blood pressure and risk (16–19). Furthermore, in some studies the systolic blood pressure (SBP) is a better predictor than diastolic blood pressure (DBP) (7, 9, 11), whereas in others the reverse has been found (10). To further complicate the situation, several workers have demonstrated U- or J-shaped relations between blood pressure and risk (20–27). The relation between blood pressure and cardiovascular risk seems to be more complex in the elderly and could at least in part be the result of selection mechanisms during earlier years (28, 29). Most of our knowledge on this issue has been provided by observational studies on mainly middle-aged people and by trials studying the effects of antihypertensive therapy in the elderly. Thus, several studies demonstrated an increased risk of cardiovascular disease in relation to high blood pressure in younger elderly (6–8, 26), whereas the risk seems to decline with age in the older elderly (12, 14).

In the early studies on severe malignant hypertension, the benefits of treatment were obvious in middle-aged hypertensives. As milder forms of hypertension were treated, the effects were no longer so clear, and a need was felt for properly designed placebo-controlled studies. Some randomized, controlled trials carried out in young or middle-aged hypertensives contained groups of patients aged 60 and older (30–37); subgroup analyses of these elderly hypertensives showed an outcome in favor of active blood pressure-lowering treatment. Several randomized, controlled trials followed, which had recruited only elderly hypertensives (38–43). The Swedish Trial in Old Patients with Hypertension (STOP-Hypertension) (44) was one of them. The outcome of all was in favor of treatment with antihypertensive drugs (38–44). Before STOP-Hypertension, however, no effect of antihypertensive treatment had been shown in those aged 75 and older (40).

The overall *aim* of STOP-Hypertension was to investigate the effects and consequences of antihypertensive treatment in elderly hypertensives on morbidity and mortality, blood pressure, side effects, and laboratory variables.

II. MATERIAL AND METHODS

The STOP-Hypertension was a multicenter study carried out at 116 health centers (out of 846) throughout Sweden, where hypertensive men and women aged 70 to 84 years were randomly allocated double-blind administration of active hypertensive therapy or placebo. Patients were included consecutively if they were willing to participate (and gave informed consent) and had untreated or treated essential hypertension (Table 1). The entry criteria were that on three separate occasions, the SBP was 180 mm Hg or above with a DBP of at least 90 mm Hg, or that the DBP was above 105 mm Hg irrespective of the systolic pressure during a 1-month placebo run-in phase in previously untreated patients. The run-in phase was preceded by a 1 to 6 month washout period in previously treated patients.

Recruitment took place between November 14, 1985 and October 31, 1990. The number of patients recruited was 1627, of whom 812 (mean age 75.7, SD 3.7) were randomly allocated to active treatment and 815 (mean age 75.6, SD 3.7) to placebo (Table 2). The average follow-up time when primary endpoints were considered was 25 months. The study was terminated on April 8, 1991 on the advice of the safety committee; investigators were advised that all blinded medication should be discontinued. All surviving patients were recalled and examined at the end of the study. No patient was lost to follow-up.

Table 1 Inclusion Criteria

- Men and women ages 70–84
- Blood pressure on three separate occasions of SBP $\geq$ 180 mm Hg and DBP $\geq$ 90 mm Hg, or DBP $\geq$ 105 mm Hg after 1 month of placebo if untreated or 1–6 month washout if previously treated
- Informed consent

Abbreviations: SBP, systolic blood pressure; *DBP*, diastolic blood pressure.

Table 2 Baseline Characteristics of Patients in STOP-Hypertension by Treatment Group

	Placebo (n = 815)	Active (n = 812)
Mean (SD) age in yr	75.7 (3.7)	75.6 (3.7)
No. (%) aged		
70–74 yr	351 (43%)	363 (45%)
75–79 yr	331 (41%)	313 (39%)
≥80 yr	133 (16%)	136 (17%)
No. (%) female	509 (63%)	510 (63%)
Mean (SD) body mass index (kg/m^2)	26.5 (3.8)	26.7 (3.9)
Mean (SD) blood pressure (mm Hg)		
Supine systolic	195 (14)	195 (14)
Supine diastolic	102 (7)	102 (7)
Standing systolic	188 (17)	187 (17)
Standing diastolic	104 (9)	104 (9)
Mean (SD) heart rate (bpm)		
Supine	76 (11)	77 (11)
Standing	82 (11)	82 (11)
No. (%) previously treated*	416 (51%)	438 (54%)
No. (%) smokers*	58 (7%)	69 (9%)
Previous stroke†‡	36 (4.5%)	32 (4%)
Previous myocardial infarction†‡	16 (2%)	17 (2.1%)
Diabetes mellitus‡	58 (7.2%)	69 (8.6%)

* Less than 6 months before run-in period.
† More than 12 months before randomization.
‡ Based on placebo n = 808, active n = 807.
Abbreviations: SD, standard deviation; *bpm*, beats per minute.
Source: Ref. 44.

III. EXCLUSION CRITERIA

Reasons for exclusion were supine blood pressure above 230 mm Hg systolic and/or 120 mm Hg diastolic; isolated systolic hypertension (180 mm Hg or higher with diastolic below 90 mm Hg); orthostatic hypotension (more than 30 mm Hg fall in SBP on standing); contraindications to any of the drugs; myocardial infarction or a stroke during the previous 12 months; angina pectoris requiring treatment with drugs other than glyceryltrinitrate; other severe or incapacitating illnesses; or unwillingness to take part (Table 3).

Table 3 Exclusion Criteria

- Supine blood pressure above 230 mm Hg systolic and/or 120 mm Hg diastolic
- Isolated systolic hypertension (180 mm Hg or higher with diastolic below 90 mm Hg)
- Orthostatic hypotension (more than 30 mm Hg fall in systolic blood pressure on standing)
- Contraindications to any of the drugs
- Myocardial infarction or a stroke during the previous 12 months
- Angina pectoris requiring treatment with drugs other than glyceryltrinitrate
- Other severe or incapacitating illnesses
- Unwillingness to take part

Table 4

Treatment consisted of:
• Atenolol 50 mg (Tenormin®)
• Hydrochlorothiazide (HCTZ) 25 mg plus amiloride (Am) 2.5 mg (Moduretic® mite)
• Metoprolol CR 100 mg (Seloken® ZOC)
• Pindolol 5 mg (Viskén®) or the matching placebo

IV. BLOOD PRESSURE MEASUREMENTS

It was standard in Swedish clinical practice that blood pressure measurements were taken with a mercury sphygmomanometer with the subject in a supine position. Blood pressure was measured by the same observer (nurse or doctor) for each patient throughout the study after five minutes of recumbent rest and after one minute of standing, by means of a mercury sphygmomanometer. The standard cuff bladder measures 12 × 35 cm, but larger (15 × 43 cm) or smaller (9 × 25 cm) cuffs were used in patients with arm circumferences larger than 32 cm or less than 22 cm, respectively. Disappearance of the Korotkoff sounds was recorded as the DBP. The average value of two recordings in the supine position, measured to the nearest 2 mm Hg, was the main blood pressure variable upon which inclusion, changes in dosage, and so on, were determined.

A. Drugs

Treatment consisted of atenolol 50 mg (Tenormin®), hydrochlorothiazide (HCTZ) 25 mg, plus amiloride (Am) 2.5 mg (Moduretic® mite), metoprolol CR 100 mg (Seloken® ZOC), or pindolol 5 mg (Viskén®), or the matching placebo (Table 4). All drugs were given once daily. If the supine blood pressure was 160 mm Hg systolic or 95 mm Hg diastolic or above after at least two months of treatment or at any later point during the study, the diuretic was added to any of the β-blockers or vice versa. Each center was free to choose any of the four basic regimens, which then had to be maintained throughout the study. The patients were randomized to active treatment or placebo but not to the four different treatment regimens. Placebo tablets were identical in shape, taste, and color to the active medication. If supine blood pressure exceeded 230/120 mm Hg (and/or) on two subsequent visits the patient was changed to open antihypertensive treatment. After a nonfatal endpoint, a patient could continue on double-blind treatment.

V. LABORATORY VARIABLES

At randomization and at months 2, 6, 12, 24, 36, 48, and 60, blood was drawn at the health centers with the patient in a nonfasting state, and the samples were analyzed at the departments of clinical chemistry at the local hospitals to which the health centers normally refer. The following analyses were carried out with the method used in the daily routine: serum sodium (S-Na^+), serum potassium (S-K^+), serum urate (S-urate), serum creatinine (S-creatinine), blood glucose (B-glucose), blood hemoglobin (B-Hb), and total serum cholesterol (S-cholesterol) (Table 5).

Table 5

Laboratory Variables
• Serum sodium
• Serum potassium
• Serum urate
• Serum creatinine
• Blood glucose
• Blood hemoglobin
• Total serum cholesterol

VI. ADVERSE EFFECTS

At the visits 2 and 12 months after randomization, the patients were asked about adverse effects in the following structured way:

Have you experienced any of these symptoms since your last visit to the health center?

1. Have you felt more tired than usual?
2. Have you felt depressed?
3. Have you had sleep disturbances?
4. Have you felt dizzy when up walking?
5. Have you felt dizzy when standing up?
6. Has your mouth felt dry?
7. Have you been short of breath or wheezy?
8. Have your ankles been swollen at night?
9. Have you experienced chest pain when carrying out physical exercise?
10. Have you felt muscle discomfort or cramp?
11. Have your hands and/or feet felt cold frequently?
12. Have you noticed a slow heart rate?
13. Have you noticed an irregular heart beat?
14. Have you had acute, severe pain in your big toe or in any other joint?

The symptoms (if any) were graded by the patients as mild or severe.

VII. ENDPOINTS

Endpoints were evaluated by an independent endpoint committee, unaware of treatment given or blood pressure. Their evaluation was based on medical records, death certificates, and necropsy reports, as appropriate. Primary endpoints were fatal and nonfatal stroke, fatal and nonfatal myocardial infarction, and other cardiovascular death (Table 6). Stroke was defined as a persisting (longer than 24 hours) neurological deficit with sudden onset

Table 6

Primary Endpoints
• Stroke
• Myocardial infarction
• Other cardiovascular death

(excluding nonvascular causes). Myocardial infarction was defined by the presence of at least two of the following three criteria: (a) chest pain (retrosternal), lasting longer than 15 minutes and with onset within the preceding 48 hours, or pulmonary edema in the absence of known valvular disease, or syncope without hypovolemia/intoxication; (b) changes on electrocardiography (diminished R-wave amplitude or pathological Q-waves; (c) temporary rises in serum aspartate aminotransferase activity (two or more results above the reference value) with a maximum 24 hours after the onset of symptoms, or changes in serum alanine aminotransferase activity, lactate dehydrogenase isoenzyme pattern, or creatine kinase activity. The diagnosis of stroke or myocardial infarction could also be made at necropsy. Other cardiovascular death included sudden death (unexpected death within one hour of onset of symptoms and without obvious cause), fatal congestive heart failure, and fatal cardiovascular events not covered by the above definitions (such as ruptured aortic aneurysm). Endpoints considered were stroke (fatal and nonfatal) and cardiac events (fatal and nonfatal myocardial infarction, sudden death, and congestive heart failure), defined as above.

VIII. STATISTICS

All analyses were based on the intention-to-treat principle. No on-treatment analysis has been performed. For continuous variables, 95% confidence intervals (95% Cl) were determined by use of the *t*-distribution, that is, the variables were assumed to be normally distributed. Confidence intervals for proportions were calculated by usual normal distribution approximations. All tests were two sided.

IX. RESULTS AND COMMENTS

Two months after randomization into STOP-Hypertension, all patients were still undergoing single drug therapy, and active treatment and placebo had lowered supine blood pressure by 13 to 25/9 to 11 mm Hg and 7 to 8/4 to 5 mm Hg, respectively. When comparing the ''net'' effects of single drug therapy, all four regimens gave approximately the same effect on diastolic blood pressure (5.3 to 6.4 mm Hg) but HCTZ + Am was more effective in lowering systolic blood pressure (17.6 mm Hg). Pindolol tended to be more effective in lowering supine systolic blood pressure (11.4 mm Hg) than metoprolol CR or atenolol (6.3 and 7.2 mm Hg, respectively) (Table 7).

After 12 months of treatment, 65% of the actively treated patients received supplementary drugs. A majority of those starting with a β-blocker received supplementary treatment (68% to 78%), compared with those who started with the diuretic (40%). Those receiving placebo had supplementary placebo treatment in approximately 80%. After addition of supplementary treatment, there were no significant differences in blood pressure lowering between the groups, which was evident already at the 6-month visit (data not given). When adding supplementary treatment, there was a further reduction in the blood pressure by 13.6/4.9 mm Hg in the metoprolol group in which 78.1% received supplementary treatment; 15.4/4.2 mm Hg (68.3% supplement) in the atenolol group; 12.8/4.0 mm Hg (72.5% supplement) in the pindolol group; and 0.6/1.3 mm Hg (40.2% supplement) in the HCTZ + Am group.

At the last follow-up before study termination in STOP-Hypertension, the supine blood pressure was 186/96 (SD 22/10) mm Hg in the placebo group and 167/87 (SD 21/9) mm Hg in the actively treated group (difference of 19.5/8.1 mm Hg). At the end of

Table 7 Efficacy of Drug Treatment on Blood Pressure (mm Hg) and Heart Rate (beats/min) 0–2 Months. Difference Between Active and Placebo Treatment = (active [2 months] − placebo [2 months]) − (active [0]-placebo [0]); 95% CI

	Metoprolol CR	Atenolol	Pindolol	HCTZ + Am
Supine				
SBP	−6.3 (−10.7, −1.8)	−7.2 (−11.8, −2.6)	−11.4 (−16.8, −5.9)	−17.6 (−21.7, −13.6)
DBP	−5.3 (−7.4, −3.2)	−6.4 (−8.7, −4.1)	−5.9 (−8.8, −3.1)	−5.8 (−7.7, −3.9)
Heart rate	−9.4 (−12.3, −6.5)	−14.4 (−17.4, −11.4)	−7.3 (−10.8, −3.7)	−0.5 (−3.0, −2.0)
Standing				
SBP	−6.4 (−11.7, −1.1)	−7.1 (−12.9, −1.4)	−9.3 (−15.7, −2.9)	17.7 (−22.4, −13.1)
DBP	−4.9 (−7.4, −2.3)	−7.5 (−10.3, −4.7)	−7.5 (−10.9, −4.2)	−7.7 (−9.8, −5.5)
Heart rate	−9.8 (−12.9, −6.8)	−17.8 (−20.8, −14.7)	−9.7 (−13.8, −5.6)	−1.2 (−1.6, 4.0)

Abbreviations: HCTZ + Am, hydrochlorothiazide plus amiloride; *SBP*, systolic blood pressure; *DBP*, diastolic blood pressure.
Source: From Ref. 54.

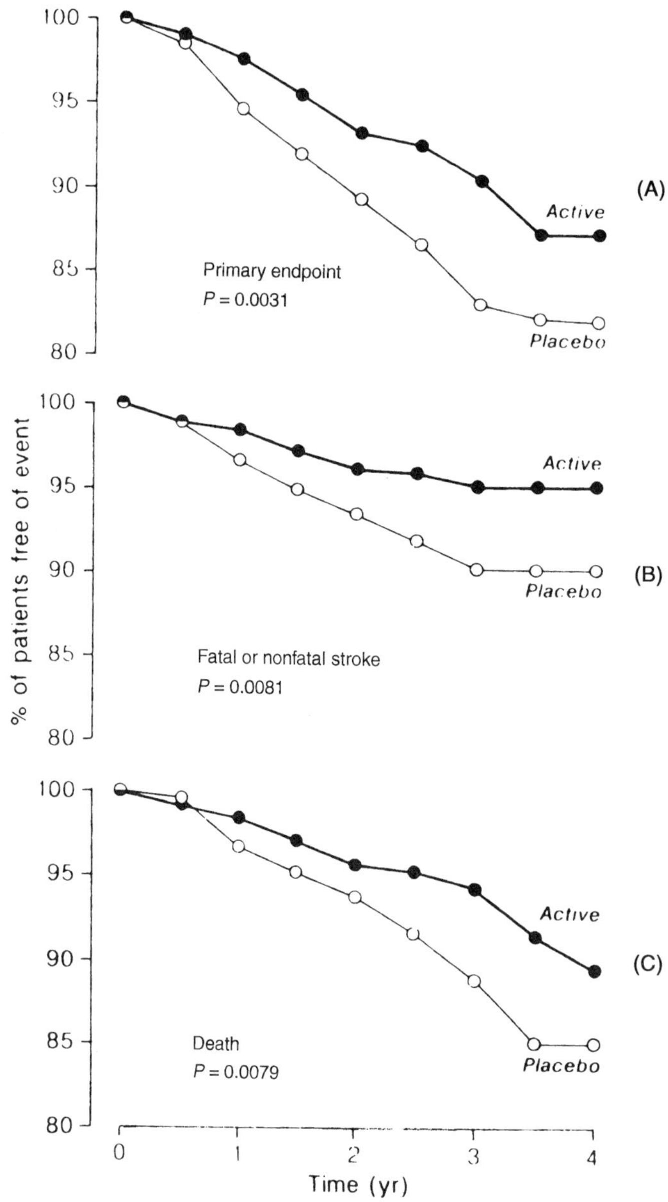

Fig. 1 Percentages of patients who have escaped a primary end point (**A**), fatal or nonfatal stroke (**B**), or death (**C**) during four years of treatment. Survival functions estimated by maximum likelihood method assuming constant hazard functions within 6-month periods; P-values apply to total study period. (From Ref. 44, used with permission.)

the study, 77% of the placebo group and 84% of the actively treated group were still taking the study medication and two-thirds of the actively treated patients received combined treatment.

The complete blood pressure goal in STOP-Hypertension (less than 160 mm Hg systolic *and* less than 95 mm Hg diastolic), at the 2-month visit, was attained by only 9% to 15% of the patients given β-blockers and 30% of those receiving HCTZ + Am. At the 12-month visit, the corresponding figures had risen from 22% to 39% and 35%, respectively.

A. Comments

Our findings clearly showed that administration of active hypertensive therapy reduced supine blood pressure substantially in comparison with placebo in hypertensive patients aged 70 to 84. Before discussing the differences in antihypertensive efficacy of the four drugs used in STOP-Hypertension, it was necessary to establish that the composition of the study groups did not differ. Before the start of the study, each health center was free to choose its basic and supplementary treatment. The 95% CIs at randomization overlapped for all four treatment regimens and their corresponding placebos. In fact, even the attained blood pressure levels after 2 months were equal for the four placebo groups. At the 2-month visit (when all patients were still on monotherapy), all four drugs were equally effective in lowering diastolic blood pressure. There were, however, considerable differences in their efficacy in lowering systolic blood pressure: as monotherapy, HCTZ + Am was more effective than the β-blockers (40% vs 68% to 78%). This finding is in accordance with the results of the Medical Research Council (MRC) trial in the elderly (42), where HCTZ + Am was found to lower systolic blood pressure better than atenolol, whereas there was no difference in the drugs' efficacy on diastolic pressure. In all patients in STOP-Hypertension, more than two-thirds of the patients were given supplementary treatment, most of them already after the 2-month visit. After addition of supplementary treatment, there was no significant difference in the lowering of blood pressure between the treatment regimens, and the attained blood pressure reduction was in line with what could be expected (39, 45, 46) (see Fig. 1).

The complete blood pressure goal of STOP-Hypertension (less than 160 and less than 95 mm Hg) was only attained in a minority of the patients at the 2-month visit. At the 12-month visit—after addition of supplementary treatment—only 22% to 35% of the patients had attained the goal. Even so, the outcome of the STOP study was satisfactory, with a considerable reduction in the incidence of cardiovascular disease in the patients receiving active treatment, as shown below.

X. ACTIVE ANTIHYPERTENSIVE TREATMENT AND MORBIDITY AND MORTALITY

Compared with placebo, active treatment significantly reduced the number of primary endpoints (94 vs 58; $P = 0.0031$), fatal and nonfatal stroke (53 vs 29; $P = 0.0081$), and total mortality (63 vs 36; $P = 0.0079$) (Table 8) (see Fig. 1).

The beneficial effects of active antihypertensive treatment were discernible at all ages studied. From life table analysis, it was evident that patients receiving active treatment had significantly fewer primary endpoints, lower morbidity and mortality from stroke, and lower total mortality than those on placebo; these effects were apparent early in the study and became more pronounced with time. Women seemed to have a better effect from the

Table 8 Primary Endpoints and Mortality by Treatment Group

	All Placebo		Active		
	No.	No. per 1000 patient-yr	No.	No. per 1000 patient-yr	Relative risk (95% CI)
Primary endpoint*					
All MI	28	16.5	25	14.4	0.87 (0.49, 1.56)
Fatal MI	6	3.5	6	3.5	0.98 (0.26, 3.66)
All stroke	53	31.3	29	16.8	0.53 (0.33, 0.86)
Fatal stroke	12	7.1	3	1.7	0.24 (0.04, 0.91)
Other CV death†	13	7.7	4	2.3	0.30 (0.07, 0.97)
Total	94	55.5	58	33.5	0.60 (0.43, 0.85)
Mortality‡					
Fatal MI	8	4.5	6	3.4	0.75 (0.21, 2.47)
Fatal stroke	15	8.4	4	2.3	0.27 (0.06, 0.86)
Sudden death	12	6.8	4	2.3	0.33 (0.08, 1.10)
Other CV death	6	3.4	3	1.7	0.50 (0.08, 2.34)
Total deaths§	63	35.4	36	20.2	0.57 (0.37, 0.87)

* Only the first endpoint to happen.
† Including sudden death.
‡ Irrespective of preceding nonfatal primary endpoint.
§ All causes.
Abbreviations: *MI*, myocardial infarction; *CV*, cardiovascular; *95% CI*, 95% confidence interval.
Source: From Ref. 44.

treatment than men, even though this difference was not statistically significant (Table 9). There was no difference in the attained blood pressure level between the two genders (data not given). During the study, 172 secondary endpoints occurred, 132 in the placebo group and 40 in the actively treated group ($P < 0.001$). These endpoints were congestive heart failure (39 vs 19), hypertension (above 230/120 mm Hg; 75 vs 10), transient ischemic attacks (9 vs 3), and angina pectoris (9 vs 8).

A. Comments

These results are at least as positive as those of previous intervention trials in young and middle-aged hypertensive patients. As well as supporting previous positive results of antihypertensive therapy in young elderly populations (38, 39), our study clearly shows

Table 9 Endpoint Rates (number per 1000 person years) According to Sex; Relative Risk; 95% Confidence Interval

	Males			Females			
	Active	Placebo	RR	Active	Placebo	RR	RR Males/RR Females (95% CI)
All mortality	23.2	49.0	0.47	18.5	27.2	0.68	0.69 (0.30; 1.59)
All stroke	25.8	31.6	0.81	11.7	31.1	0.38	2.17 (0.86; 5.42)
All MI	24.2	23.7	1.02	9.0	12.2	0.73	1.39 (0.47; 4.13)

Abbreviations: *RR*, relative risk; *95% CI*, 95% confidence interval; *MI*, myocardial infarction.
Source: From Ref. 47.

that antihypertensive treatment can be beneficial in old elderly hypertensive patients. In many previous intervention trials against various cardiovascular risk factors, there have been positive effects of treatment on particular endpoints, such as stroke morbidity or mortality, without significant effects on total mortality. Because a reduction in total mortality is as desirable a goal as an effect on individual endpoints, the highly significant reduction in total mortality obtained with active hypertensive treatment is important. Perhaps equally important is the substantial decline in stroke morbidity. Also of interest is the clear effect of active treatment on the incidence of stroke in women in the present study (11.7 vs 31.1 per 1000 person-years). In men, this effect was less impressive (25.8 vs 31.6). In the European Working Party, on High Blood Pressure in the Elderly (EWPHE) trial, the treatment effect on all cardiovascular mortality (stroke was not separated in this analysis) tended to be better in men than in women (39, 40). The same tendency was seen for stroke in the Systolic Hypertension in the Elderly Program (SHEP) study (41). In the MRC trial in the elderly, there was no difference between the sexes (42).

XI. BLOOD PRESSURE AND CARDIOVASCULAR EVENTS

It can be asked, which blood pressure variable is the most efficient predictor of stroke and cardiac event, and which linear combination of all possible combinations is the best predictor? We found DBP to be a much stronger predictor of cardiovascular disease than SBP, mean arterial pressure, pulse pressure, and postural change of blood pressure (47). We have also analyzed the predictive value of SBP alone, without the influence of DBP, and found SBP to be a very weak and nonsignificant predictor of cardiovascular disease (47).

In the whole study group (n = 1627), the risk of stroke increased by 3% per mm Hg ($P = 0.0247$) and the risk of a cardiac event increased by 2% per mm Hg ($P = 0.0376$) with increasing DBP for a given systolic pressure. For increasing SBP there was a nonsignificant decrease in stroke by 0.5% per mm Hg, and a nonsignificant increase in cardiac events by 0.2% per mm Hg for a given diastolic pressure.

A. Comments

In the present study, cardiovascular endpoints were related to the in-study DBP and not to the systolic one. This was not so in the EWPHE study, in which the opposite was found. It should be remembered, however, that the EWPHE trial recruited patients mostly from (university) clinics, 35% of whom had had a cardiovascular complication at entry (39, 40), whereas STOP-Hypertension was carried out in Swedish primary health care in patients with fewer complications at entry (Table 2). Patients in the STOP trial were also four years older and had higher blood pressure at randomization than those in the EWPHE trial.

XII. ACTIVE ANTIHYPERTENSIVE TREATMENT AND LABORATORY VARIABLES

The changes in laboratory values over time were limited (data not shown here). As expected, at the 12-month visit both serum creatinine and serum urate were slightly increased in all four groups (47). In Table 10, the relative changes in risk associated with an increase of one U (mmol/L, g/L, or μmol/L) in the laboratory variables is given; all the laboratory

Table 10 The Relative Change in Risk (%) with a 1-U Increase in the Laboratory Variable (95% CI)

Variable	Stroke	Cardiac events
S-cholesterol (mmol/L)	3.7% (−17.8%, 30.7%)	−8.3% (−25.3%, 12.5%)
S-creatinine (μmol/L)	0.1% (−0.9%, 1.1%)	0.3% (−0.5%, 1.1%)
B-glucose (mmol/L)	−5.1% (−16.4%, 7.8%)	2.8% (−5.5%, 12.0%)
B-hemoglobin (g/L)	0.8% (−1.0%, 2.7%)	0.6% (−3.5%, 4.8%)
S-potassium (mmol/L)	−4.2% (−47.3%, 74.0%)	21.8% (−24.9%, 97.4%)
S-sodium (mmol/L)	7.7% (−0.9%, 17.0%)	−1.1% (−7.5%, 5.8%)
S-urate (μmol/L)	0.1% (−0.2%, 0.4%)	0.1% (−0.1%, 0.3%)

Abbreviations: S, serum; B, blood.
Source: From Ref. 47.

variables were nonsignificant as risk factors, whereas smoking and age came out highly significant, especially for cardiac events (data not given here; for further data, see Ref. 47).

A. Comments

The present analyses clearly show that the changes in laboratory values were limited and in line with what could be expected from other studies in which diuretics have been used (38, 39, 41). Even though a majority of our actively treated patients were given a diuretic, there were no negative effects on the blood glucose values. This could be explained by the use of a potassium-sparing agent (48).

When the results of other studies in the elderly are considered, the list of contradictory results can be made long, illustrating the need for large observational studies like that of the Multiple Risk Factor Intervention Trial (MRFIT) study ($n = 356{,}222$), which gave data on middle-aged men with high precision (49). In the EWPHE study (39) comprising 822 elderly patients, 160 of whom died, there was a 14% (95% CI: 1%, 25%) decrease in total mortality for each 1-mmol/L increase in S-cholesterol. There was also an inverse trend for cardiovascular mortality ($P = 0.08$), based on 106 deaths. In the MRC trial (42), the relative risk for 1-mmol/L increase in cholesterol was 0.94 (95% CI: 0.84, 1.06) and for coronary disease, 1.27 (95% CI: 1.14, 1.41). In our own study, there was a nonsignificant decrease of −8.3% (95% CI: −25.3%, 12.5%) in cardiac events with an increase of 1-mmol/L in S-cholesterol. In contrast, another study from the Bronx of 708 old patients (mean age 82 years) with a 41-month follow-up and 213 coronary events, had a β-coefficient of 0.017 ($p < 0.005$) in a logistic regression model (50), which equals a 1.7% increase of risk per 1 mmol/L increase in S-cholesterol. In the Framingham heart study, a 1% increase in cholesterol led to a 2% increase in incidence of coronary heart disease, and this was so also for subjects aged 60 to 70 years. To reach significance in elderly subjects it was, however, necessary to increase the follow-up period from two to ten years (51). In the oldest age group of the Framingham study, the numbers were very limited and the results far from consistent; for example, there was a clear tendency toward decreasing coronary heart disease in elderly women in the highest cholesterol quintiles (52).

XIII. ACTIVE ANTIHYPERTENSIVE TREATMENT AND SIDE EFFECTS

No unexpected, serious, or previously unknown side effects were evident during the study. Fifty-eight patients on active treatment and 47 on placebo discontinued randomized treatment because of subjective side effects not classified as any specific clinical event (difference not significant). Congestive heart failure was less common in the actively treated group than placebo (19 vs 39 cases). The only significant differences found in the prevalence of symptoms at the 2-month visit (active treatment compared with placebo in monotherapy) were more dryness in the mouth (atenolol), fewer swollen ankles (metoprolol CR, HCTZ + Am), more muscle discomfort/cramp (pindolol), more reduced heart rate (atenolol), and less irregular heartbeat (HCTZ + Am). At the 12-month visit (65% with supplementary treatment), the findings were similar with a few exceptions (Table 11): there were no longer any differences in swollen ankles (metoprolol CR, HCTZ + Am), but there were more patients with cold hands and feet (atenolol).

A. Comments

Our data show that the satisfactory effect on cardiovascular morbidity and mortality was not impaired by a low tolerability of the drugs. In the EWPHE study, however, more clinical side effects were reported, especially among the 35% of patients who were given

Table 11 Difference* in Prevalence (%) of Symptoms (Mild and Severe Combined) Between Active and Placebo Groups after 12 Months of Drug Therapy (95% CI)

	Metoprolol CR	Atenolol	Pindolol	HCTZ + Am
Tired	3.3%	3.8%	−4.3%	−6.6%
	(−5.4, 12.0)	(−5.6, 13.2)	(−15.5, 6.9)	(−14.5, 1.2)
Depressed	−3.7%	3.9%	−4.3%	4.7%
	(−11.0, 3.6)	(−3.3, 11.1)	(−12.8, 4.2)	(−1.7, 11.1)
Disturbed sleep	2.9%	6.1%	4.3%	2.3%
	(−6.2, 12.0)	(−2.4, 14.7)	(−5.9, 14.5)	(−5.6, 10.2)
Dizziness	−2.5%	2.8%	4.3%	−2.3%
	(−9.7, 4.7)	(−4.6, 10.1)	(−4.9, 13.5)	(−9.0, 4.5)
Dizzy on rising	4.1%	−1.8%	−1.7%	−1.5%
	(−2.7, 10.9)	(−8.8, 5.2)	(−9.6, 6.1)	(−7.0, 4.0)
Dry mouth	4.2%	12.2%	−2.6%	0.7%
	(−4.9, 13.4)	(2.6, 21.8)	(−13.7, 8.5)	(−7.6, 9.1)
Short of breath	1.8%	5.6%	7.8%	−2.2%
	(−4.5, 8.2)	(−1.0, 12.3)	(−0.2, 15.7)	(−7.4, 2.9)
Swollen ankles	−2.8%	−2.9%	−3.4%	−2.3%
	(−9.5, 3.8)	(−9.5, 3.7)	(−12.8, 5.9)	(−7.7, 3.1)
Chest pain	1.8%	−1.2%	−2.6%	4.3%
	(−3.1, 6.7)	(−7.4, 5.0)	(−10.3, 5.1)	(−0.5, 9.0)
Muscular discomfort/cramp	2.1%	7.7%	22.4%	−2.1%
	(−5.7, 9.8)	(−0.9, 16.4)	(12.2, 32.6)	(−9.3, 5.1)
Cold hands/feet	6.7%	13.5%	0.9%	0.3%
	(−2.5, 15.9)	(3.8, 23.1)	(−9.3, 11.0)	(−7.4, 8.0)
Slow heart rate	0.2%	4.0%	0.9%	2.4%
	(−3.3, 3.7)	(0.0, 7.9)	(−0.8, 2.5)	(−0.4, 5.2)
Irregular heart rate	−3.4%	−1.2%	−2.6%	−10.0%
	(−9.0, 2.2)	(−6.5, 4.1)	(−8.0, 2.9)	(−15.4, −4.6)
Pain in big toe	−1.0%	−1.2%	1.7%	−1.0%
	(−5.2, 3.2)	(−5.0, 2.6)	(−4.4, 7.8)	(−4.1, 2.1)

Note: A negative figure indicates the symptom is more prevalent in the placebo group.
* Difference = active [12 months] − placebo [12 months].
Source: From Ref. 54.

supplementary treatment with methyldopa (44). It is interesting that so few patients in STOP-Hypertension complained of tiredness or disturbed sleep, even though the majority of the actively treated patients received β-blockers (Table 11). Significantly more patients in the group receiving pindolol, however, complained of muscle discomfort or cramp. This finding has been previously described and some suggestions for its mechanism have been made (53). In the Hypertension in Elderly Patients in Primary Care (HEP) study, there were no differences in symptoms between patients given active treatment and those given no treatment at all (38).

Finally, let us turn to some limitations of STOP-Hypertension. First, we have included relatively healthy hypertensives, as those with other, more serious cardiovascular diseases have been excluded according to the study protocol. This has been necessary because of the use of placebo in the trial. It is reasonable to believe that those with organ damage would have benefited at least as much as those without complications. Second, the studies have only been carried out during a limited period. The STOP-Hypertension study was ended for ethical reasons after a mean follow-up of only 25 months. It is difficult to say, but reasonable to believe, that the outcome would have been even better if the study had been allowed to continue for another three years as originally planned. Third, only diuretics and β-blockers were used. Therefore, STOP-Hypertension gives no information about the efficacy of the other two major groups of modern antihypertensives (angiotensin-converting enzyme-inhibitors and calcium antagonists), which may be more suitable for an individual patient because of his or her other diseases; in this age group, patients often have more than two or three diagnoses. The efficacy of these drugs has been tested in STOP-Hypertension-2. Fourth, the results are only valid for patients who fulfill the blood pressure criteria used. In STOP-Hypertension, patients had to have a SBP value at three separate visits (mean of two recordings at each visit) between 180 and 230 mm Hg with a diastolic pressure of at least 90 mm Hg, or a diastolic pressure between 105 and 120 mm Hg, irrespective of the systolic pressure. Furthermore, during this period, the patients received placebo treatment. This means that the treatment effect in STOP-Hypertension was shown in patients with relatively high blood pressure levels. Mean blood pressure at randomization was 195/102 (SD 14/7) mm Hg. Most patients who visit Swedish health centers for high blood pressure have lower blood pressure levels, and it is likely that treatment is less beneficial. Fifth, patients with other, serious noncardiovascular diseases (such as cancer) have not been included in the studies. Great care should be taken when treatment is considered in these patients.

XIV. CONCLUSION

Antihypertensive drug treatment in hypertensive men and women ages 70 to 84 confers highly significant and clinically relevant reductions in cardiovascular (especially stroke) morbidity and mortality, as well as in total mortality.

The β-blockers metoprolol CR, atenolol, and pindolol, and the diuretic combination of hydrochlorothiazide and amiloride were equally effective as single drugs in lowering DBP. There were differences in their efficacy in lowering SBP: the diuretic was more effective than the β-blockers in doing so. After addition of supplementary treatment, there were no significant differences between the groups in blood pressure lowering efficacy. The changes in laboratory values and in the prevalence of symptoms were minor for all active treatment regimens compared with placebo. Thus, the satisfactory effect on cardiovascular morbidity and mortality was not impaired by a low tolerability to the drugs.

REFERENCES

1. The Pooling Project Research Group. Relationship of blood pressure, serum cholesterol, smoking habit, relative weight and ECG abnormalities to incidence of major coronary events: final report of the Pooling Project. J Chronic Dis 1978; 31:201–306.
2. Kannel WB, Gordon T, Schwartz MJ. Systolic versus diastolic blood pressure and risk of coronary heart disease. The Framingham study. Am J Cardiol 1971; 27:335–346.
3. Uemura K. International trends in cardiovascular disease in the elderly. Eur Heart J 1988; 9(suppl D):1–8.
4. Rutan GH, Kuller LH, Neaton JD, Wentworth DN, McDonald RH, Smith WM. Mortality associated with diastolic hypertension and isolated systolic hypertension among men screened for the Multiple Risk Factor Intervention Trial. Circulation 1988; 77:504–514.
5. Collins R, Peto R, Macmahon S, Hebert P, Fiebach NH, Eberlein KA, Godwin J, Qizilbash N, Taylor JO, Hennekens CH. Blood pressure, stroke, and coronary heart disease. Part 2, Short-term reductions in blood pressure: overview of randomised drug trials in their epidemiological context. Lancet 1990; 335:827–838.
6. Holme I, Waaler HT. Five-year mortality in the city of Bergen, Norway, according to age, sex and blood pressure. Acta Med Scand 1976; 200:229–239.
7. Kannel WB, Gordon T. Evaluation of cardiovascular risk in the Framingham study. Bull NY Acad Med 1978; 54:573–591.
8. Epstein FH, Ostrander LD, Johnson BC, et al. Epidemiological studies of cardiovascular disease in a total community—Tecumseh, Michigan. Ann Intern Med 1965; 62:1170–1187.
9. Agner E. Predictive value of arterial blood pressures in old age. A ten-year prospective study of men and women born in 1897 and examined at the age of 70 and 80 years. Acta Med Scand 1983; 214:285–294.
10. Landahl S, Lernfelt B, Sundh V. Blood pressure and mortality in old age. Eleven years' follow-up of a 70-year-old population. J Hypertens 1987; 5:745–748.
11. Cullen K, Stenhouse NS, Wearne KL, Welborn TA. Multiple regression analysis of risk factors for cardiovascular disease and cancer mortality in Busselton, Western Australia 13-year study. J Chronic Dis 1983; 36:371–377.
12. Fry J. Natural history of hypertension. A case for selective non-treatment. Lancet 1974; ii: 431–433.
13. Rajala S, Haavisto M, Heikinheimo R, Mattila K. Blood pressure and mortality in the very old. Lancet 1983; ii:520–521.
14. Mattila K, Haavisto M, Rajala S, Heikinheimo R. Blood pressure and five year survival in the very old. BMJ 1988; 296:887–889.
15. Langer RD, Ganiats TG, Barrett-Connor E. Paradoxical survival of elderly men with high blood pressure. BMJ 1989; 298:1356–1357.
16. Sourander LB, Ruikka I, Kasanen A. A health survey on the aged with a 5-year follow-up. Acta Soc Med Scand 1970; suppl 3:1–41.
17. Anderson F, Cowan NR. Survival of healthy older people. Br J Prev Soc Med 1976; 30:231–232.
18. Kuramoto K, Matsushita S, Kuwajima I, Murakami M. Prospective study on the treatment of mild hypertension in the aged. Jpn Heart J 1981; 22:75–85.
19. Morgan TO, Adams WR, Hodgson M, Gibberd RW. Failure of therapy to improve prognosis in elderly males with hypertension. Med J Aust 1980; 2:27–31.
20. Lindholm L, Lanke J, Bengtsson B, Ejlertsson G, Thulin T, Scherstén B. Both high and low blood pressures risk indicators of death in middle-aged males. Isotonic regression of blood pressure on age applied to data from a 13-year prospective study. Acta Med Scand 1985; 218: 473–480.
21. Cruickshank JM, Thorp JM, Zacharias FJ. Benefits and potential harm of lowering high blood pressure. Lancet 1987; i:581–584.
22. Cruickshank JM. Coronary flow reserve and the J curve relation between diastolic blood pressure and myocardial infarction. BMJ 1988; 297:1227–1230.

23. Cruickshank JM. Coronary flow reserve and the J curve. BMJ 1989; 298:457–458.
24. Staessen J, Bulpitt C, Clement D, De Leeuw P, Fagard R, Fletcher A, Forette F, Leonetti G, Nissinen A, O'Malley K. Relation between mortality and treated blood pressure in elderly patient with hypertension: report of the European Working Party on High Blood Pressure in the Elderly. BMJ 1989; 298:1552–1556.
25. Samuelsson OG, Wilhelmsen LW, Pennert KM, Wedel H, Berglund G. The J-shaped relationship between coronary heart disease and achieved blood pressure level in treated hypertension: further analyses of 12 years of follow-up of treated hypertensives in the Primary Prevention Trial in Gothenburg, Sweden. J Hypertens 1990; 8:547–555.
26. Coope J, Warrender TS, McPherson K. The prognostic significance of blood pressure in the elderly. J Hum Hypertens 1988; 2:79–88.
27. Fletcher AE, Beevers DG, Bulpitt CJ, Butler A, Coles EC, Hunt D, Munro Faure AD, Newson R, O'Riordan PW, Petrie JC. The relationship between a low treated blood pressure and IHD mortality: a report from DHSS hypertension care computing project (DHCCP). J Hum Hypertens 1988; 2:11–15.
28. Lindholm L, Scherstén B, Thulin T. High blood pressure and mortality in the elderly. Lancet 1983; ii:745–746.
29. Burch PRJ. Ischemic heart disease: epidemiology, risk factors and cause. Cardiovasc Res 1980; 14:307–338.
30. Veterans Administration Cooperative Study Group on Anti-hypertensive Agents. A double blind control study of antihypertensive agents. I. Comparative effectiveness of reserpine, reserpine and hydralazine, and three ganglionic blocking agents, chlorisondamine, mecamyamine, and pentolinium tartrate. Arch Intern Med 1960; 106:133–148.
31. Veterans Administration Cooperative Study Group on Anti-hypertensive Agents. Effects of treatment on morbidity in hypertension. Results in patients with diastolic blood pressures averaging 115 through 129 mm Hg. JAMA 1967; 202:1028–1034.
32. Veterans Administration Cooperative Study Group on Anti-hypertensive Agents. Effects of treatment on morbidity in hypertension. II. Results in patients with diastolic blood pressures averaging 90 through 114 mm Hg. JAMA 1970; 213:1143–1152.
33. Hypertension and Detection and Follow-up Program Cooperative Group. Five-year findings of the Hypertension Detection and Follow-up Program. I. Reduction in mortality of persons with high blood pressure, including mild hypertension. JAMA 1979; 242:2562–2571.
34. Hypertension and Detection and Follow-up Program Cooperative Group. Five-year findings of the Hypertension Detection and Follow-up Program. II. Mortality by race, sex and age. JAMA 1979; 242:2572–2577.
35. Hypertension and Detection and Follow-up Program Cooperative Group. Five-year findings of the Hypertension Detection and Follow-up Program. III. Reduction in stroke incidence among persons with high blood pressure. JAMA 1982; 247:633–638.
36. Management Committee. The Australian Therapeutic Trial in Mild Hypertension. Lancet 1980; i:1261–1267.
37. Management Committee. Treatment of mild hypertension in the elderly. National Heart Foundation of Australia. Med J Aust 1981; 2:398–402.
38. Coope J, Warrender TS. Randomised trial of treatment of hypertension in elderly patients in primary care. BMJ 1986; 293:1145–1151.
39. Amery A, Birkenhäger W, Brixko P, Bulpitt C, Clement D, Deruyttere M, De Schaepdryver A, Dollery C, Fagard R, Forette F. Mortality and morbidity results from the European Working Party on High Blood Pressure in the Elderly Trial (EWPHE). Lancet 1985; i:1349–1354.
40. Amery A, Birkenhäger W, Brixko, P, Bulpitt C, Clement D, Deruyttere M, De Schaepdryver A, Dollery C, Fagard R, Forette F. Efficacy of antihypertensive drug treatment according to age, sex, blood pressure, and previous cardiovascular disease in patients over the age of 60. Lancet 1986; ii:589–592.
41. SHEP Cooperative Research Group. Prevention of stroke by antihypertensive drug treatment

in older persons with isolated systolic hypertension. Final results of the Systolic Hypertension in the Elderly Program (SHEP). JAMA 1991; 265:3255–3264.
42. Medical Research Council trial of treatment of hypertension in older adults: principal results. MRC Working Party. BMJ 1992; 304:405–412.
43. Fletcher AE. Adverse treatment effects in the trial of the European Working Party on High Blood Pressure in the Elderly. Am J Med 1991; 90(suppl 3A):42s–44s.
44. Dahlöf B, Lindholm LH, Hansson L, Scherstén B, Ekbom T, Wester P-O. Morbidity and mortality in the Swedish Trial in Old Patients with Hypertension (STOP-Hypertension). Lancet 1991; 338:1281–1285.
45. Wikstrand J, Berglund G. Antihypertensive treatment with β-blockers in patients aged over 65. BMJ 1982; 285:850.
46. Appelgate WB, Hughes JP, Vander Zwaag R. Case-control study of coronary heart disease risk factors in the elderly. J Clin Epidemiol 1991; 44:409–415.
47. Ekbom T. Risks of Hypertension in the Elderly. Lund: Studentlitteratur, 1992:1–163 (thesis).
48. Helderman JH, Elahi D, Andersen DK, Raizes GS, Tobin JD, Shocken D, Andres R. Prevention of the glucose intolerance of thiazide diuretics by maintenance of body potassium. Diabetes 1983; 32:106–111.
49. Stamler J, Wentworth D, Neaton JD. Is relationship between serum cholesterol and risk of premature death from coronary heart disease continuous and graded? Findings in 356, 222 primary screenees of the Multiple Risk Factor Intervention Trial (MRFIT). JAMA 1986; 256: 2823–2828.
50. Aronow WS, Herzig MS, Etienne F, D'Alba P, Ronquillo J. 41-month follow-up of risk factors correlated with new coronary events in 708 elderly patients. J Am Geriatr Soc 1989; 37:501–560.
51. Castelli WP, Garrison RJ, Wilson PWF, Abbott RD, Kalousdian S, Kannel WB. Incidence of coronary heart disease and lipoprotein cholesterol levels. The Framingham Study. JAMA 1986; 256:2835–2838.
52. Castelli WP, Wilson PWF, Levy D, Anderson K. Cardiovascular risk factors in the elderly. Am J Cardiol 1989; 63:12H–19H.
53. Zimlichman R, Krauss S, Paran E. Muscle cramps induced by β-blockers with intrinsic sympathomimetic activity properties: a hint of a possible mechanism. Arch Intern Med 1991; 151: 1021.
54. Ekbom T, Dahlöf B, Hansson L, Lindholm LH, Scherstén B, Wester P-O. Antihypertensive efficacy and side effects of three β-blockers and a diuretic in elderly hypertensives: a report from the STOP-Hypertension study. J Hypertens 1992; 10:1525–1530.

10

Systolic Hypertension in the Elderly Program (SHEP): The First Demonstration That Lowering Systolic Hypertension Reduced Total Stroke and All Coronary Heart Disease

JEFFREY L. PROBSTFIELD,[1] WILLIAM B. APPLEGATE,[2] KENNETH E. BERGE,[3] JEFFREY A. CUTLER,[4] BARRY DAVIS,[5] CURT D. FURBERG,[2] C. MORTON HAWKINS,[5] SARA PRESSEL,[5] ELEANOR B. SCHRON,[4] and W. McFATE SMITH[6]

The diastolic blood pressure has not been reported to be more important than the systolic in the cardiovascular complications of hypertension. No special circumstances in which the diastolic pressure is of greater importance have yet been demonstrated. Long-term aortic regurgitation with a wide pulse pressure might offer an opportunity for investigation, and in the therapeutic studies, groups of patients with the same diastolic pressure and differing systolic levels could be compared.

''If diastolic blood pressure cannot be shown to be important, why measure it at all? I discontinued the practice of repeatedly taking the diastolic blood pressure some 10–12 years ago—that is, once I have ruled out aortic valvular disease, and established that the relationship between the patient's systolic and diastolic pressure is of the usual pattern. Nevertheless, I rarely report the systolic level without being asked, What was the underneath one?'' (1).

[1] Fred Hutchinson Cancer Research Center, Seattle, Washington; [2] Wake Forest University Medical Center, Winston-Salem, North Carolina; [3] Mayo Clinic, Rochester, Minnesota; [4] National Institutes of Health, Bethesda, Maryland; [5] University of Texas, School of Public Health, Houston, Texas; [6] SRI International, Menlo Park, California.

I. INTRODUCTION

Diastolic blood pressure (DBP), as opposed to systolic blood pressure (SBP) or the combination, became the focus of cardiovascular risk assessment relatively early in the 20th century and of antihypertensive treatment trials in the 1970s (2). Clinical trials focusing on diastolic hypertension (reviewed elsewhere in this volume) showed that associated deaths from all causes and strokes could be reduced by vigorous treatment.

A renewed interest in SBP, its elevation, and associated risks was generated first by an analysis of the Build and Blood Pressure study in 1959 (3, 4). That and other studies demonstrated unequivocally that an elevation of the SBP was associated with an increase in morbidity and mortality, especially among older people (4–9). Some analyses were done with adjustments made for other risk factors (10–14). As Fisher points out, in every study where the effect of elevations of both SBP and DBP have been compared, elevations of SBP have consistently shown greater associated risk for stroke coronary heart disease (CHD), and mortality from all causes. Further, the data showed that an elevation of SBP in the presence of normal DBP (that is, isolated systolic hypertension [ISH]) was associated with an increased risk of stroke, cardiovascular disease, and mortality from any cause. Systolic Hypertension in the Elderly Program (SHEP) was the first clinical trial of antihypertensive therapy to focus on SBP and specifically ISH.

Both the SBP and DBP increase with age in men and women until the early 50s. Between the ages of 54 and 59 years, DBP plateaus and thereafter falls modestly for the remainder of life. The prevalence of elevated DBP (that is, 90 mm Hg or more), therefore, increases until the mid-50s. Elevated SBP (for example, 140 mm Hg or more) is infrequent before the age of 50, begins to rise in prevalence about age 55, and continues to increase well beyond the age of 80 (15). Further, the National Health and Nutrition Examination Survey (NHANES)-III data demonstrate that for Americans between the ages of 55 and 74, women have a slightly higher prevalence of elevated SBP than men and African-Americans have a higher prevalence than caucasians. African-American females as a race-sex group have the highest prevalence at 11.3% (15).

The SHEP pilot study (SHEP-PS) screening data demonstrated that the prevalence of ISH increased dramatically from 6% for people ages 60 to 69 years to 18% for those older than 80 years (16). Isolated systolic hypertension prevalence data, along with projections in the population growth, strongly suggested that there could be 8 million incidences of ISH in the United States alone by the year 2025.

Data from prospective epidemiological studies and insurance actuarial studies strongly suggest that ISH has an associated twofold increased risk for deaths from all cardiovascular disease, a threefold increase in risk of stroke, a twofold increase in risk of coronary heart disease (5), and a 1.7-fold increase in risk of mortality from all causes (1). These increases in risk associated with the presence of ISH are present for both middle-aged and older individuals and for both men and women. Similar findings of increased risk have been confirmed in other studies (11, 14).

A. History of SHEP

In 1973, the leadership and policy boards of the U.S. Public Health Service Hospitals and Veterans Administration Cooperative Studies trials in hypertension that had overlapping membership identified hypertension in the elderly as a high priority for clinical trial investigation (17–20). Early sample-size calculations demonstrated that a trial of approximately 4500 participants would be needed using fatal and nonfatal stroke as a primary endpoint. In 1978, an investigator-initiated application was submitted to the National Heart, Lung, and Blood Institute (NHLBI), National Institute on Aging (NIA), and the National Institute of Mental Health (NIMH). The proposed trial was to address the question of whether lowering SBP, specifically ISH, in men and women aged 60 years and older, using currently available pharmacological drugs, would significantly reduce the risks of mortality from all causes, nonfatal myocardial infarction, and nonfatal stroke. In addition, the trial was to investigate issues related to dementia and depression. An NHLBI workshop on hypertension in the elderly in January 1979 addressed issues related to the appropriate goal for SBP reduction, the optimum pharmacological regimen in the elderly, the possible impact of antihypertensive treatment on behavioral and cognitive functions, and the problem of adherence to drug regimens in the elderly. The conference concluded that a trial should be undertaken on the efficacy of drug treatment for older persons with ISH. A revised application was submitted in February 1979. Approval was recommended by the NHLBI Advisory Council after a special ad hoc panel reviewed specific protocol issues. The ad hoc review panel recommended that only those with DBP below 90 mm Hg should be included in the trial. Other concerns reviewed by that panel included the choice of study medications, their starting and maximum doses, and the potential associated adverse effects. The panel recommended that these issues be explored in a pilot study by the applicant investigative group. A final recommendation was that the institutes' contract mechanism be used in the full-scale study if the pilot study were successful (21).

The SHEP pilot study was approved by the NHLBI, NIA, and NIMH in February 1980. Investigators from five institutions comprised the steering committee (Kaiser Permanente Center for Health Research, Portland, Oregon, Washington University, St. Louis, Missouri, University of Pittsburgh, Pennsylvania, Rush Presbyterian-St. Luke's Medical Center, Chicago, Illinois; University of Alabama, Birmingham). The coordinating center was located at the University of California, San Francisco. Program staff from NHLBI participated in the planning process (21).

Objectives for SHEP-PS (22) included the following: (a) to assess the feasibility of recruiting and retaining 500 elderly participants with ISH in a long-term, double-blind, placebo-controlled trial and to estimate and compare the yield of participants for enrollment from various community groups with the use of various recruitment techniques; (b) to estimate the adherence-to-visit schedule and prescribed double-blind medication treatment regimens; (c) to estimate the efficacy of prescribed antihypertensive medications for the reduction of high SBP; (d) to estimate unwanted effects of such medication in older people; (e) to evaluate feasibility and effectiveness of periodic behavioral assessments of the participants; and (f) to develop and test methods for determination of stroke and other disease end points (22).

Recruitment of 551 participants was accomplished in about one year (16). This represented about 2% of those screened (27,299 total) who were untreated and otherwise unselected age-eligible persons. In targeted selected populations, the yields were higher. More than one-third of those screened were taking antihypertensive medications. About one-fifth of those taking antihypertensive medication were willing to discontinue their medications and were found to have ISH and were ultimately randomized.

The SHEP-PS participants kept more than 90% of their scheduled visits, and those remaining on medication took more than 90% of their assigned study drug (23). About 18.5% of the participants terminated their study medications (mostly at their own request). Alteration but continuation of the study drug regimen occurred in 7.1% of the active treatment group and 4.0% of the placebo group. Three months into the treatment regimen, 75% of those assigned to a chlorthalidone-based stepped care regimen and 34% of those assigned to placebo had achieved a 20 mm Hg reduction in their SBP (or were below 160 mm Hg) from baseline. The average reduction was 17 mm Hg in SBP (actively treated group) and 3 mm Hg in DBP. These reductions were maintained at 12, 24, and 36 months of follow-up. Although more than 50% of the cohort reported some type of symptoms, only 10% considered these troublesome and only 2% intolerable. There were changes in the mean serum potassium (lower) and uric acid (higher), but no other laboratory variables changed in the chlorthalidone-based regimen-treated group compared with the placebo-treated group. Few ectopic beats or arrhythmias were reported in either intervention group. Behavioral assessment, including evaluation of cognitive, emotional, and physical functions, was well tolerated and without logistical issues. Feasible endpoint procedures were developed for stroke and other outcome measures (22).

After successful completion of SHEP-PS recruitment and with the encouraging results from the intervention (24), NHLBI and NIA obtained approval from their respective advisory councils and a request for proposals (RFP) was solicited for both the clinical centers and the coordinating center for the full-scale study. Development of the detailed protocol was begun in 1984 (21, 25). Recruitment needed to be extended nine months (see details below). Follow-up went to the designed trial end with the monitoring boundary

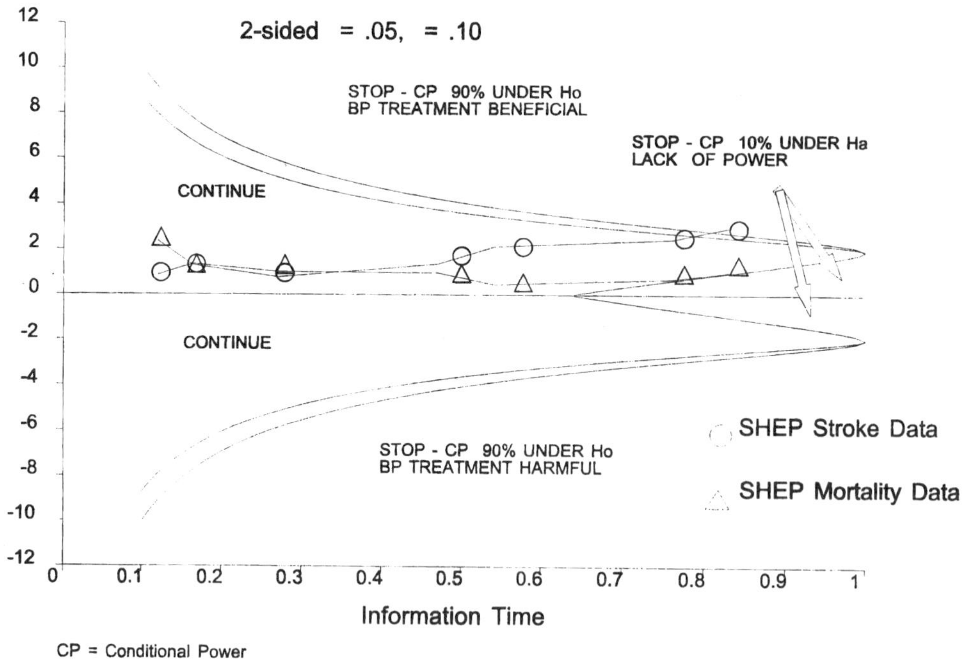

Fig. 1 Stochastic curtailment boundaries used in Systolic Hypertension of the Elderly Program (SHEP) for final coded strokes and total mortality. The last two sets of points represent the data presented at the July 1990 and December 1990 DSMB meetings. Inner boundaries represent conditional power (CP) of 80% under H_0.

for the primary outcome variable crossed only at the last regularly scheduled meeting of the Data and Safety Monitoring Board (DSMB) (Fig. 1).

II. WHY THE TRIAL WAS DONE AND THE FORMAL HYPOTHESES

A. Why

By the early 1980s, the data on disease prevalence, the mortality and morbidity associated with the condition of ISH, and expanding population at risk suggested that there was both a health condition and treatment problem of public health proportions that was developing and would continue to expand well into the 21st century. Pharmacologic studies had demonstrated an effective regimen to lower blood pressure (26). Broad interest within the scientific community had been demonstrated for investigator participation in the inquiry related to the proposed questions. Further, the successful pilot study demonstrated that an appropriate population could be identified and successfully recruited. The identified intervention regimen was successful in lowering the blood pressure and was well tolerated and associated with a low order of magnitude of adverse effects. Related questions regarding behavioral issues were possible to assess, the primary and secondary outcome measures related to the conduct of the main trial had been defined, and ascertainment was deemed feasible (21, 25).

B. Objectives and Questions Designed to be Answered in the Context of Time

1. Primary Hypothesis

The primary hypothesis to be tested in SHEP was whether long-term administration of antihypertensive therapy to older persons with ISH (SBP of 160 mm Hg or more and DBP less than 90 mm Hg) would reduce the combined incidence of fatal and nonfatal stroke during a 5-year follow-up period (21, 25). Incidence of total stroke (fatal and nonfatal) was selected as the primary endpoint because it is the major cardiovascular complication most strongly associated with level of SBP, and it is the event most conclusively affected by drug treatment of hypertension (21, 25).

2. Secondary Objectives

The SHEP investigators also aimed to assess the effect of long-term antihypertensive therapy on cardiovascular complications, including coronary events and morbidity and mortality in older people with ISH; the effect of long-term antihypertensive therapy on other selected morbidity (dementia, clinical depression, deterioration of cognitive function) and mortality from any cause; the possible adverse effects of long-term use of antihypertensive drug treatment in participants; the effect of therapy on quality-of-life indices such as hospital and nursing home admissions, days of restricted activity, level of functional impairment, and incidence of fracture of the hip, wrist, or vertebra; and the natural history of ISH in the placebo group (21, 25).

a. All CHD

Reduction in the risk of CHD, specifically nonfatal myocardial infarction (MI) and fatal CHD, had not been previously demonstrated in trials of antihypertensive treatment (27). Further, the potential benefit suggested from meta-analyses of long-term observational studies (28) was nearly double that calculated in meta-analyses from the observed effects in antihypertensive trials (27).

b. Total Mortality

Although the sample size in SHEP was of insufficient quantity to test whether death from all causes could be reduced by the proposed interventions, this outcome was interesting because of its general importance and for purposes of monitoring unexpected adverse effects (21, 25).

3. Other Analyses Not Specifically Prespecified

a. Type 2 Diabetic Participants

Diuretic and beta-blocker treatment for any indication in diabetics had been considered to be relatively contraindicated (11). Type 2 diabetic patients not requiring insulin were allowed to be randomized into the trial. Therefore, this trial would afford an opportunity to observe the effect of low-dose, diuretic-based antihypertensive treatment on major cardiovascular disease event rates in non–insulin-dependent participants compared with nondiabetic participants.

b. Prevention of Congestive Heart Failure

Heart failure is a major health problem internationally and results in approximately one million hospitalizations in the United States annually (11). Isolated systolic hypertension is specifically identified as a common antecedent to heart failure. The SHEP final results demonstrated a profound reduction in the incidence of congestive heart failure (CHF) in the actively treated group. Further analyses have focused on the impact of treatment for those with and without history of or electrocardiographic (ECG) evidence of prior MI (30).

c. Predictors of Stroke and Coronary Heart Disease

Baseline data were used to assess associated risk for stroke (31) and CHD (32, 33) in this cohort of older individuals. Variables assessed were demographic characteristics; blood pressure; history of smoking, diabetes, alcohol use and cardiovascular disease; lipid and lipoprotein variables; hematocrit; ECG abnormalities; estrogen use (women); and selected elements of the physical examination.

4. Subgroup Hypotheses

In addition to the primary and secondary hypotheses, two a priori subgroup null hypotheses were formulated and plans were made for analysis and reporting (21, 25, 34).

"The change in the incidence of total stroke due to treatment of ISH is the same in those not on antihypertensive medication at the time of initial screening as in those on such medication," and "The change in the incidence of sudden cardiac death or of cardiac death plus nonfatal myocardial infarction is the same in those with resting ECG abnormalities at baseline as in those with normal ECGs."

Although other a priori subgroup hypotheses regarding presence or absence of prior cardiovascular diseases and demographic and personal characteristics were considered, plausible expected differences in relative effects of treatment gave an estimated power of less than 50% (two-sided alpha < 0.05) (21). Therefore, these questions with calculated limited power were not included as formal subgroup hypotheses.

III. PROTOCOL SUMMARY

A. Multicenter Trial and Clinical Center Locations

In 1983, an RFP was issued by the NHLBI to identify clinical centers and a coordinating center. After following the standard competitive process, 17 clinical centers and a clinical coordinating center were identified. Despite best efforts, one of the clinical centers was unable to successfully identify and enroll participants and the center was dropped about six months into the recruitment period. Participating clinical centers included: Albert Einstein University (New York), Emory University (Atlanta), Kaiser Permanente Center for Health Research (Portland), Northwestern University (Chicago), Miami Heart Institute (Miami), Medical Research Institute (San Francisco), Robert Wood Johnson Medical School (New Brunswick), Universities of Alabama (Birmingham), California (Davis), Pacific Health Research Institute, Hawaii (Honolulu), Kentucky (Louisville), Minnesota (Minneapolis), Pittsburgh, Tennessee (Memphis), Washington University (St. Louis), Yale (New Haven) (21, 25).

B. Population

This was primarily an urban, multiethnic group of men and women from all socioeconomic groups, all of whom were 60 years of age or older (34).

1. *Entry Criteria*

The SHEP entry criteria were designed to allow inclusion of age-eligible persons meeting the blood pressure criteria and likely to be able to participate in the study, while excluding individuals with serious comorbid or other factors likely to cause problems with participation or confound the eventual results (21, 25).

a. Inclusion Criteria

Study inclusion criteria were: (a) age 60 years or older; (b) mean SBP 160 to 219 mm Hg and BDP less than 90 mm Hg (average of baseline visits 1 and 2); (c) willingness to comply with study protocol, including scheduled visits, assigned medications, and clinical laboratory; and (d) behavioral evaluations; and (e) no anticipated change in residence of more than 50 miles.

b. Exclusion Criteria

Study exclusion criteria were (21, 25): (a) evidence of atrial fibrillation or flutter, second- or third-degree atrioventricular (AV) block, multifocal ventricular premature beats (VPBs), VPBs in pairs or runs or VPBs more frequent than 10% of beats, or heart rate of less than 50 beats/min; (b) permanent pacemaker; (c) history of stroke with residual paresis or other neurological disability; (d) suspected or established significant renal dysfunction; (e) alcohol abuse (based on clinical judgment); (f) history of coronary bypass surgery or myocardial infarction within the past 6 months; (g) current treatment with insulin, anticoagulants, or drugs having antihypertensive activity; (h) uncontrolled congestive heart failure; (i) malignant neoplasm or other life-threatening disease; (j) contraindications to chlorthalidone; (k) peripheral arterial disease and evidence of ischemic tissue injury or loss; (l) dementia (based on clinical judgment); (m) residence in a nursing home; (n) history of transient ischemic attack (TIA) and carotid bruit in the appropriate location; (o) two TIAs in the same distribution; (p) malignant hypertension, past or present; and (q) treatment for known diastolic hypertension.

C. Intervention Groups, Intervention Regimen: Medications and Stepped Approach

Screenees were randomized to either active medication or placebo (Fig. 2) (21, 25). Active treatment was started the day after randomization with the low-dose diuretic, chlorthalidone (12.5 mg/day, increased as needed to 25 mg/day, maximum), to which the beta-blocker atenolol (25 mg/day increased as needed to 50 mg/day, maximum) was added, if goal SBP was not achieved. Alternatively, reserpine (0.05 or 0.10 mg/day) was used if atenolol was contraindicated. A comparable regimen using a stepped approach of placebo tablets was provided to half the participants. Chlorthalidone was selected for initial therapy because it had proven safe and effective in SHEP-PS (22) and in the older participants in the Hypertension Detection and Follow-up Program (HDFP) (22). The second agent selected for use was the once-a-day beta-blocker, atenolol. The SHEP investigators wanted an agent for which there was considerable clinical experience. Although some favored angiotensin-converting enzyme inhibitors or calcium channel blockers for the second agent, neither had been widely used at the time nor approved by the FDA for the treatment of hypertension.

D. Follow-Up

After randomization, participants returned in 4 weeks and then again 4 weeks later (21, 25). If participants were at or below SBP goal at 8 weeks, they were to return at regularly

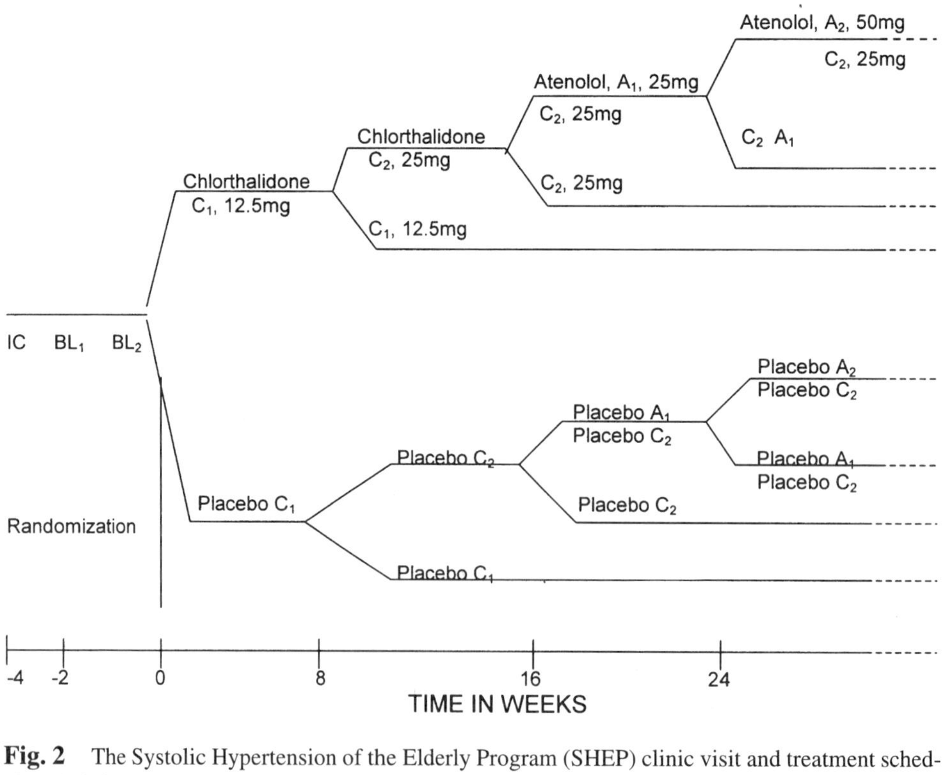

Fig. 2 The Systolic Hypertension of the Elderly Program (SHEP) clinic visit and treatment schedule. IC, initial contact; BL1 and BL2, baseline visits 1 and 2, respectively. Drug dosages are on a per-day basis. (From Ref. 21, with permission.)

scheduled quarterly visits. If goal SBP had not been reached at the end of 8 weeks, study medication (active or placebo) was increased to the maximum step or dosage. All participants were to have quarterly visits after date of randomization for measurement of blood pressure, heart rate, and body weight. For persons with persistently or severely elevated blood pressure levels, the protocol provided for the participant's own physician to select the antihypertensive drug treatment, and prescribe potassium supplements (provided by the study) for those with hypokalemia (serum potassium < 3.5 mmol/L). An interval history was also obtained, including screening for stroke and other study outcomes, as well as concomitant medication use and adverse events. A pill count and adherence self-report were done at any visit with a medication change and at 6-month intervals. Trial duration was a minimum of 4 years for every participant and averaged 4.5 years.

E. Study Organization

In addition to the 16 clinical centers, the Clinical Coordinating Center was located at the University of Texas School of Public Health in Houston (Fig. 3) (21). The Drug Distribution Center (United States Public Health Service) was located at Perry Point, Maryland. The ECG Reading Center was located at the University of Minnesota, the Central Reading Laboratory for CT Scans at Cheverly, Maryland and Houston, Texas, and the Central Clinical Laboratory determinations were done at the Smith-Kline-Beecham Laboratories in Teterboro, New Jersey. The project office was located at the Clinical Trials Branch of the Division of Epidemiology and Clinical Applications of NHLBI in Bethesda, Maryland. Study committees included a steering committee made up of the principal investigators from all of the study clinical centers, the coordinating center and the project office. The steering committee membership is listed in the Appendix. A small executive committee was charged with the day-to-day operations of the trial. An independent data and safety monitoring board (DSMB) (membership listed in the Appendix) reviewed the study data for both efficacy and safety at 6-month intervals. The DSMB used stochastic curtailment to monitor the estimate of benefit or harm demonstrated by the data. This was used to calculate the probability that a conclusion based on interim study results would remain unchanged at the trial's end, even if there were no benefits from antihypertensive treatment for the remainder of the trial (Fig. 1) (35).

F. Visit Plan

1. Study Outcomes

All study outcomes listed below, except where noted, were confirmed by a coding panel of three physicians from the Endpoint and Toxicity subcommittee blind to randomization allocation (21, 25). For neurological events, the coding panel included two neurologists. For myocardial infarction, left ventricular failure, and all causes of death the panel included at least one cardiologist. Possible adverse clinical and biochemical effects of SHEP treatments were evaluated by: (a) using a standardized questionnaire that asked participants about side effects at annual visits, at visits after administration of study drugs was started or stepped up, and at visits at which complaints were thought to be caused by SHEP medication; and (b) examining serum chemistry data from annual laboratory evaluations. The behavioral assessment included a questionnaire to detect depression and dementia, administered at baseline and semiannually. Based on specific questionnaire scores, participants were referred for expert diagnostic evaluation in accordance with American

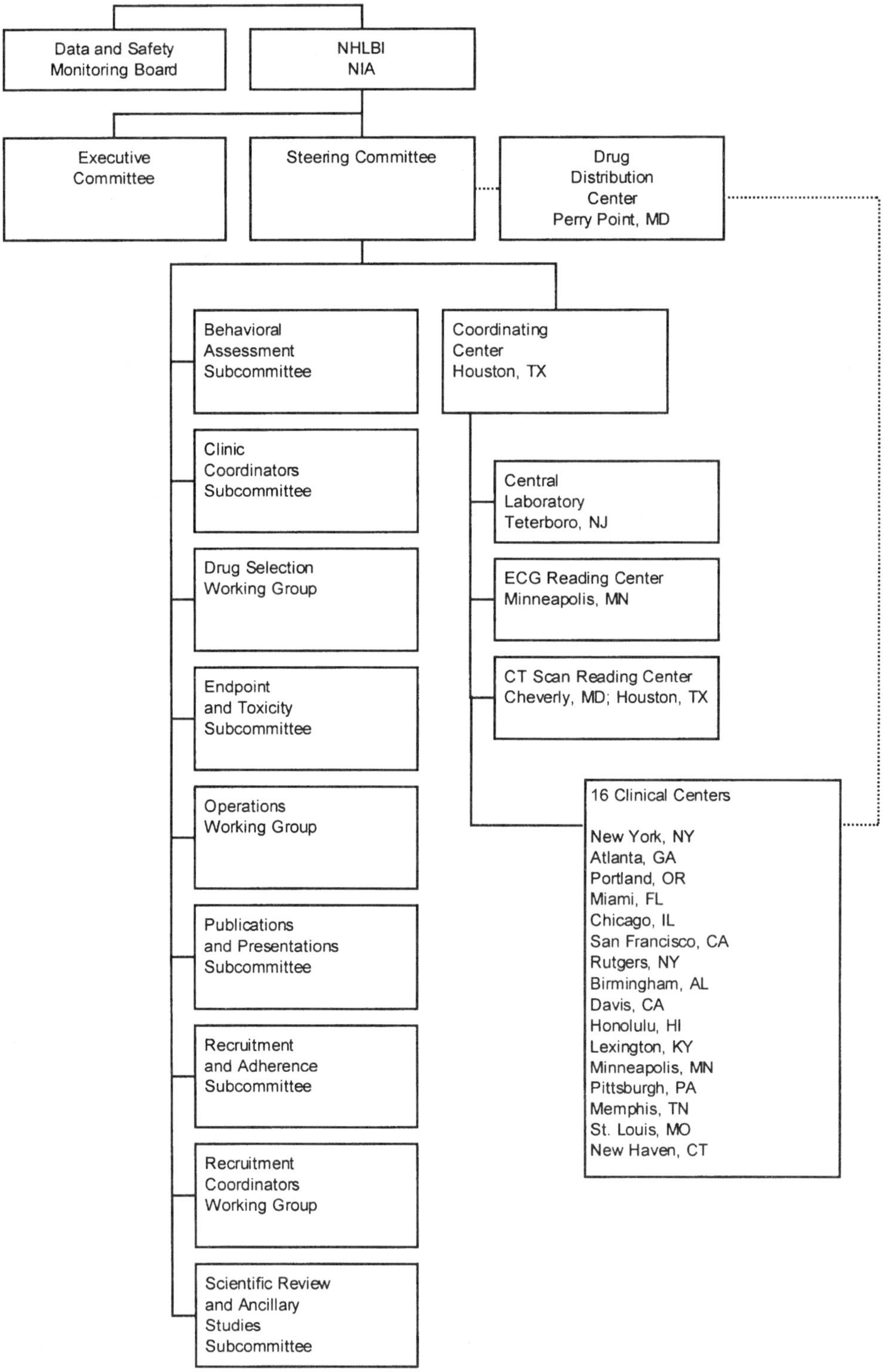

Fig. 3 Flow chart of management of Systolic Hypertension of the Elderly Program (SHEP). (From Ref. 21, with permission.)

Psychiatric Association criteria. A diagnosis of dementia had to be confirmed by the Endpoint and Toxicity subcommittee coding panel, including two neurologists. Depression was diagnosed by a psychiatrist or psychologist at each clinical center on clinical grounds and not reviewed centrally. Definitions of the primary and secondary outcome variables follow.

2. Primary Outcome Variable

The primary outcome variable was nonfatal and fatal stroke (total stroke) as determined by a specifically defined algorithm (21). Stroke was defined as rapid onset of a new neurological deficit attributed to obstruction or rupture in the arterial system. The defined deficit had to persist for at least 24 hours unless death supervened and had to include specific localizing findings confirmed at the time of neurological examination or brain scan, with no evidence of an underlying nonvascular cause. Determination of fatal stroke was based on either autopsy findings or death certificate plus data obtained at preterminal hospitalization with definite diagnosis of stroke (21).

3. Secondary Outcome Variables

a. Mortality from Any Cause

All deaths were documented by death certificate or hospital death summary (21).

b. Cause-Specific Mortality

Deaths attributable to disease categories were grouped as follows: neoplastic disease; renal disease; diabetes mellitus; gastrointestinal disease; respiratory disease; infectious disease; accidents, suicides, and homicides; and other noncardiovascular diseases (21).

c. Sudden Cardiac Death

Death occurred within 1 hour of the first evidence of acute cardiovascular symptoms or signs and unrelated to other known disease (21).

d. Rapid Cardiac Death

Death occurred within 24 hours of the first evidence of acute cardiovascular symptoms or signs and unrelated to other known disease (21).

e. Angina Pectoris

A positive Rose Questionnaire was obtained at annual visit (21).

f. Nonfatal Myocardial Infarction

There is definite ECG evidence of an acute myocardial infarction, or probable ECG evidence plus transient abnormal enzymes, or prolonged cardiac pain plus transient abnormal enzymes (21).

g. Fatal Myocardial Infarction

Defined as myocardial infarctions, as described above, that resulted in death, the death having occurred after 24 hours from the first evidence of acute cardiovascular symptoms or signs (21)

h. Left Ventricular Failure

This was defined as dyspnea or fatigue associated with a third heart sound or increased jugular venous pressure and basilar rates or increased markings on chest X-ray (21).

i. Transient Ischemic Attack

This was characterized by rapid onset of a focal neurological deficit lasting less than 24 hours, assessed to be caused by ischemia without evidence for an underlying nonvascular cause (21).

j. Coronary Artery Therapeutic Procedures

Coronary artery bypass graft or coronary angioplasty documented by submitted hospital records (21).

k. Multi-Infarct Dementia

Characterized as having a SHORT-CARE score of 4 or greater on two consecutive visits and neurological evaluation including CT scan and Haschinski score (36).

l. Clinical Depression

Depression suspected by a score of 26 or greater on the SHORT-CARE and 16 or greater on the CES-depression scale, and confirmed by a clinical examination by a psychiatrist or neurologist (37).

m. Activities of Daily Living and Social Networking

Expanded scales of physical function from basic self-care to the ability to lift heavy objects (38), and social networking specifically assessing the strength of self-support (39) were evaluated.

n. Deterioration of Cognition

Baseline and follow-up examinations of cognitive skills were assessed in all participants using the Cognitive Impairment Scale of the SHORT-CARE. This standardized test evaluates basic orientation to person, place, and time as well as general knowledge and short-term memory. A subsample of the cohort was more extensively evaluated using the following standard battery of tests: trail-making test (40, 41), digit symbol simulation test (42, 43), addition test (44), Boston naming test (45), delayed recognition span test (44), and the letter sets test (46, 47).

o. Falls and Fractures

A history of two falls in a 3-month period, and fractures of the hip, spine, and forearm were recorded on afflicted participants (21).

p. Multiple Indexes of Quality of Life

General issues of quality of life were assessed by the frequency of hospitalizations for any cause, and admission to intermediate or skilled nursing home was recorded for afflicted participants (21). In a subset of the participants, three standard quality-of-life questions were asked regarding perceptions of his or her quality of life (48–50).

q. Adverse Effects

Agents used for intervention in this study have been previously associated with such symptoms as postural hypotension, depression, asthma or bronchospasm, Raynaud's phenomenon, and serious lethargy. Other symptoms that occurred and were temporarily related to the institution of the study medications or to step-up in the dosage of one of the medications were recorded (21).

r. Renal Dysfunction

This was defined as a serum creatinine concentration greater than 265.2 μmol/L (21).

G. Description of the Blood Pressure Measurement Method

All blood pressures were taken and recorded according to a standardized method. Staff members had to be certified every 6 months on the standardized blood pressures techniques. A standardized Hawksley random-zero manometer was used for all study blood pressure determinations. The SBP was defined as the reading of the first Korotokoff sound and DBP as the reading at the last Korotokoff sound (21).

H. Participant Enrollment Goals and Screening

Before SHEP-PS, there had been little experience with recruitment of older persons to clinical trials (51). The SHEP-PS attempted to identify several recruitment strategies that were thought to facilitate the contact and screening of large numbers of older individuals. Review of the literature provided little additional information but gave no suggestion that older individuals would be more difficult to recruit than any other segment of the population.

1. Goals

The initial recruitment goal was to enroll 4800 men and women with ISH between March 1985 and February of 1987 (21, 25, 53). Each of the clinical centers had an original goal of 300 participants (except for one with a goal of 200). An overall recruitment plan was organized by the recruitment and adherence subcommittee in collaboration with the program office. The plan focused on strategies used in SHEP-PS and in a review of current recruitment literature. As recruitment and enrollment proceeded, some clinical centers encountered difficulties in enrolling their assigned numbers of participants. After review of the project enrollment and power considerations, screening was extended through September 30, 1987. Randomization was completed on January 15, 1988 (52).

Major responsibility was given to a recruitment coordinator at each of the clinical centers. That individual worked closely with the principal investigator and other staff to develop specific local recruitment plans. Staffing configuration varied widely at the clinics, depending on local considerations and strategies used (54).

Local recruitment plans were built around six major recruitment strategies (52). A national public relations campaign was augmented by specific local approaches. Local media activities included newspaper, radio, and television exposure. These media efforts were frequently coordinated with presentations by the local clinical staff to professional or lay groups. Before SHEP, mass mail campaigns had shown mixed results. The mass mailing activities of SHEP have been described in detail (54). Sophisticated approaches were developed for the handling of large numbers of personalized letters mailed to a wide variety of mailing list sources. Timeliness of mailings and management of the responses to distributed letters became highly developed skills. Some clinical centers were also able to efficiently use volunteers to aid the recruitment effort at substantial cost savings (55). Mass screening activities at a variety of locations (such as malls, hospital outpatient facilities, and health fairs) and individual chart reviews of populations considered to have high prevalence of ISH were also useful strategies (54).

2. Screening

Although blood pressure determinations from three prerandomization visits were used to determine eligibility in SHEP-PS, it was recognized that blood pressures from two screening visits were as efficient at screening and identifying those with ISH for the full-scale study (56). For persons not receiving antihypertensive drugs who had a first SBP reading greater than 150 mm Hg, two more readings were taken. When the mean of the last two readings was between 160 and 219 mm Hg for SBP and less than 100 mm Hg for DBP, the person was eligible for the first baseline visit (56).

Individuals receiving antihypertensive medication at initial contact who had SBPs between 130 and 219 mm Hg and DBPs less than 85 mm Hg and who were free of major illness were eligible for a drug withdrawal procedure. They were asked to obtain agreement to participate in the study from their primary care physician and to sign an informed consent form for current medication withdrawal. They were then monitored at multiple drug evaluation visits during a 2- to 8-week period to determine blood pressure eligibility without their usual medication (21).

The baseline phase consisted of two visits. Eligibility was determined based on study inclusion and exclusion criteria. When the average of four seated blood pressure measurements, two at each of two visits, was between 160 and 219 mm Hg for SBP and less than 90 mm Hg for DBP, the participant was eligible for the trial. Persons were excluded on the basis of history or signs of specified major cardiovascular diseases. Other major diseases, such as cancer, alcoholic liver disease, established renal dysfunction, with competing risk for the SHEP primary endpoint or the presence of medical management problems, were also exclusions. Screenees also underwent a physical examination and a 12-lead ECG was done, with a 2-minute rhythm strip (21, 25).

Those remaining eligible at the second baseline visit underwent behavioral assessment (including cognition, mood, and activities of daily living), signed an additional informed consent form for participation in the trial, and had blood drawn (21).

I. Randomization and Stratification

At the completion of the second baseline visit, after verification of eligibility, screenees were randomly allocated by the coordinating center to one of two treatment groups. Randomization was stratified by clinical center and by antihypertensive medication status at baseline. Restricted randomization using blocks of variable sizes was used to ensure that the sample sizes of the two groups remained relatively equal throughout recruitment (21).

J. Variables Evaluated at Follow-Up Visits

The SHEP participants were followed up monthly until SBP reached the goal or until the maximum level of stepped-care treatment was reached. All participants had quarterly visits from the date of randomization, at which time they underwent measurement of blood pressure (average of two readings), heart rate, body weight, general medical history, and a detailed review of medication use (prescribed and over-the-counter). At semiannual visits, standardized questionnaires were administered to screen for depression and dementia. Annual visits also included (a) a detailed medical history; (b) a complete physical examination; (c) selected laboratory tests; and (d) behavioral assessment. An ECG was also done at the second, fourth, and final annual visit. Other visits were scheduled when indicated, such as SBP above the goal, SBP or DBP above the escape criteria (see below), low serum potassium concentration (< 3.2 mmol/L), or as requested by the clinician or participant. Blood pressure readings, observed at the clinical center, above a priori escape criteria, despite maximal stepped-care therapy, were an indication for prescribing known active drug therapy. Escape criteria included SBP greater than 240 mm Hg at a single visit, DBP greater than 115 mm Hg at a single visit, sustained SBP greater than 220 mm Hg, or sustained DBP greater than 90 mm Hg (21, 25).

When adverse conditions occurred that were considered drug related, the dosage of the study medication could be reduced or therapy could be discontinued. Whenever the dosage was reduced or therapy was discontinued, consideration was given to resuming study drug therapy when it appeared safe, when the participant's blood pressure was above goal, and when the participant agreed (21, 25).

K. Sample Size

A sample size of 4800 participants was estimated for SHEP (53). This number was based on the following assumptions:

1. The primary endpoint would be fatal plus nonfatal stroke.
2. The average follow-up was to be five years.
3. Based on the SHEP pilot study experience, 5-year total stroke rate in the placebo group would be 7.75%.
4. The proportion of participants assigned to active medication who stop their study medication will be 7% in year one and 3.5% in years two through five.
5. The proportion of participants assigned to placebo who are given antihypertensive medication will be 9% in year one and 4.5%, 5.0%, 5.5%, and 6.0% in each of the next four years, respectively.
6. The expected reduction in total stroke incidence for the active group compared with the placebo group after accounting for the crossover rates decreases from 40% to 32%.
7. Based on U.S. vital statistics data, the competing risk of nonstroke death will be 15.4% for the five years.
8. A two-tailed significance level (alpha) of 0.05 and a power of 0.90 would be used. These assumptions and estimations yielded a sample size of 4800 hypertensives, aged 60 and older (21, 25, 57).

L. Statistical Methods

The primary hypothesis was assessed with the log rank test using time to first stroke. Cumulative event rates were calculated using life table methods. Relative risks and percentage differences were calculated by proportional hazard regression analyses using the entire duration of follow-up. All analyses were by treatment assignment at randomization. Subgroup hypotheses were tested by the proportional hazards model using the appropriate interaction term (21, 25, 34, 57).

IV. RESULTS

A. Population Screening

Altogether 447,921 individuals aged 60 years and older were identified and contacted at 16 clinical centers; 11.6% met initial criteria, and 2.7% completed baseline visit one. Of

Table 1 Screening and Recruitment Data (age > 60 years; SBP ≥ 160 mm Hg; DBP < 90 mm Hg)

	Numbers	Percent
Screened, all sources	447,921	100
Screened, BP eligible	52,139	11.6
No medications	19,842	4.4
1st clinic visit (CV-1)	11,919	22.9
Eligible for CV-2	7,644	64.1
2nd clinic visit (CV-2)	6,929	90.6
Eligible	4,827	69.7
Randomized	4,736	98.1

Abbreviations: *SBP*, systolic blood pressure; *DBP*, diastolic blood pressure.

those individuals, 64% were eligible for baseline visit two; of those, 70% were eligible for randomization; of those, 88% were randomized. Only 1% of those screened were ultimately randomized into SHEP, whereas 2% of those screened were eligible in SHEP-PS. The difference in enrollment proportion between the pilot and full-scale study remains unexplained but was the major reason for delayed recruitment of the sample size in the full-scale trial. Staff experience in clinical trials, especially for the recruitment coordinator, was identified as a key ingredient to the success of individual clinical centers (54).

The mass mailing effort at the 14 centers that used this strategy involved sending more than 3.4 million letters. These produced 4.3% responses to the clinical centers. Although mass screening was a very low yield procedure for study enrollment, the most effective locations for mass screening were where meals for older individuals were offered. Senior citizen centers, social security offices, and libraries also provided comparatively good yields for study enrollment (54).

B. Baseline Comparability of Treatment Groups

The baseline characteristics of the population have been completely described (58). Stratified randomization by antihypertensive drug treatment status at initial contact and by center produced two SHEP groups (active treatment and placebo) comparable at baseline (Table 2). Mean age of the participants was 72 years; 57% were women, and 14% were African-American. Included among the Caucasians were 204 Asians (5% of Caucasians), 84 Hispanics (2% of Caucasians), and 41 classified as ''other'' (1% of Caucasians). Of all participants, 1.4% reported a history of stroke and 5% reported a history of myocardial infarction. On physical examination, 7% had carotid bruits. About 61% had an ECG abnormality. As a group, the cohort was overweight with a body mass index averaging 27.5 kg/m (34). Fewer than 1% had cognitive impairment, and about 11% manifested symptoms of depression based on standardized questionnaire criteria. Only 5% reported limitation in activities of daily living. Mean SBP was 170.3 mm Hg; mean DBP was 76.6 mm Hg (34).

C. Outcomes Intervention Groups

1. *Visit and Medication Adherence by Treatment Group*

Of the 2365 participants randomized to active treatment, 98.6% continued attendance at clinic visits throughout, 90% were on active treatment at four years and ascertainment of

Table 2 Baseline Characteristics of Randomized SHEP Participants by Treatment Group*

Characteristic	Active	Placebo	Total
No. randomized	2365	2371	4736
Age, y-average†	71.6 (6.7)	71.5 (6.7)	71.6 (6.7)
60–69	41.1	41.8	41.5
70–79	44.9	44.7	44.8
≥80	14.0	13.4	13.7
Race-sex %‡			
African-American men	4.9	4.3	4.6
African-American women	8.9	9.7	9.3
Caucasian men	38.8	38.4	38.6
Caucasian women	47.4	47.7	47.5
Education, y†	11.7 (3.5)	11.7 (3.4)	11.7 (3.5)
Blood pressure, mm Hg†			
Systolic	170.5 (9.5)	170.1 (9.2)	170.3 (9.4)
Diastolic	76.7 (9.6)	76.4 (9.8)	76.6 (9.7)
Antihypertensive medication at initial contact, %	33.0	33.5	33.3
Smoking, %			
Current smokers	12.6	12.9	12.7
Past smokers	36.6	37.6	37.1
Never smokers	50.8	49.6	50.2
Alcohol use, %			
Never	21.5	21.7	21.6
Formerly	9.6	10.4	10.0
Occasionally	55.2	53.9	54.5
Daily or near daily	13.7	14.0	13.8
History of myocardial infarction, %	4.9	4.9	4.9
History of stroke, %	1.5	1.3	1.4
History of diabetes, %	10.0	10.2	10.1
Carotid bruits, %	6.4	7.9	7.1
Pulse rate, beats/min†§	70.3 (10.5)	71.3 (10.5)	70.8 (10.5)
Body-mass index, kg/m^2†	27.5 (4.9)	27.5 (5.1)	27.5 (5.0)
Serum cholesterol, mmol/L			
Total	6.1 (1.2)	6.1 (1.1)	6.1 (1.1)
High-density lipoprotein	1.4 (0.3)	1.4 (0.4)	1.4 (0.4)
Depressive symptoms, %‖	11.1	11.0	11.1
Evidence of cognitive impairment, %¶	0.3	0.5	0.4
No limitation of activities of daily living, %§	95.4	93.8	94.6
Baseline electrocardiographic abnormalities, %#	61.3	60.7	61.0

* SHEP indicates the Systolic Hypertension in the Elderly Program.

† Values are mean (SD).

‡ Included among the Caucasians were 204 Asians (5% of Caucasians), 84 Hispanics (2% of Caucasians), and 41 classified as "other" (1% of Caucasians).

§ $P < .05$ for the active treatment group compared with the placebo group.

‖ Depressive symptom scale score of 7 or greater.

¶ Cognitive impairment scale score of 4 or greater.

One or more of the following Minnesota codes: 1.1 to 1.2 (Q/QS), 3.1 to 3.4 (high R waves), 4.1 to 4.4 (ST depression), 5.1 to 5.4 (T wave changes), 6.1 to 6.8 (AV conduction defects), 7.1 to 7.8 (ventricular conduction defects), 8.1 to 8.6 (arrhythmias), and 9.1 to 9.3 and 9.5 (miscellaneous items).

Source: From Ref. 34, with permission.

primary outcome was possible in all but five participants at trial completion. For those 2371 participants randomized to placebo, 98% continued clinic attendance throughout, 58.8% remained untreated at four years, and stroke status was not determined in only five participants at completion of the trial (34).

2. Blood Pressure Response of the Intervention Groups

Treatment effect on blood pressures for the two groups is described in Table 3. A differential of −14 mm Hg in SBP was observed at one year of follow-up for those on active treatment, was at −11.5 mm Hg at four years (which occurred for all surviving participants), and was still at −11.1 mm Hg for those who achieved five years of follow-up. The differential in DBP was −3.9 mm Hg at one year for those on active treatment and −3.4 at five years (34).

3. Fatal and Nonfatal Stroke

With a mean follow-up on all participants of 4.5 years, incident fatal and nonfatal stroke was diagnosed in 103 participants in the active treatment group and 159 participants in the placebo group (Table 4). The separation of the two treatment groups is plotted in a Kaplan-Meier plot (Fig. 4) and shows clear separation as early as about six months after the initiation of treatment. By life table analyses, 5-year cumulative stroke rates were 5.2 per 100 participants for the active treatment group and 8.2 per 100 participants for the placebo group. The cumulative rates for the total period of follow-up (70 months) were 5.5 per 100 participants for the active treatment group and 9.2 per 100 participants for the placebo group. Based on proportional hazards regression analysis, relative risk was 0.64 (95% confidence interval [CI], 0.50–0.82; $2p = 0.0003$). This reduction in risk was observed regardless of the active treatment regimen (61). The absolute reduction in 5-year risk of stroke incidence rates was 30 events per 1000 participants. There were few stroke deaths—10 in the active treatment group and 14 in the placebo group (34).

Table 3 Mean Systolic and Diastolic Blood Pressures by Treatment Group and Year of Follow-Up

Year	Active	Blood Pressure, mm Hg* placebo	Difference (active–placebo)
	Systolic Blood Pressure		
Baseline	170.5 (9.5)	170.1 (9.2)	+0.4
1	142.5 (15.7)	156.5 (17.3)	−14.0
2	141.8 (17.1)	154.4 (18.7)	−12.6
3	142.4 (17.2)	155.0 (20.0)	−12.6
4	143.1 (18.0)	154.6 (19.8)	−11.5
5	144.0 (19.3)	155.1 (20.9)	−11.1
	Diastolic blood pressure		
Baseline	76.7 (9.6)	76.4 (9.8)	+0.3
1	69.5 (9.9)	73.4 (12.1)	−3.9
2	68.2 (10.9)	72.3 (12.0)	−4.1
3	68.0 (10.6)	72.1 (12.3)	−4.1
4	67.2 (11.6)	71.2 (12.6)	−4.0
5	67.7 (10.2)	71.1 (12.8)	−3.4

* Values are mean (SD).
Source: From Ref. 34, with permission.

Table 4 Total (Nonfatal Plus Fatal) Stroke Rates by Treatment Group and Year of Follow-Up*

Year	Starting no.	No. of events†	No. unavailable for follow-up	Cumulative stroke rate (SE), per 100 participants
		Active Treatment Group		
1	2365	28	0	1.2 (0.2)
2	2316	22	0	2.1 (0.3)
3	2264	21	0	3.0 (0.4)
4	2153	18	0	4.0 (0.4)
5	1438	13	5	5.2 (0.5)
6‡	613	1	0	5.5 (0.6)
		Placebo Group		
1	2371	34	0	1.4 (0.2)
2	2308	42	0	3.2 (0.4)
3	2229	22	2	4.2 (0.4)
4	2131	34	2	6.0 (0.5)
5	1393	24	1	8.2 (0.7)
6	584	3	0	9.2 (0.9)

* For the active treatment group compared with the placebo group, χ^2(1 df) = 12.90, P = .0003; relative risk, 0.64 (95% confidence interval, 0.50 to 0.82).
† There were 103 total events (96 nonfatal and 10 fatal) in the active treatment group and 159 (149 nonfatal and 14 fatal) in the placebo group. Three participants in the active treatment group and four participants in the placebo group had both a nonfatal and a fatal stroke. Only the first event (nonfatal) was counted in the total number of events and in calculation of the cumulative stroke rate.
‡ The last stroke occurred during the 67th month of follow-up.
Source: From Ref. 34, with permission.

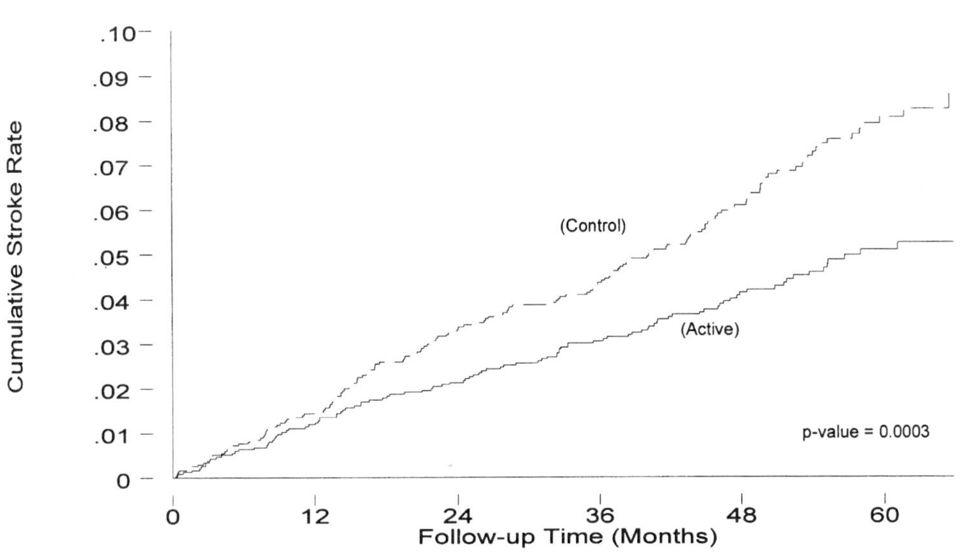

Fig. 4 Cumulative fatal plus nonfatal stroke rate per 100 participants in the active treatment (*solid line*) and placebo (*broken line*) groups during the Systolic Hypertension in the Elderly Program. (From Ref. 34, with permission.)

4. Impact of Age, Race, and Sex

Stroke incidence was lower in those randomized to active treatment than in those randomized to placebo for all baseline age groups: 60 to 69 years, 34 versus 47 events; 70 to 79 years, 48 versus 74 events; and 80 years and older, 21 versus 38 events. A favorable effect of active treatment was also noted for three of the four major race-sex groups: Caucasian men, 39 versus 64 events; Caucasian women, 48 versus 66 events; and African-American women, 7 versus 21 events. The apparent lack of any trend for the small number of African-American men was based on few events (nine vs eight events) (2).

5. Impact of Baseline Blood Pressure on Primary Outcome Response

With proportional hazards regression using SBP as a continuous variable, trend in stroke incidence for the active treatment compared with the placebo group prevailed irrespective of baseline SBP (34).

6. First Ischemic Cerebrovascular Event

Total first cerebrovascular ischemic events were reduced by 33% (158 vs 231, 95% CI 0.55–0.83).

7. Coronary Heart Disease

The incidence of confirmed fatal and nonfatal coronary events was reduced by 27% in the active treatment group (104 vs 141; 95% CI, 0.57–0.94) (Table 5). Silent myocardial infarction occurred in 66 participants (31 active treatment vs 35 placebo) (data not shown). These events added to the fatal and nonfatal coronary heart disease events gives 135 versus 176 total clinical coronary events (RR = 0.77, 95% CI, 0.62–0.96). All coronary heart disease events (including coronary artery bypass surgery and angioplasty)—nonfatal plus fatal—numbered 140 for the active treatment group and 184 for the placebo. By proportional hazards regression analysis, there were 25% fewer total coronary events in the active treatment group, with the 5-year absolute benefit estimated at 16 events per 1000 participants (34).

Using time-dependent life table regression with adjustment for several variables, the relative risks for CHD events for those using chlorthalidone plus either atenolol (1.04; 95% CI 0.58–1.87) or reserpine (0.93; 95% CI 0.29–2.96) versus those using chlorthalidone alone were similar. The strong suggestion from these analyses is that the beneficial effects seen in SHEP on the CHD outcome measure were the result of the lowering of blood pressure rather than a specific benefit attributable to a specific agent (59).

8. Mortality from All Causes and Cause-Specific Mortality

The number of deaths during the 70 months of follow-up was lower in the active treatment group than in the placebo group for mortality from all causes (213 vs 242 deaths), total cardiovascular causes (90 vs 112 deaths), and total coronary causes (59 vs 73 deaths) (range of relative risks, 0.80–0.87) (Table 5). The difference observed in total deaths from CHD was largely the result of the difference in the number of fatal myocardial infarctions. As in the analysis for stroke and CHD, the relative risk for death was similar regardless of the active treatment intervention regimen (55). The number of deaths from neoplastic disease, second only to cardiovascular disease as a main cause of mortality for SHEP participants, was similar (77 vs 77) for the active treatment and placebo groups. Nearly

Table 5 Morbidity and Mortality by Cause and Treatment Group

No. of events	Active treatment group (n = 2365)	Placebo group (n = 2371)	Relative risk (95% confidence interval)*
Stroke	96	149	0.63 (0.49–0.82)
Transient ischemic attack	62	82	0.75 (0.54–1.04)
Myocardial infarction†	50	74	0.67 (0.47–0.96)
Coronary artery bypass graft	30	47	0.63 (0.40–1.00)
Angioplasty	19	22	0.86 (0.47–1.59)
Left ventricular failure	48	102	0.46 (0.33–0.65)
Renal dysfunction	7	11	—
Fatal Events			
Total deaths	213	242	0.87 (0.73–1.05)
Total cardiovascular	90	112	0.83 (0.60–1.05)
Stroke	10	14	0.71 (0.31–1.59)
Total coronary heart disease	59	73	0.80 (0.57–1.13)
Sudden death (< 1 h)	23	23	1.00 (0.56–1.78)
Rapid death (1–24 h)	21	24	0.87 (0.48–1.56)
Myocardial infarction	15	26	0.57 (0.30–1.08)
Other cardiovascular	21	25	0.87 (0.49–1.55)
Left ventricular failure	9	8	—
Other	12	17	0.71 (0.35–1.46)
Total noncardiovascular	109	103	1.05 (0.80–1.38)
Neoplastic disease	77	77	0.96 (0.70–1.31)
Renal disease	2	2	—
Diabetes mellitus	0	1	—
Gastrointestinal disease	2	3	—
Respiratory disease	5	4	—
Infectious disease	11	8	—
Accident, suicide, homicide	5	5	—
Other noncardiovascular	7	3	—
Indeterminate cause‡	14	27	—
Combined Endpoints			
Nonfatal myocardial infarction or coronary heart disease death	104	141	0.73 (0.57–0.94)
Fatal or nonfatal stroke, nonfatal myocardial infarction, or coronary heart disease death	199	289	0.67 (0.56–0.80)
Coronary heart disease§	140	184	0.75 (0.60–0.94)
Cardiovascular disease‖	289	414	0.68 (0.58–0.79)

* Relative risk assessments were done for all types of events except those with fewer than 20 events and indeterminate cause of death.

† Nonfatal myocardial infarction does not include silent myocardial infarction.

‡ Results of death certificate coding for indeterminate causes according to the ninth revision of the International Classification of Diseases, Adapted, were as follows: stroke, two in the active treatment group and three in the placebo group; myocardial infarction, one in the placebo group; left ventricular failure, one in the placebo group; other cardiovascular disease, seven in the active treatment group and 10 in the placebo group; neoplasm, one in the active treatment group; respiratory disease, one in the placebo group; renal disease, one in the active treatment group; infectious disease, three in the placebo group; other noncardiovascular disease, one in the active treatment group and five in the placebo group; and unknown or no death certificate, one in the active treatment group and four in the placebo group.

§ Coronary heart disease includes definite nonfatal or fatal myocardial infarction, sudden cardiac death, rapid cardiac death, coronary artery bypass graft, and angioplasty.

‖ Cardiovascular disease includes definite nonfatal or fatal myocardial infarction, sudden cardiac death, rapid cardiac death, coronary artery bypass graft, angioplasty, nonfatal or fatal stroke, transient ischemic attack, aneurysm, and endarterectomy.

Source: From Ref. 34, with permission.

twice as many (14 vs 27) deaths from indeterminate cause occurred in the placebo group, a finding that remains unexplained (34).

9. Quality of Life

Findings from the extensive quality-of-life evaluation in SHEP have been described in detail (60). The SHEP cohort overall exhibited a decline over time in activities of daily living, particularly the more strenuous ones, and some decline in certain leisure activities. Although there was a slightly positive effect on several measures favoring treatment, the overwhelming finding was that mood, cognitive function, basic self-care, and moderate leisure activity were remarkably stable for both the active and placebo groups throughout the entire study (60).

During the trial, 14% of participants in the active treatment group and 15% in the placebo group met study questionnaire referral criteria for expert evaluation of possible depression. For more than 75% of these people referral was completed; the main reason for failure to achieve referral was participant refusal. Of participants in the two groups, 104 (4.4%) randomized to the active treatment group and 112 (4.7%) randomized to placebo had a confirmed diagnosis of depression (34).

Hospitalizations for any reason were recorded for 1027 active treatment group participants (1976 admissions) and 1086 placebo group participants (2204 admissions). Skilled or intermediate care nursing home admissions were recorded for 52 participants (58 admissions) in the active treatment group and 58 placebo group participants (65 admissions) (34).

10. Dementia

About 4% of persons in the active treatment and placebo groups met questionnaire referral criteria for expert evaluation of possible dementia. For more than 90% of these individuals, referral to a psychiatrist or neurologist was completed; the main reason for failure to achieve referral was participant refusal. Thirty-seven participants (1.6%) receiving active treatment and 44 (1.9%) receiving placebo had a diagnosis of dementia made and confirmed by the coding panel (34).

11. A Priori Subgroup Hypotheses

a. Antihypertensive Drug Status at Initial Contact

One of the two SHEP subgroup hypotheses was related to the effects of active treatment on participants receiving and not receiving antihypertensive medication at initial contact. Randomization was stratified by whether participants were receiving antihypertensive medication at initial contact. For the subgroup not receiving antihypertensive medication at initial contact, relative risk of stroke for active treatment compared with placebo was 0.69 (95% CI, 0.51–0.95). For participants receiving antihypertensive treatment at initial contact, relative risk for stroke was 0.57 (95% CI, 0.38–0.85) (34).

b. Impact of Baseline ECG Abnormalities and Risk of Sudden or Rapid Death or Nonfatal Myocardial Infarction and Coronary Death

The second SHEP a priori subgroup hypothesis dealt with the relationship between the incidence of nonfatal myocardial infarction and coronary death, and the incidence of sudden and rapid death to treatment assignment and the presence or absence of ECG abnormalities at baseline. For the subgroup of participants free of baseline ECG abnormalities, the relative risk of nonfatal myocardial infarction plus coronary death for active treatment compared with placebo was 0.83 (95% CI, 0.53–1.29). There were few events for the endpoint of sudden and rapid death: 15 in the active treatment group and 10 in the placebo group. For participants with baseline ECG abnormalities, the relative risk of nonfatal myocardial infarction plus coronary death was 0.69 (95% CI, 0.50–0.94). For the endpoint of sudden and rapid death, there were 29 events in the active treatment group and 36 in the placebo group. The data support that benefit for these coronary endpoints is associated with active treatment for those with or without ECG abnormalities at baseline (34).

12. *Stroke Type and Severity*

Types of strokes and their severity have been described in detail (61). Table 6 shows that strokes of all subtypes were reduced by the SHEP therapeutic regimen except the ischemic atherosclerotic subtype and those that could not be identified (at minimum) as of either ischemic or hemorrhagic etiology. Further, if a person is being treated with antihypertensive therapy but has a stroke, the size and resulting disability (as measured by days of reduced activity or by the number of days in bed) appears to be reduced (data not shown) (61).

13. *Incidence of Congestive Heart Failure*

New episodes of congestive heart failure occurred in 55 participants in the active treatment group and 105 participants in the placebo group (RR = 0.51; 95% CI 0.37–0.71) (34) (Table 7). The estimate of treatment benefit suggests that the number of persons who would need to be treated to prevent one episode of heart failure is 48. Older participants, men, and those with higher SBP at baseline or a history of ECG evidence of myocardial infarction at baseline had a yet higher risk of developing congestive heart failure. Among

Table 6 Incidence of First Stroke by Type and Subtype and Treatment Group

	Number of participants		Differences between active treatment and placebo participants	
	Active	Placebo	Risk ratio	95% Confidence interval
Total SHEP participants	2365	2371		
All first strokes	103	159	0.63	0.49 to 0.81
Ischemic strokes	85	132	0.63	0.48 to 0.82
Lacunar	23	43	0.53	0.32 to 0.88
Embolic	9	16	0.56	0.25 to 1.27
Atherosclerotic	13	13	0.99	0.46 to 2.15
Other/unknown	40	60	0.64	0.43 to 0.96
Hemorrhagic strokes	9	19	0.46	0.21 to 1.02
Subarachnoid	1	4	0.25	0.03 to 2.26
Intraparenchymal	8	15	0.52	0.22 to 1.22
Unknown type strokes	9	8	1.05	0.40 to 2.73

Note: Risk ratios indicate likelihood of a first stroke occurring in an active treatment participant, using the placebo participant as a reference (equal to 1.00). Values are adjusted for age, race, sex, years of education, baseline body mass index, systolic and diastolic blood pressure, history of diabetes, smoking, and the prerandomization use of antihypertensive agents.

Table 7 Uncorrected Relative Risk of Developing Heart Failure and Corrected Relative Risks for Baseline Variables in SHEP Participants with and Without History of ECG Evidence of Myocardial Infarction at Baseline

	Uncorrected				Corrected	
					History or ECG evidence of MI (n = 492)	No history or ECG evidence of MI (n = 4185)
HF Events	Placebo, no. (%) (n = 2371)	Active drug therapy, no. (%) (n = 2365)	Relative risk (95% confidence interval)	*P* Value	Relative risk (95% confidence interval)	Relative risk (95% confidence interval)
Nonfatal HF	102 (4.3)	48 (2.0)	0.46 (0.33–0.65)	<.001	0.15 (0.05–0.47)	0.56 (0.38–0.82)
Nonfatal hospitalized HF	75 (3.2)	38 (1.6)	0.50 (0.34–0.74)	<.001	0.21 (0.07–0.70)	0.60 (0.39–0.94)
Fatal and nonfatal HF	105 (4.4)	55 (2.3)	0.51 (0.37–0.71)	<.001	0.19 (0.06–0.53)	0.61 (0.42–0.88)
Fatal and hospitalized nonfatal HF	79 (3.3)	45 (1.9)	0.57 (0.34–0.81)	.002	0.24 (0.08–0.72)	0.67 (0.44–1.02)
Cardiac mortality and nonfatal hospitalized HF	162 (6.8)	113 (4.8)	0.69 (0.54–0.87)	.002	0.41 (0.20–0.82)	0.68 (0.51–0.91)
Cardiovascular mortality and nonfatal hospitalized HF	174 (7.3)	123 (5.2)	0.70 (0.55–0.88)	.002	0.38 (0.19–0.76)	0.70 (0.53–0.91)

Note: Cardiac mortality includes sudden death, rapid death, myocardial infarction, HF, and other cardiovascular disease mortality.
Cardiovascular mortality includes cardiac mortality and fatal stroke.
Relative risk controlled for treatment assignment group, age, sex, race, body mass index, current smoking, history of diabetes, cholesterol, education (> high school vs not), presence of carotid bruits, systolic blood pressure, diastolic blood pressure > 1 drink/wk of alcohol, and uric acid.
Abbreviations: *MI*, myocardial infarction; *ECG*, electrocardiogram; *HF*, heart failure.

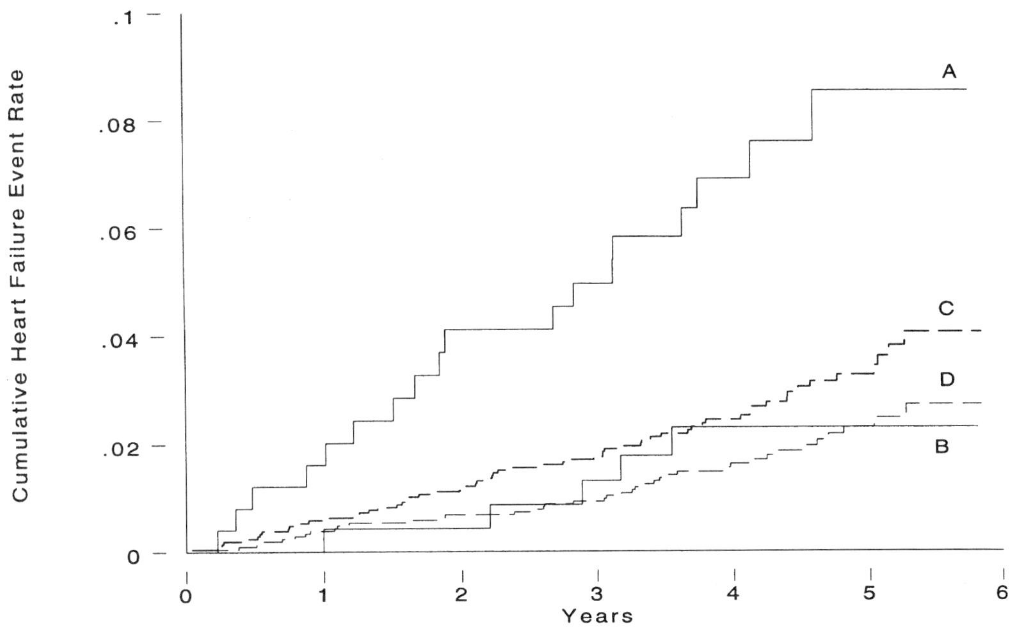

Fig. 5 Occurrence of fatal and hospitalized nonfatal heart failure in the active therapy and placebo groups of the Systolic Hypertension in the Elderly Program among participants who had a history or electrocardiographic evidence of myocardial infarction (MI) at baseline and among those who did not have a history, or electrocardiographic evidence, of MI at baseline. Line A indicates placebo group (patients with a history of MI at baseline); line B, active therapy group (patients with a history of MI at baseline); line C, placebo group (patients with no history of MI at baseline); line 4, active therapy group (patients with no history of MI at baseline). (From Ref. 30, with permission.)

those with a history of, or ECG evidence of, a prior myocardial infarction, the relative risk = 0.19 (95% Cl, 0.06–0.53) was even more substantial (30) (Fig. 5).

V. IMPLICATIONS OF SHEP

An extensive discussion of the implications of SHEP results has been previously published (61). A brief summary follows.

A. Treatment of Isolated Systolic Hypertension

Older people with ISH as defined by the SHEP trial should be identified and treated. The high prevalence of CVD, particularly, stroke and CHD, in older individuals suggests that, using the data from SHEP in 1999 (NHLBI Fact Book) annual prevention of 67,500 strokes, 59,700 CHD, and 120,000 major cardiovascular events would occur. Because of the crossover (33% of those assigned to placebo) to active medication that occurred, the estimates of treatment benefit from the SHEP data are likely an underestimate of the true benefit. Further, the generalizability of the SHEP findings of risk reduction is underscored by consistency of the data across three age strata, four race-sex strata, three baseline blood pressure strata, three baseline serum cholesterol strata, in patients both on and off antihypertensive medication at initial contact and in those with and without baseline ECG abnormalities.

B. Is There a High-Risk Subgroup Among the Elderly with ISH for Whom This Treatment Should Be Target?

The data strongly suggested that there was not a high-risk subgroup and that the findings were applicable to those who fit the inclusion-exclusion criteria used for identification of the SHEP cohort.

C. Are the SHEP Findings Extrapolatable to Other Strata of the Population with ISH?

The presence of comorbid conditions such as previous myocardial infarction, previous stroke, presence of diabetes mellitus, or ECG abnormalities does not appear to preclude the potential benefits of treatment, although some of these conditions will make treatment more difficult. Application of the treatment used in SHEP to those with stage 1 ISH (>140 but <160 mm Hg) seems reasonable because of the associated risk of that condition, but proof of benefit for this group is lacking. Similarly, those who are younger have not had a direct test of the question, but an inference of benefit seems reasonable.

D. Was a J-Shaped Curve for Coronary Mortality Observed in the SHEP Trial?

Evidence for a J-shaped curve for coronary mortality suggesting higher mortality for those at the lowest DBP levels was lacking in SHEP. In fact a reduction of 27% in coronary mortality occurred in the SHEP active treatment group despite a reduction from a mean baseline DBP blood pressure of 77 to 68 mm Hg. Also there was no J-shaped curve related to the SBP. Similar findings were evident for risk of stroke and mortality from all causes.

E. How Far Should SBP Be Lowered?

Systolic blood pressure is an even more powerful predictor than DBP of cardiovascular events, stroke, CHD, and mortality from all causes. Benefits of lowering the SBP to at least 140 mm Hg are clear from the SHEP data. Further, the strong suggestion is that even though an increased DBP may be lowered below 90 mm Hg as a result of treatment, the persistence of an elevated SBP warrants further treatment. Although benefit can be suggested to occur from attained SBPs lower than 140 mm Hg, this remains unproven.

F. Is ISH Unique from a Pharmacotherapeutic Perspective?

There is nothing to suggest from either the pathophysiology of ISH or the response to various drug treatments obtained from previous pharmacological trials that the treatment of ISH is unique. Although the results of SHEP were obtained with low-dose chlorthalidone as the step 1 and principal agent, the results of this trial should not be interpreted as limiting the choice of agents for the treatment of ISH.

G. Is the SHEP Regimen the Preferred Approach to Treating ISH?

The striking 36% risk reduction in stroke and the 27% overall risk reduction in CHD incidence in SHEP, the absence of any overall adverse effect on mortality, and only minor effects on biochemical variables or clinical signs and symptoms, and the demonstrated benefit of therapy in people with baseline ECG abnormalities all challenge the validity of previous concerns expressed regarding the risk/benefit of diuretic treatment. Further, the reduction of events type 2 diabetic participants and the magnitude of the reduction of events in those with CHF further support the intervention used in SHEP. Whatever the reasons for the prior uncertainty about the mix of benefit and risk, the positive experience in SHEP underscores the efficacy of low-dose diuretics as antihypertensive therapy.

H. Are the Results Attributable to a Protective Effect of Atenolol?

Analyses strongly suggest that the benefits for reduced risk of stroke and CHD are related to the reduction of blood pressure and are not attributable to any agent (38). Specifically, the effects observed in risk reduction were not enhanced by the use of either atenolol or reserpine.

I. What About the Newer Classes of Antihypertensive Agents?

The SHEP study was not designed to answer questions about the newer antihypertensive agents. At the time of its publication, there was no direct evidence for the efficacy of other agents in the treatment of either ISH or increases in SBP. See further comment below.

J. Do the SHEP Results Have Any Implications for Preferred Drug Treatment Regimens for DBP Hypertension?

Although SHEP gave no direct evidence about this issue, other trials, particularly Syst-Eur (63) and STOP-Hypertension-2 (64) have been subsequently published. Their findings provided important evidence regarding the choice of agents in those with diastolic hypertension or in those with mixed SBP and DBP increases. Documentation that the low-dose diuretic regimen used in SHEP is inexpensive is without question.

VI. CONCLUSIONS

The SHEP was landmark trial (65). Its implications and influence continue to permeate the medical and public health communities. It was the first trial to establish that the treatment of ISH, specifically in people older than age 60, reduced the incidence of total stroke and the traditional endpoint of all CHD (nonfatal MI and CHD death) (34). These reductions were clearly present for both men and women, for all ages included in the trial, and for all blood pressure levels included in the trial, regardless of whether one had been previously treated for hypertension or had abnormalities in a baseline ECG. The trial design and population recruited were extensively described (21, 25, 52, 57, 66–71) before the final results were published.

Nearly 50 papers have now been published from the SHEP database. The following is a brief summary of the published SHEP papers not discussed elsewhere in this manuscript. They are described as four clusters: the effect of the trial intervention, description of baseline variables, natural history studies using either part or all of the SHEP cohort, and studies describing various aspects of clinical trial methodology.

Subsequent reports to the final results paper have described the effect of the trial intervention on: trial outcomes in type 2 diabetic patients (29), trial outcomes as they relate to achieved DBP (adjusted for baseline risk factors) (72), trial outcomes in participants with mild renal dysfunction (73), trial outcomes in those with demonstrated peripheral atherosclerosis, stroke subtypes, and disability (61) an array of outcomes related to congestive heart failure (27), echocardiographically determined left ventricular mass (74), Holter-derived left ventricular ectopic activity (75, 76) progression of carotid stenosis determined by ultrasonography (77), a broad panel of quality-of-life measures (60), various biochemical variables (lipids, glucose, creatinine, uric acid, and potassium) (78), and levels of serum bone-related biochemical variables in elderly African-Americans (79).

Prevalence of baseline variables for the SHEP cohort were described including: prevalence of postural hypotension (80), reduced ankle-arm blood pressure index (81, 82), increased levels of Lp(a) and its relationship to lower extremity arterial disease (83), carotid stenosis (84, 85), and positive Osler's maneuver among screenees (86). Reports were also published regarding Doppler-echocardiographically determined cardiac structure and function (87), systemic vascular hemodynamics (88), and baseline levels of serum bone-related biochemical variables in elderly African-Americans (89).

Reports dealing with the natural history of disease processes in the SHEP cohort include: prognostic significance of asymptomatic (baseline) carotid bruits on stroke (90), prognostic significance of various baseline variables (including traditional CHD risk factors) on development of stroke (28), CHD (32, 33) and lower extremity arterial disease (low AAI) (91), the relationship of decreased ankle-arm blood pressure index and morbidity and mortality (92), the increased frequency of all cardiovascular events for those with demonstrated carotid stenosis or lower extremity arterial disease (93), the relationship of increased pulse pressure and the occurrence of stroke and mortality of all causes (94), clinical depression as associated with an increased risk of stroke, CHD, and death from all causes (95), and demographically based frequency of use of cardiovascular interventions (96).

Generic clinical trials methods have been described in the following areas: comparability of blood pressure measurements (ambulatory and random zero) (97), importance of and logistical approaches to mass mailing (33), importance of experienced clinical trials staff in trials conduct (33), contribution of lay volunteers to trial conduct (55), assessment of trial participant satisfaction (98), assessment of treatment effect using a single integrative outcome measure (99), shaping of screening rules using inclusion criteria (34), and clinical trials monitoring (28).

The major criticism of the trial has been that it gave no guidance for the use of the newer antihypertensive agents. Results of trials looking at the effects of newer agents have subsequently been reported and are described elsewhere in this volume.

Accomplishments attributable to a single trial are frequently difficult to assign, but the major ones related to SHEP outcomes appear to be that the treatment of ISH for the reduction of total stroke and a variety of other CVD endpoints was firmly established. The SHEP study was also the first demonstration that treatment of hypertension could result in a reduction in CHD. The SHEP findings clearly changed the guidelines for the treatment of hypertension as demonstrated by the changes that occurred in the Joint National Committee (JNC) III–VI (100–103). Many of the current recommendations, not only for the treatment of ISH but for the more generic approach to the treatment of hypertension with the low-dose diuretic stepped-care approach, are at least in part tied to the observations first made in SHEP.

Questions left with incomplete answers are always present when trials are finished. The optimal control of blood pressure is still incompletely understood. The controversy that arose from the analysis of the HDFP data regarding whether there was an increase in CHD mortality with DBP reduced to lower levels (below 85) remains unresolved. No such controversy was raised regarding the reduction of elevated SBP. The SHEP participants had a mean DBP level of 77 mm Hg at randomization. Those in the active treatment group had a mean DBP level of 68 mm Hg at trial's end. Yet the first reduction in the traditional CHD endpoint was observed in the total SHEP cohort. Although evidence supporting a J-shaped curve in the SHEP cohort was lacking at the analysis for the final results paper, subsequent analyses have suggested that caution about the aggressiveness of treatment be taken in those individuals who are older than age 80 and for whom DBP goes below 60 mm Hg during active intervention. Many remained unconvinced regarding the presence or absence of a J-shaped curve for CHD outcomes and the degree of DBP lowering by the available data. Subsequently, the Hypertension Optimal Treatment (HOT) trial was performed to directly test the question (104). Results from that trial have not convincingly answered the question of optimal lowering of DBP.

It has been nearly a decade since the SHEP trial first reported its results. The multiple subsequent papers expanding on the original report giving further details on the benefits of treating ISH and describing various aspects of clinical trials methodology have been described above. The conclusions and implications have been reinforced and expanded by other antihypertensive trials.

VII. TAKE-HOME MESSAGE FOR THE PRIMARY CARE PROVIDER

The primary care provider should actively identify those individuals with ISH. The SHEP study data clearly demonstrate that ISH should be treated in older patients, and probably middle-aged individuals as well. The target blood pressure is at least lower that 150 mm Hg and perhaps as low as 140 mm Hg. Diabetes mellitus, other comorbid conditions and the presence of ECG abnormalities are not contraindications to therapy. Significant numbers of strokes, CHD, and all major cardiovascular events, including CHF, will be prevented. For those who are treated and still have strokes, the post-stroke residua appear to be less severe than for those not treated. All data from this study strongly support the SHEP treatment approach as safe, well tolerated, not associated with any increase in mortality, depression, dementia, or reduction in quality of life, and a low order of clinical- or laboratory-defined adverse events. The principal therapeutic agent used in this trial of stepped-care approach to ISH was low-dose chlorthalidone, although the suggestion is that blood pressure lowering rather than the choice of therapeutic agent is the crucial issue associated with risk reduction. In summary, the treatment of ISH is effective, simple, safe, and inexpensive.

APPENDIX

Several of the SHEP researchers and key advisors are no longer living. Shirley Arch (1919–1987), Nemat O. Borhani (1926–1996), Fred I. Gilbert (1920–1995), Lot B. Page (1923–1990), Rose Stamler (1922–1998), and Philip Weiler (1940–1991).

The research on which this publication is based was supported by HHS contracts; NO-HC-48052-48058 and NO-HC-48060-48069 from the National Heart, Lung, and Blood Institute and the National Institute on Aging.

The Systolic Hypertension in the Elderly Program Data and Safety Monitoring Board members who monitored the SHEP and advised the National Heart, Lung, and

Blood Institute and National Institute on Aging regarding its progress include the following: James Hunt, MD, Chairman, University of Tennessee, Memphis; C.E. Davis, PhD, University of North Carolina, Chapel Hill; Raymond W. Gifford, MD, Cleveland (Ohio) Clinic Foundation; Millicent W. Higgins, MD, National Heart, Lung, and Blood Institute; Adrian M. Ostfeld, MD, Yale University School of Medicine, New Haven, CT; John W. Rowe, MD, Mt. Sinai Medical Center, New York, NY; K Warner Schaie, MD, Pennsylvania State University, State College PA; Herman A. Tyroler, MD, University of North Carolina, Chapel Hill, Jack P. Whisnant, MD Mayo Clinic, Rochester, MN; Joseph A. Wilber, MD, Atlanta, GA.

The SHEP Steering Committee members and the principal investigators in the trial include the following:

Chairman: Kenneth G. Berge, MD (Mayo Clinic, Rochester MN)

Clinical Centers: *Bronx*: M. Donald Blaufox, MD; *Atlanta*: W. Dallas Hall, MD; *Portland, OR*: Thomas M. Vogt, MD, MPH; *San Francisco*: William McFate Smith, MD, MPH; *Miami*: Fred Walburn, PhD; *Chicago*: David Berkson, MD; *Honolulu*: Helen Petrovitch, MD; *Piscataway*: John B. Kostis, MD; *Birmingham*: Richard M. Allman, MD; *Davis*: Nemat O. Borhani, MD, MPH; *Lexington*: Gordon P. Guthrie, Jr, MD; *Minneapolis*: Richard H. Grimm, MD, PhD; *Pittsburgh*: Lewis H. Kuller, MD, DrPH; *Memphis*: William B. Applegate, MD, MPH; *New Haven*: Henry R. Black, MD.

Coordinating Center (University of Texas School of Public Health), Houston: C. Morton Hawkins, ScD; Barry R. Davis, MD, PhD.

National Heart, Lung, and Blood Institute, Bethesda: Jeffrey L. Probstfield, MD

National Institute on Aging, Bethesda: Evan Hadley, MD

The 16 clinical centers of the cooperative group, eight coordination and service centers, their institutions, coinvestigators and senior staff were as follows: *Bronx*: Albert Einstein College of Medicine; William H. Frishman, MD; Gail Miller, RN; Maureen Magnani, RN; Sylvia Smoller, PhD; Zirel Sweezy; *Atlanta*: Emory University; Sandy Biggio, RN, BSN; Margaret Chiappini, RN, BSN; Cori Hamilton; Margaret Huber, RN, BSN; Gail McCray; Deanne J. Unger, RNC, BSN; Gary L. Wollam, MD; *Portland, OR*: Kaiser Permanente; Merwyn R. Greenlick, PhD; Stephanie Hertert; Patty Karlen, RN; Marlene McKenzie, RN, MN; Marcia Nielsen, RN, MN; Kathy Reavis, RN; *San Francisco*: Medical Research Institute; Leonard Syme, PhD, Philip Frost, MD, Geri Bailey, RN, Ann Slaby, Jacqueline Smith, RN; *Miami*: Miami Heart Institute; Maria Canosa-Terris, MD; Garcia Garrison, RN; Melissa Jones; Jeff Raines, PhD; Naldi Ritch; Avril Sampson, MD; Elisa Serantes, MD; Susan Surette; *Chicago*: Northwestern University; Flora Gosch, MD; Joseph Harrington; Patricia Hershinow, RN; Josephine Jones; Angeline Merlo; Jeremiah Stamler, MD; *Honolulu*: Pacific Health Research Institute; Sandra Akina, RN; J. David Curb, MD, MPH; Fred I. Gilbert, MD; Mary Hoffmeier, RN; Lei Honda-Sigall, RN; *Piscataway*: Robert Wood Johnson Medical School; Nora Cosgrove, RN; Susan Krieger, RN; Clifton R. Lacy, MD; *Birmingham*: Ralph E. Allen, PA-C; Donna M. Berden, MD; Lisa Carlisle; Vanessa P. Cottingham; Laura Farley, RN; Julia Hall; Glenn H. Hughes, PhD; Phillip Johnson; Linda Jones, CRNP; Laverne Parr; Pat Pierce; Harold W. Schnaper, MD; *Davis*: University of California; Patty Borhani; Alfredo Burlando, MD; Frances LaBaw, RN; Marshall Lee, MD; Sheila Lame; Susan Pace, RN; *Lexington*: University of Kentucky; Jenny Brown; Jimmie Brumagen, RN; Ellen Christian, PA-C; Lynn Hanna, PA-C; Arlene Johnson, PhD; Jane Kotchen, MD; Theodore Kotchen, MD; William Markesbery, MD; Rita Schrodt, RN; John C. Wright, MD; *Minneapolis*: University of Minnesota;

Julie Levin; Mary Perron, RN; Alice Stafford; *Pittsburgh*: University of Pittsburgh; Shirley Arch (deceased); Gale Rutan, MD; Betsy Gahagan, RN; Jerry Noviello, PhD; *Memphis*: University of Tennessee; Laretha Goodwin, RN, MBA; Stephen T. Miller, MD; Amelia Rose, RN; Alice Wallace, RN; *St. Louis*: Washington University; Great H. Camel, MD; Sharon Carmody; Jerome Cohen, MD; Judith Jensen, RN; Elizabeth Perry; *New Haven*: Yale University; Diane Christianson, RN; Janice A. Davey, MSN; Charles K. Francis, MD; Linda Loesche; *Houston*: University of Texas; William S. Fields, MD; Darwin R. Labarthe, MD, PhD; Lemuel A. Moye, MD, PhD; Sara Pressel, MS; Richard B. Shekelle, PhD; *Teterboro, NJ*: Central Chemical Laboratory MetPath Laboratories; S. Raymond Gambino, MD; Arlene Gilligan; Joseph E. O'Brien, MD; Nicholas Scalfratto; Elana Sommers; *Minneapolis*: Electrocardiographic Laboratory Center, University of Minnesota; Richard Crow, MD; Margaret Bodellan; Ronald Prineas, MBBS, PhD; *Baltimore*: Computed Tomogram Reading, University of Maryland; L. Anne Hayman, MD; C. V. G. Krishna Rao, MD; *Perry Point, MD*: Drug Distribution Center, US Public Health Service; Richard Moss; *Washington, DC*: Health Care Financing Administration; William Merashoff; *Bethesda*: National Heart, Lung, and Blood Institute; Eleanor Schron, MSN, RN; Jeffrey A. Cutler, MD, MPH; Curt Furberg, MD, PhD; Edward Lakatos, PhD; Janet Wittes, PhD; C. Eugene Harris; Linda Gardner; Thomas P. Blaszkowski, PhD; Clarissa Wittenberg, MSW; *Bethesda*: National Institute on Aging, David Curb, MD, MPH; Jack Guralnik, MD, PhD; Lot Page, MD (deceased); Teresa Radebaugh, ScD; Stanley Slater, MD; Richard Suzman, PhD.

ACKNOWLEDGMENTS

Supported by HHS Contracts; NO-HC-48052-48058 and NO-HC-48060-48069 from the National Heart, Lung, and Blood Institute and the National Institute on Aging.

REFERENCES

1. Fisher CM. The ascendancy of diastolic blood pressure over systolic. Lancet 1985; 2:1349–1350.
2. Janeway, TC. Important contributions to clinical medicine during the past thirty years from the study of human blood pressure. Bull Johns Hopkins Hosp 1915; 26:341–350.
3. Gubner RS Systolic hypertension: a pathogenetic entity. Am J Cardiol 1962; 773–776.
4. Build and Blood Pressure Study. Vol 1. Chicago: Society of Actuaries, 1959.
5. Stamler J. Lectures on Preventive Cardiology. New York: Grune & Stratton, 1967.
6. Kannel WB, Dawber TR, Sorlie P, Wolf PA. Components of blood pressure and risk of atherothrombotic brain infarction: the Framingham study. Stroke 1976; 7:327–331.
7. Colandrea MA, Friedman GD, Nichaman MZ, Lynd CN. Systolic hypertension in the elderly. An epidemiologic assessment. Circulation 1970; 41:239–245.
8. Abernethy J, Borhani NO, Hawkins CM, Crow R, Entwisle G, Jones JW, Maxwell MH, Langford H, Pressel S. Systolic blood pressure as an independent predictor of mortality in the Hypertension Detection and Follow-up Program. Am J Prev Med 1986; 2:123–132.
9. Curb JD, Borhani NO, Entwisle G, Tung B, Kass E, Schnaper H, Williams W, Berman R. Isolated systolic hypertension in 14 communities. Am J Epidemiol 1985; 121:362–370.
10. Shekelle RB, Ostfeld AM, Klawans HL, Jr. Hypertension and risk of stroke in an elderly population. Stroke 1974; 5(1):71–75.
11. Stamler J, Neaton JD, Wentworth DN. Blood pressure (systolic and diastolic) and risk of fatal coronary heart disease. Hypertension 1989; 13(5 suppl):12–12.

12. Dyer AR, Stamler J, Shekelle RB, Schoenberger JA, Farinaro E. Hypertension in the elderly. Med Clin North Am 1977; 61:513–529.
13. Garland C, Barrett-Connor E, Suarez L, Criqui MH. Isolated systolic hypertension and mortality after age 60 years. A prospective population-based study. Am J Epidemiol 1983; 118: 365–376.
14. Rutan GH, Kuller LH, Neaton JD, Wentworth DN, McDonald RH, Smith WM. Mortality associated with diastolic hypertension and isolated systolic hypertension among men screened for the Multiple Risk Factor Intervention Trial. Circulation 1988; 77:504–514.
15. Blood Pressure of Adults by Race and Area: United States, 1976–80. National Center for Health Statistics, 1986.
16. Vogt TM, Ireland CC, Black D, Camel G, Hughes G. Recruitment of elderly volunteers for a multi-center clinical trial: the SHEP pilot study. Control Clin Trials 1986; 7:118–133.
17. Veterans Administration Cooperative Study on Antihypertensive Agents. Effects of treatment on morbidity in hypertension. Results in patients with diastolic blood pressures averaging 115 through 129 mm Hg. JAMA 1967; 202:1028–1034.
18. Veterans Administration Cooperative Study on Antihypertensive Agents. Effects of treatment on morbidity in hypertension. II. Results in patients with diastolic blood pressure averaging 90 through 114 mm Hg. JAMA 1970; 213:1143–1152.
19. Veterans Administration Cooperative Study on Antihypertensive Agents. Effects of treatment on morbidity in hypertension. III. Influence of age, diastolic pressure, and prior cardiovascular disease; further analysis of side effects. Circulation 1972; 45:991–1004.
20. Smith WM. Treatment of mild hypertension: results of a ten-year intervention trial. Circ Res 1977; 40(5 suppl 1):I98–105.
21. Borhani NO, Applegate WB, Cutler JA, Davis BR, Furberg CD, Lakatos E, Page L, Perry HM, Smith WM, Probstfield JL. Systolic Hypertension in the Elderly Program (SHEP). Part 1: rationale and design. Hypertension 1991; 17(3 suppl):2–15.
22. Hulley SB, Furberg CD, Gurland B, McDonald R, Perry HM, Schnaper HW, Schoenberger JA, Smith WM, Vogt TM. Systolic Hypertension in the Elderly Program (SHEP): antihypertensive efficacy of chlorthalidone. Am J Cardiol 1985; 56:913–920.
23. Black DM, Brand RJ, Greenlick M, Hughes G, Smith J. Compliance to treatment for hypertension in elderly patients: the SHEP pilot study. Systolic Hypertension in the Elderly Program. J Gerontol 1987; 42(5):552–557.
24. Perry HM, Jr, McDonald RH, Hulley SB, Smith WM, Furberg CD, Greenlick MR, Kuller LH, Schnaper HW, Schoenberger JA, Vogt TM. Systolic Hypertension in the Elderly Program, Pilot Study (SHEP-PS): morbidity and mortality experience. J Hypertens Suppl 1986; 4:S21–S23.
25. SHEP Cooperative Research Group. Rationale and design of a randomized clinical trial on prevention of stroke in isolated systolic hypertension. The Systolic Hypertension in the Elderly Program (SHEP) Cooperative Research Group. J Clin Epidemiol 1988; 41:1197–1208.
26. Morledge JH, Ettinger B, Aranda J, McBarron F, Barra P, Gorwit J, Davidov M. Isolated Systolic Hypertension in the Elderly: a placebo-controlled, dose-response evaluation of chlorthalidone. J Am Geriatr Soc 1986; 34:199–206.
27. Collins R, Peto R, MacMahon S, Hebert P, Fiebach NH, Eberlein KA, Godwin J, Qizilbash N, Taylor JO, Hennekens CH. Blood pressure, stroke, and coronary heart disease. Part 2, short-term reductions in blood pressure: overview of randomised drug trials in their epidemiological context. Lancet 1990; 335:827–838.
28. MacMahon S, Peto R, Cutler J, Collins R, Sorlie P, Neaton J, Abbott R, Godwin J, Dyer A, Stamler J. Blood pressure, stroke, and coronary heart disease. Part 1, prolonged differences in blood pressure: prospective observational studies corrected for the regression dilution bias. Lancet 1990; 335:765–774.
29. Curb JD, Pressel SL, Cutler JA, Savage PJ, Applegate WB, Black H, Camel G, Davis BR,

Frost PH, Gonzalez N, Guthrie G, Oberman A, Rutan GH, Stamler J. Effect of diuretic-based antihypertensive treatment on cardiovascular disease risk in older diabetic patients with isolated systolic hypertension. Systolic Hypertension in the Elderly Program Cooperative Research Group. JAMA 1996; 276:1886–1892. Published erratum. JAMA 1997; 277:1356.

30. Kostis JB, Davis BR, Cutler J, Grimm RH, Jr, Berge KG, Cohen JD, Lacy CR, Perry HM, Jr, Blaufox MD, Wassertheil-Smoller S, Black HR, Schron E, Berkson DM, Curb JD, Smith WM, McDonald R, Applegate WB. Prevention of heart failure by antihypertensive drug treatment in older persons with isolated systolic hypertension. SHEP Cooperative Research Group. JAMA 1997; 278:212–216.
31. Davis BR, Vogt T, Frost PH, Burlando A, Cohen J, Wilson A, Brass LM, Frishman W, Price T, Stamler J. Risk factors for stroke and type of stroke in persons with isolated systolic hypertension. Systolic Hypertension in the Elderly Program Cooperative Research Group. Stroke 1998; 29:1333–1340.
32. Frost PH, Davis BR, Burlando AJ, Curb JD, Guthrie GP, Isaacsohn JL, Wassertheil-Smoller S, Wilson AC, Stamler J. Coronary heart disease risk factors in men and women aged 60 years and older: findings from the Systolic Hypertension in the Elderly Program. Circulation 1996; 94:26–34.
33. Frost PH, Davis BR, Burlando AJ, Curb JD, Guthrie GP, Isaacsohn JL, Wassertheil-Smoller S, Wilson AC, Stamler J. Serum Lipids and incidence of coronary heart disease. Findings from the Systolic Hypertension in the Elderly Program. Circulation 1996; 94:2381–2388.
34. SHEP Cooperative Research Group. Prevention of stroke by antihypertensive drug treatment in older persons with isolated systolic hypertension. Final results of the Systolic Hypertension in the Elderly Program (SHEP). SHEP Cooperative Research Group. JAMA 1991; 265: 3255–3264.
35. Davis BR, Wittes J, Pressel S, Berge KG, Hawkins CM, Lakatos E, Moye LA, Probstfield JL. Statistical considerations in monitoring the Systolic Hypertension in the Elderly Program (SHEP). Control Clin Trials 1993; 14:350–361.
36. Gurland B, Golden RR, Teresi JA, Challop J. The SHORT-CARE: an efficient instrument for the assessment of depression, dementia and disability. J Gerontol 1984; 39:166–169.
37. Radloff LS. The CES-D scale: a self-report depression scale for research in the general population. Appl Psych Meas 1977; 1:385–401.
38. Branch LG, Katz S, Kniepmann K, Papsidero JA. A prospective study of functional status among community elders. Am J Pub Health 1984; 74:266–268.
39. Branch LG. Established Populations for Epidemiologic Studies of the Elderly. Resource Data Book. Bethesda, MD: National Institutes of Health, No. 86-2443, 1986:33–55.
40. Reitan RM. Investigations of the validity of Halstead's measure of biological intelligence. Arch Neurol Psychiatr 1955:475.
41. Bull T. The Halstead-Reitan neuropsychology battery. Handbook of Clinical Neuropsychology. New York: Wiley-Interscience, 1981:577–607.
42. Wechsler D. Wechsler Adult Intelligence Scale Manual. New York: Psychological Corp., 1955.
43. Wechsler D. The Measurement and Appraisal of Adult Intelligence. Baltimore: Williams & Wilkins, 1958.
44. Vitaliano PP, Breen AR, Albert MS, Russo J, Prinz PN. Memory, attention and functional status in community residing Alzheimer's type dementia patients and optimally health aged individuals. J Gerontol 1984; 34:58–64.
45. Kaplan E, Goodglass H, Weintraub S. Boston Naming Test. Philadelphia: Lea & Febiger, 1983.
46. Shaie KW. The Seattle Longitudinal Study: a 21-Year Exploration of Psychometric Intelligence in Adulthood. Longitudinal Studies of Adult Psychological Development. New York: Guilford Press, 1983.

47. Ekstrom RB, French JW, Harman HH, Dermen D. Kit of Factor-Referenced Cognitive Tests. Princeton, NJ: Educational Testing Service, 1976.
48. Andrews FM, Withey SB. Social Indicators of Well-being: Americans' Perception of Life Quality. New York: Plenum Press, 1976.
49. Gurin G, Veroff J, Field S. Americans View Their Mental Health. New York: Basic Books, 1960.
50. Mossey JM, Havens B, Roos NP, Shapiro E. The Manitoba longitudinal study on aging: description and methods. Gerontologist 1981; 21:551–558.
51. Hunninghake DB, Darby CA, Probstfield JL. Recruitment experience in clinical trials: literature summary and annotated bibliography. Control Clin Trials 1987; 8:6S–30S.
52. Petrovitch H, Byington R, Bailey G, Borhani P, Carmody S, Goodwin L, Harrington J, Johnson HA, Johnson P, Jones M. Systolic Hypertension in the Elderly Program (SHEP). Part 2: screening and recruitment. Hypertension 1991; 17(3 suppl):II16–II23.
53. Lakatos E. Sample size determination in clinical trials with time-dependent rates of losses and noncompliance. Control Clin Trials 1986; 7(3):189–199.
54. Cosgrove N, Borhani NO, Bailey G, Borhani P, Levin J, Hoffmeier M, Krieger S, Lovato LC, Petrovitch H, Vogt T, Wilson AC, Breeson V, Probstfield JL. Mass mailing and staff experience in a total recruitment program for a clinical trial: the SHEP experience. Systolic Hypertension in the Elderly Program. Cooperative Research Group (in process citation). Control Clin Trials 1999; 20:133–48.
55. Hertert S, Bailey G, Cottinghan V, Carmody S, Egan D, Johnson P, Probstfield J. Community volunteers as recruitment staff in a clinical trial: the Systolic Hypertension in the Elderly Program (SHEP) experience. Control Clin Trials 1996; 17:23–32. Published erratum appears in Control Clin Trials 1996; 17(3):271.
56. Wittes J, Lakatos E, Black D, Geraci B, Davis BR, Moye LA, Probstfield JL. Selecting screening criteria for clinical trials: an example from the systolic hypertension in the elderly program. Control Clin Trials 1999; 20:121–132.
57. Wittes J, Davis B, Berge K, Cohen JD, Grimm RH, Jr, Hawkins CM, Kuller L. Systolic Hypertension of the Elderly Program (SHEP). Part 10: analysis. Hypertension 1991; 17(3 suppl):II162–II167.
58. Black HR, Unger D, Burlando A, Wright JC, Pressel SL, Allen R, McDonald RH, Surath H. Systolic Hypertension in the Elderly Program (SHEP). Part 6: baseline physical examination findings. Hypertension 1991; 17(3 suppl):II77–101.
59. Kostis JB, Berge K, Davis BR, Hawkins CM, Probstfield JL, for the SHEP Cooperative Research Group. Effect of atenolol and reserpine on selected events in the Systolic Hypertension in the Elderly Program (SHEP). Am J Hypertens 1995; 8:1147–1153.
60. Applegate WB, Pressel S, Wittes J, Luhr J, Shekelle RB, Camel GH, Greenlick MR, Hadley E, Moye L, Perry HM, Jr. Impact of the treatment of isolated systolic hypertension on behavioral variables. Results from the Systolic Hypertension in the Elderly Program. Arch Intern Med 1994; 154:2154–2160.
61. Perry HM, Price TR, Davis B, Applegate WB, Brass L, Fields W, Guralnick J, Kuller L, Pressel, S, Wallech F, Probstfield JL, for the Systolic Hypertension in the Elderly (SHEP) Cooperative Research Group. Effect of treating isolated systolic hypertension on incidence, (case fatality and disability) of specific types of stroke: The Systolic Hypertension in the Elderly Program. In press.
62. The SHEP Cooperative Research Group. Implications of the Systolic Hypertension in the Elderly Program. Hypertension 1993; 21:335–343.
63. Staessen JA, Fagard R, Thijs L, Celis H, Arabidze GG, Birkenhager WH, Bulpitt CJ, de Leeuw PW, Dollery CT, Fletcher AE, Forette F, Leonetti G, Nachev C, O'Brien ET, Rosenfeld J, Rodicio JL, Tuomilehto J, Zanchetti A. Randomised double-blind comparison of placebo and active treatment for older patients with isolated systolic hypertension. The Systolic Hypertension in Europe (Syst-Eur) Trial Investigators [see comments]. Lancet 1997; 350: 757–764.

64. Hansson L, Lindholm LH, Ekbom T, Dahlof B, Lanke J, Schersten B, Wester PO, Hedner T, de Faire U. Randomised trial of old and new antihypertensive drugs in elderly patients: cardiovascular mortality and morbidity the Swedish Trial in Old Patients with Hypertension-2 study. Lancet 1999; 354(9192):1751–1756.
65. Holme I, Ekelund LG, Hjermann I, Leren P. Quality-adjusted meta-analysis of the hypertension/coronary dilemma. Am J Hypertens 1994; 7(8):703–712.
66. Vogt TM, Schron E, Pressel S, Wasserthiel-Smoller S, Eddleman EE, Miller S, Stamler J. Systolic Hypertension in the Elderly Program (SHEP). Part 3: sociodemographic characteristics. Hypertension 1991; 17(3 suppl):II24–II34.
67. Curb JD, Lee M, Jensen J, Applegate W. Systolic Hypertension in the Elderly Program (SHEP). Part 4: baseline medical history findings. Hypertension 1991; 17(3 suppl): II35–II61.
68. Labarthe DR, Blaufox MD, Smith WM, Lacy CR, Schnaper H, LaBaw F, Mascioli S, Davey J, Lakatos E. Systolic Hypertension in the Elderly Program (SHEP). Part 5: baseline blood pressure and pulse rate measurements. Hypertension 1991; 17(3 suppl):II62–II76.
69. Hall WD, Davis BR, Frost P, Hoffmeier M, O'Brien JE, Pace S, Page L, Schneider KA, Stamler J. Systolic Hypertension in the Elderly Program (SHEP). Part 7: baseline laboratory characteristics. Hypertension 1991; 17(3 suppl):II102–II122.
70. Kostis JB, Prineas R, Curb JD, Lee M, Berkson D, Raines J, Frishman W, Francis CK, Sheffield T. Systolic Hypertension in the Elderly Program (SHEP). Part 8: electrocardiographic characteristics. Hypertension 1991; 17(3 suppl):II123–II151.
71. Weiler PG, Camel GH, Chiappini M, Greenlick MR, Hughes GH, Luhr JC, Moye LA, Mungas D, Perron M, Peters MH. Systolic Hypertension of the Elderly Program (SHEP). Part 9: behavioral characteristics. Hypertension 1991; 17(3 suppl):II152–II161.
72. Somes GW, Pahor M, Shorr RI, Cushman WC, Applegate WB. The role of diastolic blood pressure when treating isolated systolic hypertension. Arch Intern Med 1999; 159:2004–2009.
73. Pahor M, Shorr RI, Somes GW, Cushman WC, Ferrucci L, Bailey JE, Elam JT, Applegate WB. Diuretic-based treatment and cardiovascular events in patients with mild renal dysfunction enrolled in the systolic hypertension in the elderly program. Arch Intern Med 1998; 158: 1340–1345.
74. Ofili EO, Cohen JD, St. Vrain JA, Pearson A, Martin TJ, Uy ND, Castello R, Labovitz AJ. Effect of treatment of isolated systolic hypertension on left ventricular mass. JAMA 1998; 279:778–780.
75. Kostis JB, Lacy CR, Hall WD, Wilson AC, Borhani NO, Krieger SD, Cosgrove NM. The effect of chlorthalidone on ventricular ectopic activity in patients with isolated systolic hypertension. The SHEP Study Group. Am J Cardiol 1994; 74:464–467.
76. Kostis JB, Allen R, Berkson DM, Curb JD, Davey J, Grimm RH, Hall WD, Lacy CR, Lee M, Miller S. Correlates of ventricular ectopic activity in isolated systolic hypertension. SHEP Cooperative Research Group. Am Heart J 1994; 127:112–121.
77. Sutton-Tyrrell K, Wolfson SK, Jr, Kuller LH. Blood pressure treatment slows the progression of carotid stenosis in patients with isolated systolic hypertension. Stroke 1994; 25: 44–50.
78. Savage PJ, Pressel SL, Curb JD, Schron EB, Applegate WB, Black HR, Cohen J, Davis BR, Frost P, Smith W, Gonzalez N, Guthrie GP, Oberman A, Rutan G, Probstfield JL, Stamler J. Influence of long-term, low-dose, diuretic-based, antihypertensive therapy on glucose, lipid, uric acid, and potassium levels in older men and women with isolated systolic hypertension: The Systolic Hypertension in the Elderly Program. SHEP Cooperative Research Group. Arch Intern Med 1998; 158:741–751.
79. Perry HM, Jensen JK, Kaiser FE, Horowitz MP, Perry HM, Jr, Morley JE. The effects of thiazide diuretics on calcium metabolism in the aged. J Am Geriatr Soc 1993; 41(8):818–822.
80. Applegate WB, Davis BR, Black HR, Smith WM, Miller ST, Burlando AJ. Prevalence of

postural hypotension at baseline in the Systolic Hypertension in the Elderly Program (SHEP) cohort. J Am Geriatr Soc 1991; 39:1057–1064.

81. Newman AB, Sutton-Tyrrell K, Rutan GH, Locher J, Kuller LH. Lower extremity arterial disease in elderly subjects with systolic hypertension. J Clin Epidemiol 1991; 44:15–20.
82. Newman AB, Sutton-Tyrrell K, Kuller LH. Lower extremity arterial disease in older hypertensive adults. Arterioscler Thromb 1993; 13:555–562.
83. Sutton-Tyrrell K, Evans RW, Meilahn E, Alcorn HG. Lipoprotein (a) and peripheral atherosclerosis in older adults. Atherosclerosis 1996; 122:11–19.
84. Sutton-Tyrrell K, Alcorn HG, Wolfson SK, Jr, Kelsey SF, Kuller LH. Predictors of carotid stenosis in older adults with and without isolated systolic hypertension. Stroke 1993; 24: 355–361.
85. Franklin SS, Sutton-Tyrrell K, Belle SH, Weber MA, Kuller LH. The importance of pulsatile components of hypertension in predicting carotid stenosis in older adults. J Hypertens 1997; 15:1143–1150.
86. Wright JC, Looney SW. Prevalence of positive Osler's manoeuver in 3387 persons screened for the Systolic Hypertension in the Elderly Program (SHEP). J Hum Hypertens 1997; 11: 285–289.
87. Pearson AC, Gudipati C, Nagelhout D, Sear J, Cohen JD, Labovitz AJ. Echocardiographic evaluation of cardiac structure and function in elderly subjects with isolated systolic hypertension. J Am Coll Cardiol 1991; 17(2):422–430.
88. Pasierski T, Pearson AC, Labovitz AJ. Pathophysiology of isolated systolic hypertension in elderly patients: Doppler echocardiographic insights. Am Heart J 1991; 122(2):528–534.
89. Perry HM, III, Miller DK, Morley JE, Horowitz M, Kaiser FE, Perry HM, Jr, Jensen J, Bentley J, Boyd S, Kraenzle D. A preliminary report of vitamin D and calcium metabolism in older African Americans. J Am Geriatr Soc 1993; 41(6):612–616.
90. Shorr RI, Johnson KC, Wan JY, Sutton-Tyrrell K, Pahor M, Bailey JE, Applegate WB. The prognostic significance of asymptomatic carotid bruits in the elderly. J Gen Intern Med 1998; 13(2):86–90.
91. Newman AB, Sutton-Tyrrell K, Vogt MT, Kuller LH. Morbidity and mortality in hypertensive adults with a low ankle/arm blood pressure index. JAMA 1993; 270:487–489.
92. Sutton-Tyrrell K, Alcorn HG, Herzog H, Kelsey SF, Kuller LH. Morbidity, mortality, and antihypertensive treatment effects by extent of atherosclerosis in older adults with isolated systolic hypertension. Stroke 1995; 26:1319–1324.
93. Newman AB, Tyrrell KS, Kuller LH. Mortality over four years in SHEP participants with a low ankle-arm index. J Am Geriatr Soc 1997; 45:1472–1478.
94. Domanski MJ, Davis BR, Pfeffer MA, Kastantin M, Mitchell GF. Isolated systolic hypertension: prognostic information provided by pulse pressure. Hypertension 1999; 34:375–380.
95. Wassertheil-Smoller S, Applegate WB, Berge K, Chang CJ, Davis BR, Grimm R, Jr, Kostis J, Pressel S, Schron E. Change in depression as a precursor of cardiovascular events. SHEP Cooperative Research Group (Systoloc Hypertension in the Elderly). Arch Intern Med 1996; 156:553–561.
96. Bearden D, Allman R, McDonald R, Miller S, Pressel S, Petrovitch H. Age, race, and gender variation in the utilization of coronary artery bypass surgery and angioplasty in SHEP. SHEP Cooperative Research Group. Systolic Hypertension in the Elderly Program. J Am Geriatr Soc 1994; 42:1143–1149.
97. Rutan GH, McDonald RH, Kuller LH. Comparison of ambulatory and clinic blood pressure and heart rate in older persons with isolated systolic hypertension. Am J Hypertens 1992; 5(12 Pt 1):880–886.
98. Schron EB, Wassertheil-Smoller S, Pressel S. Clinical trial participant satisfaction: survey of SHEP enrollees. SHEP Cooperative Research Group. Systolic Hypertension in the Elderly Program. J Am Geriatr Soc 1997; 45:934–938.
99. Brittain E, Palensky J, Blood J, Wittes J. Blinded subjective rankings as a method of assessing

treatment effect: a large sample example from the Systolic Hypertension in the Elderly Program (SHEP). Stat Med 1997; 16:681–693.
100. The 1984 Report of the Joint National Committee on Detection, Evaluation, and Treatment of High Blood Pressure. Arch Intern Med 1984; 144(5):1045–1057.
101. The 1988 Report of the Joint National Committee on Detection, Evaluation, and Treatment of High Blood Pressure. Arch Intern Med 1988; 148(5):1023–1038.
102. Joint National Committee on Detection, Evaluation and Treatment of High Blood Pressure. The fifth report of the Joint National Committee on the Detection, Evaluation, and Treatment of High Blood Pressure (JNC V). Arch Intern Med 1993; 153:154–183.
103. The sixth report of the Joint National Committee on prevention, detection, evaluation, and treatment of high blood pressure. Arch Intern Med 1997; 157(21):2413–2446. Published erratum. Arch Intern Med 1998; 23; 158:573.
104. Hansson L, Zanchetti A, Carruthers SG, Dahlof B, Elmfeldt D, Julius S, Menard J, Rahn KH, Wedel H, Westerling S. Effects of intensive blood-pressure lowering and low-dose aspirin in patients with hypertension: principal results of the Hypertension Optimal Treatment (HOT) randomised trial. HOT Study Group. Lancet 1998; 351:1755–1762.
105. Hansson L, Lindholm LH, Ekbom T, Dahlof B, Lanke J, Schersten B, Wester P-O, Hedner T, de Faire U, for the STOP-Hypertension-2 study group. Randomised trial of old and new antihypertensive drugs in elderly patients: cardiovascular mortality and morbidity the Swedish Trial in Old Patients with Hypertension-2 study. Lancet 1999; 354:1751–1756.
106. Amery A, Birkenhager W, Brixko P, Bulpitt C, Clement D, Deruyttere M, De Schaepdryver A, Fagard R, Forette F, Forte J. Glucose intolerance during diuretic therapy in elderly hypertensive patients. A second report from the European Working Party on High Blood Pressure in the Elderly (EWPHE). Postgrad Med J 1986; 62:919–924.
107. Donahue RP, Abbott RD, Wilson PWF. Effect of diuretic use on the development of diabetes mellitus. Horm Metab Res (suppl 1) 1991; 22:46–48.
108. Blohme G, Lapidus L, Lissner L, Lundgren H. Diabetes incidence in users and non-users of antihypertensive drugs in relation to serum insulin, glucose tolerance and degree of adiposity. J Intern Med 1992; 231:583–588.
109. Levy D, Larson MG, Vasan RS, Kannel WB, Ho KK. The progression from hypertension to congestive heart failure. JAMA 1996; 275(20):1557–1562.

11

Medical Research Council Trial of Treatment of Hypertension in Older Adults

COLIN T. DOLLERY

University of London, London, England

I. BACKGROUND

During the last 2 decades, interest in treating diseases of older people has increased. The risk of cardiovascular diseases, especially stroke, rises steeply with advancing age, but most of the earlier randomized, controlled trials of antihypertensive therapy excluded patients older than ages 60 to 65 at entry. The reasons for doing so were never well articulated. However, it was probably believed that both the medical and economic benefits were limited, coupled with concern that adverse effects might be more prominent in the elderly.

Several factors changed medical attitudes. The publication of a number of randomized, controlled trials of antihypertensive therapy in patients younger than age 65 demonstrated a reduction in stroke approaching 50%, whereas the adverse effects of the treatments used in these trials were modest. Increasing life expectancy and recognition of the medical and economic burden of nonfatal stroke began to focus attention on the possibility of prevention.

The successful Medical Research Council (MRC) trial of treatment in mild hypertension in patients ages 35 to 64 set the stage for a similar study in older patients (1). The trial in the elderly used a number of assets from the earlier trial, especially the national network of collaborating general (family) practices. The working party that supervised the trial had a substantial common membership, and the trial was again coordinated by the MRC Epidemiology and Medical Care Unit at Northwick Park Hospital, Harrow (2).

The design of the elderly trial was heavily influenced by the earlier mild hypertension trial. Men and women ages 65 to 74 years were recruited by screening the age and sex registers of the collaborating family practices. The same two classes of drugs—a beta-adrenergic blocker and a diuretic—were used, although the chemical entities were different and the relative doses were lower. The use of 10 mg of bendrofluazide daily in the MRC mild hypertension trial had caused appreciable reduction of the serum potassium level, and evidence suggested that the dose-response curve to diuretics was relatively flat. For this reason, a combination of amiloride and hydrochlorothiazide (Moduret-25) was used for the diuretic arm. In the earlier trial, practolol was (fortunately) rejected in favor of propranolol because of limited experience of practolol's use. In the elderly trial, atenolol was chosen because a beta-1 selective drug was thought to cause fewer side effects, and there was already substantial experience of its use.

II. PATIENTS AND METHODS

Calculations suggested that the trial would require 5000 men and women ages 65 to 74 to be followed up for 5 years to detect a 30% reduction in the rate of fatal and nonfatal stroke between the active and placebo groups at a 2% level of significance with a power of 90%. As in the mild hypertension trial, the numbers were calculated on the basis of the active group as a whole rather than the individual therapeutic regimens. In retrospect, as both trials suggested that there might be differences in outcome between the two active treatments unrelated to their effect on blood pressure, it is a pity that the trial was not increased in size to give sufficient power for the comparison between active drugs. Cost, however, was an important consideration.

A. Patient Selection

Recruitment took place over 5 years starting in March 1982 (Table 1).

The population was identified from the age-sex registers of 226 group practices participating in the MRC General Practice Research Framework throughout England, Scotland, and Wales: 184,653 invitations for screening were sent and 125,861 people (68%) attended. Three sitting blood pressure measurements were recorded by a specially

Table 1 Screening and Recruitment

Invited for screening	184,653
Attended for screening	125,861
Systolic BP 160–209 mm Hg Diastolic BP < 115 mm Hg	20,389
Remained within trial limits after three run-in visits	8,832
After physician BP check referred for entry examination	4,961
Entered trial	4,396

Abbreviation: *BP*, blood pressure.

trained trial nurse using a Hawksley random zero sphygmomanometer, on which the zero offset can only be read after the blood pressure has been recorded. The mean of the second and third systolic readings was calculated. The person entered the run-in stage of the trial if the systolic pressure lay between 160 and 209 mm Hg and the diastolic pressure was less than 115 mm Hg. 20,389 individuals (10% of those attending screening) fulfilled these criteria. If the systolic pressure was less than 160 mm Hg the person was reassured and if the diastolic was greater than 115 mm Hg the person was referred to his or her general practitioner for consideration of treatment.

Looking back 17 years after the trial was designed, these pressure criteria appear high. However, there was concern that the lability of systolic pressure in the elderly related to the decreased elasticity of the aorta might mean that a narrower band of entry pressure would leave a high proportion of the patients below the trial limits by the end of the run-in period.

B. Run-In Period and Criteria for Entry into Main Trial

1. *Screening*

A relatively complex blood pressure rescreening procedure was used before entry to the trial proper. Patients attended for three run-in visits 1, 4, and 8 weeks after screening. At each visit, the sitting blood pressure was measured three times by the nurse, using the same method as for the screening visit, and the mean of the second and third readings was calculated as before. If the overall mean of the three mean run-in blood pressures still lay within the trial limit, the subjects (n = 8832) attended to have their blood pressures measured by a doctor.

2. *Trial Entry*

If the doctor confirmed that the pressures remained within the trial limits, an appointment was made for a trial entry physical examination and a further reading of blood pressure. In retrospect, it would probably have been better to rely entirely on the nurse's readings because the ''white coat effect'' of the medical examination gave an entry pressure that was higher than the usual level in these individuals. Subjects with a mean systolic pressure of 210 mm Hg or more, recorded over two visits, were ineligible for the trial and further management was left to their general practitioners, 4961 of those screened, who remained within the trial limits, were referred for the entry examination.

At this examination, the patient completed a questionnaire concerning cardiovascular and other symptoms, smoking, and previous treatment for hypertension, gout, asthma, or diabetes. Urine was tested for glucose and protein; blood was taken for measuring total serum cholesterol, urea, creatinine, electrolyte, and glucose concentrations, and a 12-lead electrocardiogram was recorded.

Several exclusion criteria were required largely because of known adverse effects of one or another of the main active treatment regimens (Table 2).

After the inclusion and exclusion criteria had been applied, 4396 patients (3.5% of those screened) gave informed consent and entered the trial. Some commentators have expressed concern that this degree of selection may have impaired the feasibility of extrapolating the results to the general population. Undoubtedly, one effect of multiple exclusion criteria is to select a population that is, in other respects, of above-average health and less likely to suffer morbid events. This is a problem common to almost all large randomized controlled trials.

Table 2 Inclusion and Exclusion Criteria

Inclusion Criteria	Exclusion Criteria
• Men and women aged 67–74 years, selected from age/sex registers in family practice • Systolic BP—160–209 mm Hg • Diastolic BP < 115 mm Hg • Maintained through three run-in visits taken by a specially trained nurse and a check by a physician	• Known or suspected secondary hypertension • Already taking antihypertensive drug(s) • Heart failure • Myocardial infarction or stroke within the preceding 3 months • Current treatment for angina pectoris • Impaired renal function • Diabetes mellitus • Serum potassium of <3.4 mmol/L or >5.0 mmol/L • Asthma • Cancer • Other serious intercurrent disease

Abbreviation: BP, blood pressure.

C. Treatment Regimens and Dose Titration

A small dose-ranging study was carried out with two strengths of the diuretic regimen, 5 mg of amiloride and 50 mg of hydrochlorothiazide or 2.5 mg of amiloride and 25 mg of hydrochlorothiazide, combined in a single commercial tablet once daily (Moduretic or Moduret-25). The effects of the two doses were indistinguishable and all patients on active diuretic therapy were transferred to the lower dose in 1985.

Patients were randomized to one of four treatment regimens as described in Table 3.

Each patient was assigned a target systolic blood pressure (150 or 160 mm Hg), depending on the mean systolic pressure after the run-in period (mean $<$ 180 mm Hg, target $\leq$ 150 mm Hg; mean $\geq$ 180 mm Hg, target $\leq$ 160 mm Hg). There was no goal diastolic pressure. Drug regimens for those on active treatment were modified by the coordinating center if blood pressure had not responded after 12 weeks or if target pressure had not been achieved after 6 months. The change needed most often was an increase in

Table 3 Trial Treatment Regimens

Initial treatment	1. Amiloride 2.5 mg with hydrochlorothiazide 25 mg in a single tablet 2. Matching placebo 3. Atenolol 50 mg daily 4. Matching placebo
At 12 weeks, if no initial response or above target systolic BP (150 mm Hg or 1600 mm Hg) at 6 months	Step 1 Increase atenolol to 100 mg daily Step 2 Amiloride 2.5 mg with hydrochlorothiazide 25 mg in a single tablet, plus atenolol 50 mg daily Step 3 Add nifedipine (standard formulation) up to 20 mg daily (10 mg bd) Step 4 Rarely, if these measures were insufficient other drugs could be added

Abbreviation: *BP*, blood pressure; *bd*, twice a day.

atenolol to 100 mg daily, in 225 patients. When further reduction in blood pressure was necessary, the other active trial drug was used to supplement the drug allocated by randomization. After this, the calcium channel blocker, nifedipine, was used in doses of up to 20 mg daily. Other supplementary drugs were also allowed.

D. Trial Design

The trial was randomized, placebo controlled, and single blind. Randomization was in stratified blocks of eight within each sex and clinic. Patients did not know which treatment group they were in, but the doctors and nurses did. The single-blind design may have had some effect on withdrawals because of side effects, but the Hawksley random zero sphygmomanometer was used to minimize bias in taking pressure readings.

E. Long-Term Follow-Up

Patients who entered the trial were followed up fortnightly for 4 weeks, then monthly up to 3 months, and every 3 months until the end of the trial. At each visit, blood pressure was measured twice in the sitting position by a specially trained nurse. If the mean blood pressure at any visit during the main trial reached or exceeded 115 mm Hg diastolic or 210 mm Hg systolic, the patient was recalled 2 weeks later. If either of these pressures were sustained on active trial treatment, the general practitioner managed further treatment outside the trial protocol. Patients whose blood pressure equaled or exceeded the upper limits on any three nonconsecutive occasions were similarly managed.

F. End Points

1. Terminating Events

Each terminating event was evaluated by an assessor who was blind to the treatment regimen. All available documentation was reviewed, including copies of general practitioners' notes, hospital inpatient or outpatient notes, electrocardiographic recordings, necropsy findings, and death certificates. Strokes and coronary events were classified using World Health Organization criteria. Data on terminating events were analyzed every 5000 patient years and were reviewed by an independent monitoring and ethics committee. Table 4 lists the trial-terminating events.

2. Death from Any Cause

All the patients in the trial were "flagged" at the NHS central register to ensure notification of death if they died in the United Kingdom, which was likely to be the case in this

Table 4 Trial Terminating Events

• Death from any cause	
• Stroke	(fatal or nonfatal)
• Coronary event	(fatal or nonfatal MI; sudden, presumed cardiac, death; dissection of aorta).

Abbreviation: *MI*, myocardial infarction.

age group. Patients who died after defaulting from treatment continued to be reported in this way (and reporting of deaths continued after the formal trial ended).

3. Stroke

A fatal or a nonfatal stroke was a trial-terminating event.

4. Coronary Event

This included both fatal and nonfatal myocardial infarction, sudden death presumed to have a coronary cause, deaths resulting from hypertension, or to rupture or dissection of an aortic aneurysm.

If a patient had a nonfatal event followed by a fatal event in the same category, only the fatal event was included in the analyses (19 strokes and 22 coronary events). If a person had two events in different categories (13 patients)—for example, a nonfatal stroke then a coronary event (fatal or nonfatal)—both were included.

G. Statistical Management

The initial analysis was on an intention-to-treat basis according to the primary randomization. Both placebo groups were combined for analytical purposes and, for the main analysis, so were the two active regimens.

The relation of several baseline characteristics and treatment with primary event outcomes were further investigated by logistic regression.

H. Cognitive Assessment

There was some concern that reduction of blood pressure, or drug side effects, might have an adverse effect on cognitive function and, conversely, there was a possibility that reduction of blood pressure might lessen the risk of vascular dementia. For this reason a substantial, representative fraction of the patients ($n = 2584$) in the trial was invited to take part in a longitudinal assessment of cognitive function. The patients completed the Paired Association Learning Test (PALT) and the Trial-Making Test (TMT) five times over the duration of the trial. The PALT measures the ability to learn a pair of matched words and recall one when prompted by the other. It tests associative memory. The TMT measures the speed with which the subject can join up with a pencil a sequence of letters and numbers scattered over a piece of paper.

The trial nurses questioned patients every 3 months and asked them to list all the medication they were taking, and these data were used to assess whether other commonly used medications such as nonsteroidal anti-inflammatory drugs (NSAIDs) or medicines taken for indigestion might influence the rate of change of cognitive function. In the trial, 1545 of the patients were surveyed for dementia, and a substudy was made of the cases ascertained to investigate factors that might influence progression into dementia.

III. RESULTS

The original objective was to accumulate 25,000 patient years of observation by recruiting 5000 patients and following up with them for 5 years. As only 4396 patients were recruited, the trial was allowed to continue to an average follow-up time of 5.8 years, thus achieving 25,355 patient years of observation.

The treatment groups were well matched by the randomization with the mean age ranging from 70.2 to 70.4 years and the body mass index from 26.1 to 26.8 kg/m^2. The men had very similar blood pressures in each of the groups—183/91–92 mm Hg. The average systolic blood pressures of the women were slightly higher but well matched across the groups, ranging from 186/90–91 mm Hg. Among the men, 21% to 24% were smokers, but among the women the figures were lower at 13% to 15%.

A. Course of Blood Pressure

The doctors' entry records of systolic and diastolic blood pressure measurements were higher by 10/3 mm Hg than the nurses' run-in values. After entry, the systolic and diastolic pressures fell immediately in all groups, probably partly because of the loss of the ''white coat effect'' (Fig. 1). The largest fall in systolic pressure was in the diuretic group in the first 3 months. More patients randomized to receive β-blocker required supplementary

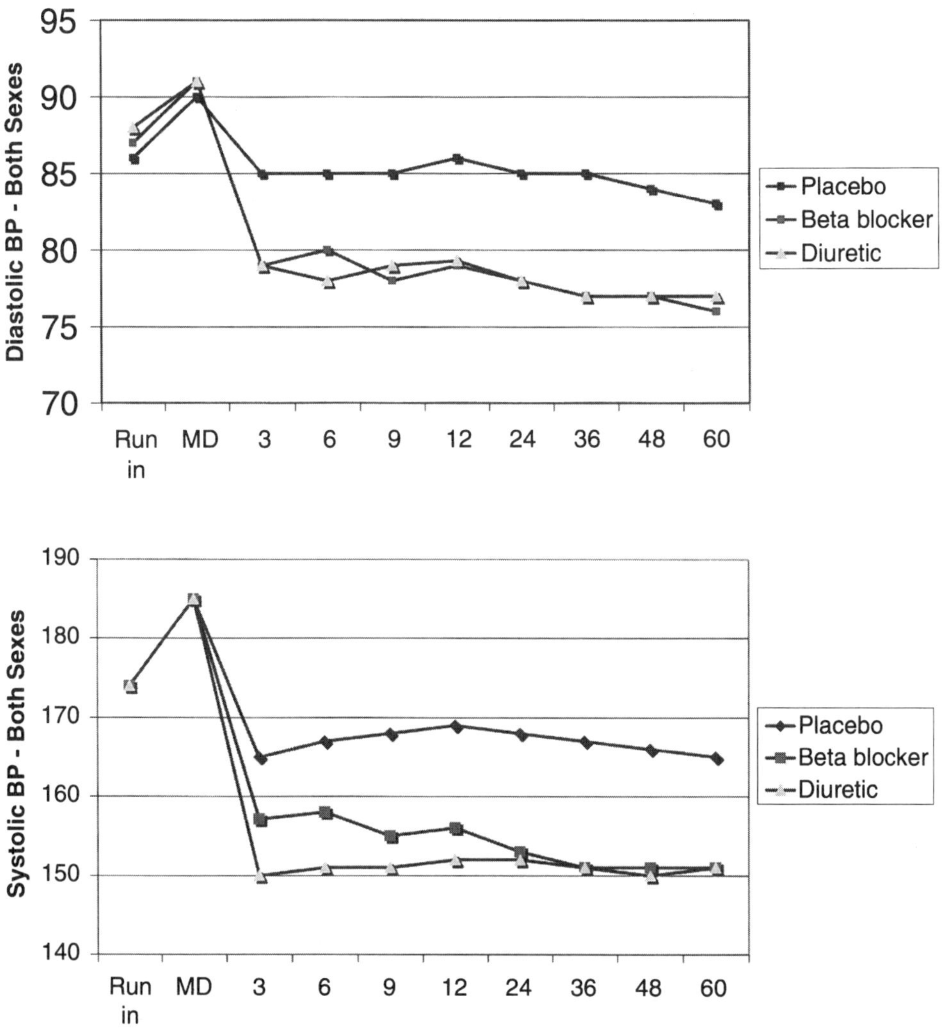

Fig. 1 Mean systolic and diastolic blood pressure in patients treated with placebo, beta adrenergic blockade, or diuretic. Note the rise in pressure due to the ''white coat effect'' at the time of the physician's examination; run-in values were taken by nurses.

drugs than those randomized to diuretic (52% β-blocker vs 38% diuretic at 5 years). This partly explains why the differences in blood pressure between diuretic and β-blocker groups became smaller as the trial progressed.

B. Withdrawals from Randomized Treatment

The main reasons for withdrawal of patients from randomized treatment were adverse reactions to treatment or poor blood pressure control. One hundred sixty patients were withdrawn from the diuretic group because of major side effects and one for inadequate control while in the β-blocker group, 333 were withdrawn because of side effects, and 12 for inadequate control. In the placebo group, 82 were withdrawn because of side effects and 175 because of inadequate control. The side effects that were severe enough to warrant withdrawal largely reflected the known pharmacological properties of the primary treatment regimens (Table 5).

Over the 5½ years, 25% of the patients were lost to follow-up. Loss from follow-up occurred progressively throughout the trial, so that the loss in patient years of treatment was about half this figure. If a tagged patient died, this was reported by the NHS central register to the trial coordinating center but no further information about nonfatal events was available in those who defaulted. The cumulative percentages of people who stopped taking their randomized treatment, including both those withdrawn but continuing on follow-up and those lost to follow-up, were 48% of the diuretic group, 63% of the β-blocker group, and 53% of the placebo group. The difference between the two active regimens largely reflects the greater incidence of side effects with the beta-blocker. By the end of the trial, there were about 6300 patient-years in each of the four randomly allocated treatment groups. In the diuretic group, treatment accounted for 69% of the patient-years, including supplementation by the β-blocker for 11% of the time. Corresponding percentages for those allocated to the β-blocker were 55% and supplementation with diuretic for 16%. In the placebo groups, 69% of the patient-years were spent on placebo treatment, with 6% of the time on either of the active treatments. Some critics of the trial appear to have confused withdrawal from randomized treatment (with continued follow-up) with

Table 5 Withdrawals from Randomized Treatment Because of Side Effects in Rates per 1000 Patient-Years

	Diuretic	Beta-blocker	Placebo
Glucose intolerance	6.9*	5.8*	2.7
Gout	4.4*	0.0	0.1
Muscle cramps	5.2*	1.0	0.1
Nausea	7.4*	4.1	1.1
Dyspnea	0.8	22.9*	1.1
Raynaud's	0.6	11.3*	0.3
Headache	2.5	7.2*	1.1
Dizziness	7.4*	10.6*	1.2
Lethargy	4.1	19.1*	2.0
Inadequate BP control (number)	n =1	n = 12	n = 175

Abbreviation: *BP*, blood pressure.
* Significant difference from placebo.

the much smaller proportion who were lost to follow-up (about 13% of total patient years). Even in the latter case, deaths were notified by the OPCS.

C. Terminating Events

1. Stroke

The total number of fatal and nonfatal strokes was significantly reduced in patients randomized to active treatment (101 active vs 134 placebo, $P = 0.04$) with a reduction in rates of 25% (95% confidence interval, 3% to 42%). The reduction in fatal strokes was confined to the diuretic group (2.5 per 1000 patient-years diuretic, 3.3 per 1000 patient-years for both beta-blocker and placebo groups). Nonfatal strokes were reduced in both active treatment groups, but the reduction was greater in the diuretic-treated patients (4.7 per 1000 patient-years on diuretic, 5.6 per 1000 patient-years on beta-blocker and 7.4 on placebo) (Fig. 2 and Table 6).

2. Coronary Events

Coronary events were less common in patients randomized to active treatment (128 events) than in those receiving placebo (159, $P = 0.08$), with a reduction in rates of 19% (−2% to 36%) (Fig. 2). The reduction in coronary events was confined to the bendrofluazide-treated group. The rates for fatal and nonfatal coronary events combined were 12.7 per

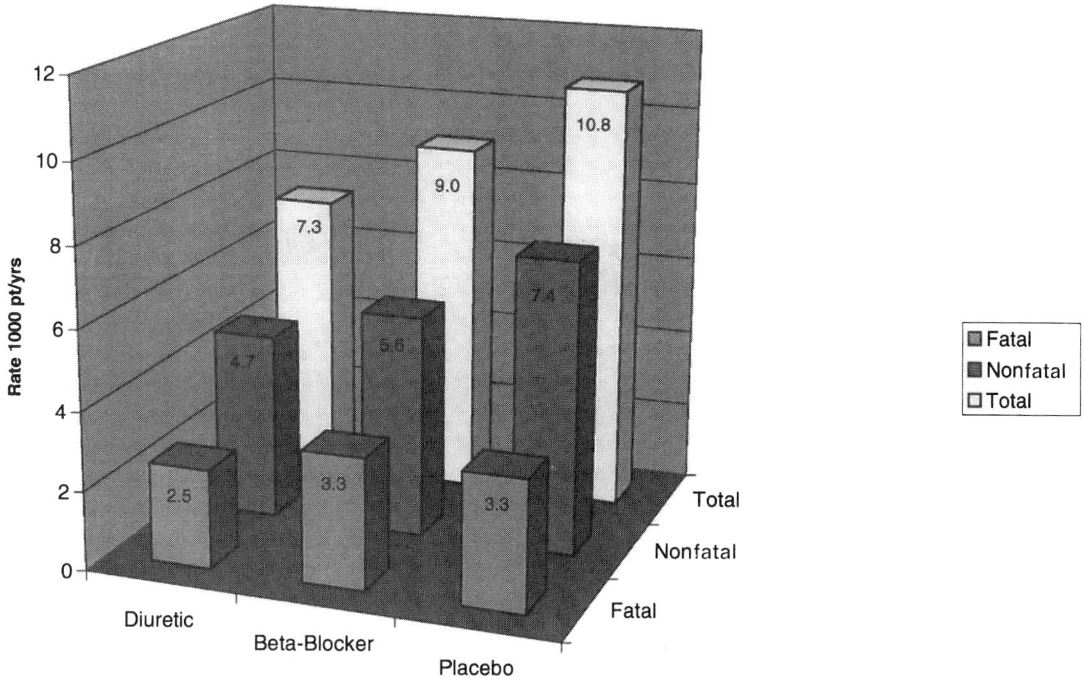

Fig. 2 Incidence of fatal, nonfatal, and strokes by treatment regimen. The treatment effect was most marked in the diuretic treated patients.

Table 6 Principal Results

Event	Active treatment	Placebo	*P* value
Stroke	101	134	0.04
Coronary	128	159	0.08
All CV events	258	309	0.03
All deaths	301	315	ns

Abbreviation: *CV*, cardiovascular.

1000 patient-years in the placebo group, 12.8 per 1000 patient-years in the placebo group but only 7.7 per 1000 patient-years in the bendrofluazide group (Fig. 3 and Table 6).

3. *All Cardiovascular Events*

The total number of cardiovascular events was significantly reduced on active treatment (258 vs 309 placebo, $P = 0.03$) with a 17% (2% to 29%) reduction in rates. Of these events, 235 (41%) were strokes and 287 (51%) were coronary episodes (Table 6).

4. *Mortality*

All-cause mortality was similar in the treated and placebo groups (23.9 [treated] vs 24.7 [placebo] per 1000 patient-years) (Fig. 3). Deaths from cardiovascular causes were slightly fewer in the active treatment group than the placebo group (161 vs 180 placebo), but both

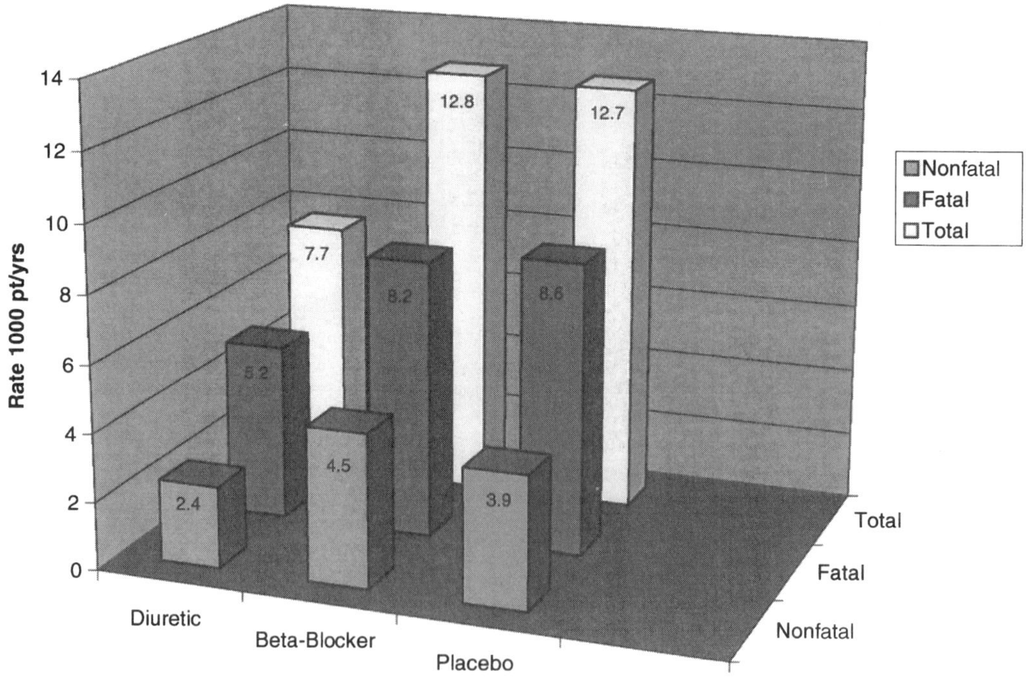

Fig. 3 Incidence of fatal, nonfatal, and total coronary events by treatment regimen.

groups had similar numbers of deaths from noncardiovascular causes (140 vs 135) and from cancer (108 vs 99). The difference between the total number of deaths in the diuretic and β-blocker-treated patients approached statistical significance ($P = 0.07$), with a 19% reduction in mortality in the diuretic group (Fig. 4 and Table 6).

5. Cancer Mortality

There was a difference between the sexes in deaths from cancer; 74 men receiving active treatment and 47 receiving placebo died of cancer compared with 34 women receiving active treatment and 52 receiving placebo (interaction test between treatment and sex ($P = 0.002$). Twenty-one of these patients had a history of cancer at entry to the trial (four receiving diuretic; six β-blocker and 11 placebo. Omitting these patients did not substantially alter the statistical significance of the interaction test. The excess mortality from cancer in men was more pronounced in the β-blocker group than the diuretic group, which gave rise to some concern in the trial steering committee. Review of the site and type of tumor showed no organ or system clustering, except for cancer of the lung/bronchus, which affected 14 men randomized to β-blocker compared with eight in the diuretic group and 11 in the placebo group.

6. Sex Differences

Besides the sex difference in cancer mortality already noted, the main differences between the sexes was in coronary events, which were reduced by 30% in men but unaltered in women. The reduction in stroke was similar in both sexes (Table 7).

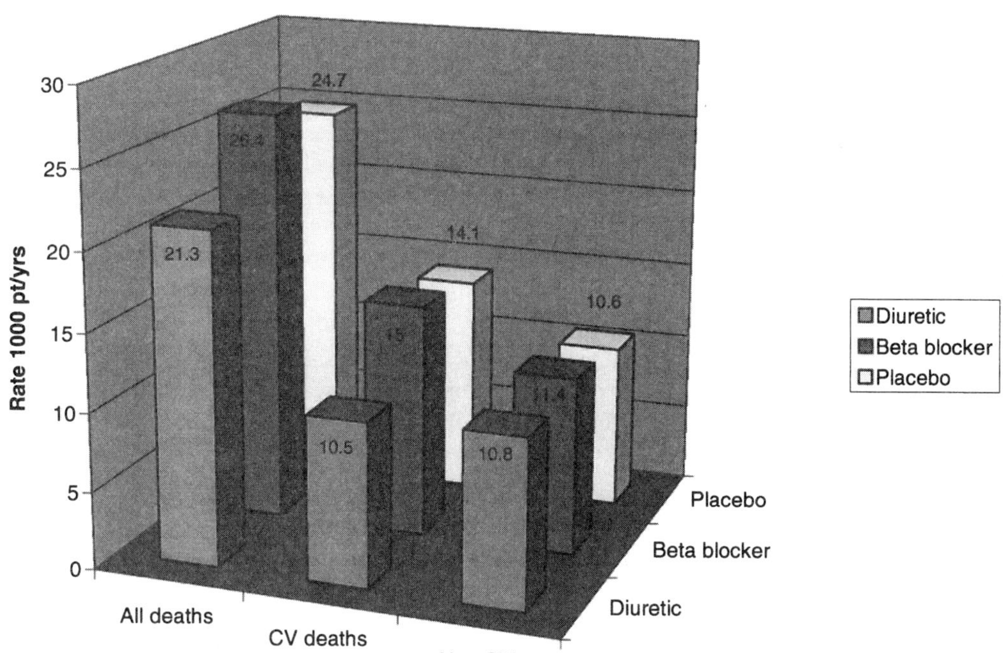

Fig. 4 Cardiovascular, noncardiovascular, and total mortality by treatment regimen.

Table 7 Percentage Reduction in Events, by Sex

	Men	Women
Stroke	−21.3%	−27.0%
Coronary events	−30.0%	−0.0%
All CV events	−21.1%	−9.2%
CV deaths	−20.8%	+10.5%
Non-CV deaths	+48.0%	−34.4%
Cancer deaths	+60.4%	−34.8%
All deaths	+4.0%	−12.8%

Abbreviation: *CV*, cardiovascular.

7. Tobacco Smoking

The majority of the patients in the trial were nonsmokers. There were 5405 patient-years of smokers and 20,038 of nonsmokers. The stroke rate was similar in smokers and nonsmokers, 10.9 and 10.7 per 1000 patient-years respectively. However, the reduction in stroke was confined to nonsmokers, with the greatest effect in diuretic-treated patients (−46.7%) compared with beta-blocker-treated patients (−26.1%).

The coronary event rate was nearly twice as high in smokers as nonsmokers (21.9 vs 11.47 per 1000 patient-years). The reduction in coronary events was virtually confined to the diuretic-treated group and was similar in smokers and nonsmokers: 42% and 37.7%, respectively. The total death rate was substantially higher in smokers compared with nonsmokers, 36.2 versus 21.6 per 1000 patient-years.

8. Per-Protocol (On-Treatment) Analysis

As it is likely that some specific pharmacological effects of treatment are only manifest while the patient is taking the designated drug, a secondary analysis was made of deaths in those patients who were still taking the drug to which they were randomized. The results were similar to the intention-to-treat analysis. The cardiovascular death rate was 6.5 per 100 patient-years on the diuretic, 11.5 per 1000 patient-years on the beta-blocker and 9.9 per 100 patient-years on placebo. These rates are lower than the corresponding intention-to-treat rates (10.5, 15.0 and 12.8, respectively), but populations that continue with assigned treatment differ in important respects from those that do not.

9. Cardiovascular Risk Factors

In the original trial publication, logistic regression analysis was used to relate status at entry to subsequent trial events. The risk of stroke was related to entry diastolic blood pressure, sex, age, and ischemic changes on the electrocardiogram, but this result may have been influenced by the effect of treatment. The risk of a major coronary event was predicted by male sex, cholesterol concentration, ischemic electrocardiographic changes, and smoking. Only the diuretic group showed a significant reduction in risk when the groups were adjusted for entry risk factors.

The factors predicting total deaths were sex, age, smoking, and ischemic changes on electrocardiography. An inverse association with total cholesterol did not reach statistical significance. The reduction in total mortality in the diuretic group also failed to achieve significance after allowing for baseline characteristics.

10. Cognitive Assessment

Of the patients in the trial, 2584 were invited to take part in a longitudinal assessment of cognitive function. The patients completed the PALT and the TMT five times over the duration of the trial. The TMT scores may have been influenced by learning effects, as there was an average 9 second improvement in the test result over the 54 months of the trial, whereas the PALT declined by an average of one point over the same period (3).

The factors identified as being associated with PALT decline were advancing age, male sex, residence in a rural area, depression, and low intelligence. Women appeared to be more adversely affected by smoking and advancing age than men (4).

11. Dementia

Of the patients in the trial, 1545 were surveyed for dementia and 50 cases were identified of which 31 were probably suffering from Alzheimer's disease. They were compared with 223 matched controls from the same general practice populations. A family history of dementia was strongly predictive for dementia as a whole (odds ratio 4.36) and for Alzheimer's disease (odds ratio 4.69). Among individuals with a negative family history, cardiovascular risk factors such as ischemic changes on the electrocardiogram, systolic hypertension, and cigarette smoking, approached but did not achieve statistical significance as predictors of the onset of dementia. The authors suggested that there might be a form of nonfamilial vascular dementia that was distinct from multi-infarct dementia (5).

12. Treatment and Dementia

There was no clear evidence in the trial that treatment of hypertension slowed the onset of dementia, but the number of nonfamilial cases was small. The trial data were also examined to investigate whether other drugs might affect progression to dementia based on the 3-monthly questioning about other medication made by the trial nurses. These data were used to test the hypothesis that use of nonsteroidal anti-inflammatory drugs might influence the rate of cognitive decline, as has been proposed in studies of elderly people (6, 7). The frequency of NSAID use was divided into three strata: (a) not used, (b) used on 25% of assessments, (c) used on more than 25% of assessments. Sixty-one percent never used NSAIDs, 19% took them but on less than 25% of assessments, and 20% on more than 25%. At least three data points were available in 88% of patients.

Having adjusted for other factors, the use of NSAIDs was significantly associated with change in PALT score with time, in favor of the NSAID users. The protective effect diminished with increasing age and was lost by the age of 74 years. There was no change in TMT score related to NSAID use. Anti-indigestion drugs were also examined but they had no effect on either PALT or TMT.

It is unclear whether the NSAID effect resulted from prevention of microthrombi or emboli in the cerebral circulation or whether it is caused by an anti-inflammatory effect in the central nervous system.

IV. DISCUSSION

The three main target organs of hypertension are the brain, the heart, and the kidney. Mild to moderate hypertension does not usually lead to serious impairment of renal function, unless there is underlying chronic renal disease, and this discussion will concentrate on the effects of treatment on the brain and heart.

A. Brain Function

1. Stroke

The MRC elderly trial contained few surprises in relation to stroke. Actively treated patients had a 25% reduction in stroke ($P = 0.04$) and the trial size calculations had been based on a 30% reduction. Although the percentage reduction in stroke in the elderly trial was materially less than in the earlier MRC trial in younger patients (45%), the number of strokes saved per 1000 patient-years was higher because of the much higher stroke rates in the elderly patients (14.1 and 8.5 per 1000 patient-years in men and women respectively vs 2.6 per 1000 patient-years in the two sexes combined in the mild trial). Thus in the mild trial, one stroke was saved per 833 patient-years of treatment, whereas in the elderly it was one per 370 patient-years. In the Systolic Hypertension in the Elderly Program (SHEP), the 5-year incidence of stroke was 5.2 per 100 participants for active treatment versus 8.2 per 100 for placebo (relative risk 0.64, $P = .0003$).

It is possible that these results understate the true benefit because patients whose blood pressure consistently exceeded 115 mm Hg diastolic or 210 mm Hg systolic were managed outside the trial protocol. As a result, 6% of the placebo patient-years were spent on one or another of the active treatments and only 69% of the placebo patient-years were spent on placebo. Millar and Lever (8, 9) attempted to calculate the effect of the transfer to active treatment of the patients randomized to placebo in the MRC mild hypertension trial in which 12% were withdrawn because the diastolic pressure exceeded 109 mm Hg. They plotted a regression curve of screening systolic pressure against stroke rate and used this to predict the risk for those who were withdrawn. The authors also used the blood pressure at 3 months into the trial to adjust for the ''white coat'' effect of the entry medical examination on the blood pressure. Using both assumptions, they postulated that the number of patient-years of treatment required to prevent one stroke in a truly hypertensive patient might be substantially less than that reported in the trial (as low as 240 patient-years). However, so many factors are exceptional in a well-run randomized controlled trial (screening out high-risk patients, meticulous supervision, motivated patients, etc.) compared with the ebb and flow of normal clinical practice that such adjustments must be treated with considerable caution.

Another issue raised by both MRC trials was whether there was a real difference between the two active regimens. In each case, the diuretic patients fared better than those randomized to beta-adrenergic blockade, although the specific drugs used were different.

These data suggest that the diuretic may have a 2.57- to 1.94-fold advantage over the beta-blocker which, if true, would be of considerable clinical significance. Blood pressure

Table 8 Stroke Rate Per 1000 Patient-Years in the MRC Hypertension Trials

	Diuretic	Beta-blocker	Placebo
''Mild''	0.8	1.9	2.6
''Elderly''	7.3	9.0	10.8
	Stroke Rate as Percentage of Placebo Rate		
''Mild''	30.8	73.1	100.0
''Elderly''	67.6	83.3	100.0

control was slightly less with the beta-blocker than with the diuretic, but this could not explain a difference of this magnitude. Moreover, other studies, with different beta-blockers, did not replicate this finding.

The International Prospective Primary Prevention Study in Hypertension (IPPPSH) compared a beta-blocker-containing (oxprenolol) with a non-beta-blocker-containing antihypertensive regimen in 6357 hypertensive men and women with moderate to severe hypertension (10). There was no significant difference in outcome in the two groups (11, 12). The Heart Attack Primary Prevention in Hypertension (HAPPHY) study compared patients treated with beta-blockers, mainly metoprolol and atenolol, with diuretics and showed no significant difference between them (13). The HAPPHY study was terminated, but the Metoprolol and Atenolol Prevention in Hypertension (MAPHY) study, which was mainly the metoprolol subgroup of HAPPHY, continued for a longer period (14). The risk for coronary events was significantly lower in patients on metoprolol than in patients on diuretics, 14.3 versus 18.8 cases/1,000 patient-years with a relative risk of 0.76 (95% confidence interval 0.58–0.98). This study created some unease because of its slightly checkered history, although it conformed more to expectations in relation to beta-blockade and coronary heart disease. There seem to be three possible explanations for the different results in the studies that compared diuretics and beta-blockers: (a) the difference observed between beta-blockers and diuretics in both MRC studies was pure chance, (b) the difference was real but metoprolol is different from propranolol or atenolol, and (c) the MAPHY result was also chance. The HAPPHY result is consistent with there being a difference between metoprolol and atenolol. Although it is best to be extremely cautious about such interpretations the possibility of additional pharmacological properties of beta-adrenergic blocking drugs contributing to the effect should not be dismissed. However, it appears inherently more probable that the effects of blood pressure reduction on hypertensive vascular disease would be related more to the magnitude of pressure reduction than to ancillary properties of the drug.

2. Dementia

Although it has received less attention, the effects of high blood pressure and antihypertensive therapy on the rate of decline of cognitive function in the elderly could be of considerable importance. On general principles, it might be anticipated that there would be a causal relationship between hypertension and multi-infarct dementia and that reduction of blood pressure might prevent the onset of dementia in some patients. A counter-argument is that hypertensive patients with cerebrovascular disease might have reached the limit of vascular autoregulation in some territories, and reduction of perfusion pressure might impair cognitive function. It would be possible for both hypotheses to be true in different circumstances.

The evidence is inconclusive (15). In one case-control study in African Americans, raised systolic blood pressure was negatively correlated with dementia (16), although advanced age, low educational attainment, history of myocardial infarction, and recent cigarette smoking were positively correlated. In the MRC elderly trial, systematic cognitive function testing in a large subset of the patients did not reveal any evidence of deterioration in the TMT, and the fall in the PALT score was small (4, 17). Decline in the PALT was associated with advanced age, male sex, rural residence, depression, and low intelligence (4). Some of the test results (TMT) improved, but this was probably more the result of learning to do them better than to treatment. In the Syst-Eur trial, evidence was obtained that dementia might be prevented by antihypertensive therapy, but the numbers involved were small (18). There is more substantial evidence that multiple emboli from atrial fibrillation are associated with cognitive decline (19).

B. Cardiac Function

1. *Coronary Disease and Myocardial Infarction*

The second major finding of the MRC elderly trial was a 19% reduction in coronary events ($p = 0.08$). This finding has been replicated in a number of other studies in older hypertensive patients. The SHEP trial included patients with systolic hypertension (160 to 219 mm Hg) aged 60 years and older who were randomized to either step care (first step with chlorthalidone and second with atenolol) or to placebo. For the secondary endpoint of clinical nonfatal myocardial infarction plus coronary death, the relative risk was 0.73 (20). The European Working Party on High Blood Pressure in the Elderly compared a diuretic-based regimen with placebo in 840 elderly hypertensive patients. Cardiovascular mortality was reduced in the actively treated group (−38%, $P = 0.023$), because of a reduction of cardiac deaths (−47%, $P = 0.048$), but the reduction of cerebrovascular mortality (−43%, $P = 0.15$) was not significant (21). The Syst-Eur trial, a study of 4695 elderly patients with systolic hypertension, which used nitrendipine as first-line therapy with enalapril as the second step, also showed a reduction in both stroke and cardiac events (23). The HOT study suggest that low dose aspirin should also be part of the regime in elderly hypertensives unless there is a specific contraindication and it is interesting to note the additional favorable effect of NSAIDs upon cognitive function in the MRC trial.

There has been controversy about the effects of different types of pharmacological action upon the incidence of coronary disease in treated hypertensives. It was anticipated that beta-adrenergic blockade would have a more favorable effect than diuretic-based regimens because of the proven efficacy of beta-blockade after myocardial infarction. A trend in that direction, which did not reach significance, was seen in the MRC mild hypertension trial but none was seen in the elderly trial in which the benefit was entirely in the diuretic-treated group (Table 9).

A controversy has raged about the safety of calcium ''L'' channel antagonists in patients with ischemic heart disease (22). The Syst-Eur trial, whose main active treatment was the dihydropyridine calcium channel blocker, nitrendipine showed a beneficial effect upon stroke (−44%) and a reduction in all cardiac endpoints (26%) compared with placebo (23). The HOT study, which compared two active therapy regimens based on the dihydropyridine, felodipine, showed a very low incidence of morbid events (24). The balance of evidence does not support there being a general risk attached to calcium antagonists (24, 25) but there may be one for fast-absorbed, short-acting calcium antagonists administered to patients with severe coronary artery disease.

Table 9 Coronary Events (Rate per 1000 Patient-Years)

	MRC mild trial			MRC elderly trial		
	Diuretic	Beta-blocker	Placebo	Diuretic	Beta-blocker	Placebo
Fatal	2.8	2.2	2.3	5.2	8.2	8.6
Nonfatal	2.8	2.6	3.2	2.4	4.5	3.9
All	5.6	4.7	5.5	7.7	12.8	12.7

2. *Heart Failure*

The MRC trial did not analyze specific data about the incidence of heart failure. A particularly interesting finding in the SHEP study was the reduction by about half in fatal and nonfatal heart failure with 105 of 2371 patients on placebo versus 55 of 2365 on active treatment (26). The EWPHE trial also showed a marked reduction in the incidence of heart failure.

These findings are consistent with epidemiological data showing a rapidly rising incidence of heart failure with age and a high early mortality with about one third of patients dying within 2 years of onset (27). The two most common predisposing conditions are hypertension and coronary artery disease (28–30). There is, of course, the possibility that some of the apparent benefit, particularly of diuretic-based regimens, is false in that some of the overt clinical manifestations of heart failure are relieved but not the underlying pathology. The favorable effect on mortality suggests, however, the benefit is real and not just symptomatic. It will be particularly interesting to see the effects of angiotensin-converting enzyme inhibitors and angiotensin II receptor antagonists in the elderly in view of their favorable effects in heart failure (31, 32).

C. Adverse Effects

1. *All-Cause Mortality*

All-cause mortality was not significantly altered in the MRC elderly trial. The rates per 1000 patent-years for diuretic, beta-blocker, all active treatment, and placebo were 21.3, 26.4, 23.9, and 24.7 respectively. In the MRC mild hypertension trial, the rates for all active treatment and placebo were 5.8 and 5.9 per 1000 patient-years respectively. The lack of effect on all-cause mortality was disappointing, particularly in the elderly trial. One possible explanation might be that treatment increased mortality from noncardiovascular causes while decreasing cardiovascular deaths. In the elderly trial, there was some concern because of an increased incidence of cancer in male atenolol-treated patients but scrutiny of other (nonrandomized) populations of hypertensive patients treated with atenolol did not show any cause for concern (33, 34). All antihypertensive drugs cause some symptoms in some patients. In recent years, substantial efforts have been made to quantitate the symptom burden and the effects of treatment upon activities of daily living (35). Overall, the incidence of severe effects appear to be small, although the frequency with which drugs are switched in family practice suggests that mild to moderate symptoms, such as cough on angiotensin-converting enzyme inhibitors, headache on calcium antagonists, and fatigue on beta-blockers, are common. In the MRC elderly trial, the drugs used are generally considered to cause a low incidence of symptomatic side effects but even so, 160 patients were withdrawn from the diuretic group and 333 from the beta-blocker group because of side effects. These are substantial numbers, bearing in mind that there were only about 1100 patients in each actively treated group and patients were kept on the original randomized treatment if possible.

More serious adverse effects were rare, but there has been some concern about the safety of thiazide diuretics both in relation to provocation of ventricular arrhythmia and predisposing to diabetes mellitus. A subgroup analysis in the Multiple Risk Factor Intervention study (MRFIT) suggested that a diuretic might predispose to cardiac events (36), but neither of the MRC placebo-controlled trials showed any supportive evidence apart from a moderate increase in the incidence of ventricular ectopics in an intensively monitored subgroup. The dose of bendrofluazide used in the first MRC trial, 10 mg, was in retrospect rather high. A variant on the argument has been to say that the trial results might have been even better if a postulated adverse myocardial effect of thiazides could have been avoided, but this argument was deployed mainly against the trials in patients younger than age 60 in whom the beneficial effects upon coronary heart disease were less than anticipated.

There is good evidence that thiazides can be diabetogenic in some circumstances and diuretics may have an adverse effect in patients who have already developed diabetes (37). There was evidence of decreased glucose tolerance in the EWPHE, diuretic-based, trial. But this problem appears to be dose related, and Berglund found no adverse effects on glucose metabolism of a low dose of a thiazide over 10 years (38). In the same study several patients developed glucose intolerance on propranolol. Overall this appears to be much less of a problem than once feared.

V. CONCLUSION

The MRC trial of treatment of hypertension in the elderly demonstrated a significant reduction in stroke, cardiac, and all cardiovascular events. The benefits of treatment were greater in the diuretic-treated group than in those randomized to the beta-blocker. Many patients suffered mild drug-related symptoms that necessitated a change in treatment, particularly in the beta-blocker group. There was no deterioration of cognitive function as a result of treatment, and evidence was obtained that incidental use of nonsteroidal anti-inflammatory drugs might have some protective effect against dementia.

ACKNOWLEDGMENTS

I am particularly grateful to Drs. Tom Mead, Pat Brennan, and Anthony Mann, all of whom were involved in the original trial, for helpful discussions. This trial was only made possible by the efforts of the family practitioners and nurses of the 226 practices in the MRC general practice research framework who took part in this study. To them most of the the credit should be given.

The members of the MRC working party were:

Professor Sir Stanley Peart (chairman), Mr. P.J. Brennan, Mr. P. Broughton, Professor Sir Colin Dollery, Dr. M.F. Hudson, Dr. A.F. Lever, Dr. T.W. Meade, Professor G.A. Rose, Dr. G. Greenberg, Professor S.J. Pocock.

The members of the monitoring and ethics committee were:

Professor M.J. Healy, Professor P.S. Sever, Professor J.D. Swales.

Data were reviewed and analyzed by:

P.J. Brennan, D.C. Webster, H.C. Wilkes.

Endpoint assessment was made by:

Professor H. Tunstall-Pedoe.

REFERENCES

1. Medical Research Council Working Party. MRC trial of treatment of mild hypertension: principal results. Br Med J 1985; 291:97–104.
2. Medical Research Council Working Party. Medical Research Council trial of treatment of hypertension in older adults: principal results. Br Med J 1992; 304:405–412.

3. Prince M, Rabe-Hesketh S, Brennan P. Do antiarthritic drugs decrease the risk of cognitive decline? An analysis based on data from the MRC Treatment Trial of Hypertension in Older Adults. Neurology 1998; 50:374–379.
4. Prince M, Lewis G, Bird A, Blizard R, Mann A. A longitudinal study of factors predicting change in cognitive test scores over time, in an older hypertensive population. Psychol Med 1996; 26:555–568.
5. Prince M, Cullen M, Mann A. Risk factors for Alzheimer's disease and dementia: a case-control study based on the MRC elderly hypertension trial. Neurology 1994; 44:97–104.
6. Rozzini R, Ferrucci L, Losonczy, K, Havlik, RJ, and Guralnik, JM. Protective effect of chronic NSAID use on cognitive decline in older persons. J Am Geriatr Soc 1996; 44:1025–1029.
7. Stewart WF, Kawas C, Corrada M, Metter EJ. Risk of Alzheimer's disease and duration of NSAID use. Neurology 48:626–632.
8. Millar JA, Isles CG, Lever AF. Blood pressure, ''white-coat'' pressor responses and cardiovascular risk in placebo-group patients of the MRC Mild Hypertension trial. J Hypertens 1995; 13:175–183.
9. Millar JA, Lever AF. Effect of sex-related changes in blood pressure at entry to the MRC trial on prediction of cardiovascular risk. Clin Exp Pharmacol Physiol 1994; 21:167–169.
10. Bolli P, Buhler FR, McKenzie JK. Smoking, antihypertensive treatment benefit, and comprehensive antihypertensive treatment approach: some thoughts on the results of the International Prospective Primary Prevention Study in Hypertension. J Cardiovasc Pharmacol 1990; (suppl 16) 7:S77–S80.
11. The IPPPSH Collaborative Group. Cardiovascular risk and risk factors in a randomized trial of treatment based on the beta-blocker oxprenolol: the International Prospective Primary Prevention Study in Hypertension (IPPPSH). J Hypertens 1985; 3:379–89.
12. The IPPPSH Collaborative Group. Myocardial infarctions and cerebrovascular accidents in relation to blood pressure control. J Hypertens Suppl 1985;(suppl 3) 3:S513–S518.
13. Wilhelmsen L, Berglund G, Elmfeldt D, Fitzsimons T, Holzgreve H, Hosie J, et al. Beta-blockers versus diuretics in hypertensive men: main results from the HAPPHY trial. J Hypertens 1987; 5:561–572.
14. Wikstrand J, Warnold I, Tuomilehto J, Olsson G, Barber HJ, Eliasson K, et al. Metoprolol versus thiazide diuretics in hypertension. Morbidity results from the MAPHY Study. Hypertension 1991; 17:579–588.
15. Phillips SJ, Whisnant JP. Hypertension and the brain. The National High Blood Pressure Education Program. Arch Intern Med 1992; 152:938–945.
16. Gorelick PB, Brody J, Cohen D, Freels S, Levy P, Dollear W, et al. Risk factors for dementia associated with multiple cerebral infarcts. A case-control analysis in predominantly African-American hospital-based patients. Arch Neurol 1993; 50:714–720.
17. Mann A. Hypertension: psychological aspects and diagnostic impact in a clinical trial. Psychol Med Monogr Suppl 1984; 5:1–35.
18. Forette E, Seux ML, Staessen JA, Thijs L, Birkenhager WH, Babarskiene MR, Babeanu S, Bossini A, Gil-Extremera B, Girerd X, Laks T, Lilov E, Moisseyev V, Toumilheto J, Vanhanen H, Webster J, Yodfat Y, Fagard R. Prevention of dementia in randomised double-blind placebo-controlled Systolic Hypertension in Europe (Syst-Eur) trial. Lancet 1998; 352:1347–1351.
19. Kilander L, Andren B, Nyman H, Lind L, Boberg M, Lithell H. Atrial fibrillation is an independent determinant of low cognitive function: a cross-sectional study in elderly men. Stroke 1998; 29:1816–1820.
20. SHEP Co-operative Research Group. Prevention of stroke by antihypertensive drug treatment in older persons with isolated systolic hypertension. Final results of the Systolic Hypertension in the Elderly Program (SHEP). JAMA 1991; 265:3255–3264.
21. Amery A, Birkenhager W, Brixko P, Bulpitt C, Clement D, de LP, et al. Influence of hypotensive drug treatment in elderly hypertensives: study terminating events in the trial of the Euro-

pean Working Party on High Blood Pressure in the Elderly. J Hypertens Suppl 1985; (suppl 3) 3:S501–S511.
22. Furberg CD, Psaty BM, Meyer JV. Nifedipine. Dose-related increase in mortality in patients with coronary heart disease. Circulation 1995; 92:1326–1331.
23. Staessen JA, Fagard R, Thijs L, Celis H, Birkenhager WH, Bulpitt CJ, et al. Subgroup and per-protocol analysis of the randomized European Trial on Isolated Systolic Hypertension in the Elderly. Arch Intern Med 1998; 158:1681–1691.
24. Abascal VM, Larson MG, Evans JC, Blohm AT, Poli K, Levy D. Calcium antagonists and mortality risk in men and women with hypertension in the Framingham Heart Study. Arch Intern Med 1998; 158:1882–1886.
25. Messerli FH. Safety of calcium antagonists: dissecting the evidence. Am J Cardiol 1996; 78: 19–23.
26. Kostis JB, Davis BR, Cutler J, Grimm-RH J, Berge KG, Cohen JD, et al. Prevention of heart failure by antihypertensive drug treatment in older persons with isolated systolic hypertension. SHEP Co-operative Research Group. JAMA 1997; 278:212–216.
27. Kannel WB, Belanger AJ. Epidemiology of heart failure. Am Heart J 1991; 121:951–957.
28. Stokes J, Kannel WB, Wolf PA, D'Agostino RB, Cupples LA. Blood pressure as a risk factor for cardiovascular disease. The Framingham Study—30 years of follow-up. Hypertension 1989; 13:I13–I18.
29. Kannel WB. Epidemiological aspects of heart failure. Cardiol Clin 1989; 7:1–9.
30. Ho KK, Pinsky JL, Kannel WB, Levy D. The epidemiology of heart failure: the Framingham Study. J Am Coll Cardiol 1993; 22:6A– 13A.
31. The SOLVD Investigators. Effect of enalapril on survival in patients with reduced left ventricular ejection fractions and congestive heart failure. N Engl J Med 1991; 325:293–302.
32. Garg R, Yusuf S. Overview of randomized trials of angiotensin-converting enzyme inhibitors on mortality and morbidity in patients with heart failure. Collaborative Group on ACE Inhibitor. JAMA 1995; 273:1450–1456.
33. Fletcher AE, Beevers DG, Bulpitt CJ, Coles EC, Dollery CT, Ledingham JG, Palmer AJ, Petrie JC, Webster J. Cancer mortality and atenolol treatment. BMJ 1993; 306:622–623
34. Hole DJ, Hawthorne VM, Isles CG, McGhee SM, Robertson JW, Gillis CR, Wapshaw JA, Lever AF. Incidence of and mortality from cancer in hypertensive patients. BMJ 1993; 306: 609–611.
35. Bulpitt CJ, Fletcher AE. Quality of life and the heart: evaluation of therapeutic alternatives. Br J Clin Pract Symp Suppl 1994; 73:18–22.
36. Freis ED. The cardiotoxicity of thiazide diuretics: review of the evidence. J Hypertens Suppl 1990; 8:S23–S32.
37. Warram JH, Laffel LM, Valsania P, Christlieb AR, Krolewski AS. Excess mortality associated with diuretic therapy in diabetes mellitus. Arch Intern Med 1991; 151:1350–1356.
38. Berglund G, Andersson O, Widgren B. Low-dose antihypertensive treatment with a thiazide diuretic is not diabetogenic. A 10-year controlled trial with bendroflumethiazide. Acta Med Scand 1986; 220:419–424.

12

The Treatment of Mild Hypertension Study (TOMHS): Design and Additional Analyses

RICHARD H. GRIMM, Jr., RONALD J. PRINEAS, JOSEPH ROEL, and GREG GRANDITS

University of Minnesota, Minneapolis, Minnesota

I. INTRODUCTION

Hypertension is one of the most commonly occurring medical conditions in the U.S. It affects one in four adults; hypertension clinic visits are the most common reason to visit a physician. Since the mid-1960s, a large number of clinical trials have conclusively established that lowering blood pressure prevents cardiovascular disease (1, 2). Trials have also established the benefits of lowering systolic pressure in older patients (3–6). Clearly, lowering high blood pressure is one of the most effective interventions currently delivered in primary care medicine.

However, past hypertension trials have also reported results that suggest the type of antihypertensive drug prescribed may contribute to outcomes independently from lowering blood pressure. In fact, antihypertensive mortality/morbidity adverse effects have been attributed to specific drugs used in clinical trials. The Multiple Risk Factor Intervention Trial (MRFIT) observed a higher rate of sudden death and fatal/nonfatal coronary disease in a subgroup of special intervention men; those with baseline electrocardiographic (ECG) abnormalities treated with high-dose diuretics (50–100 mg daily of hydrochlorothiazide and chlorthalidone) compared with usual care (community care) (7). More recently, serious concerns have emerged that suggest possible harmful effects of dihydropyridine calcium channel blockers (8–10).

Concerns about differential effects by type of drug were the main impetus in designing the Treatment of Mild Hypertension Study (TOMHS). The TOMHS was an NHLBI investigator-initiated grant carried out by four medical centers: the University of Minnesota (clinical center, administrative center, and data coordinating center), the Rush-Presbyterian Medical School in Chicago, the University of Pittsburgh, and the University of Alabama in Birmingham (11).

The TOMHS was originally designed as a two-phase study. Phase I was conducted between 1986 and 1993 in 902 stage I diastolic hypertensives. The primary goal of phase I was to estimate the open label drug treatment rate in the placebo-plus-lifestyle group compared with active treatment (Fig. 1), and the feasibility of using as treatment arms these active drugs, in conjunction with lifestyle advice. Phase II was designed to address the question: does treatment reduce cardiovascular disease (CVD) in patients with stage 1 hypertension and does type of drug treatment affect CVD risk?

A. Methods

The TOMHS was a randomized double-blind placebo-controlled study comparing five active drugs with one another and placebo for long-term hypertension care. All participants

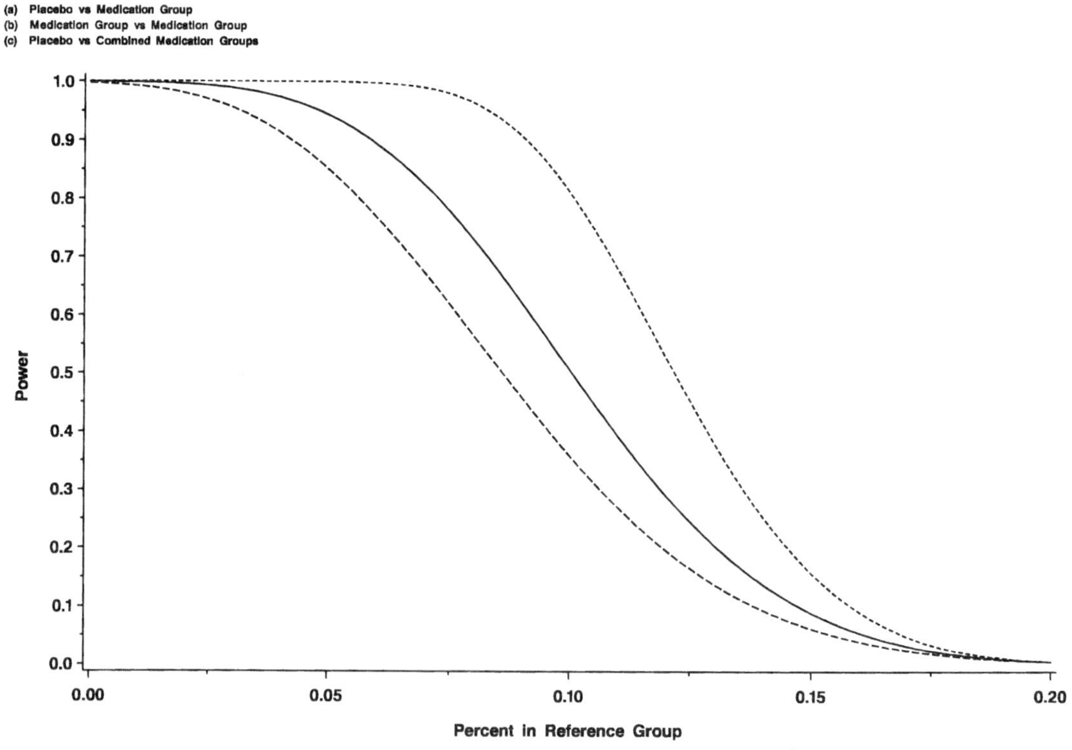

Fig. 1 Power curves for endpoint: Percent for whom Step 1 treatment is discontinued [$n = 125$ (medication groups); $n = 215$ (placebo group)].

also received intensive lifestyle intervention including weight loss, dietary sodium and alcohol reduction, and increased leisure time physical activity (12). The following questions were addressed:

1. Do the drug-treated groups differ from placebo or from each other with respect to measures of drug tolerance, BP change, quality of life, lipoprotein, biochemistries, reported side effects, sexual function, and ECG and echocardiographic changes over 4 years? For these measures, the study power was about 0.90 to detect clinically meaningful differences in these measures. Clinically meaningful measures were defined as a diastolic BP change of 3.5 mm Hg, a 15% difference in participants who remained on step 1 therapy, a 0.5 quality of life (QL) unit difference, and a 19 g difference between groups in left ventricular mass on ECG. The TOMHS drug schedule including step and dose are shown in Table 1.

2. The second question was: does drug treatment combined with lifestyle changes reduce 4-year incidence of cardiovascular morbidity and mortality compared with lifestyle intervention alone? Phase I was not adequately powered for this endpoint, although CVD morbidity and mortality were ascertained.

Inclusion criteria included men and women ages 45 to 69 with stage I diastolic hypertension defined as a diastolic pressure between 90 and 99 mm Hg averaged over three eligibility visits. Participants on medication at the initial screen could be eligible if they could be weaned off their medication and, over 12 weeks (five visits) of observation, have diastolic pressures between 85 and 99 mm Hg. Further details of inclusions and BP entry criteria are published in the final result paper (13). The TOMHS phase I inclusions and exclusions are provided in Table 2. The actual specific fatal and nonfatal and the clinical events are shown in Table 3.

B. Randomization

Recruitment was carried out over 18 months. Participants were assigned to treatment using a block randomization method stratifying for clinical center and use of BP drugs at screen 1. There were eight strata altogether with an allocation ratio to the six treatment

Table 1 TOMHS Drug Schedule

Step 1			Step 2		
Acebutolol	Dose 1	400 mg qd	Chlorthalidone	Dose 1	15 mg qd
	Dose 2	400 mg bid		Dose 2	15 mg bid
Amlodipine	Dose 1	5 mg qd	Chlorthalidone	Dose 1	15 mg qd
	Dose 2	5 mg bid		Dose 2	15 mg bid
Chlorthalidone	Dose 1	15 mg qd	Enalapril	Dose 1	5 mg qd
	Dose 2	15 mg bid		Dose 2	5 mg bid
Doxazosin	Dose 1	2 mg qd	Chlorthalidone	Dose 1	15 mg qd
	Dose 2	2 mg bid		Dose 2	15 mg bid
Enalapril	Dose 1	5 mg qd	Chlorthalidone	Dose 1	15 mg qd
	Dose 2	5 mg bid		Dose 2	15 mg bid
Placebo	Dose 1		Chlorthalidone	Dose 1	15 mg qd
	Dose 2			Dose 2	15 mg bid

Abbreviation: *TOMHS*, Treatment of Mild Hypertension Study.

Table 2 TOMHS Inclusions/Exclusions

Inclusions	
Ages 45 to 69	
Stage 1–2 diastolic hypertension	
Exclusions	
Do not meet BP criteria	
Stratum 1	74%
Stratum 2	22%
On more than one type antihypertensive drug	11%
Inability to obtain technically acceptable echocardiogram	5%
Rose angina	3%
>50% of meals eaten away from home	2%
Unwilling to make dietary changes	2%
Clinical evidence of CVD	<1%
Life-threatening illness	<1%
ECG hypertrophy (LVH)	<1%

Abbreviations: *TOMHS*, Treatment of Mild Hypertension Study; *CVD*, cardiovascular disease; *LVH*, left ventricular hypertrophy.

Table 3 TOMHS Phase II Primary Endpoint

Fatal
1. Death from CHD
2. Death from other CVD including stroke
3. Death from other causes

Nonfatal
1. Nonfatal MI (clinical criteria)
2. Nonfatal MI (serial ECG)
3. Nonfatal stroke
4. Congestive heart failure
5. Surgery for aortic aneurysm
6. Coronary artery bypass graft
7. Coronary angioplasty
8. Administration of thrombolytic agents for possible MI
9. Hospitalization for unstable angina
10. Definitive ''hard'' ECG-LVH (MN code 3.1 + 4.1 − 4.3 or 5.1 − 5.3)
11. Impaired renal function (serum creatinine ≥2.0 mg/dl and at least a doubling from baseline)

Endpoints were selected as fatal events, and nonfatal events were ordered by severity hierarchy. All these events increase risk for CVD mortality. Only one event was counted per participant on the final endpoint measure.
Abbreviations: *TOMHS*, Treatment of Mild Hypertension Study; *CHD*, coronary heart disease; *CVD*, cardiovascular disease; *ECG*, electrocardiogram; *MI*, myocardial infarction.

groups of 1.7 : 1 : 1 : 1 : 1 : 1. The largest allocation was to placebo. This was done to increase power for comparing each drug group to placebo. All patients provided written informed consent in a form approved by the human subject review boards of each participating institution.

During planning, a drug selection committee chose the study drugs. Treatment groups were (a) placebo (n = 234); (b) acebutolol (beta-blocker, n = 132); (c) amlodipine (dihydropyridine calcium channel blocker, n = 131); (d) chlorthalidone (diuretic, n = 136); (e) doxazosin (alpha 1 antagonist, n = 134); and (f) enalapril (angiotensin-converting enzyme [ACE] inhibitor, n = 135). Amlodipine and enalapril were used in the maleate form to allow all drugs to fit into identical capsules. Because all drugs fit into #3 capsules, except for acebutolol, the study was done ''double-dummy'' with participants taking 2 capsules (one #3, one #00) daily. Initial doses of drugs were amlodipine 5 mg, chlorthalidone 15 mg, doxazosin 2 mg (after an initial 1-month dosing of 1 mg given h.s.), enalapril 5 mg, and acebutolol 400 mg. All were given once daily. The dose was doubled if BP increased to prespecified levels: (a) diastolic blood pressure (DBP) ≥95 mm Hg on three successive visits; (b) DBP ≥105 mm Hg on a single visit. Participants were seen at follow-up visits every 3 months for 4 to 5.5 years depending on the date of randomization. Figure 2 shows the study design.

At the initiation of the TOMHS, ambulatory 24-hour ECG monitoring and echocardiographic measurements (echo) were included as measures to study the feasibility of performing these measurements as routine for documenting specific endpoints for the

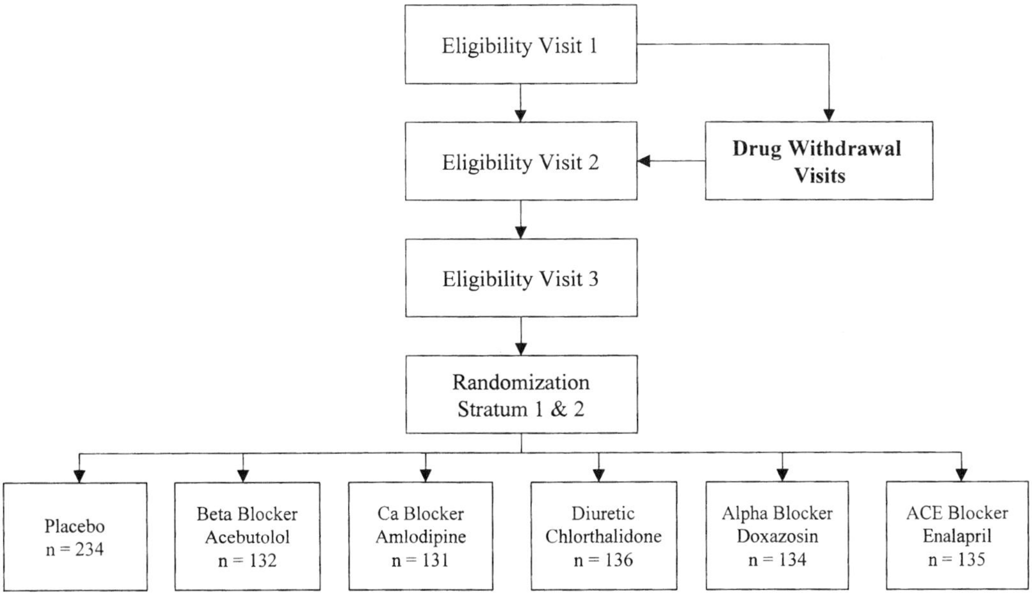

Fig. 2 TOMHS design. All participants were between 45 and 69 years, had diastolic blood pressures between 90 and 99 mm Hg, were free of coronary heart disease, and received nonpharmacological treatments for weight loss, sodium reduction, and physical activity.

study and to compare these endpoints between treatment groups. The resting ECG was also included for routine measurement to determine specific endpoints for the study. Resting ECG, echo, and 24-hour ECGs were recorded at baseline, 3 months, and annually.

1. Echocardiography

Left ventricular (LV) measurements were obtained at end diastole. End diastolic measurement criteria included both the American Society of Echocardiography (ASE) and the Penn conventions. The ASE convention uses a leading edge measurement with end diastole identified at the beginning of the QRS complex of the simultaneously recorded ECG (14). The Penn convention excludes endocardial or epicardial surfaces in the measurement of wall thickness and includes endocardial surfaces in the LV dimension measurement (15). End diastole is defined as the peak of the R wave of the QRS complex. The LV measurements included interventricular septal thickness at end diastole ($IVST_d$), the posterior wall thickness at end diastole (PWT_d), and LV internal dimension at end diastole ($LVID_d$). From the diastolic measurements, LV wall mass (LVM) was calculated from the Penn convention, according to the equation of Devereux and Reichek (15), by the formula $LVM = 1.04([IVST_d + PWT_d + LVID_d]^3 - [LVID_d]^3) - 13.6$ g. The LV mass index (LVMI, grams per square meter [g/m^2]) was calculated by dividing LV mass by body surface area (BSA): BSA (m^2) = 71.84 [height (cm)]$^{0.725}$ [weight (kg)]$^{0.425}$. Diagnostic criteria for LV hypertrophy using LV mass index (g/m^2) were $\geq$134 g/m^2 for men and $\geq$110 g/m^2 for women, representing the sex-specific 97th percentile of a previously published reference standard in a normal population (18), both based on Penn convention measurements.

Echocardiograms were obtained with the participant lying in a modified left lateral decubitus position with the head angled at 30° from the horizontal. Recordings were made at the end of expiration, if possible, using a Kontron Sigma ISC sonographic recorder with a 3.5 MHz transducer. Strip chart recordings were made on a fiberoptic L585 Honeywell recorder on light-sensitive paper at 50 mm/s. M-mode study of the left ventricle for determination of LV mass was accomplished by using a cursor from the two-dimensional image of the parasternal short-axis view of the left ventricle at the level of the tips of the mitral valve leaflets. At least five cycles were recorded for analysis. Tracings were read by one of two physician readers. Inter- and intrareader reliability for LV mass was assessed throughout the study. Intrareader correlations for LV mass were 0.93 and 0.89 for each of the two physician readers. Based on 222 recordings for each of the two physician's readers, interreader correlation was 0.83 with a mean difference between readers of 8 g and a standard deviation of 34 g.

2. Electrocardiography

a. *Resting ECG*

The ECG data were collected by using a standardized procedure for lead placement and ECG recording. The ECG recorder acquired 12 leads simultaneously for 10 seconds. The ECG data were transmitted from each of four clinical sites to the Edmonton computer ECG center for processing, analysis, and storage. Twelve-lead ECG signals were processed by using a special computer algorithm (NOVACODE), which systematically assigns the Minnesota Code and provides continuous 12-lead ECG amplitude and duration measurements (21). These computer measurements were used to define the following eight ECG-LV hypertrophy criteria sets: Sokolow-Lyon (22), Cornell voltage (23), Cornell voltage-duration product (23), Casale/Devereux (24), Rautaharju ECG (25), Romhilt-Estes point score (26), sum of 12-lead voltage, and 12-lead voltage-duration product (23).

b. Holter Monitoring

The routinely collected Holter recordings were received and processed at the Minnesota ECG coding center. The ambulatory ECG recorder used in TOMHS was a real-time ambulatory ECG recorder designed to detect changes in an individual's ECG waveform pattern, including irregularities of the heartbeat, fast or slow heart rates, abrupt pause, ventricular ectopy, and abnormal deviations of the ST segment. Ten-second samples of these ECG patterns or rhythm changes plus a systematic 10-second sample every 45 minutes were recorded and stored in solid-state memory. This method examines and reports on, but does not produce a wave-form recording of, *each* detected abnormality; rather, it provides the user with a number of ECG examples to document its performance. Up to 124 10-second 2-channel strips can be stored during a 24-hour period. A statistical editing procedure was performed by a trained technician who determined whether the monitor-annotated finding was correct. In this procedure, false-positive and false-negative rates for each category of detected event were determined and the monitor's count was adjusted accordingly.

All episodes of ST segment depression and ventricular premature beats were measured and rates were calculated. The ST segment depression was coded if there were 1 or more minutes of recording with ST depression of at least a Minnesota code of 4-1-1 or 4-1-2. Severe ST depression was defined as 10 or more minutes of ST depression with at least one Minnesota Code of 4-1-1 or 4-1-2.

C. Results

Over 18 months, 11,914 persons were screened and 902 were randomized. Table 4 provides baseline characteristics for the 902 participants by ethnicity and sex. Additional details of baseline characteristics are published elsewhere (28). Overall average age was 54.8 years, 61% were male, 20% were black, 11% were current smokers, 61% at initial

Table 4 Baseline Characteristics by Gender and Ethnicity

Baseline	White women (n = 233)	Black women (n = 112)	White men (n = 492)	Black men (n = 65)
Age (years)	55	53.7	55	54
Weight (lb)	163.2	175.6	200.3	196.2
BMI (kg/m^2)	28.1	29.8	29.1	28.3
Urinary sodium (mEq/24 h)	131.7	158.4	173.4	173.7
Alcohol users (%)	72.3	58.2	77.2	64.1
Drinks/week for users	3.6	3	5.7	6.8
Current cigarette smokers (%)	8.6	20.5	7	32.3
On BP drugs at initial visit (%)	66.1	63.4	59.6	47.7
Systolic pressure (mm Hg)	141.7	141.2	140.1	136.4
Diastolic pressure (mm Hg)	90	90.5	90.8	90.6

Abbreviation: *BP*, blood pressure.

screening. Two clinical centers, the Rush-Presbyterian and University of Alabama, recruited most of the black participants. Women made up 64% of blacks.

All participants were followed up a minimum of 4 years, average follow-up was 4.4 years, the range was 4 to 5.5 years. Attendance at follow-up visits was excellent: 90.6% for the quarterly visit and 92.8% for all four annual visits. There were no significant differences in attendance between treatment groups. Only five participants were counted as dropouts (<1%) because they attended no follow-up visits. Follow-up rates were similar by ethnic and gender group (91.3% white, 87.4% African-American, 91.2% men, 89.5% women).

Figures 3 to 5 show changes in lifestyle factors over 4 years by race. Overall participants achieved an average weight loss of −7.97 lb., −10.1 mEqL 8-hour urinary sodium, 376 kcal/day increase in leisure physical activity and a −1.1 drinks/week reduction in self-reported alcohol intake (data not shown). All groups lost weight: black women lost the least amount of weight, 3.6 lb, and white men the most, 9.9 lb, black men lost 4.4 lb, and white women 6.4 lb (data not shown).

Success with lifestyle intervention varied by age (Table 5). Men and women 60 years of age and older tended to have more success compared with younger participants.

Figure 6 shows the drug adherence status by treatment group over 4 years. At 1 year, 83.9% of those on active drugs were still taking their assigned step 1 medication, and this fell to 72.4% at 4 years. Also, use of open-label drugs (not step 1) was 5.9% at 12 months with all active versus 17.1% at 48 months. Amlodipine and acebutolol had the highest percentage of patients on step 1 and the lowest on open-label drugs at the 48-month visits. The placebo-treated participants had 81% on capsules at 12 months, but this proportion had dropped to 58.5% at 48 months. This group also had the highest percent (32.9%) on open-label drug treatment at 48 months, which was largely the result of being

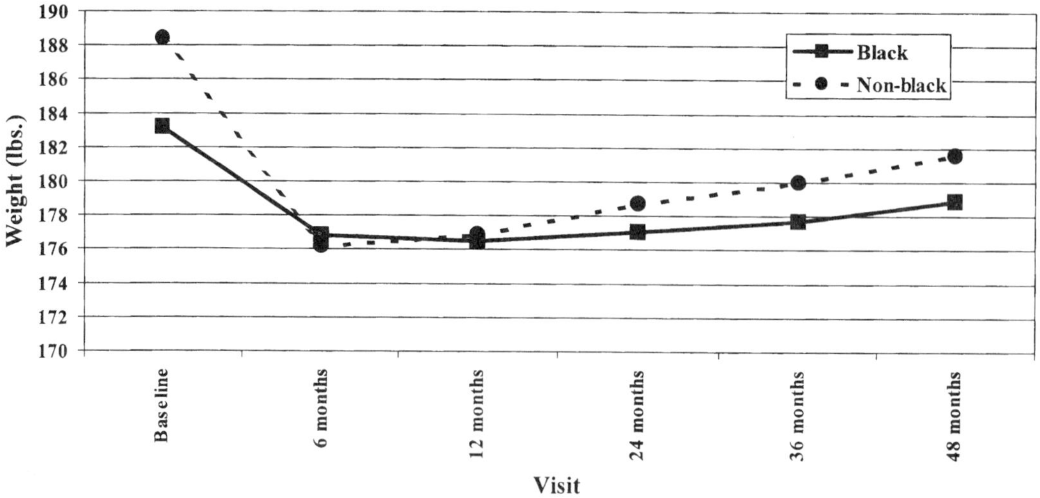

Fig. 3 Weight changes between blacks (baseline $n = 177$) and nonblacks (baseline $n = 725$) from baseline to 48 months.

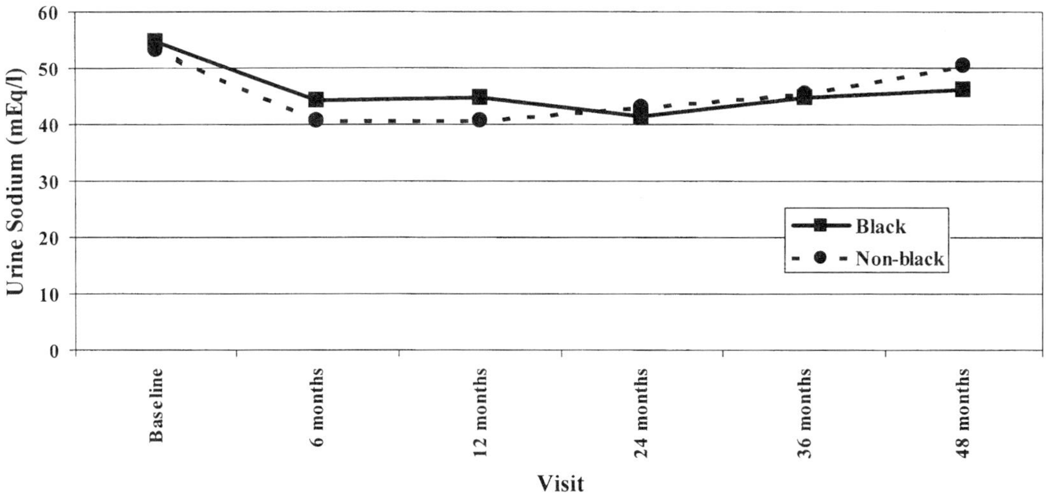

Fig. 4 Urine sodium changes for blacks (baseline $n = 177$) and nonblacks (baseline $n = 725$) from baseline to 48 months.

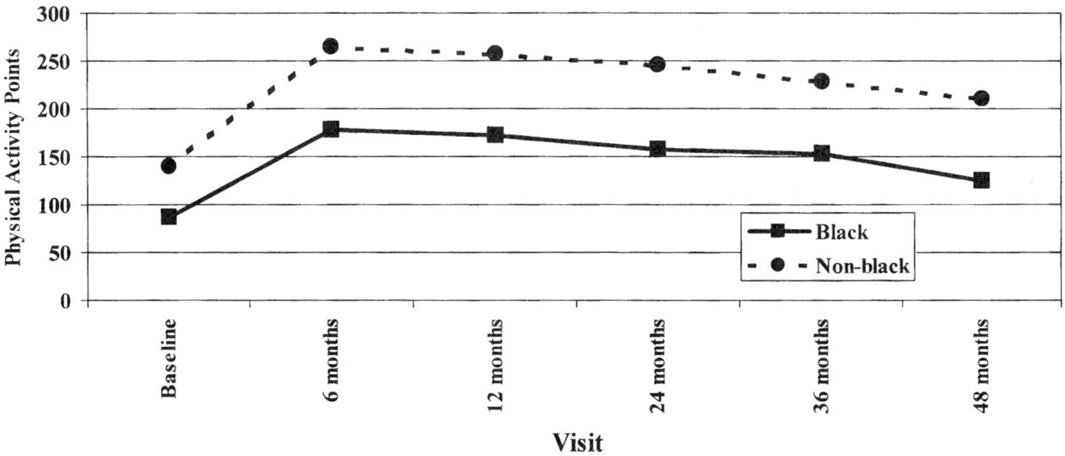

Fig. 5 Physical activity levels for blacks (baseline $n = 177$) and nonblacks (baseline $n = 725$) from baseline to 48 months (one physical activity point equals 4 kcal).

Table 5 Average Response to Lifestyle Modification over 48 Months by Treatment Group and Age for TOMHS Participants

	All active		Placebo		Total	
	<60	≥60	<60	≥60	<60	≥60
Change in weight	−7.3	−10.0	−6.9	−9.3	−7.2	−9.8
Change in drinks/week	−1.1	−1.0	−0.6	−1.8	−1.0	−1.2
Change in activity points	100.2	104.8	65.7	96.0	91.1	102.6
Change in urinary Na	−9.5	−11.8	−9.3	−14.7	−9.4	−12.5
N	487	171	175	59	662	230

Abbreviation: *TOMHS*, Treatment of Mild Hypertension Study.

put on active drug as a result of higher clinic blood pressure, or more commonly, by their private physician.

Figure 7 shows the changes in systolic and diastolic pressure by treatment group. Lifestyle only (placebo) lowered systolic pressure by 8.6 mm Hg. Among the drugs, acebutolol, amlodipine, and chlorthalidone were slightly better in lowering systolic pressure, compared with doxazosin and enalapril. Figure 8 shows systolic change by ethnic group

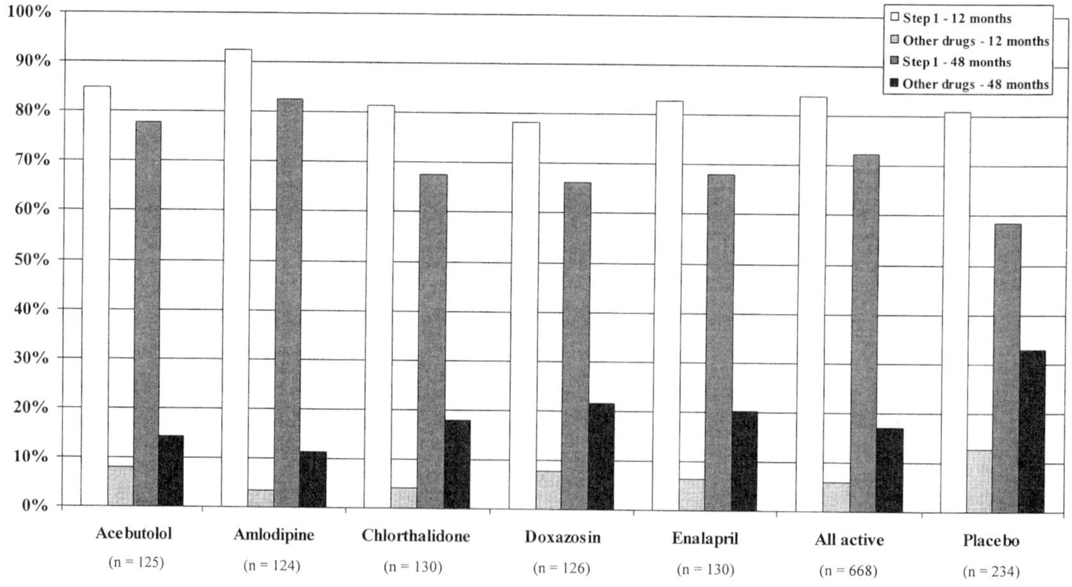

Fig. 6 Percent of participants taking step-1 medication and on other drugs at the 12-month and 48-month visits.

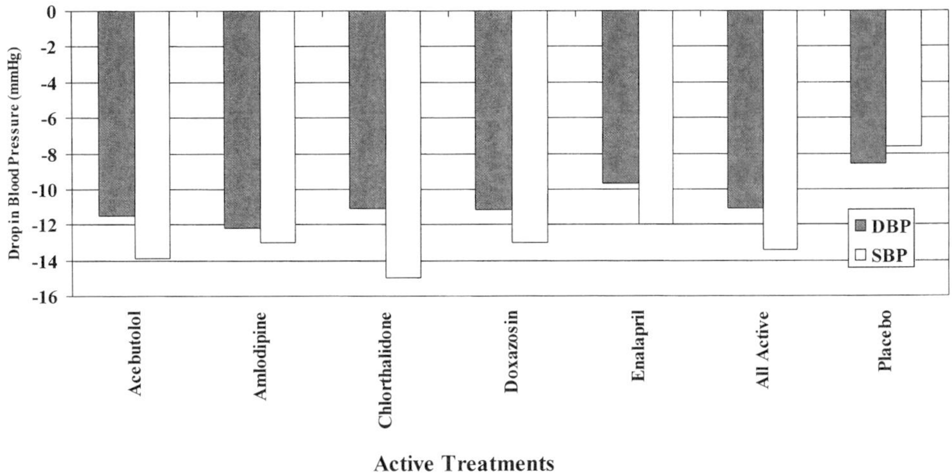

Fig. 7 Change in systolic and diastolic blood pressure from baseline to 48 months by treatment group.

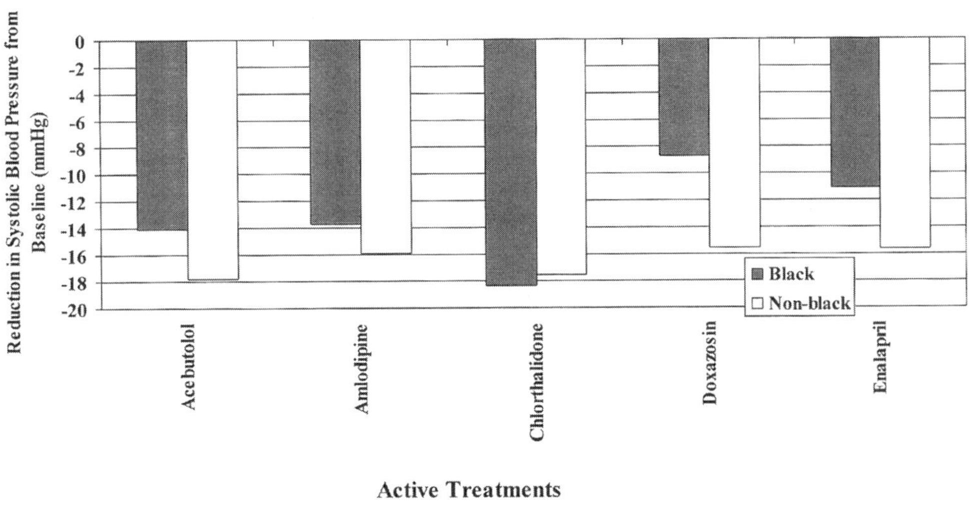

Fig. 8 Change in systolic blood pressure, averaged over 48 months, for black and nonblack participants.

Table 6 Mean Change in Selected Chemistries by Treatment Group

	Acebutolol		Amlodipine		Chlorthalidone		Doxazosin		Enalapril		All active		Placebo				
Measurement	Mean	SE	Mean	SE	Mean	SE	Mean	SE	Mean	SE	Mean	SE	Mean	SE	*P*(5)*	*P*(4)	*P*(1)
Glucose	−1.60	0.98	−1.40	0.76	−0.85	0.99	−1.83	1.33	−1.26	1.14	−1.39	0.47	−0.79	0.95	0.916	0.870	0.461
Potassium	−0.01	0.04	−0.07	0.03	−0.38	0.04	−0.04	0.03	0.06	0.03	−0.9	−0.02	−0.02	0.02	0.000	0.000	0.008
Calcium	−0.16	0.03	−0.12	0.03	−0.06	0.03	−0.22	0.03	−0.17	0.03	−0.09	0.02	−0.13	0.02	0.000	0.000	0.955
Uric acid	0.15	0.07	−0.21	0.06	0.51	0.07	−0.15	0.07	−0.13	0.07	+0.03	0.03	0.01	0.05	0.000	0.000	0.851
Creatinine	−0.01	0.01	−0.05	0.01	−0.06	0.01	−0.05	0.01	−0.05	0.01	−0.05	0.00	−0.05	0.01	0.003	0.002	0.645
Alk Phos	1.31	1.08	9.83	1.25	2.21	1.08	5.57	1.18	6.53	1.33	−0.13	0.02	8.47	0.94	0.000	0.000	0.002
Sodium	−0.61	0.24	−0.07	0.28	−0.83	0.24	−0.36	0.22	−0.80	0.24	0.03	0.03	−0.46	0.17	0.766	0.705	0.575
Chloride	−2.44	0.25	−2.02	0.23	−4.31	0.27	−1.87	0.24	−2.55	0.20	0.01	0.05	−2.40	0.17	0.000	0.000	0.147
Albumin	−0.08	0.01	−0.04	0.02	−0.06	0.01	−0.09	0.02	−0.08	0.02	−0.05	0.00	−0.05	0.01	0.003	0.017	0.023
WBC	−0.02	0.10	0.04	0.11	0.23	0.09	−0.21	0.08	0.08	0.09	−0.05	0.01	0.06	0.06	0.026	0.030	0.217
Plate/1000	13.27	3.13	26.09	2.96	19.40	2.97	6.90	3.33	22.69	3.14	5.06	0.54	13.69	2.13	0.000	0.000	0.214
N	131		127		132		132		133		655		232				

* All *P* values adjusted for clinic, stratum, and baseline level.

over 48 months. Whites overall experienced a greater reduction in pressure; however, within group, order of pressure response to specific drugs was similar among blacks and whites, although acebutolol was the best in whites versus chlorthalidone in blacks.

D. Laboratory

Table 6 shows changes from baseline in biochemistries and complete blood count results averaged over 4 years by treatment group. Chlorthalidone was associated with a 0.38 mEq/L reduction in serum potassium, and enalapril showed a slight increase of +0.06 mEq/L. Alkaline phosphatase increased in participants taking amlodipine. White blood cell count (WBC) increased with chlorthalidone by +230 cells, and decreased on doxazosin by −210 cells. Platelet counts increased most with amlodipine and enalapril, least with doxazosin. Figure 9 plots the change in serum potassium over 4 years, comparing chlorthalidone with other drugs and placebo. At 12 and 48 months, 2.4% and 3.4% of the chlorthalidone participants were taking supplemental KCl.

Serum creatinine was measured at baseline and then every 6 months over the duration of the study. By 12 months, serum creatinine fell in most groups including placebo (Fig. 10). There was a trend for serum creatinine to continue to fall over the 48 months of observation. One group, acebutolol (a beta-blocker), experienced significantly less lowering in serum creatinine, although even this group experienced a reduction in creatinine compared to baseline.

Lipid changes with diet and drug have been published elsewhere (29). A summary of lipid changes by group is shown in Table 7. Weight loss was strongly associated with lowering of LDL-C and triglycerides with increases in HDL-C (data not shown). The doxazosin group experienced the most favorable lipid changes with reductions in LDL-C, TG, and the most favorable change was in the HDL-C total cholesterol ratio. An unex-

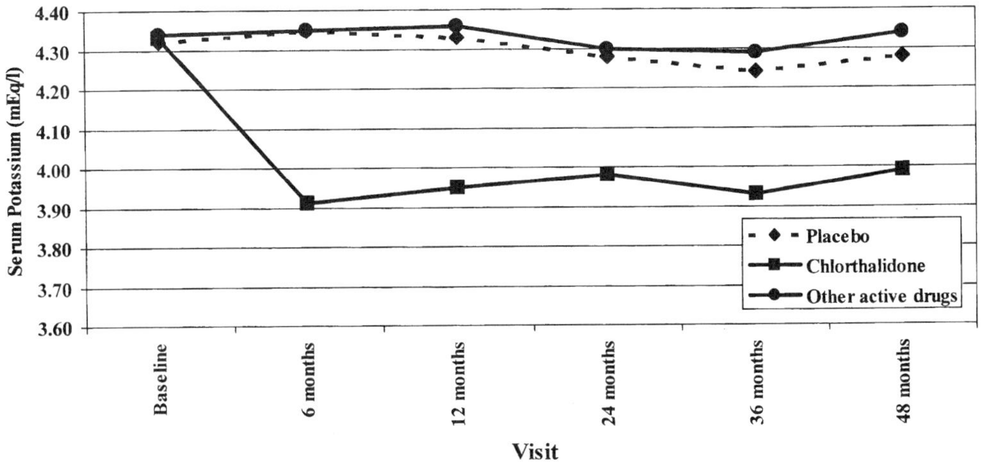

Fig. 9 Changes in barium potassium from baseline to 48 months with the chlorthalidone, placebo, and other active drugs.

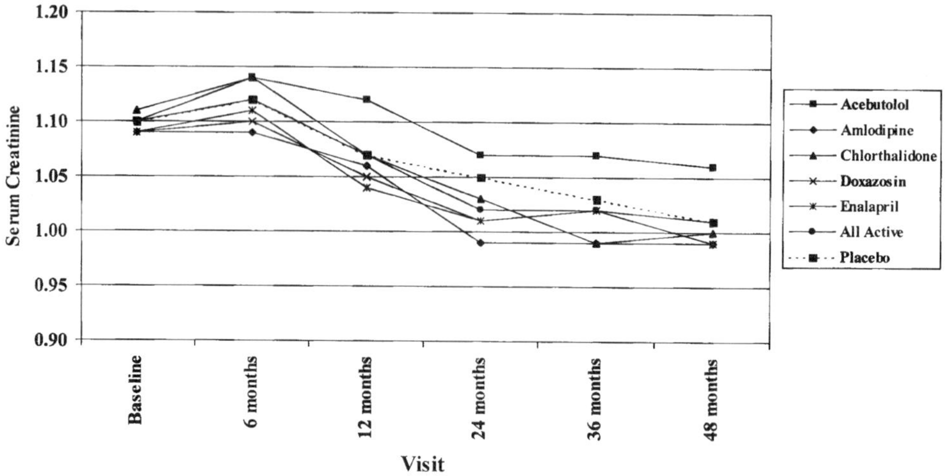

Fig. 10 Average serum creatinine at baseline through 48 months by treatment group.

pected result was that the acebutolol-treated participants also experienced a significant reduction in LDL-C.

Fasting plasma insulin was measured on all participants who attended the 48-month visit. Table 8 shows the level of fasting insulin by study group. It is reasonable to expect that the study groups had similar baseline insulins. The highest insulin was observed in the placebo group. The lowest insulin was with doxazosin $P = <0.01$ vs. placebo. It is noteworthy that the beta-blocker acebutolol also had a significantly lower insulin compared to placebo. It is of interest to note that when all drugs were combined and compared to placebo, fasting insulin was significantly lower in all drugs compared to placebo.

E. "Side Effects"/QL

Table 9 shows the percent of participants with a new or worsening condition from baseline in commonly reported symptoms by treatment group at 48 months. Of the total reported symptoms, 86% were classified as "mild" (not interfering with daily activities), 12% moderate (some interference with daily activities), and 2% severe (not able to do daily activities, with hospitalization). These percentages of levels of severity were essentially identical in patients taking placebo or active drugs, men and women, and whites and blacks.

Table 10 provides a summary of QL measures that have been published previously (30). Quality of life improved in all groups over 4 years. Improvements in QL were strongly related to weight loss (data not shown). The larger the weight loss, the greater the improvement in QL. Changes in QL were also related to level of change in systolic and diastolic blood pressure averaged over 4 years (adjusted for weight change).

Sexual function was assessed in men and women and detailed results have been previously published (31). There was no relationship of treatment to incidence of sexual

Table 7 Baseline Plasma Lipids and Average Change, Averaged Over 4 Years of Follow-Up

Plasma lipid	Acebutolol	Amlodipine	Chlorthalidone	Doxazosin	Enalapril	PLCB	*P* value
Total cholesterol							
Baseline, mean (sd)	233.2 (40.6)	229.1 (40.9)	229.7 (38.2)	228.8 (37.8)	225.7 (36.4)	225.3 (37.4)	
Average change	−11.7 (2.0)	−6.7 (2.3)	−4.5 (1.8)	−13.8 (2.0)	−8.0 (1.8)	−5.1 (1.3)	<0.001
LDL-C							
Baseline, mean (sd)	162.9 (35.4)	160.0 (37.3)	159.8 (34.4)	158.0 (35.2)	153.6 (33.5)	156.8 (33.1)	
Average change	−10.6 (2.0)	−5.1 (2.1)	−3.6 (1.9)	−11.3 (1.9)	−5.9 (1.9)	−3.6 (1.1)	0.004
HDL-C							
Baseline, mean (sd)	43.9 (12.7)	43.5 (10.6)	43.5 (11.2)	44.7 (10.9)	43.9 (12.5)	42.8 (11.9)	
Average change	0.2 (0.5)	2.0 (0.5)	2.1 (0.6)	2.4 (0.5)	2.6 (0.6)	1.4 (0.4)	0.01
(HDL-C/total) × 100							
Baseline, mean (sd)	19.1 (5.4)	19.5 (5.5)	19.3 (5.3)	19.8 (4.9)	19.7 (5.5)	19.3 (5.7)	
Average change	1.2 (0.3)	1.5 (0.3)	1.4 (0.3)	2.0 (0.4)	1.9 (0.3)	1.2 (0.2)	<0.001
Triglycerides							
Baseline, mean (sd)	131.9 (67.7)	128.0 (71.0)	131.9 (79.6)	130.5 (65.4)	141.3 (102.5)	128.8 (70.8)	
Average change	−6.4 (4.4)	−18.4 (3.9)	−14.7 (5.0)	−24.9 (4.1)	−23.6 (5.7)	−14.5 (3.0)	<0.001

Abbreviations: *PLCB*, placebo; *LDL*, low-density lipoprotein; *HDL*, high-density lipoprotein.

Table 8 Fasting Insulin at 48 Months by Treatment Group

	Insulin	
	Mean	SD
Acebutolol n = 119	9.60	5.24
Amlodipine n = 112	10.23	9.20
Chlorthalidone n = 115	10.68	8.39
Doxazosin n = 118	8.53	5.53
Enalapril n = 117	10.60	6.48
All active n = 581	9.92	7.13
Placebo n = 205	11.60	7.91
P(5)* = 0.012	*P*(4) = 0.109	*P*(1) = 0.006

* All *P* values adjusted for clinic, stratum, and baseline level.
Abbreviation: *SD*, standard deviation.

dysfunction in women. In men at 24 months, chlorthalidone was associated with more erectile dysfunction (failure to obtain and maintain erections) compared with placebo. Other drugs were similar to placebo for new incidence of erectile dysfunction. A separate analysis was carried out in the 65 men who reported erectile dysfunction at baseline and their status at 24- and 48-month visits. Erectile dysfunction had remitted in 54% at 24 months, and 57% at 48 months in men in the placebo group. This was similar to remission in each of the active drug groups except that all 8 of the men on doxazosin who reported dysfunction at baseline reported return of function at the 24-month visit (*P* .04 vs placebo), and 7 of 8 at 48 months (*P* .16 vs placebo).

1. *Echocardiography*

The baseline measurements showed a substantial proportion of left ventricular hypertrophy (LVH), with 12.7% of the men with an LVMI $\geq$134g/m^2 and 19.5% of the women with an LVMI $\geq$110g/m^2 for women. The LVMI was significantly, positively, and independently correlated with systolic blood pressure, body mass index, smoking, and urinary sodium secretion (33–36). Table 11 shows that mean LVMI decreased in successive visits through 4 years of follow-up for all treatment groups in TOMHS. Mean decrease ranged from 34 g for participants given chlorthalidone to 23 g for participants given enalapril (34). Table 12 shows the significant difference in LVMI reduction among the five treatment groups and that the reduction in LVMI for participants taking chlorthalidone was significantly greater than for those in the enalapril and the acebutolol treatment groups. The reduction in urinary sodium over 48 months was significantly and independently associated with a reduction in LVMI (35).

2. *Electrocardiography*

Table 13 shows the incidence of resting ECG findings by treatment group for the 4-year period of the study. Incidence of ischemic codes, ST segment depression, tall R waves, and ECG LVH had significantly lower 4-year incidence among the treatment groups than among those receiving placebo. Frequent ventricular premature beats (VPB, >10/hour) were present in approximately 13% of all participants at baseline, with slight increase in

Table 9 Percent TOMHS Participants Who Attended the 48-Month Visit Who Reported a Worsening or New Condition Since Baseline

Condition	Acebutolol n-126	Amlodipine n-114	Chlorthalidone n-116	Doxazosin n-121	Enalapril n-120	Placebo n-206	All groups	Among active	All active drugs vs placebo
Drowsiness	5.6	7.9	7.8	9.1	15	10.7	0.16	0.1	0.5
Tiredness	14.3	14.9	19.8	24.0	25	20.4	0.16	0.1	0.84
Faintness when standing	7.9	4.4	11.2	7.4	9.2	9.7	0.53	0.43	0.5
Itchy skin	4.8	9.6	6.9	9.1	12.5	12.1	0.2	0.25	0.12
Skin rash	10.3	7.9	9.5	5.8	11.7	7.3	—	—	—
Headaches	19.0	20.2	18.1	26.4	29.2	26.2	0.18	0.15	0.28
Ears ringing	16.7	15.8	12.9	15.7	14.2	15.0	0.94	0.87	0.93
Stuffy nose	26.2	26.3	25.0	30.6	33.3	31.1	0.61	0.53	0.5
Dry mouth	4.8	7.0	3.4	10.7	9.2	6.8	0.21	0.13	0.9
Cough	11.9	7.9	10.3	17.4	25.8	15.5	0.002	0.001	0.8
Heart beating fast	8.7	8.8	8.6	12.4	13.3	12.6	0.6	0.53	0.43
Chest pain	9.5	7.9	10.3	9.1	13.3	12.6	0.7	0.72	0.34
Joint pain	35.7	40.4	34.5	34.7	45.0	41.3	0.45	0.39	0.47
Swelling of feet	5.6	10.5	12.1	8.3	10.0	7.3	0.52	0.54	0.35
Muscle cramps	9.5	12.3	18.1	11.6	17.5	13.1	0.34	0.23	0.77
Waking up early	12.7	15.8	17.2	18.2	14.2	24.3	0.08	0.78	0.004
Feeling depressed	12.7	8.8	6.9	8.3	15.0	13.6	0.2	0.17	0.24

Abbreviation: *TOMHS*, Treatment of Mild Hypertension Study.

Table 10 Mean Change from Baseline in QL Indices Averaged Over All Follow-Up Visits for All Active Drugs Combined (Plus Lifestyle) and Placebo (Plus Lifestyle)

	All Active (n = 653)		Placebo (n = 230)		
QL index	Mean	SE	Mean	SE	*P* value active vs placebo
General health	1.26	0.16	0.98	0.25	0.10
Energy or fatigue	0.95	0.10	0.67	0.17	0.03
Mental health	2.14	0.23	1.43	0.43	0.01
General functioning	−0.03	0.06	−0.32	0.10	0.01
Satisfaction with physical abilities	0.38	0.03	0.25	0.05	0.07
Social functioning	0.12	0.03	−0.12	0.06	0.004
Social contacts	0.09	0.06	0.15	0.11	0.75
Global QL statistic	450.10	5.65	420.31	9.39	0.007

Abbreviation: *QL*, quality of life.

prevalence at successive annual visits (Table 16). The 4-year incidence of frequent VPB on Holter was approximately 22% for all treatment groups combined, and not significantly different between drug- and placebo-treated groups (28).

3. *Holter Monitoring*

At baseline, 16.9% of the drug treatment participants and 24.5% of the placebo group showed severe ST segment depression on the Holter. Over 4 years there was a decrease in the percent of participants with severe ST segment depression in all treatment groups. Tables 14 and 15 show comparisons of treatment of ST segment and severe ST segment depression. The incidence of ST segment depression was significantly less among participants receiving acebutolol than those in the placebo group, chlorthalidone group, enalapril group, or doxazosin group (ST depression). For severe ST depression, the incidence among those in the acebutolol group was significantly less than that among the chlorthalidone and enalapril participants (Table 17).

F. Combined Fatal and Nonfatal Cardiovascular Events

Although phase I was not powered for cardiovascular endpoints, a composite endpoint was developed that included the hierarchy shown in Table 3. Because phase I participants were to be included in phase II, this was the a priori-stipulated endpoint. To examine the effect of active drug treatment plus lifestyle compared with placebo (lifestyle only), all active drug groups were combined (n = 668) and compared with the 234 participants on placebo. Figure 11 shows systolic blood pressure change from baseline over 4 years in the active drug group and placebo. Throughout the study, the active drug systolic blood pressure was about 124 mm Hg and placebo was 133 mm Hg (diastolic 78 and 82 mm Hg, respectively) ($P < 0.001$). Incidence of major CV events was examined by group, and the active drug group experienced an incidence of 31% reduction compared with

Table 11 Average LVMI (g/m^2) from the Echocardiogram at Baseline, 3, 12, 24, 36, and 48 Months by Treatment Group

	Acebutolol		Amlodipine		Chlorthalidone		Doxazosin		Enalapril		All active		Placebo	
Visit	N	Mean	N	Mean	N	Mean	N	Mean	N	Mean	N	Mean	N	Mean
Baseline	119	101.2	122	96.3	130	105.3	128	101.2	125	102.6	624	101.4	218	102.3
3-Months	121	92.6	114	91.3	120	92.3	120	94.0	120	92.9	595	92.7	211	91.7
12-Months	109	95.1	107	86.4	115	89.7	119	92.4	111	94.4	561	91.6	199	95.0
24-Months	114	88.7	108	82.4	113	84.7	115	86.1	109	87.4	559	85.9	187	87.7
36-Months	119	91.3	99	85.1	99	87.6	114	90.5	103	90.6	534	89.2	168	89.8
48-Months	103	88.7	91	84.2	95	90.0	98	89.5	94	89.9	481	88.5	153	87.3

Abbreviation: *LVMI*, left ventricular mass index.

Table 12 Summary of Longitudinal Analysis Through 48 Months of LVMI (g/m²)

	Treatment effect vs placebo			
	Beta	SE (Beta)	Z (Stat)	*P* Value
Acebutolol	1.03228	1.55868	0.66	0.5078
Amlodipine	−1.64350	1.57900	−1.04	0.2979
Chlorthalidone	−3.50904	1.53853	−2.28	0.0226
Doxazosin	−0.23975	1.52647	−0.16	0.8752
Enalapril	1.41984	1.56359	0.91	0.3638
P (5 df) = 0.0490				
P (4 df) = 0.0287				
P (1 df) = 0.5894				
Significant contrasts ($P < 0.01$)				
Chl < Ace				
Chl < Ena				

Abbreviation: *LVMI*, left ventricular mass index.

placebo (P = .21). These groups were also compared for major and minor cardiovascular events (Fig. 12). Combined major and minor CVD events showed a similar reduction in the active drug group vs. placebo 34% (P = 0.03).

II. DISCUSSION

Phase I results of TOMHS produces strong support for the aggressive treatment of stage I hypertension. The six-group randomized, parallel, placebo-controlled study involving five different active drugs, placebo, and lifestyle for all participants followed up for several years is unique. This is in contrast to the majority of past hypertension trials that were often designed to provide the safety and efficacy data needed for drug approval. Phase III and IV trials usually have a smaller sample size with placebo or active drug comparisons and study durations of 10 to 16 weeks. Such studies are inadequate for making treatment decisions for a condition treated for a lifetime once drugs are started. The TOMHS has several features that overcome these limitations: (a) a parallel design comparing six treatment groups including placebo; (b) double-blind; (c) longer duration, 4 to 5.5 years; (d) lifestyle management. These features have provided a data set giving us a different perspective on the treatment of hypertension. Lifestyle intervention in TOMHS was very successful. The success was accomplished using an intensive intervention program involving both group and individual sessions. The sessions were conducted by highly trained, skilled, and experienced nutritionists. The TOMHS established that lifestyle management, weight loss, sodium and alcohol reduction, and increased physical activity can be successful and partially maintained, and these changes will result in an 8% to 10% reduction in systolic and diastolic blood pressure. This is a similar reduction to that observed with drugs used as monotherapy (without lifestyle advice). There is little regression to the mean in the BP lowering because baseline

Table 13 Incidence of Resting ECG Abnormalities Through 48 Months by Treatment Group for TOMHS Participants

	ACE		AML		CHL		DOX		ENA		All ACT		PLA				
ECG Abnormalities	No.	%	No.	%	No.	%	No.	%	No.	%	No.	%	No.	%	*P* Val (5 DF)	*P* Val (4 DF)	*P* Val (1 DF)
Any major abnormality*	13	10.2	6	4.8	11	9.0	9	7.0	8	6.5	47	7.5	28	12.7	0.155	0.531	0.022
Any abnormality†	37	44.6	33	35.1	33	39.8	32	34.8	36	40.4	171	38.8	51	37.5	0.513	0.346	0.798
Q-waves (1X)	4	3.2	10	8.1	8	6.3	8	6.3	12	9.3	42	6.7	12	5.6	0.393	0.322	0.590
R-waves (3X)	18	15.5	4	3.4	2	1.8	8	6.5	4	3.4	36	6.1	24	11.7	0.000	0.000	0.006
ST-depression (4X)	6	4.6	1	0.8	3	2.4	4	3.0	4	3.1	18	2.8	14	6.2	0.176	0.521	0.024
T-waves (5X)	22	19.0	14	11.9	20	17.7	16	13.6	14	12.1	86	14.8	45	22.3	0.064	0.391	0.011
Ischemic codes (ISC) (4.1–4.1, 5.1–5.3)	22	17.9	10	8.3	12	10.4	12	9.7	11	9.2	67	11.1	38	18.4	0.018	0.152	0.005
A-V conduction defect (6X)	10	7.9	8	6.3	7	5.5	11	8.7	11	8.4	47	7.4	16	7.1	0.942	0.864	0.926
Ventricular conduction defect (7X)	20	17.9	9	7.6	23	19.7	10	8.1	15	12.4	77	13.0	19	9.3	0.008	0.012	0.169
Miscellaneous (9X)	3	2.3	4	3.1	2	1.6	2	1.5	2	1.5	13	2.0	9	3.9	0.639	0.894	0.120
ST elevation (92)	5	3.8	2	1.6	2	1.5	2	1.5	3	2.3	14	2.1	5	2.2	0.836	0.738	0.982
LVH (3.1 + ISC code)	2	1.5	0	0.0	2	1.6	2	1.5	0	0.0	6	0.9	9	3.9	0.054	0.430	0.003
LVH (3.1–3.3 + ISC code)	7	5.4	0	0.0	2	1.6	3	2.3	0	0.0	12	1.9	11	4.8	0.009	0.007	0.017

P value calculated using Logrank test.

* MN Code 1.1, 1.2 (except 1.2.6 or 1.2.8), 4.1, 4.2, 5.1, 5.2 or (3.1 + an ischemic code).

† Any Minnesota code.

Abbreviation: *ECG*, electrocardiogram; *TOMHS*, Treatment of Mild Hypertrophy Study; *ACE*, acebutolol; *AML*, amlodipine; *CHL*, chlorthalidone; *DOX*, doxazosin; *ENA*, enalapril; *ACT*, active; *PLA*, placebo.

Table 14 Summary of Longitudinal Analysis Through 48 Months of Follow-Up Percent with ST-Segment Depression in the Ambulatory ECG

	Treatment effect vs placebo			
	Beta*	SE (Beta)	Z (Stat)	*P* value
Acebutolol	−10.14	3.150	−3.22	0.001
Amlodipine	−2.70	3.208	−0.84	0.400
Chlorthalidone	4.11	3.206	1.28	0.200
Doxazosin	−0.14	3.153	−0.04	0.966
Enalapril	5.40	3.203	1.69	0.092
P(5 df) = <0.001				
P(4 df) = <0.001				
P(1 df) = 0.76				
Significant contrasts ($P < 0.01$)				
Ace < Chl, Dox, Ena, Pla				

* Positive value indicates higher value for active group compared to placebo.
Abbreviations: *ECG*, electrocardiogram; *Ace*, acebutolol; *Chl*, chlorthalidone; *Dox*, doxazosin; *Ena*, enalapril; *Pla*, placebo.

entry pressures were made up of the average of the second and third eligibility visits. The combination of lifestyle plus drugs lowers pressure an additional 5%, and there were no major differences in pressure lowering between drugs. However, at the low doses used in TOMHS, enalapril and doxazosin did not lower BP as much as the other drugs.

All five drugs in TOMHS were well tolerated over 4 to 5.5 years and were effective for lowering blood pressure. The TOMHS patients' blood pressures remained under control using the lowest dose (step one, dose one) of the TOMHS. Blacks and whites responded similarly in rank order to BP lowering by type of drug although blacks in general were not as successful making the lifestyle changes. This suggests that there are no major, clinically relevant differences in BP response using the different TOMHS drugs.

The TOMHS side effect data were collected in a standardized manner with an effort to collect complete information. Most side effects were classified as "mild," that is, they did not interfere with daily activities (86%). Side effects generally were reported with similar rates in the placebo and active therapy groups. This suggests that the ubiquitous concerns about drug-related side effects with the classes of drugs used in TOMHS are likely overstated. The improvement in QL in the combined drug group compared with placebo also leads to this conclusion.

It is noteworthy that low-dose diuretic chlorthalidone performed well in lowering pressure with minimal adverse serum lipid and potassium effects. These results underscore the advisability of using low-dose diuretics in the management of hypertension. In more recent trials, low-dose diuretics have consistently been impressive in reducing CVD mortality and morbidity (2–4).

Table 15 Percent with Severe ST Depression from the 24-Hour ECG at Baseline, 3, 12, 24, 36, and 48 Months by Treatment Group

	Acebutolol		Amlodipine		Chlorthalidone		Doxazosin		Enalapril		All active		Placebo	
Visit	N	%	N	%	N	%	N	%	N	%	N	%	N	%
Baseline	131	22.1	129	16.3	131	17.6	131	14.5	130	13.8	652	16.9	229	24.5
3-Months	127	15.0	118	13.6	128	19.5	128	16.4	126	15.9	627	16.1	219	14.6
12-Months	123	11.4	115	13.0	121	19.8	124	14.5	121	19.8	604	15.7	207	16.9
24-Months	122	8.2	115	9.6	118	18.6	122	13.1	118	16.9	595	13.3	199	14.6
36-Months	120	10.0	107	13.1	110	16.4	119	10.9	113	14.2	569	12.8	190	15.3
48-Months	122	9.0	105	14.3	107	16.8	115	12.2	108	16.7	557	13.6	183	13.1

Table 16 Average % VPB >10/Hour from the 24-Hour Electrocardiogram at Baseline, 3, 12, 24, 36, and 48 Months by Treatment Group

	Acebutolol		Amlodipine		Chlorthalidone		Doxazosin		Enalapril		All active		Placebo	
Visit	N	Mean	N	Mean	N	Mean	N	Mean	N	Mean	N	Mean	N	Mean
Baseline	131	6.11	129	8.53	130	19.23	131	17.56	130	13.85	651	13.06	229	15.28
3-Months	127	5.51	118	12.71	128	19.53	128	18.75	126	15.87	627	14.51	219	10.96
12-Months	123	8.13	115	13.04	121	20.66	124	16.94	121	14.05	604	14.57	207	14.01
24-Months	122	9.02	115	12.17	118	25.42	122	14.75	118	15.25	595	15.29	199	15.08
36-Months	120	13.33	107	15.89	110	17.27	119	21.01	113	18.58	569	17.22	190	20.00
48-Months	122	10.66	105	15.24	107	22.43	115	14.78	108	18.52	557	16.16	183	20.22

Table 17 Summary of Longitudinal Analysis Through 48 Months of Percent with Severe* ST Depression on the Ambulatory ECG

	Treatment effect vs. placebo			
	Beta	SE (Beta)	Z (Stat)	*P* value
Acebutolol	−3.02	2.440	−1.24	0.215
Amlodipine	0.99	2.486	0.04	0.690
Chlorthalidone	6.75	2.487	2.71	0.007
Doxazosin	3.33	2.449	1.36	0.174
Enalapril	6.12	2.486	2.46	0.014
$P(5\text{ df}) = 0.001$				
$P(4\text{ df}) = 0.002$				
$P\ (1\text{ df}) = 0.12$				
Significant contrasts ($P < 0.01$)				
Ace < Chl, Ena				
Ch1 < Pla				

* Severe ST depression = 10 or more minutes of ST depression (see text).
† Positive value indicates higher value for active group compared with placebo.
Abbreviations: *ECG*, electrocardiogram; *Ace*, acebutolol; *Chl*, chlorthalidone; *Ena*, enalapril, Pla, placebo.

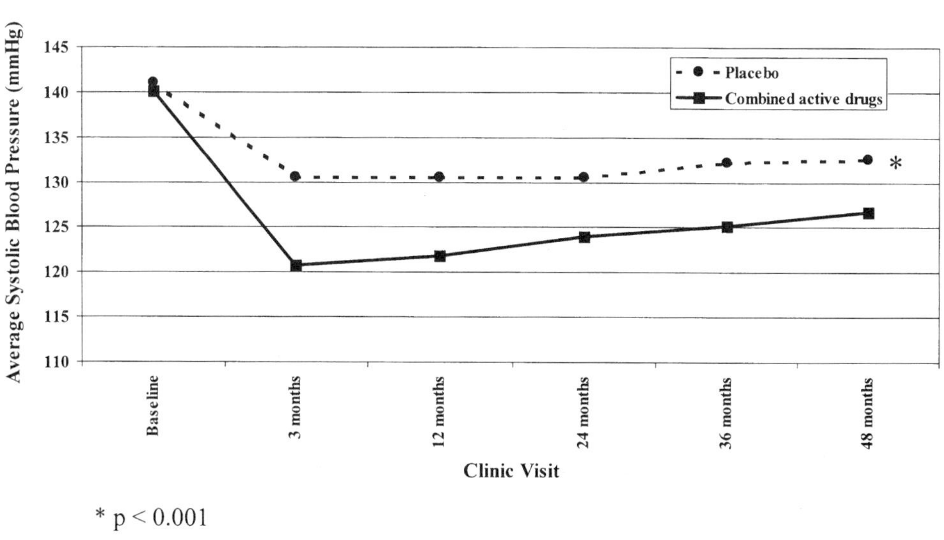

Fig. 11 Systolic blood pressure change from baseline to 3 months and annual clinic visits, for placebo ($n = 234$) and combined active drugs ($n = 668$).

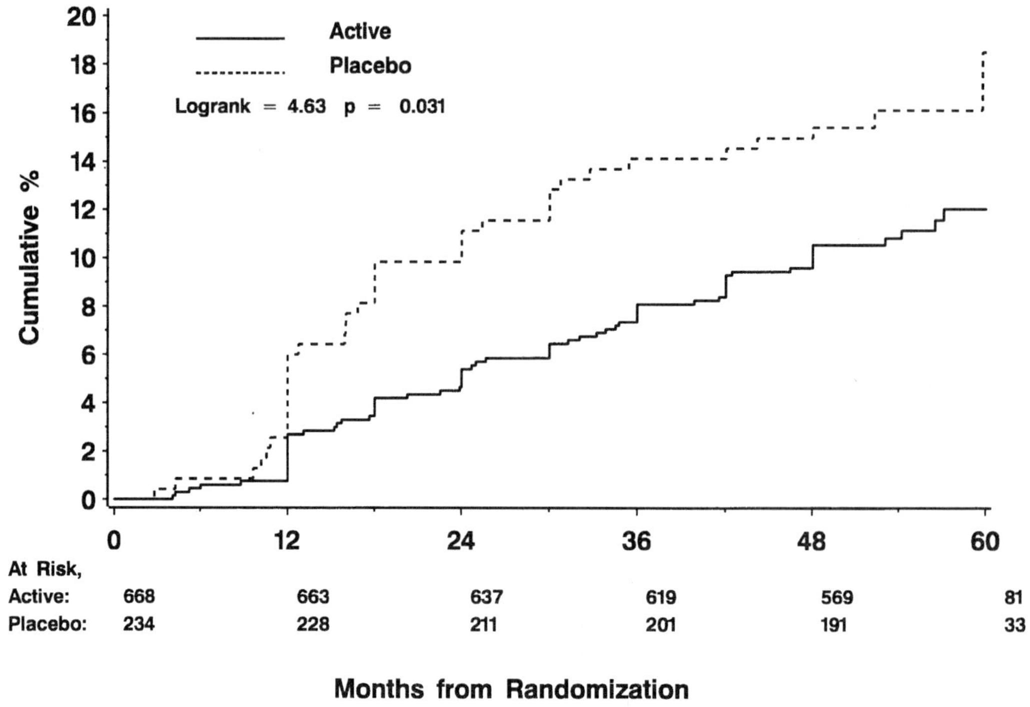

Fig. 12 Cumulative major plus other clinical events minus active vs. placebo.

The TOMHS phase I results have provided important new insights into the management of stage I hypertension. The data provide convincing support for the benefit of aggressive lowering of pressure in this group using combined lifestyle/drug intervention. The results of the TOMHS and HOT trials (13, 37) should make physicians reconsider their approach to the management of hypertension by more frequent use of drug therapy with lifestyle change, and by considering concerns about drug side effects and QL in proper perspective. Although phase II of TOMHS was not carried out, data from TOMHS and the VA monotherapy trial were used in planning the design and conduct of the ongoing NHLBI-sponsored Antihypertensive and Lipid Lowering to Prevent Heart Attack Trial (ALLHAT) (38, 39). The ALLHAT is examining the important question concerning the role of type of antihypertensive drug and effectiveness in lowering fatal and nonfatal CHD.

To date in the United States, we have provided inadequate treatment and control for hypertension. The NHANES III data showed that only about 50% of hypertensives were taking medications, and only 27% were controlled (39). The results of TOMHS and other recent trials should make physicians reconsider their approach in the management of hypertension. Physicians need to be more active in the use of drug therapy combined with lifestyle advice, and side effect and QL concerns should be placed in proper perspective.

REFERENCES

1. Collins R, Peto R, MacMahon S. Drug treatment of hypertension: an overview of the unconfounded randomized trials in the context of observational epidemiology. Lancet 1990; 335: 827–838.
2. The Sixth Report of the Joint National Committee on Prevention, Detection, Evaluation, and Treatment of High Blood Pressure. Arch Intern Med 1997; 157:2414–2446.
3. The SHEP Cooperative Research Group. Prevention of stroke by antihypertensive drug treatment in older persons with isolated systolic hypertension: final results of the systolic hypertension in the elderly program (SHEP). JAMA 1991; 265:3255–3264.
4. Dahlöf B, Lindholm LH, Hansson L, Schersten B, Ekbom T, Wester PO. Morbidity and mortality in the Swedish Trial in Old Patients with Hypertension (STOP-Hypertension). Lancet 1991; 338:1281–1285.
5. MRC Working Party. Medical research council trial of treatment of hypertension in older adults: principal results. BMJ 1992; 304:405–412.
6. Stassen JA, Ambridge GG, Birkenhager WH. Morbidity and mortality in the European Trial on Isolated Systolic Hypertension. Lancet 1997; 350:757–764.
7. Multiple Risk Factor Intervention Trial Research Group. Multiple risk factor intervention trial—risk factor changes and mortality results. JAMA 1982; 248:1465–1477.
8. Furberg CD, Psaty BM, Meyer JV. Nifedipine: dose-related increase in mortality in patients with coronary heart disease. Circulation 1995; 92:1326–1331.
9. Estacio RO, Jeffers, BW, Hiatt WR. The effect of nisoldipine as compared with enalapril on cardiovascular outcomes in patients with non-insulin dependent diabetes and hypertension. N Engl J Med 1998; 338:645–652.
10. Borhani NO, Mercuri M, Borhani PA. Final outcome results of the multicenter isradipine diuretic atherosclerosis study (MIDAS): a randomized uncontrolled trial. JAMA 1996; 276: 785–791.
11. Stamler J, Prineas RJ, Neaton JD. Background and design of the new U.S. trial on diet and drug treatment of "mild" hypertension. Am J Cardiol 1987; 59:516–606.
12. Elmer PJ, Grimm RH, Laing B. Lifestyle intervention: results of the treatment of mild hypertension study (TOMHS). Prev Med 1995; 24:378–388.
13. Neaton JD, Grimm RH, Prineas RJ, Stamler J, Grandits G, Elmer PJ, Cutler JA, Flack JM, Schoenberger JA, McDonald R, Lewis C, Liebson PR. Treatment of Mild Hypertension Study: final results. JAMA 1993; 270:713–724.
14. Sahn DJ, DeMaria A, Kisslo J, Weyman A. Committee on M-Mode Standardization of the American Society of Echocardiography: recommendations regarding quantification in M-mode echocardiography: results of a survey of echocardiographic measurement. Circulation 1978; 58:1072–1083.
15. Devereux RB, Reichek N. Echocardiographic determination of left ventricular mass in man. Circulation 1977; 55:613–618.
16. Levy D, Savage DD, Garrision RJ, Anderson KM, Kannel WB, Castelli WP. Echocardiographic criteria for left ventricular hypertrophy: the Framingham Heart Study. Am J Cardiol 1987; 59:956–960.
17. Ditchey RV, Schuler G, Peterson KL. Reliability of echocardiographic and electrocardiographic parameters in assessing serial changes in left ventricular mass. Am J Med 1981; 70: 1042–1050.

18. Devereux RB, Lutas EM, Casale RN, Kligfield P, Eisenberg RR, Hammond IW, Miller DH, Reis G, Alderman MH, Laragh JH. Standardization of M-mode echocardiographic left ventricular anatomic measurements. J Am Coll Cardiol 1984; 4:1222–1230.
19. Savage DD, Garrision RJ, Kannel WB, Levy D, Anderson SJ, Stokes J, Feinleib M, Castelli WP. The spectrum of left ventricular hypertrophy in a general population sample: the Framingham Study. Circulation 1987; 75(suppl I):I-26–I-33.
20. Henry WL, Clark CE, Epstein SE. Asymmetric septal hypertrophy (ASH): echocardiographic identification of the pathognomonic anatomic abnormality of IHSS. Circulation 1973; 47:225–233.
21. Rautaharju PM, MacInnis PJ, Warren JW. Methodology of ECG interpretation in the Dalhousie program: novacode ECG classification procedures for clinical trials and population health surveys. Meth Inform Med 1986; 29:362–370.
22. Sokolow M, Lyon T. Ventricular complex in left ventricular hypertrophy as obtained by unipolar precordial and limb leads. Am Heart J 1949; 37:161–186.
23. Molloy JM, Okin PM, Devereux RB, Kliggfield P. Electrocardiographic detection of left ventricular hypertrophy by the simple QRS voltage-duration product. J Am Coll Cardiol 1992; 5:1180–1186.
24. Devereux RB, Casale PN, Eisenberg RR, Miller DH, Kligfield P. Electrocardiographic detection of left ventricular hypertrophy using echocardiographic determination of left ventricular mass as the reference standard: comparison of standard criteria, computer diagnosis and physician interpretation. J Am Coll Cardiol 1984; 3:82–87.
25. Rautaharju PM, La Croix AZ, Savage DD. Electrocardiographic estimate of left ventricular mass versus radiographic cardiac size and the risk of cardiovascular disease mortality in the epidemiologic follow-up of the first national health and nutrition examination survey. Am J Cardiol 1988; 62:59–66.
26. Romhilt DW, Estes EH. A point score system for the ECG diagnosis of left ventricular hypertrophy. Am Heart J 1968; 75:752–758.
27. Prineas RJ, Crow R, Blackburn H. The Minnesota Code Manual of Electrocardiographic Findings. Littleton MA: John Wright—PSG, 1982.
28. Mascioli SR, Grimm RH, Neaton JD. Characteristics of participants at baseline in the treatment of mild hypertension study (TOHMS). Am J Cardiol 1990; 66:32c–35c.
29. Grimm RH, Flack J, Grandits GA. Long-term effects on plasma lipids of diet and drugs to treat hypertension. JAMA 1996; 275:1549–1556.
30. Grimm RH, Grandits GA, Cutler JA. Relationships of quality of life measures to long term lifestyle and drug treatment of mild hypertension study. For the TOMHS Research Group. Arch Intern Med 1997; 157:638–648.
31. Grimm RH, Grandits GA, Prineas RJ. Long-term effects on sexual function of five antihypertensive drugs and nutritional hygienic treatment in hypertensive men and women. Treatment of Mild Hypertension Study (TOMHS). Hypertension 1997; 29:8–14.
32. Liebson PR, Grandits G, Prineas R, Dianzumba S, Flack JM, Cutler JA, Grimm RH, Stamler J. Echocardiographic correlates of left ventricular structure among 844 mildly hypertensive men and women in the Treatment of Mild Hypertension Study (TOMHS). Circulation 1993; 87:476–485.
33. Liesbon PR, Prineas RJ, Grimm RH. Regression of left ventricular mass in the treatment of hypertension: successes and carcatsd. Prev Cardiol 1998; spring:24–32.
34. Liebson PR, Grandits GA, Dianzumba S, Prineas RJ, Grimm RH, Neaton JD, Stamler J. Comparison of five antihypertensive monotherapies and placebo for change in left ventricular mass in patients receiving nutritional-hygienic therapy in the Treatment of Mild Hypertension Study (TOMHS). Circulation 1995; 91:698–706.
35. Prineas RJ, Grimm R, Grandits G, Liebson P, Neaton J, Stamler J, Elmer P, Cutler J, Rautaharju P. The effect of dietary sodium and body weight on echocardiographic measures of left

ventricular mass among treated hypertensive men and women: four year change in the TOMHS Study. Nieren-und Hochdruckkrankheiten 1994; 23(suppl 1):S14–S21.

36. Hypertension Detection and Follow-up Program Cooperative Group. Five year-findings of the hypertension detection and follow-up program: reduction in mortality of persons with high blood pressure, including mild hypertension. JAMA 1979; 242:2562–2571.
37. Hansson L, Zanchetti A, Carruthers SG. Effects of intensive blood pressure lowering and low dose aspirin in patients with hypertension: principal results of the hypertension optimal treatment (HOT) randomized trial. Lancet 1998; 351:1755–1762.
38. Davis BR, Cutler JA, Gordon DJ. Rationale and design for the antihypertensive and lipid lowering treatment to prevent heart attack trial (ALLHAT). AJH 1996; 9:342–360.
39. Burt VL, Cutler JA, Higgins M. Trends in the prevalence, awareness, treatment, and control of hypertension in the U.S. adult population: data from the health examination surveys, 1960 to 1997. Hypertension 1995; 26:60–69.

13

Department of Veterans Affairs Cooperative Study on Monotherapy of Hypertension

BARRY J. MATERSON

University of Miami, Miami, Florida

DOMENIC J. REDA

Hines VA Hospital, Hines, Illinois

I. INTRODUCTION

Dr. Edward D. Freis assembled the first major Veterans Administration (VA) Cooperative Study Group on Antihypertensive Agents. He is renowned for proving that oral drug treatment of hypertension conferred a major benefit by reducing the damaging impact of hypertension on target organs (1). When that study was planned in 1960, the prevailing wisdom was that "benign essential" hypertension should not be treated at all! Dr. Freis subsequently organized and conducted a series of cooperative studies that made significant contributions to our understanding of hypertension and its therapy. The studies were always organized to provide information to practicing physicians in their care of hypertensive patients. Most of the study groups involved seven VA centers with two seven-center groups operating simultaneously on different projects.

The Department of Veterans Affairs Cooperative Study Group on Antihypertensive Agents (participants are listed in Section XIII) started planning for its largest cooperative study in September 1984. Fourteen (later 15) VA medical centers would follow the same protocol with the intention to enroll 1400 patients. It required more than 2 years for the approval process, funding, training, drug acquisition, and packaging and shipping of drugs and study forms to the 14 original participating VA medical centers. Patient intake began on October 10, 1986, and the first patient was randomized to the Titration Phase on November 19, 1986. A fifteenth medical center (Dallas) joined the group 2 weeks later. The study progressed relatively smoothly, although multiple site visits, special trouble shooting, and additional training sessions were required. Annual study group meetings were of considerable value in maintaining the integrity of the study. The progress of the study was continuously monitored by an internal executive committee, an external data monitoring board that had the power to recommend to the chief of the program that the study be stopped if necessary, and the central human rights committee. The patient intake period ended on September 30, 1989, and the last patient completed follow-up on September 30, 1990. The first major manuscript (2–4) was published in the New England Journal of Medicine on April 1, 1993. An additional 16 manuscripts based on this data set have been published and at least three more are pending.

II. PRIMARY OBJECTIVE

The primary objective of this study was to determine the blood pressure lowering efficacy, ability to maintain blood pressure control, and incidence of medical terminations of different classes of antihypertensive agents used as single-drug therapy (monotherapy). The six drug classes (and representative drug) selected were: β-adrenergic blocking agents (atenolol), angiotensin converting enzyme inhibitors (captopril), central α_2-agonists (clonidine), calcium antagonists (diltiazem-SR), thiazide diuretics (hydrochlorothiazide), and peripheral α_1-blocking agents (prazosin).

III. SECONDARY OBJECTIVES

There were five secondary objectives:

1. To determine whether patient characteristics such as age, race, body weight, serum and urinary electrolytes, and baseline plasma renin activity are associated with response or nonresponse to various classes of antihypertensive agents, and to formulate guidelines for the practicing physician to select a monotherapy regimen likely to be successful in lowering blood pressure in a patient with a given set of characteristics.
2. To determine the incidence of side and adverse effects for the different classes of antihypertensive drugs.
3. To determine the short- and long-term effects of different classes of antihypertensive drugs on selected cardiovascular or metabolic variables: (a) left ventricular function and thickness, (b) changes in serum lipids, (c) serum and urine electrolytes, and (d) fasting glucose.
4. To evaluate those patients who do not achieve goal blood pressure with the drug to which they were randomized by means of a pilot trial in which those patients will be randomly assigned to treatment with an alternative single antihypertensive agent.
5. To evaluate those patients who do not achieve goal blood pressure with either the first or second assigned single antihypertensive drug in a pilot trial wherein patients will be treated with a combination of the first and second antihypertensive drug.

IV. PRIOR HYPOTHESES

A. Stepped-Care Algorithm

Early randomized clinical trials in the United States and Europe established the concept and utility of a stepped-care algorithm for treatment of hypertension (5). In general, patients were to be started on therapy with a thiazide diuretic. If the maximum drug dose failed to control the blood pressure, a second drug (usually a sympatholytic such as reserpine) was to be added and titrated to effect. If this failed, a third drug (usually a vasodilator such as hydralazine) was to be added and titrated to effect. Finally, guanethidine could be added to the three other drugs, if necessary.

Although effective, this algorithm was criticized because of its rigidity, need to titrate drugs to potential toxicity, and lack of firm basis in the physiology of hypertension. As newer drugs, such as beta-blockers, peripheral selective alpha-blockers, angiotensin-converting enzyme inhibitors, and calcium antagonists became available, clinical evidence mounted supporting alternative regimes (6).

B. Age and Racial Differences in Response to Drug Therapy

At the time planning for the monotherapy study was initiated in the fall of 1984, the VA Cooperative Study Group on Antihypertensive Agents had already demonstrated that propranolol was an equivalent first-step agent to hydrochlorothiazide in white patients (7) and captopril was an effective monotherapy in white patients with mild hypertension (8, 9). The group had also discovered that black (African-American) patients responded much less well than whites to monotherapy with propranolol or captopril. Other extant data indicated that younger and older patients responded differently to different drugs (10).

These observations led the group to test prospectively the efficacy of the different classes of drugs in a sufficiently large group to observe the effect of patient characteristics such as age, race, and the interaction of age and race on the response to these drugs.

C. Plasma Renin Profiling

Plasma renin activity was established by Laragh and colleagues (11) as an important physiologic measure to determine the underlying mechanism of hypertension. Plasma renin profiling was used by that group to classify patients with hypertension. They proposed that plasma renin profiling be used routinely to help in the selection of antihypertensive therapy. The VA Cooperative Study Group had determined that the plasma renin profile did not accurately predict response to either hydrochlorothiazide or propranolol (12). We, therefore, included baseline plasma renin profiles in this study to test the ability of the profile to predict response to each of the six study drugs.

D. Adverse Metabolic Effects of Thiazide Diuretics

The metabolic effects of thiazide diuretics on plasma lipids, lipoproteins, potassium, and glucose were known to be potentially harmful when high doses of the diuretics were used for a short term (13). These metabolic perturbations were used as a reason by many practitioners for avoiding the use of diuretics for the treatment of their hypertensive patients. We had an opportunity to test very low doses of hydrochlorothiazide over the long term (1 to 2 years).

E. Regression of Left Ventricular Hypertrophy

There was relatively little information available in human subjects on the effect of various antihypertensive drugs on the regression of left ventricular hypertrophy (LVH). Animal studies demonstrated regression of LVH with captopril (14), but it was thought that thiazide diuretics would not have a beneficial effect. We had an opportunity to establish baseline left ventricular mass and posterior wall thickness by performing echocardiograms and to determine change from baseline after short- and long-term treatment with the six antihypertensive drugs.

F. Established Drug Doses

The prevailing practice at the time this study was designed was to use much larger doses of antihypertensive medication than is the practice today. The VA Group had used as much as 200 mg of hydrochlorothiazide daily and 640 mg of propranolol daily in an earlier trial (7). Hydrochlorothiazide was generally used at 50 to 100 mg and atenolol at 50 to 100 mg daily. These doses of atenolol were associated with a significant incidence of bradycardia. Although not a stated objective of this study, we decided to test 12.5 mg of hydrochlorothiazide and 25 mg of atenolol as initial doses.

V. PROTOCOL

A. Entry and Baseline

All patients signed an informed consent document before entering the study. The study protocol and consent form had been previously reviewed by a central human studies committee and the institutional review boards at each of the participating medical centers. After considerable debate, a decision was made to include only men in the study because of the very small number of women in the veteran population at the time.

This protocol did not require the imposition of rigorous nonpharmacological therapy. Nevertheless, the study centers routinely counseled patients on limitation of sodium intake, achieving ideal body weight, limiting ethanol intake, and not smoking. Patients were not entered into the trial if they were in the process of making substantive lifestyle changes.

The basic design of this prospective, randomized, double-blind study is displayed in Figure 1. Ambulatory veterans who met the inclusion criteria (Table 1) entered the 4- to 8-week washout phase during which they received single-blind placebo tablets. Baseline laboratory studies were performed during this period, as were electrocardiogram (ECG), echocardiogram, plasma lipid and lipoprotein determinations, and plasma renin profile. Patients who were compliant by pill count and who met the entry blood pressure (BP) criteria (average of three readings on each of the last two visits) were randomly allocated to double-blind treatment with one of the six drugs listed in Table 2 or placebo. The blind was preserved by means of a double-dummy technique. Every patient received two bottles of coded medication at each visit. One contained active drug and the other contained placebo; those patients allocated to the placebo group were given placebo in both bottles. The placebo pills or capsules were identical to the matching active drug.

B. Drug Titration and Subsequent Phases

Drug ordering, repackaging, and distribution were handled by the clinical research pharmacist (Carol Fye) at the Cooperative Studies Program Clinical Research Pharmacy Coor-

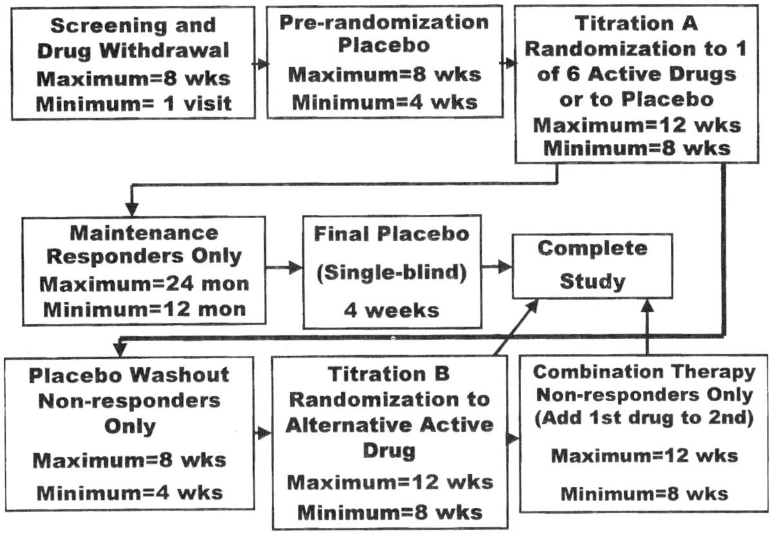

Fig. 1 Protocol and flow chart of the VA Monotherapy of Hypertension Study.

dinating Center in Albuquerque, New Mexico. She devised a method of packaging the various blinded medications so that the risk of an error in distributing the correct drug or drug dose was reduced almost to zero. She also acted as the liaison with the various pharmaceutical companies and negotiated the donation of a specific drug with matching placebo for each drug class. Neither the chairman of the study nor the clinicians involved participated in this process.

Blinded medication was titrated over the 8- to 12-week titration phase to achieve a goal BP of less than 90 mm Hg without adverse effects on two successive clinic visits. Patients who achieved goal BP then entered a maintenance phase for up to 2 years. At the end of the maintenance phase, patients were converted back to single-blind placebo and were seen in 1 month.

To avoid a potential first-pass hypotensive response to prazosin, a blister pack with a 2-week supply of prazosin (or matching placebo) was issued to the patient. The first four doses were 1-mg tablets to be taken initially at bedtime and then twice daily. This was followed by 2-mg tablets to be taken twice daily. Subsequent supplies of prazosin or its placebo were issued in bottles, as were the other medications.

To avoid rebound hypertension from sudden discontinuation of clonidine, patients who were taking the medium or high dose (or its placebo) were issued a 2-week blister card that accomplished blinded down-titration and discontinuation over 1 week. No discontinuation protocol for atenolol was established because of its long half-life.

Patients who failed to achieve goal BP were entered into a pilot substudy. They were randomly reassigned to one of the six active drugs. However, they could not be reassigned to the same active drug that they had taken during the first phase. Patients who achieved goal BP after titration with the second drug were deemed to have completed the trial; they did not enter a maintenance phase. Those who failed to achieve goal BP on the second drug were entered into a combination phase in which they continued to take the active second drug, and the active first drug was carefully added. Patients who achieved

Table 1 Inclusion and Exclusion Criteria Used at Screening

- Inclusion criteria
  - Ambulatory male veteran who has passed his 21st birthday
  - Untreated diastolic BP 95–109 mm Hg or that BP after placebo washout
  - No exclusions
  - Signed informed consent
- Exclusion criteria
  - Known hypersensitivity or reaction to any of the study drugs
  - History or current evidence of hypertensive retinopathy greater than K-W-B ii
  - History of cerebral or subarachnoid hemorrhage
  - Atherothrombotic stroke or myocardial infarction within 6 months of entry into this study
  - Symptomatic ischemic heart disease
  - Atrial fibrillation or any other cardiac dysrhythmia that would preclude accurate blood pressure measurement or is indicative of serious underlying heart disease
  - History of congestive heart failure as evidenced by at least two of the following four criteria: recent dyspnea or orthopnea not of pulmonary origin; ventricular diastolic gallop (S_3); basal pulmonary rales; evidence of congestive heart failure on chest X-ray
  - Bradycardia of <50 beats per min
  - Greater than first degree heart block
  - Serum creatinine >2.0 mg/dL
  - Collagen vascular disease other than rheumatoid arthritis
  - Surgically curable or other secondary forms of hypertension
  - Malignancies or other diseases likely to be fatal or disabling within 3 years
  - History or evidence of a nonsituational, clinically important mental depression confirmed by a psychiatrist (or other organic/functional forms of mental dysfunction of a chronic type)
  - Drug abuse, severe alcohol abuse, or severe organic brain disease
  - Adult bronchial asthma, past or present, or chronic obstructive lung disease with wheezing
  - Diabetes mellitus requiring treatment with insulin
  - Hyperlipidemia with cholesterol >300 mg/dL in two separate blood samples after at least a 12-hour fast or of sufficient severity to require treatment with medication
  - When the physician believes that it is not clinically advisable to discontinue current antihypertensive medication
  - Treatment with a drug or drugs that are contraindicated as concomitant medication for this protocol, that are used by the patient on a chronic basis because of clinical reasons or disease state, and from which the patient cannot be withdrawn
  - Failure of diastolic BP to rise to or above 95 mm Hg by 8 weeks after withdrawal from prior antihypertensive medication
  - Diastolic BP is above 109 mm Hg
  - Systolic BP is above 199 mm Hg
  - Patient withdraws consent or fails to return for rescreening

Abbreviation: *BP*, blood pressure.

goal BP were deemed to have completed the study; those that failed were removed from further participation.

C. Blood Pressure Determination and Definitions

All reported BP readings were the average of three determinations made with the patient seated, his arm supported at heart level, his back supported in the chair, and after at least a 5-minute rest. Clinic personnel were trained and tested in BP determination techniques before the initiation of the trial. The inclusion BP was the screening BP and was required

Table 2 Medications and Dose Titration for Monotherapy of Hypertension Study*

Drug	Low dose	Medium dose	High dose
Atenolol	25	50	100
Captopril	**25**	**50**	**100**
Clonidine	**0.2**	**0.4**	**0.6**
Diltiazem-SR	**120**	**240**	**360**
Hydrochlorothiazide	12.5	25	50
Prazosin	**4**	**10**	**20**

* All doses are given in milligrams. Drugs and doses in bold type were administered in divided doses, twice daily.
Abbreviation: *SR*, the slow release preparation of diltiazem.

to be in the range of 95 to 109 mm Hg, inclusive. The baseline BP was the mean of the BP averages at the last two visits of the prerandomization period. To qualify for randomization, the baseline BP had to be in the range of 95 to 109 mm Hg, and the two-visit averages used to calculate the baseline BP could not differ by more than 6 mm Hg. Goal BP was the mean of the averages of the last two visits of the titration phase being less than 90 mm Hg. Treatment response was defined as having achieved goal BP during the titration phase without adverse drug effects. Treatment success was defined as having a treatment response and then maintaining BP of less than 95 mm Hg without adverse drug effects until the end of the first year of the maintenance phase. It was permissible to titrate the study drug to maximum dose during the maintenance phase, if necessary, to maintain BP at less than 95 mm Hg.

D. Adverse Events Monitoring and Removal from the Study

Patients were monitored for adverse drug events by the clinic staff on each visit. They used both a preprinted form that included known adverse effects associated with each of the drugs and asked open-ended questions seeking new symptoms or changes since the last visit.

Patients could be removed from the study for administrative reasons such as moving to a new location, having a job that interfered with the clinic visits, or other personal reasons for declining continued participation. The latter reason was scrutinized to be certain it was not a surrogate for dissatisfaction resulting from an adverse drug reaction. All removals from the study that were not clearly administrative were deemed to be medical. These were divided into adverse drug reactions, BP exceeding the defined safety limits, and other medical reasons. Diastolic BP safety limits were an average of three readings higher than 114 mm Hg at any one visit, average higher than 109 mm Hg at two consecutive visits, or average higher than 99 mm Hg on three consecutive visits during the maintenance phase. An average systolic BP higher than 199 mm Hg at any one visit required removal.

Criteria for removing a patient from the study are listed in Table 3. Information about all patients removed from the study was referred to the study chairman. He reviewed the information while blinded to the randomly assigned drug and determined whether the removal was for medical or administrative reasons. If medical, he then determined whether the removal was for an adverse drug effect, BP above the safety limits, or other medical reason. Whenever there was doubt, the decision was made against the blinded drug.

Table 3 Criteria for Discontinuing Protocol Therapy

1. Severe adverse effects from a study drug.
2. Development of hypertensive retinopathy greater than K-W group II.
3. Development of cerebral or subarachnoid hemorrhage.
4. Development of atherothrombotic stroke or myocardial infarction.
5. Development of symptomatic ischemic heart disease.
6. Development of atrial fibrillation or any other cardiac dysrhythmia that would preclude accurate blood pressure measurement or is indicative of serious underlying heart disease.
7. Development of congestive heart failure as evidenced by at least two of the following:
   a. Dyspnea or orthopnea not of pulmonary origin.
   b. Ventricular diastolic gallop (S_3).
   c. Basal pulmonary rales.
   d. Evidence of congestive heart failure on chest X-ray.
8. Development of symptomatic bradycardia (<50 beats/min).
9. Development of greater than first degree heart block.
10. Serum creatinine greater than 2.0 mg/dL and 50% higher than baseline.
11. Development of collagen vascular disease other than rheumatoid arthritis.
12. Development of a malignancy or other disease likely to be fatal or disabling within 3 years.
13. Development of a nonsituational clinically important mental depression confirmed by a psychiatrist (or other organic/functional forms of mental dysfunction of a chronic type).
14. Drug abuse, severe alcohol abuse, or development of severe organic brain disease.
15. Development of adult bronchial asthma or chronic obstructive lung disease with wheezing.
16. Development of diabetes mellitus that cannot be controlled without insulin.
17. Hyperlipidemia of sufficient severity to require treatment with medication.
18. Proteinuria greater than 1 g per 24 hours (determined from 24-hour urine sample).
19. Neutrophils less than 1000/cu mm (differential obtained when WBC is less than 5000/cu mm).
20. Considered in the best interest of the patient by the investigator.
21. The patient cannot be withdrawn from a contraindicated concomitant medication.
22. Unrelated intercurrent illness that renders the patient unable to continue the study.
23. Interruption of treatment for more than 21 days.
24. Death.
25. Patient requests termination.
26. Patient moved, lost to follow-up for more than 1 month beyond the last scheduled visit, or unreliable.
27. Diastolic BP greater than 114 mm Hg on any one visit.
28. Diastolic BP greater than 109 mm Hg on two consecutive visits.
29. Systolic BP greater than 199 mm Hg on any one visit.
30. Diastolic BP greater than 99 mm Hg on three consecutive visits during maintenance phase.
31. The patient displays moderate adverse effect and BP is above goal during maintenance phase.
32. The patient displays moderate adverse effect on the lowest level of the study medication during maintenance phase.

Abbreviations: *WBC*, white blood cell count; *BP*, blood pressure.

E. Plasma Renin Profiling

Plasma renin profiling was accomplished by collecting an 8:00 AM blood sample from the patient into a tube containing potassium-EDTA. The sample was centrifuged at room temperature, the plasma carefully separated then quick frozen in a dry ice-acetone mixture. The frozen samples were shipped to a central laboratory at the Boston VA Medical Center (Dr. Hamburger). An aliquot from a contemporaneous 24-hour urine collection was frozen and mailed to the same laboratory. Plasma renin activity was determined by a modification of the Haber method (15). Plasma renin profile was determined by using a nomogram distribution of plasma renin activity versus 24-hour urine sodium excretion. Urine sodium, potassium, creatinine, and protein were measured in this central laboratory. Urine collections were made during the prerandomization phase, the initial titration phase, and at the 12- and 24-month visits in the maintenance phase.

F. Lipid and Lipoprotein Analysis

Blood was collected from patients for plasma lipid and lipoprotein profiles after they had fasted for 14 hours. The blood was collected in a tube containing EDTA and the plasma was separated. It was shipped chilled, but not frozen, to a central laboratory in Washington, D.C. (Dr. Lakshman). Samples were processed by techniques developed by the National Institutes of Health and monitored with controls from the Centers for Disease Control and Prevention quality control program (16). Samples were collected during the prerandomization and initial titration phases and at 12 and 24 months in the maintenance phase.

G. Echocardiograms

Echocardiograms (two-dimensional and M-mode) were performed on as many patients as possible during the prerandomization phase. The tapes of the echocardiograms were sent to a central laboratory in Washington, D.C. (Dr. Gottdiener) for blinded analysis. If a baseline tracing could not be obtained, or if it were of unacceptable quality, no further echocardiograms were performed on those patients. The analytical methodology is reported in detail in the relevant publications (17, 18).

VI. SAMPLE SIZE ANALYSIS AND POWER ESTIMATES

Biostatisticians, particularly Domenic J. Reda and Dr. William G. Henderson, were involved from the beginning and throughout the study. The conduct of the study was coordinated through the Cooperative Studies Program Coordinating Center at the Hines, Illinois Veterans Affairs Hospital. The center provided administrative, budgetary, biostatistical, and data processing support.

Based on data from prior VA cooperative studies on hypertension, the planning committee made the following assumptions. Under the null hypothesis, the percentage of patients in each group remaining in the study after 1 year of maintenance and maintaining BP control will be 25%. A spread of more than 15% (17.5% to 32.5%) across treatment groups is clinically important. Similarly, the percentage of patients classified as treatment responders in the titration A phase is expected to be 30%, with a spread of 15% (22.5% to 37.5%) considered clinically important. The medical termination rate is expected to be 3% with a spread of more than 6% (0 to 6%) considered to be clinically important.

For each outcome measure, the test of the null hypothesis will be a Chi-square test of homogeneity for a 2 × 7 contingency table using $\alpha = 0.05$ as the criterion for statistical significance.

A method developed by Lachin (19) was used to estimate the sample size requirement.

$$N = \frac{\lambda(\mu, \alpha, \beta)}{\tau}$$

where λ is the noncentrality parameter of the Chi-square distribution with μ degrees of freedom, probability (type I error) $= \alpha$ and probability (type II error) $= \beta$; and τ, the effect size reduces to

$$\tau = \frac{1}{r} \sum \delta_{i1}^2/(\alpha_1(1 - \alpha_1))$$

where

α_1 = marginal expectation of the first column under H_0
r = number of rows
δ_{i1} = difference between the conditional expectations under H_0 and H_1 for the cell in row i and column 1.

For the primary outcome measure, we considered three alternative hypotheses that would satisfy the assumptions of the Planning Committee. We expressed the possible percentage of patients completing 1 year of maintenance under each alternate hypothesis and the corresponding effect size in the following table.

Alternate hypothesis	Effect size	Percentage of patients in each treatment group maintaining BP control after 1 year of maintenance						
		1	2	3	4	5	6	7
A_1	.026	.325	.325	.325	.250	.175	.175	.175
A_2	.013	.325	.300	.275	.250	.225	.200	.175
A_3	.009	.325	.250	.250	.250	.250	.250	.175

Based on prior studies, moderate variability in the treatment effects across randomized groups (alternate hypothesis A_2) was considered to be the most reasonable assumption.

The following table gives the treatment group percentages under the most reasonable alternative hypothesis and the effect size for the two secondary outcome measures of the primary objective.

Outcome measure	Effect size	Treatment group						
		1	2	3	4	5	6	7
Medical terminations	.014	.00	.01	.02	.03	.04	.05	.06
Efficacy in titration A phase	.012	.225	.250	.275	.300	.325	.350	.375

A sample size of 1400 randomized patients is estimated to provide power of 0.90 when alpha = .05 to detect the stated differences in the percentage of patients remaining on the study after 1 year of maintenance and maintaining BP control. This sample size also provided power of 0.88 for comparison of the goal BP rate during the titration phase and power of 0.93 for comparison of medical termination rates.

Assuming a prerandomization exclusion rate of 10%, a phase A dropout rate of 10%, and a maintenance dropout rate of 17%, we expected the number of patients in each phase of the study as shown in the following chart:

Main study		
Enter study	1555	
Excluded	155	(10%)
Randomized to titration A	1400	(90%)
Terminated	140	(10%)
Randomized to pilot study	840	(60%)
Advanced to maintenance	420	(30%)
Terminated	70	(17%)
Completed study	350	(83%)
Pilot study		
Enter titration B phase	840	
Terminated	84	(10%)
Achieved goal BP?	252	(30%)
Randomized to combination	504	(60%)
Terminated	50	(10%)
Completed combination	454	(90%)

To detect differences in titration A phase individual side effect rates, with the expected rate at 3% and a doubling of the rate considered to be clinically important, the power calculation would be identical to that developed for the rate of medical terminations. Therefore, with alpha = .05 and the sample size = 1400, the power would be .93.

In maintenance, if the expected rate of an individual side effect is 5%, and a doubling of the rate is considered clinically important, setting alpha = .05 and the expected sample size = 420 (30% of randomized patients entering maintenance) would yield a power of .70 to detect such differences. If the entry rate to maintenance is 40%, that is, 560 patients achieve goal BP in titration A, the power would increase to .85.

VII. ELIGIBILITY CRITERIA

Table 1 displays the inclusion and exclusion criteria that were applied at the time of screening patients for this study.

VIII. MAIN RESULTS

Of the 1635 patients who entered this study, we successfully randomized 1292 to one of the seven treatment groups (2–4). The four age by race groups were younger whites (n = 246; mean ± SD; age 51 ± 7 years), younger blacks (n = 291; age 49 ± 9), older whites (n = 408; age 66 ± 4), and older blacks (n = 330; age 66 ± 4). Younger was defined as less than age 60. Observed response rates to monotherapy were much higher than expected, averaging nearly 60% compared with the anticipated 30%. There were significant differences in the percentage of patients achieving goal BP at the end of the titration phase with each drug. For the overall group, diltiazem was highest with 75% (n = 185); placebo was lowest at 33% (n = 187). There were also significant differences in the achievement of goal BP and actual reduction in BP for each drug in the age by race subgroups. The more clinically important changes were in those 745 patients who achieved goal BP and entered the maintenance phase. Of these, 145 withdrew during the first year of maintenance and 65 thereafter.

Their results at the end of 1 year of maintenance are presented in Figure 2. Note that these are the corrected figures and are somewhat different from those originally published. While reviewing the database for another paper, we discovered that an error had been made in one line of computer code. When this error was corrected (3, 4) the maintenance data actually improved, although there were some minor hierarchical changes. Only the maintenance data were effected. In brief, younger and older blacks responded best to diltiazem, younger whites responded best to atenolol and captopril (and poorly to hydrochlorothiazide), and older whites responded well across the drug groups. Although the

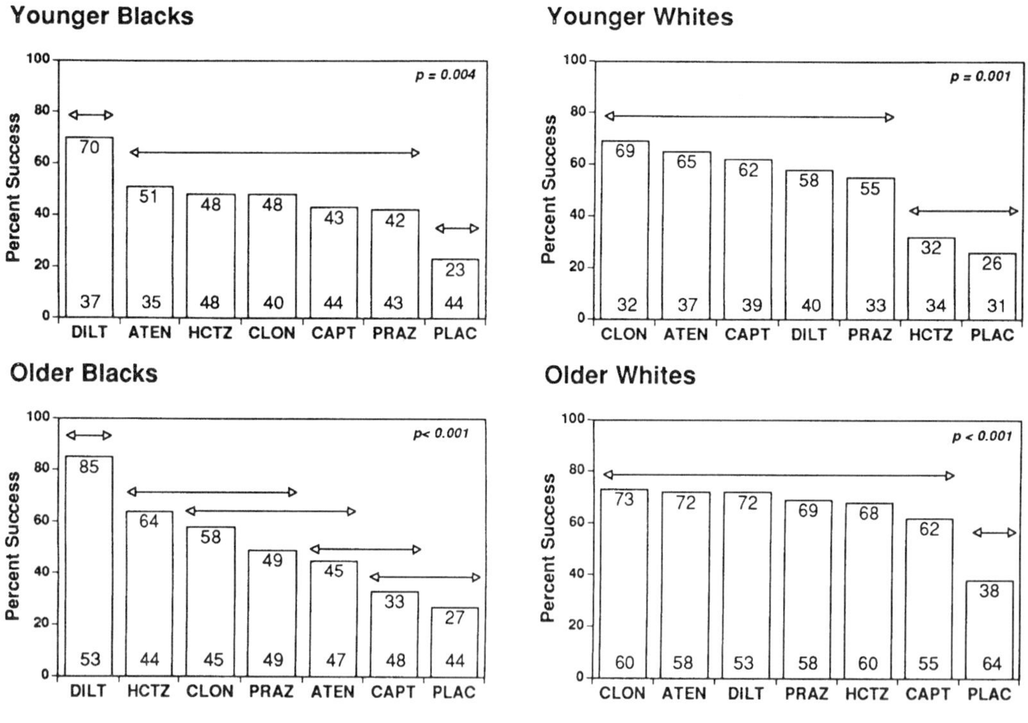

Fig. 2 Percent success for each of the age by race subgroups in the VA Monotherapy of Hypertension Study. Success was defined as having achieved goal diastolic blood pressure (<90 mm Hg without adverse effects) for two consecutive visits at the end of the titration period and having diastolic blood pressure <95 mm Hg through 1 year of the maintenance period. Younger was defined as <60 years old. *Abbreviations*: *ATEN*, atenolol; *CAPT*, captopril; *CLON*, clonidine; *DILT*, diltiazem-SR; *HCTZ*, hydrochlorothiazide; *PLAC*, placebo; *PRAZ*, prazosin. The horizontal arrows group the drugs whose effects do not differ from each other by >15%. (From Ref. 4, used with permission.)

success rate with clonidine was high, we did not list that drug as a first-line choice because of the high incidence of adverse effects.

There were differences in the dose level at which response was achieved (Fig. 3). For hydrochlorothiazide, 48 of 107 responders (45%) responded at 12.5 mg; 49% of responders to atenolol did so at the 25-mg dose, but captopril and diltiazem tended to require the full dose for about one third of the responders.

Withdrawals for adverse drug effects were highest for prazosin (13.8%), followed by clonidine (10.1%), diltiazem (6.5%), placebo (6.4%), captopril (4.8%), atenolol (2.2%), and hydrochlorothiazide (1.1%). It is noteworthy that the two drug classes recommended as first-line choices in the absence of special indications by the sixth report of the Joint National Committee (JNC VI) (20) had the lowest withdrawal rate. There were also differences in drug-induced withdrawal in the age by race subgroups. Prazosin (15.2%) was highest among the younger whites compared with hydrochlorothiazide (2.9%) and captopril (2.6%). Prazosin (19.0%) and clonidine (16.7%) were the highest in older whites compared with atenolol and hydrochlorothiazide (both 1.7%). The highest withdrawal rates in older blacks were for diltiazem (12.2%) and prazosin (11.3%), even though diltiazem was the most effective. The highest withdrawal rate in younger blacks was for placebo (6.8%).

There was also a drug differentiation for discontinuation because the BP safety limits were exceeded. These were highest for placebo (7.5%), followed by captopril (6.1%), hydrochlorothiazide (4.6%), atenolol (3.7%), clonidine (3.1%), prazosin (1.9%), and none for diltiazem.

In summary, this study demonstrated that age by race interaction was a valid predictor of response to a single drug used for treatment of stage 1–2 hypertension. It further

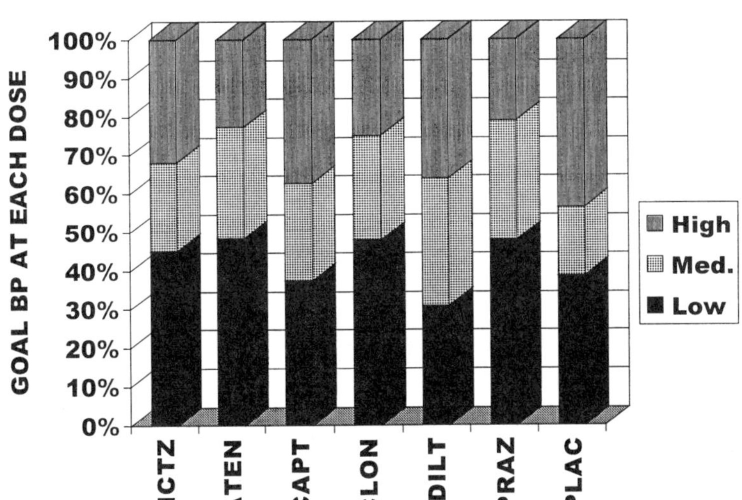

Fig. 3 Percentage of patients who achieved goal diastolic blood pressure (<90 mm Hg on the last two visits of the titration period without adverse drug effects) on the low, medium, and high dose of each drug. The dose schedule is displayed in Table 2. The abbreviations are the same as in Figure 2. Patients who received hydrochlorothiazide, atenolol, clonidine, and prazosin tended to respond to the low dose, whereas captopril, diltiazem, and placebo required the high dose. (From Ref. 2.)

validated the efficacy of 12.5 mg of hydrochlorothiazide and 25 mg of atenolol as initial doses.

IX. SECONDARY RESULTS

A. Response to Alternate Monotherapy

Of the 1292 patients randomized to monotherapy, 745 (57.7%) achieved goal BP and entered the maintenance phase, 137 were removed from the study for a variety of reasons, and 410 failed to respond to the initial drug. These patients were then placed on single-blind placebo and followed up every 2 weeks for a maximum of 8 weeks until their BP rose to baseline levels or they exceeded the BP safety limits (21). Fifty-eight of these patients were removed from the study during washout and the remaining 352 were randomly allocated to an alternate active single drug. Placebo was not permitted in this phase for safety and ethical reasons.

The response rate was surprisingly high—49.1%—in a group of patients who were selected by having failed initial monotherapy. The overall drug results are displayed in Figure 4. With the exception of atenolol and captopril, all sequential responses were within 10% of the initial response. Black (46.4%) and white (54.0%) patients had a similar response, but younger patients (37.6%) did not respond as well to the random second monotherapy as did the older patients (58.5%). Adverse effects were remarkably low.

The importance of this study was that it validated the concept of sequential monotherapy as a possible alternative to stepped-care. It also demonstrated that there is no important disadvantage to being exposed to a different second monotherapy when the first effort has failed.

B. Combination Phase

Of the 179 patients who either failed to respond to the second monotherapy or dropped out of the study, 102 were eligible for the combination phase (22). There was no placebo

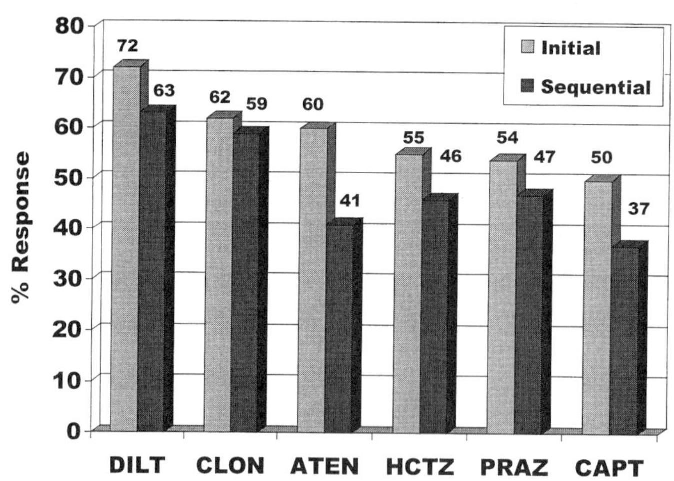

Fig. 4 Percentage response (diastolic blood pressure <90 mm Hg at the end of the titration period) achieved by each of the initial drugs compared with that achieved by each of the sequential single drugs. All of the patients who received the sequential drug had failed to achieve a response to an initial drug. Abbreviations are the same as in Figure 2. (From Ref. 21, with permission.)

washout period. The first drug was carefully added to the second drug until goal BP was achieved by 59 (57.8%) of this group. When these responders were added to those from the first and second monotherapy trials, 82.8% of the original 1105 patients exposed to active treatment responded (intention to treat).

There were 15 combination pairs with n = 2 to 14. Almost all combinations produced at least an additive effect compared with the results with either monotherapy. Atenolol plus captopril was the least effective (−3.7/−9.0 mm Hg). Combinations that included hydrochlorothiazide were more effective than those that did not. The response rate with hydrochlorothiazide was 77% systolic and 69% diastolic compared with that without hydrochlorothiazide: 46% systolic ($p = 0.002$) and 51% diastolic ($p = 0.067$). The effect was greater for systolic pressure (−22.4 ± 10.4 vs −17.8 ± 19.3 mm Hg) than for diastolic pressure (−14.1 ± 6.6 vs −13.6 ± 9.1 mm Hg).

Because of the higher than expected response rates in the initial and alternate monotherapy phases, the number of patients entering the combination phase was much less than expected. Thus, it was difficult to make comparisons among individual combinations or to report results by age–race subgroup.

C. Lessons from Combination Therapy

In the above analysis of combination therapy, we ignored the order in which the drugs were given and did not provide a detailed age-by-race analysis for each combination. We subsequently posed the question as to whether there is an ordering effect (23, 24). We found two types. In the first type, there were different results for each drug in the pair, but the result of the combination was the same regardless of which drug was administered first. For example, prazosin had only a 6% response rate in patients who had not achieved a response with diltiazem as the initial drug, diltiazem had a 22% response rate in patients who had not achieved goal blood pressure on prazosin, but the combinations yielded the same total responses (86% and 84%) regardless of order. The second type of ordering effect produced a different end result of the combination. For example, captopril plus diltiazem had an 88% response rate compared with diltiazem plus captopril (97%). No ordering effects were observed in combinations in which one of the drugs was either hydrochlorothiazide or prazosin. We published a detailed analysis of each combination order (n = 30) by race and by age group; the numbers were too small to consider age by race interaction. There were ordering differences in each subset, but it is difficult to project these to an overall population based on the small sample size.

D. Proteinuria

We had the opportunity to perform 24-hour urine collections on all patients in this study. Of the 1635 patients with hypertension who entered the study, 27 (1.7%) were found to have proteinuria higher than 1000 mg/day (25). We were able to obtain follow-up information on 19 of these patients and found six with identifiable renal disease. One had focal segmental sclerosis and went on to end-stage renal failure; three had type II diabetes mellitus, one had asymptomatic renal calcifications, and one had asymptomatic proteinuria that was not further characterized. Five of the 19 patients developed serum creatinine above 3.5 mg/dl, but the rest remained below 2.0 mg/dl over the 6 to 9 years of follow-up. There were significant associations between proteinuria and obesity ($P = 0.02$) and higher systolic blood pressure ($P = 0.05$).

A very important observation was that there were no significant changes in urinary protein excretion within or between the drugs, including placebo. Specifically, there was no increase observed with captopril. Of 18 patients removed from the study because of new onset of proteinuria, four had been taking hydrochlorothiazide, three each placebo, diltiazem SR, and prazosin, two each clonidine and atenolol, and one captopril.

An important conclusion of this study was that there were no data to support the contention that captopril was associated either with an increase in urinary protein excretion or the de novo development of proteinuria.

E. Importance of Obesity, Age, and Race for LVH

The subset of patients from whom echocardiographic studies were obtained provided a substantial database for a series of secondary studies. M-mode and 2-D tracings were obtained in the participating medical centers and sent to the central laboratory in Washington (Dr. John Gottdiener) where they were processed blind to drug and demographic information. Calculations were made using both the American Society of Echocardiography (ASE) and Cornell-Penn conventions to avoid controversy. The Framingham method of indexing to body height rather than body surface area was also used. Inter- and intraobserver variation was low. The database for the first observational study (17) was 692 men whose blood pressure averaged 153/100 mm Hg at baseline. The overall acquisition rate was 72%, and the proportion of technically acceptable studies was 75%.

Left ventricular hypertrophy was prevalent: 63% by Framingham and 46% by Cornell criteria, but it was not more prevalent in blacks than whites. This was in contrast to ECG criteria by which LVH was present in 31% of blacks and 10% of whites. The most striking correlation of LVH was with body mass index ($r = 0.329$; $P < 0.0001$); it was weaker with systolic blood pressure ($r = 0.186$; $P < 0.0001$). As seen in Figure 5, obesity magnifies the relationship between systolic blood pressure and LVH.

F. Differential Drug Effects on Regression of LVH

Observation of the effects of the individual drugs on regression of LVH provided the basis for a seminal publication (26). There were 93 to 100 analyzed echocardiograms in each drug class at baseline, 61 to 73 at 8 weeks, and 28 to 52 at 1 year. Regression of established LVH had been observed with most antihypertensive drugs when a short-term (4 to 8 weeks) ''snapshot'' was used. This was true in our study as well. All drugs showed at least some reduction in LV mass at 8 weeks in the highest tertile (>350 g at baseline), although diltiazem (−48 g) and prazosin (−54 g) were significantly greater than the other drugs. The picture was different, however, at 1 year. The greatest regression of LV mass in the highest tertile was effected by hydrochlorothiazide (−66 g), followed by captopril (−45 g) and atenolol (−37 g), whereas prazosin showed no change (+1 g), clonidine −13 g, and diltiazem −21 g. The changes for each of the tertiles by drug at 1 year are depicted in Figure 6.

These findings are significant in that they suggest a possible mechanism for the documented beneficial effect of hydrochlorothiazide on cardiac morbidity and mortality in hypertensive patients.

G. Left Atrial Size: Obesity, Race, and Age

Our echocardiographic studies permitted observations on the left atrium in addition to those on the left ventricle (18). Similar to the observations on the left ventricle, this study demonstrated a strong positive relationship between increasing body mass and left atrial

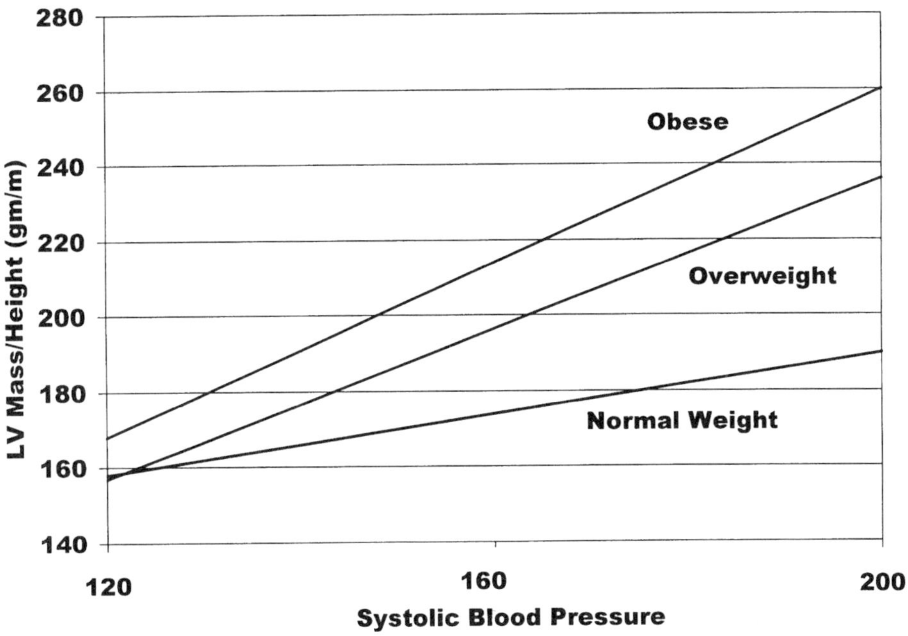

Fig. 5 Effect of obesity on relation between systolic blood pressure and left ventricular (LV) mass. Body weight categories are normal for body mass index (BMI) ≤ 27 kg/m^2, overweight for BMI 27 to 30 kg/m^2, obese for BMI >30 kg/m^2. (From Ref. 17, with permission.)

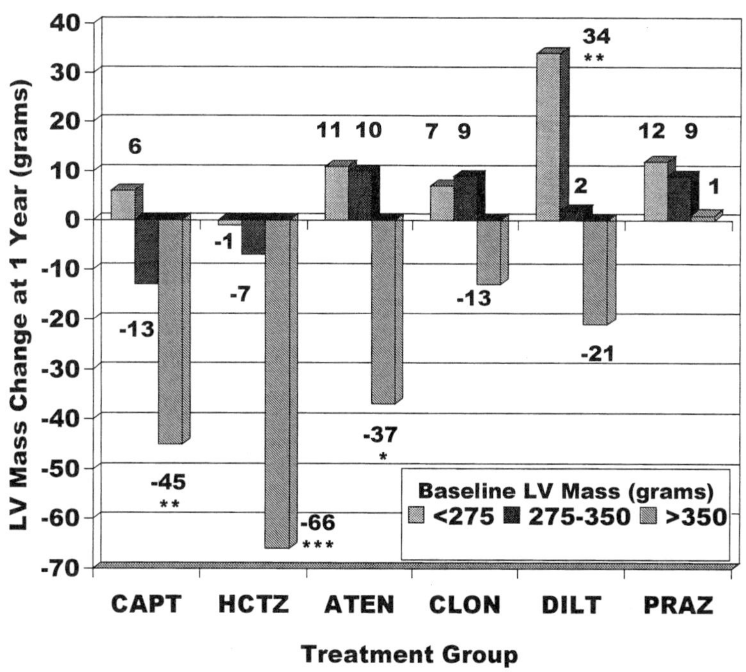

Fig. 6 Change in left ventricular (LV) mass from baseline values with single-drug therapy at 1 year by pretreatment LV mass tertile. For highest tertile of pretreatment LV mass, significant reductions were seen for hydrochlorothiazide, captopril, and atenolol. For lowest tertile, increases were associated with diltiazem. $*P < .05$, $\dagger P < .01$, $\ddagger P < .001$ vs baseline. (From Ref. 25, with permission.)

size. Left ventricular mass did not correlate with left atrial mass in normal-weight men, but there was a positive correlation in obese patients. In addition, older white men were found to have greater left atrial size than older black men. These findings are of significance because of the relationship of increased left atrial size with the incidence of atrial fibrillation and embolic stroke.

H. Regression of Left Atrial Size

Our large echocardiographic database allowed us to analyze the effect of the six antihypertensive drugs on the size of the left atrium, analogous to the study on regression of LV hypertrophy (27). The results, unadjusted for covariates, at 8 weeks, one year and two years are depicted in Figure 7. As with LVH, the best results were seen with hydrochlorothiazide. The data were then adjusted for covariates and the group was stratified by normal or enlarged left atrial size at baseline. In the normal baseline group, only hydrochlorothiazide effected a reduction in left atrial size. In the abnormal group (Fig. 8), left atrial size diminished significantly from baseline with hydrochlorothiazide, atenolol, clonidine, and diltiazem at 1 year and for all treatments at 2 years. At 2 years, the reduction effected by hydrochlorothiazide was significantly greater from that effected by captopril and prazosin. There are no data as yet that specifically demonstrate that reduction of left atrial size decreases morbidity and mortality. Nevertheless, such reduction should remove a clinically important risk factor for atrial fibrillation and embolic stroke. Furthermore, the reduction in left atrial hypertrophy most likely occurs *pari passu* with regression of LVH.

I. Systolic Function

The echocardiographic database allowed Sadler and colleagues (28) to investigate systolic function in hypertensive patients with concentric remodeling (normal LV mass index with high ratio of wall thickness to LV cavity radius). Controls were hypertensive patients with normal geometry. They demonstrated that 28% of the patients with concentric remodeling fell below the 95% confidence interval (CI) for controls for the regression of percent endocardial fractional shortening versus circumferential stress. A similar regression of percent midwall fractional shortening against circumferential stress showed that 42% of the patients with concentric remodeling fell below the 95% CI for hypertensive patients with normal geometry. Obesity did not influence these relationships. The data indicate that it is the increased relative wall thickness (RWT) rather than hypertrophy, per se, that accounts for decreased systolic function in these patients.

J. Plasma Lipid and Lipoprotein Profiles: Racial Differences

Studies from our central lipid laboratory (Dr. Raj Lakshman) yielded two major publications. The first of these looked at the effect of race, age, obesity, blood pressure, smoking and drinking history on baseline (off antihypertensive medications), fractionated plasma lipids, and lipoproteins (29). Table 4 shows the racial differences at baseline. Black patients had a lower cardiovascular risk profile based on these data than did whites. Triglycerides decreased whereas high-density lipoprotein (HDL) cholesterol and HDL subtypes increased with age. High-density lipoprotein, HDL subclasses, and apolipoprotein A_1 increased significantly with increasing alcohol consumption. Increased HDL_2 had not been known to be an effect of alcohol consumption. Such an increase would add a cardioprotec-

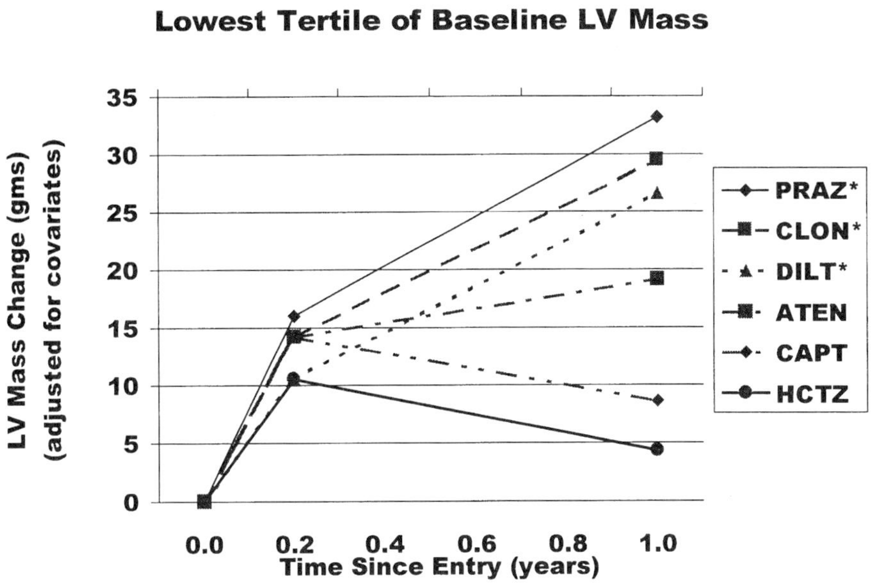

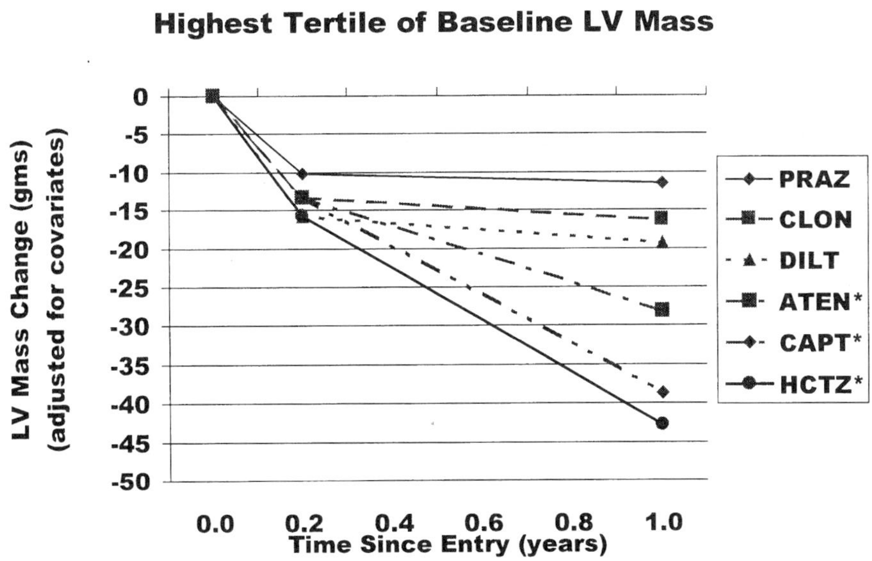

Fig. 7 Left ventricular (LV) mass changes over time adjusted for patient covariates. For the lowest tertile of baseline LV mass, prazosin (PRAZ), clonidine (CLON), and diltiazem-SR (DILT) were associated with significant increase of LV mass over 1 year. For the highest tertile of baseline LV mass, hydrochlorothiazide (HCTZ), captopril (CAPT), and atenolol (ATEN) are associated with significant reductions in LV mass. An asterisk denotes statistically significant differences from baseline. (From Ref. 25, with permission.)

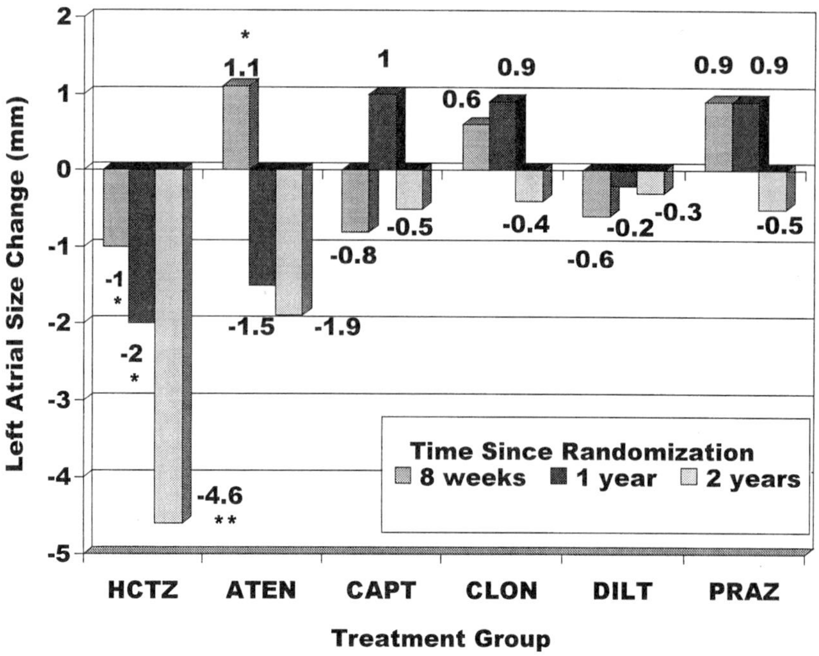

Fig. 8 Serial changes in left atrial size during 2 years of treatment, unadjusted for effects of covariates. Only hydrochlorothiazide was associated with statistically significant decreases in left atrial size from baseline at all three measurement intervals. Atenolol was associated with significant increase in left atrial size at 8 weeks and a trend toward decrease in left atrial size at 1 and 2 years. $^*P < 0.05$; $^{**}P = 0.002$. (From Ref. 26, with permission.)

Table 4 Racial Differences in Plasma Lipid and Lipoprotein Profiles*

Plasma	Whites	Blacks	Racial difference
Component	(n = 622)	(n = 594)	(*P* value)
Tryglycerides	153 ± 103	116 ± 100	<0.001
Total cholesterol	205 ± 37	204 ± 37	0.547
LDL cholesterol	130 ± 36	130 ± 38	0.788
HDL cholesterol	45 ± 11	52 ± 14	<0.001
HDL_2 cholesterol	11 ± 8	15 ± 11	<0.001
Apo A_1	112 ± 23	121 ± 29	<0.001
Apo B	77 ± 19	75 ± 21	0.069
HDL/LDL	0.40 ± 0.38	0.47 ± 0.61	0.018
HDL_2/LDL	0.11 ± 0.24	0.15 ± 0.37	0.031
HDL_2/HDL_3	0.34 ± 0.35	0.41 ± 0.32	<0.001
HDL/TC	0.23 ± 0.07	0.26 ± 0.09	<0.001
Apo A_1/Apo B	1.55 ± 0.52	1.79 ± 1.97	<0.001

* Concentration (mg/100 mL).

After an initial washout period of 4 weeks, plasma lipids and lipoproteins were determined in the plasma samples of the indicated number of veterans. Values are expressed as mean ± SD.

Abbreviations: Apo, apolipoprotein; *HDL*, high-density lipoprotein; *LDL*, low-density lipoprotein; *TC*, total cholesterol.

tive effect. Increasing obesity weakened the beneficial effects of alcohol on these lipids. Therefore, not only does obesity correlate with higher cardiovascular risk from its negative effect on plasma lipids and lipoproteins, but it also truncates any beneficial effect of moderate alcohol consumption.

K. Differential Drug Effects on Plasma Lipids and Lipoproteins Profiles

We had the opportunity to compare the effects of each of the six antihypertensive monotherapies on plasma lipids and lipoprotein profiles over time (30). Most earlier studies that had demonstrated an adverse effect (increasing cardiovascular risk profile) of diuretics and beta-blockers used high drug doses and reported a short-term cross-sectional profile. In this landmark study, the expected adverse response to hydrochlorothiazide was seen at 8 weeks only in nonresponders but not at 8 weeks or at 1 year in responders to hydrochlorothiazide. No long-term adverse lipid effects were seen with atenolol. Indeed, none of the six drugs showed a long-term adverse effect on plasma lipids or lipoprotein profile.

L. Age by Race Subgroup versus Plasma Renin Profile to Predict Response to Monotherapy

Our main results had demonstrated that the age by race interaction was a valid means of predicting the response to antihypertensive monotherapy. Plasma renin profiling is another method that can be used to select an initial drug. We had also performed plasma renin profiles on each of our study patients so that we were able to compare the two methods (31). In a logistic regression analysis, baseline diastolic blood pressure had the largest effect (stage 1 hypertension was more predictive for response to monotherapy than stage 2), followed by the age by race interaction. The addition of plasma renin profiling did not further contribute. The age by race interaction was somewhat superior to plasma renin profiling and, of course, is without cost.

M. Effects of Antihypertensive Drugs on Heart Rate Changes

Another inexpensive but often ignored physical parameter is the heart rate (32). Palatini and Julius (33) have called attention to the multitude of associations high heart rate has with hypertension and other cardiovascular risk factors. We evaluated the heart rate changes associated with each of the six drugs and placebo over 2 years. In general, heart rate changes from baseline to the end of titration tended to persist over the 2 years of observation, although there were further slight decreases for hydrochlorothiazide and placebo (Fig. 9). When the baseline heart rates were classified by the Framingham heart rate quartiles, all drugs except atenolol effected a slight increase in the lowest heart rate quartile, and all drugs decreased the heart rate in the highest quartile (Fig. 10). We validated the clinical data with a subset of heart rates determined from electrocardiograms taken at those same time periods.

N. Resistance to Antihypertensive Therapy in the Stroke Belt

Six of the 15 VA Medical Centers that participated in this study were located in or near the Stroke Belt, an area of the southeast United States that has a disproportionately higher

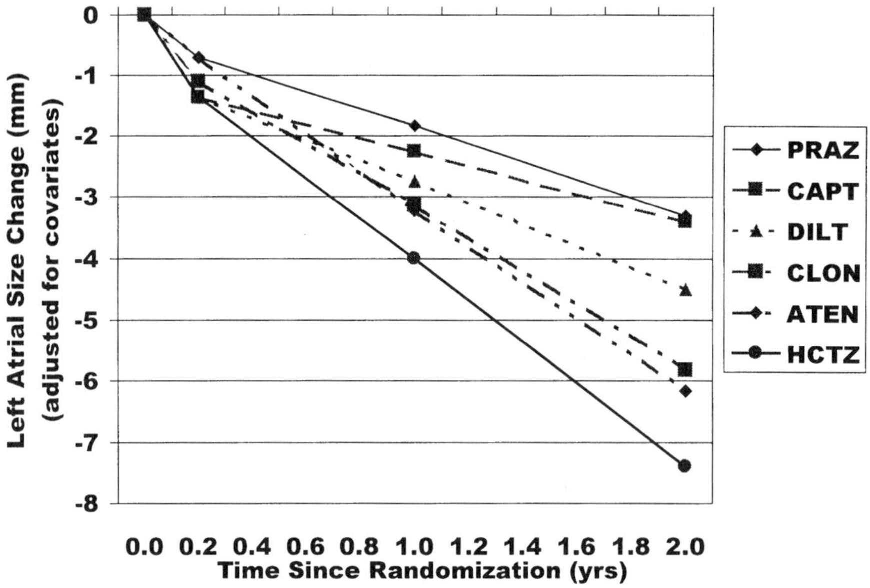

Fig. 9 Estimated changes in left atrial size during 2 years of treatment, adjusted for effects of covariates. For patients with enlarged left atrial size at baseline, reduction in left atrial size at 2 years with hydrochlorothiazide was significantly different from captopril and prazosin. Compared with baseline, left atrial size decreased significantly with hydrochlorothiazide, atenolol, clonidine, and diltiazem at 1 year and for all treatments at 2 years. (From Ref. 26, with permission.)

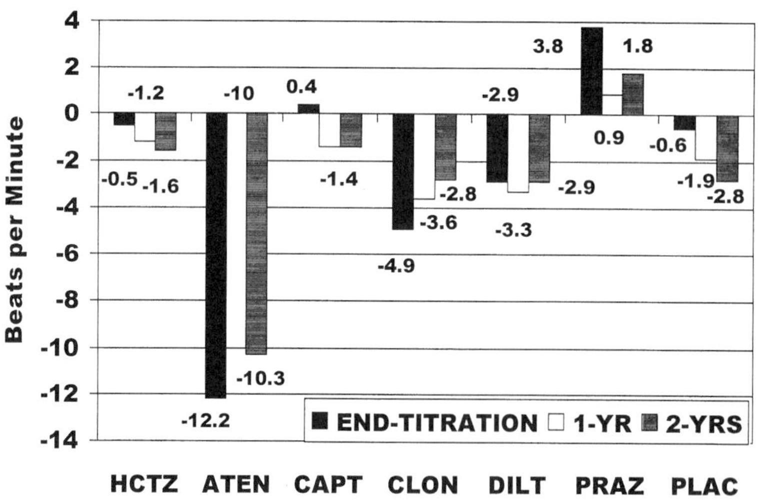

Fig. 10 Changes in heart rate (beats per minute) at end-titration, 1 year, and 2 years for each of the six active drugs and placebo. Abbreviations are the same as in Figure 2.

rate of stroke than the rest of the country. Cushman et al. (34) compared the demographic data from patients within and outside of the Stroke Belt.

Independent of race, Stroke Belt patients were younger, had lower serum potassium, urine potassium excretion, alcohol intake, and plasma renin activity, and higher blood pressure, body mass index, heart rate, and left ventricular mass. Patients residing in the Stroke Belt were less likely to achieve treatment success at 1 year than those outside the Stroke Belt (49% vs 65%). There were numerous drug differences based on race and geographic location. For example, black patients in the Stroke Belt responded less to captopril, compared with the nearly equal response of white patients in the Stroke Belt and both races out of the Stroke Belt.

O. Placebo Response

We had the opportunity to evaluate the ''therapeutic'' response to blinded placebo in this trial as well as adverse drug effects attributed to the placebo (35). The placebo response was particularly high in the older white group. Discontinuations from the trial resulting from perceived adverse drug reaction from patients randomly allocated to placebo were at the median of the seven treatment regimens. Prazosin, clonidine, and diltiazem were higher, whereas captopril, atenolol, and hydrochlorothiazide were lower.

X. DISCUSSION

A. Why Was the Trial Done?

Please refer to the Introduction and Prior Hypothesis sections above.

B. What Questions Was It Designed to Answer in Context of the Times in Which It Was Performed?

Please refer to the Prior Hypothesis section above.

C. How Has This Trial Influenced or Failed to Influence Clinical Practice?

To the best of our knowledge, there have been no systematic attempts to evaluate the specific impact of this study on clinical practice. There was considerable media publicity regarding the initial blood pressure findings of this study. A number of slide sets and other educational materials were generated and sent to community and academic physicians. Many symposia, lectures, and conferences both at the community and academic/scientific level were conducted. It is possible that the favorable findings of this study regarding diltiazem effects on blood pressure control contributed to the increase in use of calcium antagonists. It is also possible that the less favorable results for hydrochlorothiazide in blood pressure control of younger whites contributed to the further decline in the use of thiazide diuretics in hypertension. Nevertheless, studies suggest that physician prescribing habits have not been greatly influenced by the recommendations of the Joint National

Committee on Prevention, Detection, Evaluation, and Treatment of High Blood Pressure. It would be rather presumptuous, given the lack of evidence, to assume that the VA Monotherapy of Hypertension Study had a greater influence on the selection of initial drug therapy in stage 1 hypertension.

XI. DESCRIPTION AND ANALYSIS

A. Strengths

The major strengths of this VA Cooperative Study are the rigor with which it was conducted and analyzed, the large database generated, and the freedom from outside interference.

The biostatistical support center at Hines VA Hospital near Chicago was involved from the inception and throughout the analysis, writing, and publication of all papers that derived from the study. A central cooperative studies evaluation committee reviewed the study. The initial protocol had to achieve a sufficiently high scientific rank from this independent review committee to be funded for planning. The planning involved the statisticians and physician experts in hypertension and conduct of clinical trials. A research pharmacist also participated in the planning. She ultimately designed the double-dummy blinding scheme, and solved the formidable packaging and shipping logistics. She provided a buffer between the pharmaceutical companies that agreed to donate study drug and matching placebo and those responsible for the operation of the study protocol. The study was monitored in many ways. The various local and central institutional review boards met periodically; the central board reviewed study safety data and interviewed randomly selected patients to be certain there were no human rights violations. The data monitoring board had full access to all data and was responsible for recommending that the study could continue. Executive and study group committees also met for problem-solving and training purposes. Problem-solving visits were made to the study sites when required.

Of course, one of the major advantages was to be able to assemble 15 experienced local groups that could follow an identical protocol and operate in medical centers that were very much alike despite their individual characteristics. This permitted the acquisition of a sample size sufficiently robust to address the study objectives adequately.

The VA Cooperative Studies are free from commercial influence. All data are collected in the clinics and sent directly to the biostatistical support center. All data analysis is performed there and the blind is maintained. Decisions on publication of data are made by the executive committee and do not require the approval of a sponsor.

B. Weaknesses

The major potential weakness for a VA study is that it might not be generalizable to the population at large. This was particularly worrisome in that no women were included in the trial. Nevertheless, data from other VA studies have proven to be generalizable and other studies seem to support the results of this trial. We are not aware of any data that show a gender difference in response to specific medications. Indeed, extant data suggest the opposite conclusion.

The two racial groups were white Americans and black African-Americans. Blacks from the Caribbean, Central and South America, and Africa were not represented and no conclusions can be drawn about their antihypertensive monotherapy response from this study. Only 17 Asians were included in the study, certainly not a sufficient database for conclusions. Our largest Hispanic group was Puerto Rican. There are large cultural differences between Spanish-speaking peoples of different nationalities, so we cannot extrapolate these data to all people designated as Hispanic.

A study of this type is not a replica of a community-based office practice. All of the patients were seen in a hospital-based ambulatory clinic that was devoted to hypertension screening, treatment, and research. Patients were selected for specific criteria, including the ability to cooperate fully in the trial. Compliance with the protocol was assessed by pill counts and other determinations of reliability. Before randomization, patients who were not fully compliant were reinstructed and, if still noncompliant, were removed from the study. Nevertheless, one of the goals of the VA study group was to provide data to practicing physicians, and past studies have done that very well.

The study was not in any way designed to provide information on morbidity or mortality related to the six drug classes or placebo. A mortality study would have required a much larger sample size and would have been difficult to conduct even within a large health care system such as the VA. However, Antihypertensive and Lipid-Lowering Treatment to Prevent Heart Attack Trial (ALLHAT) is such a study in progress. Two members of the VA Cooperative Study Group on antihypertensive agents were advisors to the ALLHAT planning committee, and one is coordinating the numerous VA medical centers that are participating in ALLHAT.

Finally, this study was not designed to provide new information into physiological mechanisms. Such studies generally need to be focused on the specific mechanistic hypothesis and can usually be performed using a much smaller sample size.

C. What Did This Study Accomplish?

This study demonstrated that the practicing physician can make a rational first choice of a single drug to treat stage 1–2 hypertension based only on the patient's age and race. No special laboratory studies are necessary.

Hydrochlorothiazide 12.5 mg and atenolol 25 mg are rational first-step doses for monotherapy. These lower doses have a reasonable chance of therapeutic success and are associated with fewer adverse effects.

Hydrochlorothiazide effects regression of established left ventricular hypertrophy without loss of left ventricular function. Furthermore, it effects regression of left atrial hypertrophy.

Hydrochlorothiazide does not perturb serum lipids or lipoproteins to any clinically important degree.

Hydrochlorothiazide greatly enhanced the therapeutic efficacy of nondiuretic drugs. Combinations that included hydrochlorothiazide tended to be more efficacious than the combination of two nondiuretic drugs.

Captopril was not associated with new-onset proteinuria in this study.

D. What Did This Study Fail to Accomplish?

This study was not designed as a morbidity or mortality trial, and we cannot make any statement about either potential beneficial or harmful effect on cardiovascular risk.

We did not fulfill our goal of having a multifactorial algorithm for selection of the initial antihypertensive drug. The most powerful factor was the baseline blood pressure; the target audience is the group with stage 1 hypertension. Age and race together are the next most powerful factors. No other demographic factor added further discrimination to the system.

Despite the robust database, the number of subjects was not large enough to allow us to drill down to even greater levels of detail.

XII. CONCLUDING COMMENTS

The Cooperative Studies Program of the Department of Veterans Affairs Medical Research Service was able to sponsor this highly productive study for about $3 million. It has generated new data on the predictive value of the age by race interaction, lower drug doses and the improved safety of those lower doses, and unexpected benefits in terms of regression of left ventricular and left atrial hypertrophy. The database generated is still open to further analysis as the participating investigators and their colleagues invent new relevant questions to pose. The data-generating phase of this study has long ended, but the analysis and interpretation phase still has a long way to go.

ACKNOWLEDGMENTS

This study was supported by the Cooperative Studies Program of the Department of Veterans Affairs Medical Research Service. We gratefully acknowledge the supply of drugs and their matching placebos by CIBA-GEIGY (hydrochlorothiazide), ICI Pharma (atenolol), E.R. Squibb & Sons, Inc. (captopril), Boehringer Ingelheim Pharmaceuticals, Inc. (clonidine), Marion Merrell Dow, Inc. (diltiazem), and Pfizer Labs Division (prazosin). We also gratefully acknowledge a grant of unrestricted funds to Friends of Medical Research, Inc. by Marion Merrell Dow, Inc.

The members of the Department of Veterans Affairs Cooperative Study Group on Antihypertensive Agents were: Barry J. Materson (Chairman), Richard A. Preston, Joseph Asch, Mary H. Smith, Clydie Rainey, Miami; William G. Henderson, Domenic J. Reda (biostatistician), Jean Rowe, David Williams, Mazen Abdellatif, Robert J. Anderson, Shirley Tir, Peter Finley, Roland Mais, Barbara Lizano, Dolly Koontz, Barbara Mackay, Hines, Illinois; Mike R. Sather, Carol Fye (pharmacist), Sandra Buchanan, Claude Foy, Frances Chacon, Albuquerque, New Mexico; Edward D. Freis, Ibrahim Khatri, Barbara Gregory, John Gottdiener, Aldo Notargiacomo, Raj Lakshman, Rhonda Sapp, Peter Coutlakis, Washington, D.C.; Eli A. Ramirez, Jose L. Cianchini, Alba Jimenez, San Juan, Puerto Rico; Robert J. Hamburger, Mike Tobin, Ann Pieczek, Boston, Massachusetts; Frederick N. Talmers, Chris Grant, Allen Park, Michigan; William W. Neal, Martin Henry, Dallas; Kalman C. Mezey, Barbara Luzniak, East Orange, New Jersey; Richard E. Borreson, Colleen Stewart, Houston, Texas; Narain T. Srivastava, Karen M. Cooper, Jackson, Mississippi; Lois Anne Katz, Rosemary Mannix, Manhattan, New York; William C. Cushman, Stewart Nunn, Anita McKnight, Memphis, Tennessee; Mahendr S. Kochar, Dee Trottier, Patricia Olzinski, Milwaukee, Wisconsin; H. Mitchell Perry, Jr., Deborah Berg, Larry Monahan, Judy Politte, St. Louis, Missouri; Barry Massie, Elaine Der, San Francisco, California; Bangshi Mukherji, Marion Pannone, Charlene Arnold, Kathleen Fox, Topeka, Kansas; Data Monitoring Board: Walter M. Kirkendall (Chairman), University of Texas

Medical School, Houston, Texas; William H. Gaasch, Worcester Memorial Hospital, Worcester, Massachusetts; Ray W. Gifford, Jr., Cleveland Clinic Foundation, Cleveland, Ohio; Robert F. Woolson, University of Iowa College of Medicine, Iowa City, Iowa; VA Central Office: Daniel Deykin (Chief, Cooperative Studies Program), Ping Huang, Janet Gold, Boston and Washington.

REFERENCES

1. Veterans Administration Cooperative Study Group on Antihypertensive Agents. Effects of treatment on mortality in hypertension: I. Results in patients with diastolic blood pressures averaging 115 through 129 mm Hg. JAMA 1967; 202:116–122.
2. Materson BJ, Reda DJ, Cushman WC, Massie BM, Freis ED, Kochar MS, Hamburger RJ, Fye C, Lakshman R, Gottdiener J, Ramirez EA, Henderson WG. Single-drug therapy for hypertension in men. A comparison of six antihypertensive agents with placebo. N Engl J Med 1993; 328:914–921.
3. Materson BJ, Reda DJ. Correction: single-drug therapy for hypertension in men. N Engl J Med 1994; 330:1689.
4. Materson BJ, Reda DJ, Cushman WC, for the Department of Veterans Affairs Cooperative Study Group on Antihypertensive Agents. Department of Veterans Affairs single-drug therapy of hypertension study: revised figures and new data. Am J Hypertens 1995; 8:189–192.
5. Report of the Joint National Committee on Detection, Evaluation, and Treatment of High Blood Pressure: a cooperative study. JAMA 1977; 237:255–261.
6. The Joint National Committee on Detection, Evaluation, and Treatment of High Blood Pressure. The 1984 report of the Joint National Committee on Detection, Evaluation, and Treatment of High Blood Pressure. Arch Intern Med 1984; 144:1045–1057.
7. Veterans Administration Cooperative Study Group on Antihypertensive Agents. Comparison of propranolol and hydrochlorothiazide for the initial treatment of hypertension. I. Results of short-term titration with emphasis on racial differences in response. JAMA 1982; 248:1996–2003.
8. Veterans Administration Cooperative Study Group on Antihypertensive Agents. Racial differences in response to low-dose captopril are abolished by the addition of hydrochlorothiazide. Br J Clin Pharmacol 1982; 14:97s–101s.
9. Veterans Administration Cooperative Study Group on Antihypertensive Agents. Low-dose captopril for the treatment of mild to moderate hypertension. I. Results of a 14-week trial. Arch Intern Med 1984; 144:1947–1953.
10. Materson BJ. Black-white differences in response to antihypertensive therapy. J Natl Med Assoc 1985; 77(suppl):9–13.
11. Laragh JH, Baer L, Brunner HR, Buhler FR, Sealey JE, Vaughan ED. Renin, angiotensin and aldosterone in pathogenesis and management of hypertensive vascular disease. Am J Med 1972; 52:633–652.
12. Freis ED, Materson BJ, Flamenbaum W, and the VA Cooperative Study Group. Comparison of propranolol or hydrochlorothiazide alone for treatment of hypertension. III. Evaluation of the renin-angiotensin system. Am J Med 1983, 74:1029–1041.
13. Materson BJ. Thiazides increase cardiovascular risk. Drug Therapy 1986; 16:51–55.
14. Kleber FX, Pfeffer MA, Pfeffer JM. Alterations in the electrocardiogram of spontaneously hypertensive rats by chronic antihypertensive therapy with captopril. Clin Exp Hypertens [A] 1982; 4:977–987.
15. Haber E, Koerner T, Page LB. Application of a radioimmunoassay for angiotensin 1 to the physiologic measurements of plasma renin activity in normal human subjects. J Clin Endocrinol Metab 1969; 29:1349–1355.

16. Rifkin BM, Segal S. Lipid research clinics program reference values for hyperlipidemia and hypolipidemia. JAMA 1983; 250:1869–1872.
17. Gottdiener JS, Reda DJ, Materson BJ, Massie BM, Notargiacomo A, Hamburger RJ, Williams DW, Henderson WG. Importance of obesity, race and age to the cardiac structural and functional effects of hypertension. J Am Coll Cardiol 1994; 24:1492–1498.
18. Gottdiener JS, Reda DJ, Williams DW, Materson BJ, for the Department of Veterans Affairs Cooperative Study Group on Antihypertensive Agents. Left atrial size in hypertensive men: influence of obesity, race and age. J Am Coll Cardiol 1997; 29:651–658.
19. Lachin JM. Sample size determination for r X c comparative trials. Biometrics 1997; 33:315–324.
20. The sixth report of the Joint National Committee on Prevention, Detection, Evaluation, and Treatment of High Blood Pressure. Arch Intern Med 1997; 157:2413–2446.
21. Materson BJ, Reda DJ, Preston RA, Cushman WC, Massie BM, Freis ED, Kochar MS, Hamburger RJ, Fye C, Lakshman R, Gottdiener J, Ramirez AE, Henderson WG, for the Department of Veterans Affairs Cooperative Study Group on Antihypertensive Agents. Response to a second single antihypertensive agent used as monotherapy for hypertension after failure of the initial drug. Arch Intern Med 1995; 155:1757–1762.
22. Materson BJ, Reda JD, Cushman WC, Henderson WG, for the Department of Veterans Affairs Cooperative Study Group on Antihypertensive Agents. Results of combination antihypertensive therapy after failure of each of the components. J Hum Hypertens 1995; 9:791–796.
23. Materson BJ, Reda DJ, Williams D. Lessons from combination therapy in Veterans Affairs studies. Am J Hypertens 1996; 9:187S–191S.
24. Materson BJ, Reda DJ, Williams DW, for the Department of Veterans Affairs Cooperative Study Group on Antihypertensive Agents. Effects of antihypertensive single-drug therapy on heart rate. Am J Hypertens 1999; 12:9S–11S.
25. Preston RA, Materson BJ, Reda DJ, Hamburger RJ, Smith MH, for the Department of Veterans Affairs Cooperative Study Group on Antihypertensive Agents. Proteinuria in mild to moderate hypertension: results of the VA cooperative study of six antihypertensive agents and placebo. Clin Nephrol 1997; 47:310–315.
26. Gottdiener JS, Reda DJ, Massie BM, Materson BJ, Williams DW, Anderson RJ. Effect of single-drug therapy on reduction of left ventricular mass in mild to moderate hypertension: comparison of six antihypertensive agents. The Department of Veterans Affairs Cooperative Study Group on Antihypertensive Agents. Circulation 1997; 95:2007–2014.
27. Gottdiener JS, Reda DJ, Williams DW, Materson BJ, Cushman W, Anderson RJ, for the VA Cooperative Study Group on Antihypertensive Agents. Effect of single-drug therapy on reduction of left atrial size in mild to moderate hypertension: comparison of six antihypertensive agents. The Department of Veterans Affairs Cooperative Study Group on Antihypertensive Agents. Circulation 1998; 98:140–148.
28. Sadler DB, Aurigemma GP, Williams DW, Reda DJ, Materson BJ, Gottdiener JS. Systolic function in hypertensive men with concentric remodeling. Hypertension 1997; 30:777–781.
29. Lakshman MR, Reda D, Materson BJ, Cushman WC, Kochar MS, Nunn S, Hamburger RJ, Freis ED, for the Department of Veterans Affairs Cooperative Study Group on Antihypertensive Agents. Comparison of plasma lipid and lipoprotein profiles in hypertensive black versus white men. Am J Cardiol 1996; 78:1236–1241.
30. Lakshman MR, Reda DJ, Materson BJ, Cushman WC, Freis ED, for the Department of Veterans Affairs Cooperative Study Group on Antihypertensive Agents. Diuretics and β-blockers do not have adverse effects at 1 year on plasma lipid and lipoprotein profiles in men with hypertension. Arch Intern Med 1999; 159:551–558.
31. Preston RA, Materson BJ, Reda DJ, Williams DW, Hamburger RJ, Cushman WC, Anderson RJ. Age-race subgroup compared to renin profile as predictors of blood pressure response to

antihypertensive therapy in 1031 patients: results of a VA cooperative study. JAMA 1998; 280:1168–1172.
32. Materson BJ, Reda DJ, Williams DW, for the Department of Veterans Affairs Cooperative Study Group on Antihypertensive Agents. Comparison of effects of antihypertensive drugs on heart rate: changes from baseline by baseline group and over time. Am J Hypertens 1998; 11:597–601.
33. Palatini P, Julius S. Heart rate and the cardiovascular risk. J Hypertens 1997; 15:3–17.
34. Cushman WC, Reda DJ, Perry HM Jr, Williams D, Abdellatif M, Materson BJ, for the Veterans Affairs Cooperative Study Group on Antihypertensive Agents. Regional and racial differences in response to antihypertensive medication use in a randomized controlled trial of men with hypertension in the United States. Arch Intern Med 2000; 160:825–831.
35. Preston RA, Materson BJ, Reda DJ, Williams DW. Placebo-associated blood pressure response and adverse effects in the treatment of hypertension. Observations from a Department of Veterans Affairs Cooperative Study. Arch Intern Med 2000; 160:1449–1454.

14

The Systolic Hypertension in Europe Trial

JAN A. STAESSEN, ROBERT H. FAGARD, and LUTGARDE THIJS

University of Leuven, Leuven, Belgium

I. INTRODUCTION

By 1988, several major outcome trials on antihypertensive drug treatment had been published (1–5). However, at that time, the findings in the elderly still left a wide margin of uncertainty as evidenced by the borderline significance of the effects of therapy on fatal endpoints (6). Indeed, the results of the early trials (1–5) demonstrated that antihypertensive drug treatment reduced all cardiovascular deaths by 28% ($P = 0.02$) and stroke mortality by 41% ($P = 0.03$), whereas the decreases in coronary (−28%; $P = 0.14$) and all-cause mortality (−14%; $P = 0.07$) had not reached statistical significance (6). Furthermore, until 1988, all outcome trials in hypertension had used diastolic blood pressure as the main criterion to recruit patients and to adjust treatment. This contrasted with the growing insight gained from many cross-sectional and longitudinal studies, that in older patients systolic blood pressure is the main cardiovascular risk factor, whereas diastolic blood pressure is no risk factor or may even be inversely correlated with cardiovascular outcome (7). In addition, the prevalence of isolated systolic hypertension rises curvilinearly with age. It averages 8% in sexagenarians and exceeds 25% beyond 80 years (7). Thus, isolated systolic hypertension affects a considerable proportion of all older individuals.

Against this background, in 1989, the European Working Party on High Blood Pressure in the Elderly started the placebo-controlled double-blind Syst-Eur (Systolic Hypertension in Europe) trial (8). Active treatment was initiated with the dihydropyridine calcium-channel blocker nitrendipine (9) with the possible addition of enalapril, hydrochlorothiazide, or both. In 1991 the Systolic Hypertension in the Elderly (SHEP) trial demonstrated that diuretic-based treatment prevented nonfatal stroke, myocardial infarction, and heart failure (10). In view of the remaining uncertainties with regard to the

Table 1 Study Endpoints

Endpoint	Type
Fatal and nonfatal cardiovascular endpoints	Secondary
Fatal and nonfatal stroke	Primary
Keith-Wagener stage III–IV retinopathy	Secondary
Fatal and nonfatal cardiac endpoints	Secondary
Sudden death	Secondary
Fatal and nonfatal myocardial infarction	Secondary
Fatal and nonfatal heart failure	Secondary
Dissecting aortic aneurysm	Secondary
Renal insufficiency	Secondary

treatment of isolated systolic hypertension in the elderly (11–15), the Syst-Eur trial continued after the publication of the SHEP results (10). Furthermore, the controversy on the role of calcium-channel blockers as first-line antihypertensive agents (16–19) highlighted the lack of evidence that these drugs reduce cardiovascular risk.

The primary hypothesis tested was that in older patients with isolated systolic hypertension, active treatment would reduce fatal and nonfatal stroke (Table 1). The secondary endpoints included total and cardiovascular mortality, all cardiovascular endpoints, and fatal and nonfatal cardiac endpoints. This review article reports the morbidity and mortality results in the 4695 randomized Syst-Eur patients. The trial stopped on February 14, 1997 after the second of four planned interim analyses. According to the predefined stopping rules, a significant benefit for stroke—the primary endpoint of the trial (8)—had been reached.

II. PROTOCOL

A. Study Design

The protocol of the multicenter Syst-Eur trial (8) was approved by the ethics committees of the University of Leuven and the participating centers. The trial was conducted according to the principles outlined in the Helsinki declaration (20).

Patients were recruited from 198 centers in 23 countries across western and eastern Europe. Each center kept a register of screened patients. Patients were eligible (a) if they were at least 60 years old, (b) if on single-blind placebo treatment during the run-in phase their sitting systolic blood pressure ranged from 160 to 219 mm Hg with diastolic blood pressure below 95 mm Hg, (c) if their standing systolic pressure was 140 mm Hg or more, (d) if they consented to be enrolled, and (e) if long-term follow-up was possible (Table 2). The blood pressure criteria for entry were based on the averages of six sitting and six standing readings, that is, two in each position at three baseline visits 1 month apart. Patients could not be enrolled (Table 2) if the systolic hypertension was caused by a condition for which specific medical or surgical treatment was indicated. The other exclusion criteria included: retinal hemorrhage or papilledema, heart failure, dissecting aortic aneurysm, a serum creatinine concentration at presentation of 180 μmol/L (2 mg/dL) or higher; a history of severe nose bleeds, stroke or myocardial infarction within 1 year of randomization, dementia or substance abuse, any condition prohibiting a sitting or standing position, and any severe concomitant cardiovascular or noncardiovascular disease.

Table 2 Inclusion and Exclusion Criteria

Inclusion criteria	Exclusion criteria
1. Age ≥ 60 years 2. Blood pressure* • Sitting systolic ≥ 160 mm Hg • Sitting diastolic < 95 mm Hg • Standing systolic > 140 mm Hg 3. Informed consent 4. Stable living condition with possibility of long-term follow-up	1. Secondary hypertension 2. Retinopathy grade III or IV 3. Overt heart failure 4. Dissecting aneurysm of the aorta 5. Serum creatinine ≥ 180 μmol/L 6. Myocardial infarction or stroke within 1 year of randomization 7. Severe concomitant cardiovascular or non-cardiovascular disease, e.g., cardiomyopathy, cancer, liver dysfunction, etc. 8. Dementia 9. Substance abuse 10. Severe nose bleeds 11. Any condition prohibiting a sitting or standing position 12. Poor collaboration

*Mean of six readings, i.e., two at each of three run-in visits.

Eligible patients were stratified by center, sex, and previous cardiovascular complications and randomized to double-blind treatment with active medication or placebo. Active treatment was initiated with nitrendipine. If necessary, the calcium-channel blocker was combined with or replaced by enalapril, hydrochlorothiazide, or both. The study medications were stepwise titrated and combined in an attempt to reduce the sitting systolic blood pressure by 20 mm Hg or more to less than 150 mm Hg (8). In the active treatment group, tablets with 20 mg nitrendipine, 10 mg enalapril, and 25 mg hydrochlorothiazide were used (Table 3). The dosage steps for nitrendipine were 10 mg in the evening, 10 mg twice daily, and 20 mg twice daily. For enalapril, the dosage steps were 5 mg, 10 mg, and 20 mg in the evening and for hydrochlorothiazide, 12.5 mg and 25 mg in the morning. In the control group, matching placebo tablets were used similarly. Nitrendipine

Table 3 Treatment Steps

Drugs (or matching placebos)	Dosage steps*
Nitrendipine (20 mg per tablet)	10 mg in the evening
	10 mg twice daily
	20 mg twice daily
Enalapril (10 mg per tablet)	5 mg in the evening
	10 mg in the evening
	20 mg in the evening
Hydrochlorothiazide (25 mg per tablet)	12.5 mg in the morning
	25 mg in the morning

*The study medications were titrated and combined to reach the goal blood pressure, defined as a sitting systolic blood pressure less than 150 mm Hg and a decrease in the sitting systolic blood pressure by at least 20 mm Hg in comparison with the level at entry.

was started in the evening and continued as a twice-daily drug, because this dihydropyridine has a terminal plasma half-life of 12 hours (9). In addition, starting treatment with an evening dose was expected to reduce the risk of orthostatic hypotension during daytime and to lead to a more rapid upward titration to twice-daily dosing. Indeed, patients on the starting dose of 10 mg of nitrendipine in the evening would be examined on the next clinic day at trough levels.

To facilitate the intention-to-treat analysis, patients withdrawing from double-blind treatment were maintained in open follow-up (8). During double-blind treatment and supervised open follow-up, clinic visits were scheduled at 3-month intervals. For patients withdrawing from double-blind treatment in whom regular follow-up was impossible, information on vital status, the incidence of major endpoints and other events and the use of antihypertensive medications was collected annually (nonsupervised open follow-up). Patients without any report within the year before the trial had stopped were considered to be lost to follow-up.

B. Sample Size

The original sample size calculations assumed a stroke incidence in the placebo group of 17.0 events per 1000 patient-years. Fifteen thousand patient-years, that is, 3000 patients with an average follow-up of 5 years, were required to detect a 40% change in the overall stroke incidence with a two-tailed significance of 1% and 90% power (8). On August 18, 1995 (Fig. 1), the projected number of randomized patients was attained. However, because in the early phase of the study the stroke rate in the placebo group was only 13.6 events per 1000 patient-years, the steering committee decided in January 1996 to continue recruitment through 1996 or until at least 4000 patients had been randomized.

C. Definition and Validation of Major Endpoints

The protocol (8) defined the following major endpoints: death, stroke, retinal hemorrhage or exudates, myocardial infarction, heart failure, dissecting aortic aneurysm, and renal

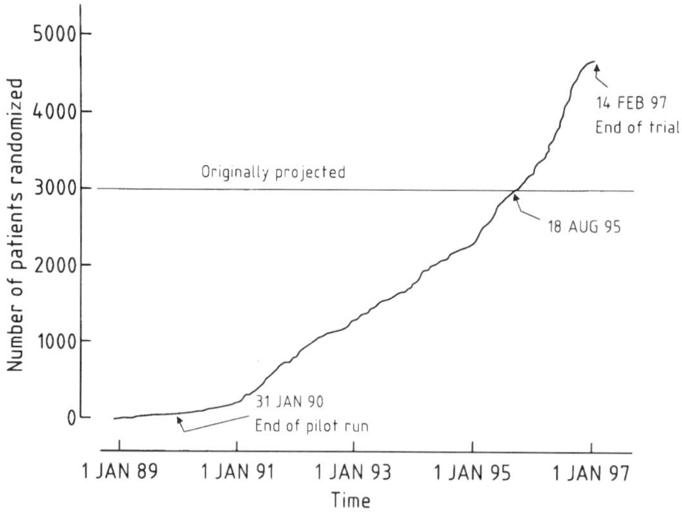

Fig. 1 Randomization of patients in the Syst-Eur trial. (From Ref. 22.)

Table 4 Definition of Major Endpoints

Inclusion criteria	Exclusion criteria
Stroke	Neurological deficit of vascular origin continuing for > 24 hours or leading to death
Retinal exudates and hemorrhage	Keith-Wagener retinopathy stages III–IV
Myocardial infarction (not including silent cases)	At least two of three disorders: typical chest pain, electrocardiographic changes, or increase in cardiac enzymes
Sudden death	Death of unknown origin occurring instantly or within 24 hours
Heart failure	Presence of each of three conditions: symptoms (dyspnea, etc.), clinical signs (ankle edema, rales, etc.), and necessity of treatment with diuretics, vasodilators, or antihypertensive drugs
Cardiac endpoints	Fatal and nonfatal myocardial infarction, sudden death, and fatal and nonfatal heart failure
Dissecting aneurysm of the aorta	Based on arteriographic, ultrasonographic, radiographic evidence or on necropsy
Cardiovascular endpoints	Fatal and nonfatal stroke, cardiac complications and other cardiovascular endpoints
Renal insufficiency	At two consecutive follow-up visits, serum creatinine ≥ 4.0 mg/dL (360 μmol/L) or doubled in comparison with the level at entry

insufficiency (Table 4). The blinded endpoint committee ascertained all major endpoints by reviewing the local patient files and other source documents, by requesting detailed written information from the investigators, or by both approaches. Diseases were coded according to the ninth (1975) revision of the International Classification of Diseases (21).

Stroke, the primary endpoint in the Syst-Eur trial, was defined as a neurological deficit with symptoms continuing for more than 24 hours or leading to death with no apparent cause other than vascular (Table 4). Typical chest pain, electrocardiographic changes, and the increase in cardiac enzymes led to the diagnosis of acute myocardial infarction, provided that at least two of these three criteria were fullfilled. Myocardial infarction did not include silent myocardial infarction. Heart failure required the presence of three conditions, namely symptoms such as dyspnea, clinical signs, such as ankle edema or rales, and the necessity to initiate treatment with diuretics, vasodilators, or antihypertensive drugs. Sudden death included any death of unknown origin occurring instantly or within an estimated 24 hours after the onset of acute symptoms as well as unattended death for which no likely cause could be established by autopsy or recent medical history. Cardiac endpoints included fatal and nonfatal heart failure, fatal and nonfatal myocardial infarction, and sudden death. Renal insufficiency was diagnosed if at two consecutive visits the serum creatinine concentration reached or exceeded 360 μmol/L (4.0 mg/dL) or had doubled in comparison with the level at randomization.

D. Other Events

All other events were checked at the coordinating office by doctors blinded with regard to the treatment group. Transient ischemic attack was defined as focal cerebral dysfunction lasting for less than 24 hours. It did not lead to the discontinuation of double-blind treatment and was therefore not an endpoint (8). The diagnosis of angina pectoris rested on suggestive chest pain with or without electrocardiographic signs of coronary ischemia, the need for coronary revascularization in the absence of acute myocardial infarction, or the indication to start treatment with nitrates. Diseases of the large (noncoronary) arteries included codes (ninth revision) (21) 433.0–433.9, 440.0–440.9, 442.0–442.9, 443.1, 443.9–444.9, and 447.0–447.9 and surgical or angioplastic procedures on these arteries, but not dissecting aortic aneurysm. Intercurrent diseases were nonfatal noncardiovascular disorders leading to hospitalization or withdrawal from double-blind treatment or supervised open follow-up. Bleeding disorders excluded cerebral and retinal hemorrhage.

Uncontrolled hypertension was a sitting blood pressure exceeding 219 mm Hg systolic or 99 mm Hg diastolic at three consecutive visits while the patients were on the maximal tolerated double-blind treatment. In January 1996, at the recommendation of the ethics committee, the upper admissible sitting systolic blood pressure at randomization was lowered to 200 mm Hg, but the maximum level during double-blind treatment was maintained at 219 mm Hg.

E. Statistical Methods

Database management and statistical analysis were performed with SAS software (SAS Institute Inc., Cary, NC) at the coordinating office of the study in Leuven, Belgium. The data were entered in duplicate with systematic quality checks at 3-month intervals. The trial was first analyzed according to an intention-to-treat principle using two-sided tests (22). A per-protocol analysis was performed later (23). Comparisons of means and proportions relied on the standard normal z-test and the χ^2-statistic. Survival curves were compared using Kaplan-Meier survival function estimates and the logrank test. Relative risk was assessed by single and multiple Cox regression (24).

A total of 250 strokes were projected to occur within 5 years. A beneficial or adverse effect could arise early in the trial. Interim analyses were planned after the accumulation of every 50 strokes (8). Asymmetric monitoring boundaries, drawn according to the O'Brien-Fleming method (25), allowed the study to stop for a beneficial effect of active treatment on total stroke at 1% probability or for an adverse effect on any major endpoint at 5% (8). At the first interim analysis in May 1995, these statistical thresholds were not attained. The second interim analysis in February 1997 showed a significant decrease of stroke in the active-treatment group, which according to the predefined stopping rules, led to the early termination of the trial.

III. PRINCIPAL MORBIDITY AND MORTALITY RESULTS BY INTENTION TO TREAT (22)

A. Patient Characteristics at Randomization

Of 8926 patients entered in the registers of screened patients, 6403 (71.7%) were enrolled in the run-in period and 4695 (52.6%) were randomized (Fig. 2). Of 8926 screened patients, 6403 (71.7%) were eligible for enrollment in the run-in period (Fig. 2); 1708 patients were not randomized because of blood pressure values (n = 570; 33.4%) or age (n = 9; 0.5%) outside the recruitment range, withdrawal of consent (n = 275; 16.1%), the presence or occurrence of cardiovascular disorders prohibiting randomization (n = 126; 7.4%), symptoms on treatment with single-blind placebo (n = 33; 1.9%), the need

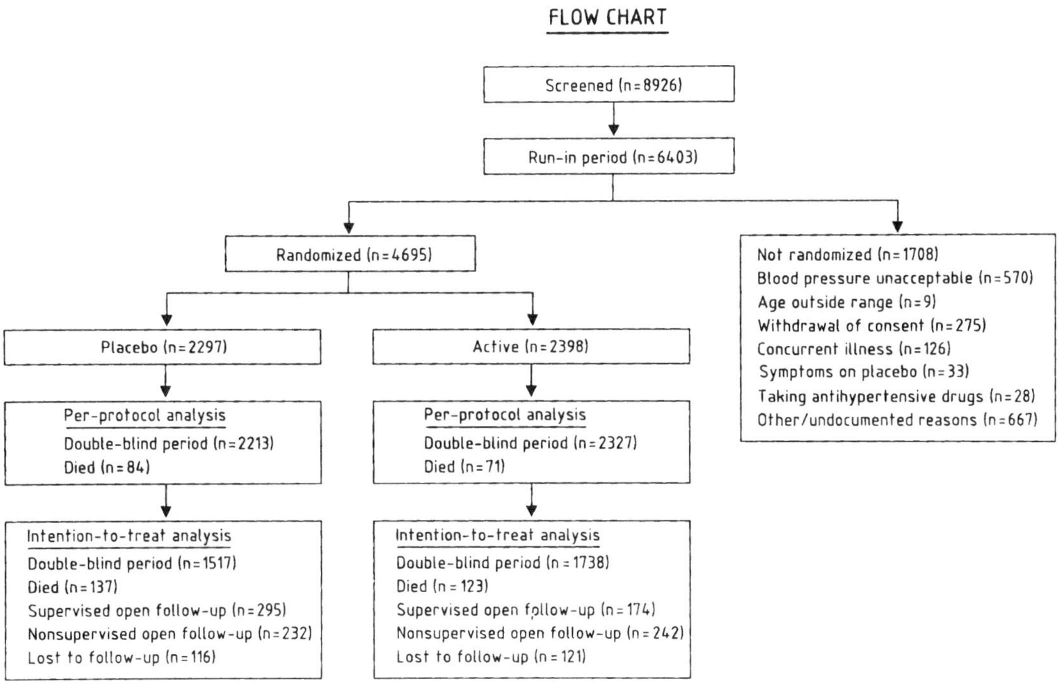

Fig. 2 Flow of patients. (From Ref. 23.)

to prescribe drugs with blood pressure-lowering action (n = 28; 1.6%), or for other undocumented reasons (n = 667; 39.1%).

Of the randomized patients, 1262 (26.9%) were recruited in Finland, 1044 (22.2%) in Bulgaria, 321 (6.8%) in the Russian Federation, 273 (5.8%) in Belgium, 227 (4.8%) in Italy, 213 (4.5%) in Israel, 210 (4.5%) in the United Kingdom, 172 (3.7%) in France, 161 (3.4%) in Estonia, 155 (3.3%) in Lithuania, 139 (3.0%) in Spain, 127 (2.7%) in Poland, and 102 (2.2%) in Romania. Fewer than 100 patients were enrolled in each of the following countries: Belorussia, the Czech Republic, Croatia, Germany, Greece, Ireland, the Netherlands, Portugal, Slovakia, and Slovenia (Table 5).

At randomization, the patients in the placebo (n = 2297) and active treatment (n = 2398) groups were similar in sex ratio, age, blood pressure, pulse rate, body mass index, serum cholesterol, the use of tobacco and alcohol, the prevalence of diabetes mellitus defined according to the World Health Organization criteria (26), previous cardiovascular complications and antihypertensive treatment (Table 6). In both groups combined, 343 (7.5%) patients, 231 men and 112 women, smoked at randomization and 525 (11.2%), 393 men and 132 women, consumed at least 1 unit of an alcoholic beverage per day.

In the two treatment groups combined, a total of 1402 (29.9%) patients showed cardiovascular complications at randomization (Table 6). Of the latter patients, 575 (41.0%) and 103 (7.4%) had symptoms or signs suggestive of coronary heart disease or cerebrovascular disease, respectively. Electrocardiographic changes compatible with left ventricular hypertrophy were present in 614 patients (43.8%). A total of 110 subjects (7.8%) showed a combination of these conditions or other vascular, retinal, or renal le-

Table 5 Patients and Centers by Country

Country	Patients	Centers
Finland	1262	21
Bulgaria	1044	16
Russia	321	11
Belgium	273	44
Italy	227	12
Israel	213	10
United Kingdom	210	9
France	172	28
Estonia	161	2
Lithuania	155	4
Spain	139	10
Poland	127	7
Romania	102	4
Netherlands	64	7
Greece	61	2
Ireland	37	1
Portugal	33	3
Belorussia	25	1
Slovenia	19	1
Czech Republic	18	1
Slovakia	18	1
Germany	10	2
Croatia	4	1
All 23 countries	4695	198

sions. Among all patients with previous cardiovascular complications, only 58 (4.1%) had a history of stroke and 163 (11.6%) a history of myocardial infarction.

B. Follow-Up

In the intention-to-treat analysis, the median follow-up of the 4695 patients was 2.0 years. Because the patients had been recruited over 8 years (Fig. 1), the follow-up of individual patients ranged from 1 to 97 months. The number of patient-years in the placebo and active treatment groups amounted to 5709 and 5995, respectively. On February 14, 1997, when the trial was stopped, 1517 patients in the placebo group were still on double-blind treatment, 295 were in supervised open follow-up, 232 in nonsupervised open follow-up, 137 had died, and 116 were lost to follow-up (Fig. 2). In the patients randomized to active treatment, these numbers were 1738, 174, 242, 123, and 121, respectively.

C. Treatment and Blood Pressure by Year of Follow-Up

At 2 years, 866 of the patients randomized to placebo and 1014 of those randomized to active treatment remained in double-blind follow-up (70.1% vs 78.8%; $P < 0.001$; Table 7). Of the actively treated patients, 856 (84.4%) were taking nitrendipine (mean daily dose 28.2 mg), 330 (32.6%) enalapril (13.8 mg/day), 164 (16.2%) hydrochlorothiazide (21.2 mg/day), and 10 (1.0%) other antihypertensive drugs. For the matching placebos in the

Table 6 Clinical Features of Treatment Groups at Randomization

Characteristic	Placebo (n = 2297)	Active treatment (n = 2398)
Mean (SD) age, y	70.2 (6.7)	70.3 (6.7)
Mean (SD) blood pressure, mm Hg		
Sitting systolic, mm Hg	173.9 (10.1)	173.8 (9.9)
Sitting diastolic, mm Hg	85.5 (5.9)	85.5 (5.8)
Standing systolic, mm Hg	169.2 (12.1)	168.8 (12.4)
Standing diastolic, mm Hg	87.4 (7.7)	87.3 (7.7)
Mean (SD) sitting heart rate, beats/minute	73.0 (8.1)	73.3 (7.9)
Mean (SD) body mass index, kg/m^2		
Men	26.3 (3.1)	26.6 (3.5)
Women	27.5 (4.4)	27.2 (4.5)
Mean (SD) serum cholesterol, mmol/L		
Total cholesterol	6.0 (1.2)	6.0 (1.2)
High-density lipoprotein cholesterol	1.4 (0.5)	1.4 (0.5)
Characteristic present at baseline, No. (%)		
Female	1520 (66.2%)	1618 (67.5%)
Previous antihypertensive medication	1083 (47.1%)	1104 (46.0%)
Cardiovascular complications	697 (30.3%)	705 (29.4%)
Diabetes mellitus*	240 (10.4%)	252 (10.5%)
Never smokers	1705 (74.2%)	1763 (73.5%)
Past smokers	427 (18.6%)	454 (18.9%)
Current smokers	164 (7.1%)	179 (7.5%)
Abstaining from alcohol	1674 (72.9%)	1724 (71.9%)
Drinking < 1 U alcohol per day	355 (15.5%)	414 (17.3%)
Drinking ≥ 1 U alcohol per day	267 (11.1%)	258 (10.8%)

*Defined according to the criteria of the World Health Organization (26).

control group, these numbers were 800 (92.4%), 477 (55.1%), 297 (34.2%), and 8 (0.9%), respectively (Table 7).

The proportion of patients started on multiple drug treatment or proceeding to open follow-up increased faster ($P < 0.001$) in the placebo than in the active treatment group (Table 7). At 2 years, nitrendipine or matching placebo was the only treatment administrated to 597 (58.9%) and 343 (39.6%) patients, respectively. Among the patients in open follow-up at 2 years, 65 (36.5%) of those randomized to active treatment and 157 (58.1%) of those in the placebo group were on antihypertensive drugs, whereas treatment status with regard to hypertension was undocumented in 88 (49.4%) and 81 (30.0%) patients, respectively.

At 2 years, in the intention-to-treat analysis, the sitting systolic/diastolic blood pressure fell on average (SD) by 13/2 (17/8) mm Hg in the placebo group and by 23/7 (16/8) mm Hg in the active treatment group (Fig. 3) and the standing blood pressure by 10/2 (18/8) mm Hg and 21/7 (17/9) mm Hg, respectively. At median follow-up, the percentage of patients who had reached the goal blood pressure was 21.4% in the placebo group and 43.5% in the active-treatment group ($P < 0.001$). At 2 years, the changes in the sitting pulse rate were 0.3 (9.0) beats per minute ($P = 0.25$) and 0.2 (8.9) beats per minute ($P = 0.54$), respectively. The between-group differences were calculated by subtracting the changes from baseline in the placebo group from the corresponding changes

Table 7 Follow-Up and Treatment Status by Randomization Group and Year of Follow-Up

	Number of patients at specified year of follow-up							
Groups	Placebo group (n = 2297)				Active treatment group (n = 2398)			
Year of follow-up	1st	2nd	3rd	4th	1st	2nd	3rd	4th
Total number	1683	1235	928	682	1758	1285	979	705
Deceased	34	51	63	61	15	41	54	54
Double-blind follow-up	1428	866	544	325	1580	1014	677	426
No double-blind drugs	5	2	2	0	2	6	2	2
1 double-blind drug	693	343	178	95	1037	597	385	216
≥ 2 double-blind drugs	725	519	358	226	537	405	283	202
Treatment unknown	5	2	6	4	4	6	7	6
Nitrendipine*†	1352	800	486	286	1407	856	571	351
Enalapril*†	677	477	330	206	471	330	223	152
Hydrochlorothiazide*†	315	297	226	150	147	164	139	104
Antihypertensive drugs‡	16	8	6	1	12	10	8	5
Open follow-up	193	270	267	253	122	178	190	181
Supervised	133	186	179	162	71	89	90	92
Nonsupervised	60	84	88	91	51	89	100	89
Antihypertensive drugs	99	157	166	156	41	65	78	86
No treatment	13	32	24	28	15	25	23	26
Treatment unknown	81	81	77	69	66	88	89	69
Lost to follow-up§	28	48	54	43	41	52	58	44

*In the placebo group, matching placebos were used. In the active treatment group, the mean daily doses (SD) of nitrendipine, enalapril, and hydrochlorothiazide were 28.2 (12.1) mg, 13.5 (6.2) mg and 21.2 (6.2) mg, respectively.

†Because many patients were on combined treatment, these numbers are not additive.

‡To bridge medical emergencies without having to break the code, antihypertensive drugs could be prescribed during the double-blind period for up to 3 consecutive months.

§Patients without follow-up data for more than 1 year.

in the active treatment group. For the sitting blood pressure, they averaged 10.1/4.5 mm Hg (95% confidence interval [CI]: 8.8 to 11.4/3.9 to 5.1 mm Hg) at 2 years and 10.7/4.7 mm Hg (CI: 8.8 to 12.5/3.7 to 5.6 mm Hg) at 4 years. The differences in pulse rate were −0.1 beats per minute (CI: −0.8 to 0.6 beats per minute) and −0.6 beats per minute (CI: −1.7 to 0.5 beats per minute), respectively.

Uncontrolled hypertension led to the withdrawal from double-blind treatment in 126 patients (5.5%) of the placebo group and 11 (0.5%) randomized to active treatment ($P <$ 0.001). Among 59 and five of these patients, the blood pressure criteria applied by the clinical investigator were less stringent than those foreseen by the protocol.

D. Major Endpoints

Cardiovascular mortality tended to be less on active treatment (−27%; CI: −48 to 2%; $P = 0.07$), but all-cause mortality was not significantly changed (Table 8). In the placebo group, the mortality rate due to stroke, heart failure, myocardial infarction, and sudden death ranged from 1.8 to 4.7 deaths per 1000 patient-years. Although mortality from these causes was less on active treatment, the confidence intervals of these changes were wide

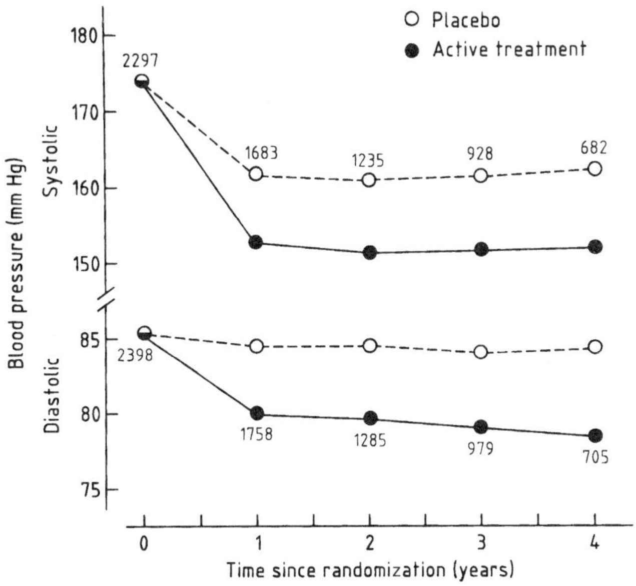

Fig. 3 Average sitting systolic and diastolic blood pressure at randomization and at yearly intervals during follow-up in the intention-to-treat analysis. The number of patients per group at each time point is also presented. (From Ref. 22.)

Table 8 Mortality by Treatment Group (Intention-to-Treat Analysis)

	Rate per 1000 patient-years (number of deaths)		Relative difference with rate in placebo group	
Cause of death	Placebo (n = 2297)	Active (n = 2398)	% rate (95% CI)	*P*
All causes	24.0 (137)	20.5 (123)	−14 (−33, 9)	0.22
Unknown cause	0.4 (2)	0.7 (4)	—	—
Cardiovascular	13.5 (77)	9.8 (59)	−27 (−48, 2)	0.07
Stroke	3.7 (21)	2.7 (16)	−27 (−62, 39)	0.33
Cardiac mortality*	9.1 (52)	6.7 (40)	−27 (−51, 11)	0.14
Heart failure	1.8 (10)	1.3 (8)	−24 (−70, 93)	0.57
Coronary mortality†	7.4 (42)	5.3 (32)	−27 (−54, 15)	0.17
Myocardial infarction	2.6 (15)	1.2 (7)	−56 (−82, 9)	0.08
Sudden death	4.7 (27)	4.2 (25)	−12 (−49, 52)	0.65
Dissecting aortic aneurysm	0.4 (2)	0.2 (1)	—	—
Pulmonary embolism	0.2 (1)	0.3 (2)	—	—
Peripheral arterial disease	0.2 (1)	0.0 (0)	—	—
Noncardiovascular	10.2 (58)	10.0 (60)	−1 (−31, 41)	0.95
Cancer	4.4 (25)	3.0 (18)	−31 (−63, 26)	0.22

*Cardiac mortality included deaths from heart failure and coronary mortality.
†Coronary mortality consisted of fatal myocardial infarction and sudden death.
Abbreviation: *CI*, confidence interval.

and did not exclude the possibility of no effect of antihypertensive drug treatment. Noncardiovascular and cancer mortality did not change significantly (Table 8).

Fatal combined with nonfatal stroke was the primary endpoint in the Syst-Eur trial. It was observed in 77 patients randomized to placebo and 47 of the active treatment group. The cumulative rates were 13.7 and 7.9 strokes per 1000 patient-years (Table 9, Fig. 4). Active treatment reduced the occurrence of total stroke by 42% ($P = 0.003$) and that of nonfatal stroke by 44% ($P = 0.007$). In the active treatment group, nonfatal cardiac endpoints decreased by 33% ($P = 0.03$). All fatal and nonfatal cardiac endpoints, including sudden death, declined by 26% ($P = 0.03$). A similar trend was observed for nonfatal heart failure (−36%; $P = 0.06$), for all cases of heart failure (−29%; $P = 0.12$) and for fatal and nonfatal myocardial infarction (−30%; $P = 0.12$) (Table 9, Fig. 4). Active treatment reduced all fatal and nonfatal cardiovascular endpoints by 31% ($P < 0.001$).

In terms of absolute benefit, at the rates observed in the Syst-Eur placebo group, treating 1000 elderly patients with isolated systolic hypertension for 5 years would prevent 29 strokes or 53 major cardiovascular events.

E. Other Events

Transient ischemic attacks were not significantly influenced by active treatment (−12%; $P = 0.62$; Table 10). The rate of all cerebrovascular events, that is fatal and nonfatal strokes and transient ischemic attacks, was 18.0 and 11.8 events per 1000 patient-years (100 and 70 cases) in the placebo and active treatment groups, respectively. Active treatment reduced ($P = 0.006$) the incidence of all cerebrovascular events by 34% (CI: −51 to −11).

Table 9 Nonfatal Endpoints Alone and Combined with Fatal Endpoints (Intention-to-Treat Analysis)

	Rate per 1000 patient-years (number of endpoints)		Relative difference with rate in placebo group	
Nature of endpoint	Placebo (n = 2297)	Active (n = 2398)	% rate (95% CI)	*P*
Nonfatal endpoints				
Stroke	10.1 (57)	5.7 (34)	−44 (−63, −14)	0.007
Retinal exudates	0.0 (0)	0.2 (1)	—	—
Cardiac endpoints	12.6 (70)	8.5 (50)	−33 (−53, −3)	0.03
Heart failure	7.6 (43)	4.9 (29)	−36 (−60, 2)	0.06
Myocardial infarction	5.5 (31)	4.4 (26)	−20 (−53, 34)	0.40
Renal failure	0.4 (2)	0.5 (3)	—	—
Fatal and nonfatal endpoints				
Stroke	13.7 (77)	7.9 (47)	−42 (−60, −17)	0.003
Cardiac endpoints*	20.5 (114)	15.1 (89)	−26 (−44, −3)	0.03
Heart failure	8.7 (49)	6.2 (37)	−29 (−53, 10)	0.12
Myocardial infarction	8.0 (45)	5.5 (33)	−30 (−56, 9)	0.12
All cardiovascular endpoints	33.9 (186)	23.3 (137)	−31 (−45, −14)	< 0.001

*Nonfatal and fatal cardiac endpoints included fatal and nonfatal heart failure, fatal and nonfatal myocardial infarction, and sudden death (see Table 4).
Abbreviation: *CI*, confidence interval.

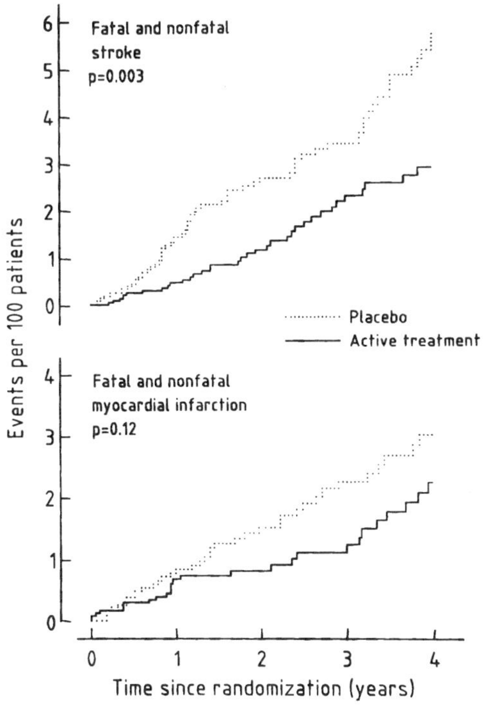

Fig. 4 Cumulative rates of fatal and nonfatal stroke and myocardial infarction by group in the intention-to-treat analysis. (From Ref. 22.)

Table 10 Other Events (Intention-to-Treat Analysis)

	Rate per 1000 patient-years (number of events)		Relative difference with rate in placebo group	
Nature of Event	Placebo (n = 2297)	Active (n = 2398)	% rate (95% CI)	*P*
Nonfatal cardiovascular events				
Transient ischemic attack	5.1 (29)	4.5 (27)	−12 (−48, 49)	0.62
Angina pectoris	23.9 (131)	18.1 (105)	−24 (−41, −2)	0.04
Peripheral arterial disease	10.2 (57)	6.9 (41)	−32 (−54, 2)	0.06
Noncardiovascular events				
Fatal and nonfatal cancer	14.7 (82)	12.4 (73)	−15 (−38, 16)	0.29
Benign neoplasm	3.0 (17)	4.0 (24)	35 (−28, 151)	0.35
Intercurrent disease*	31.4 (168)	33.1 (186)	5 (−15, 90)	0.63
Bleeding†	3.5 (20)	3.2 (19)	−10 (−52, 69)	0.74

*Intercurrent disease refers to nonfatal noncardiovascular disorders requiring admission to the hospital or withdrawal from double-blind treatment or supervised open follow-up.
†Bleeding excludes cerebral and retinal hemorrhage.
Abbreviation: CI, confidence interval.

The incidence of angina pectoris (−24%; $P = 0.04$) and peripheral arterial disease (−32%; $P = 0.06$) tended to decrease in the patients randomized to active treatment (Table 10). The occurrence of cancer, benign neoplasm and bleeding, excluding cerebral and retinal hemorrhage, was similar in the two treatment groups (Table 10). This was also the case for intercurrent diseases of noncardiovascular origin that led to hospitalization or withdrawal from double-blind treatment or supervised open follow-up. In the placebo group, 137 patients were admitted to the hospital because of noncardiovascular disorders and 145 in the active treatment group (25.3 vs 25.4 admissions per 1000 patient-years; $P = 0.95$).

IV. SUBGROUP ANALYSIS BY INTENTION TO TREAT (23)

A. Sex and Previous Cardiovascular Complications

Before randomization, the patients had been prospectively stratified by sex and previous cardiovascular complications. The trial included 1557 men (33.2%), 3138 women (66.8%), 1402 patients with previous cardiovascular complications (29.9%), and 3293 patients without such complications (70.1%).

Men and patients with cardiovascular complications at entry experienced significantly more endpoints during follow-up. However, with adjustments applied for the covariates listed in Table 11, male sex did not behave as a significant predictor of fatal and nonfatal stroke (relative hazard rate [RHR]: 1.17; CI: 0.81 to 1.70; $P = 0.40$) or of fatal and nonfatal cardiac endpoints (RHR: 1.28; CI: 0.95 to 1.17; $P = 0.10$). Further analysis showed that the benefits of active treatment were evenly distributed across the sex and cardiovascular complication groups. In multiple Cox regression, the P values for the interactions with treatment ranged from 0.62 to 0.86 for sex and 0.26 to 0.87 for cardiovascular complications.

B. Age

In single and multiple regression (Table 11), age was a strong predictor of outcome. In Cox regression (Fig. 5), with adjustments applied for the significant covariates listed in Table 11, the treatment-by-age interaction term was significant ($P = 0.009$) for total mortality (RHR: 1.04; CI: 1.01 to 1.08) and nearly significant ($P = 0.09$) for cardiovascular mortality (RHR: 1.04; CI: 0.99 to 1.09). In contrast, the treatment-by-age interaction terms for the combined fatal and nonfatal endpoints were not statistically significant.

C. Systolic and Diastolic Blood Pressure

In single Cox regression, all endpoints, with the exception of fatal and nonfatal cardiac complications, were positively correlated with systolic blood pressure. However, after adjustment for the significant covariates listed in Table 11, systolic blood pressure predicted only stroke incidence. Furthermore, for total mortality, the interaction term between treatment and systolic blood pressure was borderline significant ($P = 0.05$), suggesting greater benefit at higher initial systolic blood pressure (Fig. 5).

In single regression, a higher diastolic blood pressure was associated with lower total ($P < 0.001$) and cardiovascular ($P < 0.001$) mortality and fewer combined fatal and nonfatal endpoints (P values ranging from 0.0007 to 0.02). However, after adjustment for the significant covariates listed in Table 11, these associations weakened to a nonsignifi-

Table 11 Adjusted Relative Hazard Rates* According to Various Characteristics in the Intention-to-Treat Analysis

	Mortality		Fatal and nonfatal cardiovascular endpoints		
	Total	Cardiovascular	All	Stroke	Cardiac
Active treatment (0, 1)†	0.86 (0.67–1.10)	0.73 (0.52–1.03)[o]	0.67 (0.54–0.84)[c]	0.59 (0.38–0.79)[b]	0.71 (0.54–0.94)[a]
Male sex (0, 1)†	1.34 (1.04–1.75)[a]	1.45 (1.02–2.08)[a]	1.30 (1.03–1.64)[b]	NS ($P = 0.40$)	NS ($P = 0.10$)
Cardiovascular complications (0, 1)‡	1.86 (1.45–2.38)[c]	2.17 (1.54–3.05)[c]	1.90 (1.52–2.37)[c]	1.44 (1.00–2.07)[a]	2.27 (1.72–2.99)[c]
Age, y	1.14 (1.13–1.16)[c]	1.12 (1.10–1.15)[c]	1.09 (1.07–1.10)[c]	1.08 (1.05–1.10)[c]	1.09 (1.07–1.11)[c]
Systolic pressure, +10 mm Hg	NS ($P = 0.20$)	NS ($P = 0.51$)	NS ($P = 0.55$)	1.16 (1.00–1.34)[b]	NS ($P = 0.71$)
Eastern European extraction (0, 1)†	1.54 (1.10–2.16)[a]	NS ($P = 0.09$)	NS ($P = 0.78$)	NS ($P = 0.74$)	NS ($P = 0.72$)
Smoking (0, 1)†	2.00 (1.39–2.86)[c]	1.82 (1.10–3.01)[a]	1.79 (1.29–2.50)[c]	NS ($P = 0.58$)	2.34 (1.60–3.41)[c]

*Because the relative hazard rates were calculated by stepwise Cox regression with treatment forced into the model, they are automatically adjusted for randomization group and for all significant covariates listed in the table. Diastolic blood pressure at randomization and drinking alcohol were not independently and significantly correlated with outcome. The relative hazard rates are presented with 95% confidence interval and level of statistical significance ([o]$p = .07$; [a]$p \leq .05$; [b]$p \leq .01$; [c]$p \leq .001$). For nonsignificant (NS) covariates, the probability of entry into the model is given between parentheses.

†Dichotomous variables were coded 0 or 1, depending on whether the condition was absent or present.

‡Among the 1402 patients with cardiovascular complications at randomization, only 58 (3.4%) had a history of stroke and 163 (11.6%) a history of myocardial infarction.

§Compared with patients recruited in western European countries and Israel.

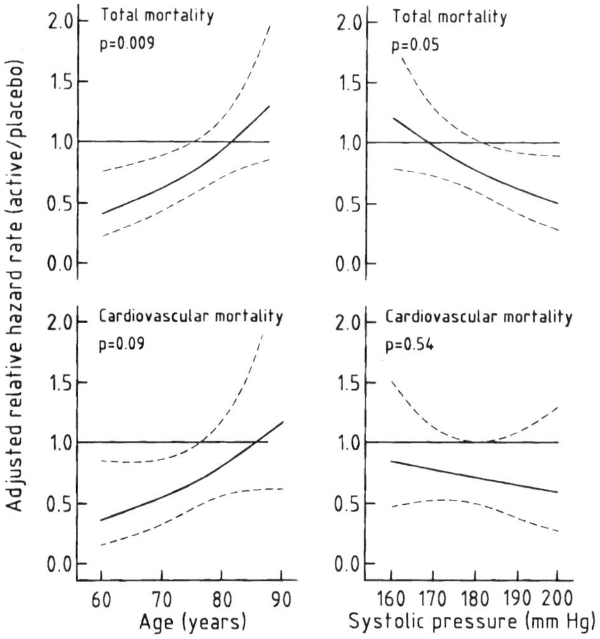

Fig. 5 Adjusted relative hazard rates of total and cardiovascular mortality according to age and initial systolic blood pressure. The hazard rates (placebo/active treatment), calculated by intention-to-treat, are presented as continuous risk functions with 95% confidence interval. P-values refer to the interaction terms between treatment and the independent predictor variable. (From Ref. 23.)

cant level (*P* values ranging from 0.16 to 0.93) and were also not influenced by treatment status. The *P* values of the interaction terms between treatment and diastolic blood pressure ranged from 0.14 to 0.82.

D. Eastern Versus Western European Extraction

Of the 4695 patients, 1994 (42.5%) had been recruited in eastern Europe. However, because of the longer follow-up of the western European patients (median: 3.2 vs 1.1 years), most deaths (210 vs 50) and nonfatal cardiovascular endpoints (170 vs 36) occurred in western European patients.

After adjustment for significant covariates (Table 11), the relative hazard rate of total mortality was significantly higher in eastern than in western Europe, including Israel. However, the treatment-by-residence interaction term was not significant ($P = 0.53$). This was also the case for cardiovascular mortality ($P = 0.08$) and for the other combined fatal and nonfatal endpoints (*P* values ranging from 0.34 to 0.61).

E. Smoking and Drinking Habits

At randomization, the median daily use of tobacco was 15 cigarettes in 231 male smokers (P_5–P_{95} interval [PI]: 3 to 50 cigarettes) and 10 cigarettes (PI: 2 to 30 cigarettes) in 112 female smokers. Both before and after (Table 11) adjustment for significant covariates, smoking predicted total and cardiovascular mortality and the combined fatal and nonfatal cardiovascular and cardiac endpoints. With adjustments applied for significant covariates (Table 11), Cox regression for stroke showed a significant interaction ($P = 0.01$) between treatment and smoking. The relative hazard rate of active versus placebo treatment was 0.47 (CI: 0.32 to 0.69) in nonsmokers but 2.75 (CI: 0.73 to 10.4) in smokers. The percentage of smokers was similar among the 124 stroke patients (n = 11; 8.9%) and the 4571 other participants (n = 332; 7.3%).

At randomization, 393 men and 132 women consumed at least 1 U of an alcoholic beverage per day, that is, one glass of beer, wine, aperitif, fortified wine, or liquor. Their median daily consumption of alcohol was 19 g (5 to 95th percentile interval [PI]: 10 to 54 g) and 14 g (PI: 10 to 36 g), respectively. Alcohol intake was not correlated with outcome either before or after (Table 11) adjustment for covariates (*P* values ranging from 0.14 to 0.64 and from 0.19 to 0.85, respectively). In multiple Cox regression, the *P* values for the interaction terms between treatment and drinking alcohol ranged from 0.16 to 0.99.

V. PER-PROTOCOL ANALYSIS (23)

Analysis by intention-to-treat reduces bias resulting from selective withdrawals. However, the intention-to-treat approach may underestimate the true effects of treatment by including all endpoints in the calculations, regardless of whether they occurred on randomized therapy or on open-label medication. In a per-protocol analysis of the Syst-Eur trial (23), the question was addressed whether the estimates of benefit remained consistent, if the analysis accounted only for the endpoints that occurred during randomized double-blind treatment.

In the per-protocol analysis (Table 12), the number of patient-years in the placebo and active treatment groups amounted to 4508 and 5166, respectively. The median follow-up was 1.7 years (range: 1 to 95 months). Of the placebo and active treatment groups, 1235 and 1285 patients had a follow-up of 2 years or more, and 866 and 1014 were still in double-blind follow-up at 2 years (70.1% vs 78.9%; $P < 0.001$). Of the actively treated patients in double-blind follow-up, 856 (84.4%) were taking nitrendipine (mean daily dose: 28.2 mg), 330 (32.6%) enalapril (13.8 mg per day) and 164 (16.2%) hydrochlorothiazide (21.2 mg per day). In the placebo group, these numbers were 800 (92.4%), 477 (55.1%), and 297 (34.2%), respectively. At median follow-up, the sitting systolic and diastolic blood pressures had fallen by 13 (16) mm Hg and 2 (7) mm Hg in the placebo group and by 25 (15) mm Hg and 7 (8) mm Hg in the active treatment group. The between-group differences in the sitting systolic and diastolic blood pressures then averaged 11.6 mm Hg (CI: 10.1 to 13.0 mm Hg) and 5.3 mm Hg (CI: 4.5 to 6.0 mm Hg), respectively.

Of the patients remaining on double-blind medication, 84 died in the placebo group and 71 in the active treatment group. The cumulative total mortality in the per-protocol analysis amounted to 18.6 and 13.7 deaths per 1000 patient-years, respectively (Table 12). Active treatment reduced total mortality by 26% ($P = 0.05$). A similar trend was observed for fatal myocardial infarction (−60%; $P = 0.08$). Although cerebrovascular (−31%; $P = 0.36$) and cardiac (−20%; $P = 0.34$) mortality were less on active treatment, the wide confidence intervals for these fatal outcomes did not exclude the possibility of no effect of antihypertensive drug treatment.

In general, the per-protocol analysis of the nonfatal endpoints and the combined fatal and nonfatal endpoints (Table 12) produced results similar to those in the intention-to-treat approach (Table 9). In the patients who remained in double-blind follow-up, active treatment reduced total stroke by 44% ($P = 0.004$) and nonfatal stroke by 48% ($P =$

Table 12 Per-Protocol Analysis

Nature of endpoint	Rate per 1000 patient-years (number of endpoints) Placebo (n = 2297)	Active (n = 2398)	Relative difference with rate in placebo group % rate (95% CI)	*P*
Mortality				
Total	18.6 (84)	13.7 (71)	−26 (−46, 0)	0.05
Cardiovascular	11.5 (52)	8.5 (44)	−26 (−51, 10)	0.13
Stroke	3.1 (14)	2.1 (11)	−31 (−69, 51)	0.36
Cardiac mortality	7.5 (34)	6.0 (31)	−20 (−51, 29)	0.34
Noncardiovascular	7.1 (32)	5.2 (27)	−26 (−56, 23)	0.20
Cancer	2.4 (11)	1.4 (7)	−44 (−78, 43)	0.20
Nonfatal endpoints				
Stroke	10.0 (45)	5.2 (27)	−48 (−68, −16)	0.005
Cardiac endpoints	12.2 (55)	8.7 (45)	−29 (−52, 6)	0.07
Heart failure	7.5 (34)	4.3 (22)	−44 (−67, −4)	0.03
Myocardial infarction	5.1 (23)	4.8 (25)	−5 (−46, 67)	0.81
Fatal and nonfatal endpoints				
Stroke	13.1 (59)	7.4 (38)	−44 (−63, −16)	0.004
Cardiac endpoints*	19.8 (89)	14.7 (76)	−26 (−45, 0)	0.05
Heart failure	8.7 (39)	5.6 (29)	−35 (−60, 5)	0.06
Myocardial infarction	7.5 (34)	5.8 (30)	−23 (−53, 26)	0.28
All cardiovascular endpoints	33.8 (152)	23.0 (119)	−32 (−46, −13)	0.001

*Nonfatal and fatal cardiac endpoints included fatal and nonfatal heart failure, fatal and nonfatal myocardial infarction, and sudden death (see Table 4).
Abbreviation: *CI*, confidence interval.

0.005). In the active treatment group, nonfatal cardiac endpoints decreased by 29% (P = 0.07). A similar trend was observed for fatal and nonfatal cases of heart failure (−35%; P = 0.06). All fatal and nonfatal cardiac endpoints, including sudden death, declined by 26% (P = 0.05). Active treatment reduced all fatal and nonfatal cardiovascular endpoints by 32% ($P < 0.001$).

In terms of absolute benefit, the per-protocol analysis suggested that at the rates observed in the placebo group, treating 1000 patients for 5 years could prevent 24 deaths or 54 major cardiovascular endpoints, that is, 29 strokes and 25 cardiac endpoints.

VI. CALCIUM-CHANNEL BLOCKADE AND CARDIOVASCULAR PROGNOSIS (27)

In the Syst-Eur trial, active treatment was initiated with the dihydropyridine calcium-channel blocker, nitrendipine (9). The controversy about possible adverse effects of calcium-channel blockers arose in 1995 (18); it was not considered in 1991 or 1992 when the ethics committee of the Syst-Eur trial and the review boards of the participating centers decided to continue the trial. However, in view of the persistent concerns about the use of calcium-channel blockers as first-line antihypertensive drugs (18,19,28–32), further analyses addressed the question whether treatment with nitrendipine (9) alone could influence prognosis.

A. Early Benefit

At 6 months, 1517 patients of the placebo group (66.0%) and 1829 of those randomized to active treatment (76.3%) were still on monotherapy with the first-line study medication. The net blood pressure reduction in the active treatment group was 7.7 mm Hg systolic (CI: 6.8 to 8.6 mm Hg) and 3.3 mm Hg diastolic (CI: 2.8 to 3.7 mm Hg). At this early moment in the trial, when most patients were still taking the first-line medication, active treatment reduced all cardiovascular endpoints by 55% (CI: 20% to 75%; $P = 0.005$), all cardiac endpoints by 62% (CI: 21 to 82%; $P = 0.007$), total mortality by 60% (CI: 17 to 81%; $P = 0.01$), and cardiovascular mortality by 62% (CI: 14 to 83%; $P = 0.02$). In contrast, the 37% (CI: −78 to 77%) reduction in fatal and nonfatal stroke was not yet significant. The reduction in all cardiovascular endpoints at 6 months was of the same order of magnitude as at 1, 2, or 4 years of follow-up, when more patients had proceeded to combined therapy (Fig. 6).

B. Matched Pairs Analysis

To ascertain that the apparent benefit conferred by nitrendipine was not the result of selection bias in the control group, the 1327 patients who remained on single nitrendipine treatment throughout the whole trial were matched by sex, age (60–69, 70–79, and ≥ 80 years), previous cardiovascular complications, and systolic blood pressure at entry (within 4 mm Hg) with an equal number of placebo patients drawn from the control group, regardless of the type of placebos taken.

At 2 years (median follow-up in the two groups), the net blood pressure reduction in the actively treated patients averaged 13.7 mm Hg systolic (CI: 11.9 to 15.5 mm Hg)

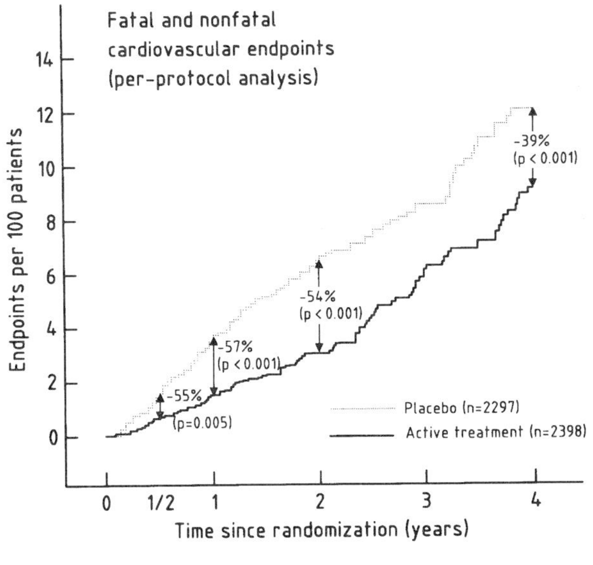

Fig. 6 Cumulative rates of all cardiovascular endpoints in the per-protocol analysis. The between-group differences in the rates are presented for various follow-up intervals. The benefit of active treatment was already significant at 6 months, when most of the 4695 randomized patients were still on monotherapy with active nitrendipine or matching placebo. (From Ref. 27.)

Table 13 Outcome in 1327 Patients on Monotherapy with Active Nitrendipine in Comparison with Matched* Placebo Patients

	Rate per 1000 patient-years (number of endpoints)		Relative difference with rate in placebo group	
Nature of endpoint	Placebo (n = 2297)	Active (n = 2398)	% rate (95% CI)	*P*
Mortality				
Total	22.0 (57)	15.9 (41)	−28 (−52, 8)	0.12
Cardiovascular	13.9 (36)	8.1 (21)	−41 (−66, 0)	0.05
Fatal and nonfatal endpoints				
Stroke	13.5 (35)	8.9 (23)	−34 (−61, 12)	0.12
Cardiac endpoints	23.2 (60)	15.5 (40)	−33 (−55, 0)	0.05
Heart failure	9.6 (25)	5.0 (13)	−48 (−73, 0)	0.05
Myocardial infarction	8.9 (23)	7.4 (19)	−17 (−55, 52)	0.55
All cardiovascular endpoints	37.5 (97)	25.2 (65)	−33 (−51, −8)	0.01

*Patients remaining on single nitrendipine treatment were matched by sex, age, previous cardiovascular complications, and systolic blood pressure at entry with patients drawn from the whole placebo group.
Abbreviation: *CI*, confidence interval.

and 5.4 mm Hg diastolic (CI: 4.5 to 6.4 mm Hg). Compared with the matched control group (Table 13), active nitrendipine reduced cardiovascular mortality by 41% ($P = 0.05$), all cardiovascular endpoints by 33% ($P = 0.01$), fatal and nonfatal cardiac endpoints by 33% ($P = 0.05$), and fatal and nonfatal heart failure by 48% ($P = 0.05$).

VII. UPDATE ON THE MORBIDITY AND MORTALITY RESULTS (33)

The Syst-Eur trial stopped after the second of four planned interim analyses, when predefined stopping rules (8) revealed that active treatment diminished the incidence of stroke, the primary endpoint. The ethics committee unanimously resolved that all endpoints that had occurred before February 14, 1997, at 5:00 PM should be included in the final analysis. The long communication lines between the coordinating office and 198 centers in 23 countries (Table 5) made the practical implementation of this recommendation very difficult. The coordinating office had to strike a delicate balance between reporting long-awaited outcome results or postponing publication until a greater number of terminating report forms had been returned. In the initial Syst-Eur report (22), 116 (5.1%) of 2297 placebo patients and 121 (5.0%) of 2398 patients randomized to active treatment were classified as lost to follow-up, because in the preceding year no report had reached the coordinating office. However, after publication of the outcome results on September 13, 1997 (22), efforts to locate all patients continued and the database was updated.

The number of patients lost to follow-up decreased to 61 (2.7%) in the placebo group and to 63 (2.6%) in the active treatment group: 1559 and 1795 patients, respectively, were in double-blind follow-up, 147 and 135 had died, 283 and 150 were in supervised open follow-up, and 247 and 255 were in nonsupervised follow-up (33). The number of patient-years accumulated in the placebo and active treatment groups increased from 5709 to 5844 and from 5995 to 6140, respectively. The greater number of endpoints available for analysis (Table 14) (33) did not affect the conclusions of the initial (22) Syst-Eur

Table 14 Update on the Morbidity and Mortality Results (Intention-to-Treat Analysis)

	Rate per 1000 patient-years (number of endpoints)		Relative difference with rate in placebo group	
Nature of endpoint	Placebo (n = 2297)	Active (n = 2398)	% rate (95% CI)	*P*
Mortality				
Total	25.2 (147)	22.0 (135)	−13 (−31, 10)	0.28
Cardiovascular	14.0 (82)	10.4 (64)	−26 (−46, 3)	0.08
Noncardiovascular	11.0 (64)	10.8 (66)	−2 (−30, 38)	0.94
Nonfatal endpoints				
Stroke	10.4 (60)	5.7 (35)	−45 (−64, −17)	0.004
Cardiac endpoints	12.8 (73)	8.8 (53)	−32 (−52, −2)	0.04
Fatal and nonfatal endpoints				
Stroke	13.9 (80)	8.0 (49)	−42 (−60, −18)	0.002
Cardiac endpoints	20.9 (119)	15.6 (94)	−25 (−43, −2)	0.03
Heart failure	8.9 (51)	6.6 (40)	−26 (−51, 12)	0.16
Myocardial infarction	8.1 (47)	5.9 (36)	−27 (−53, 12)	0.16
All cardiovascular endpoints	34.6 (194)	24.2 (145)	−30 (−44, −13)	< 0.001

Abbreviation: *CI*, confidence interval.

report (Tables 8 and 9) (22). Fatal and nonfatal cancer (change with active treatment: −12%; CI: −36 to 20%; $P = 0.42$) and bleeding episodes not including nose bleeds and cerebral and retinal hemorrhage (−9%; CI: −50 to 65%; $P = 0.96$) occurred with similar frequency in both treatment groups.

VIII. OTHER FINDINGS

A. Outcome in Diabetic and Nondiabetic Patients (34)

At randomization, 492 patients (10.5%) had diabetes (Table 6). At 2 years (median follow-up), the net differences in blood pressure between the placebo and active treatment groups were 8.6 mm Hg systolic and 3.9 mm Hg diastolic in the diabetic patients; in the 4203 patients without diabetes, these differences were 10.3 mm Hg and 4.5 mm Hg, respectively.

In diabetic patients (Fig. 7), with adjustments for possible confounders applied, active treatment reduced all-cause mortality by 55% (CI: 15 to 76%), cardiovascular mortality by 76% (CI: 33 to 91%), all cardiovascular endpoints by 69% (CI: 41 to 84%), fatal and nonfatal stroke by 73% (CI: 26 to 90%), and all cardiac endpoints by 63% (CI: 10 to 85%). In the nondiabetic patients, active treatment decreased all cardiovascular endpoints by 26% (CI: 6 to 41%) and fatal and nonfatal stroke by 38% (CI: 8 to 58%). Active treatment reduced total mortality ($P = 0.04$), cardiovascular mortality ($P = 0.02$), and all cardiovascular endpoints ($P = 0.01$) significantly more in diabetic than nondiabetic patients (34).

B. Prevention of Dementia (35,36)

Systolic hypertension increases the risk of dementia in aging people. The Vascular Dementia Project (35–37) set up in the framework Syst-Eur trial, investigated whether

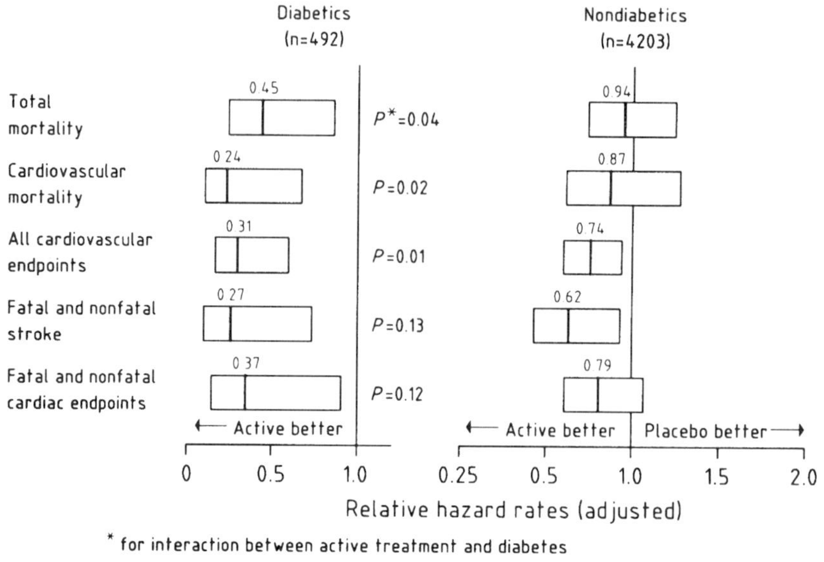

Fig. 7 Relative hazard rates of active treatment versus placebo in diabetic and nondiabetic patients with cumulative adjustments for sex, age, previous cardiovascular complications, systolic blood pressure at entry, smoking, and residence in western Europe. The *P* values refer to the treatment-by-diabetes interaction and indicate whether the treatment effect was significantly different according to the presence of diabetes at randomization. (From Ref. 34.)

antihypertensive drug treatment could reduce the incidence of dementia. At baseline and follow-up, cognitive function was assessed by the Mini Mental State Examination (MMSE) (38). If the MMSE score was 23 or less, the diagnosis of dementia was ascertained based on the Diagnostic and Statistical Manual (DSM-III-R) criteria (39), which at the start of the Syst-Eur trial in 1988 was the generally accepted standard (40–42). If the DSM-III-R criteria (39) confirmed the diagnosis of dementia, the Modified Ischemic Score (43), including a computerized tomographic brain scan, served to differentiate vascular from degenerative disease. If a brain scan could not be performed, the Hachinski Score (44) replaced the Modified Ischemic Score (43) to establish the cause of dementia.

In total, 2418 patients were enrolled in the analysis. Median follow-up by intention to treat was 2.0 years. Compared with placebo (n = 1180), active treatment (n = 1238) reduced the incidence of dementia by 50% (CI: 0 to 76%; $P = 0.05$) from 7.7 to 3.8 cases per 1000 patient-years (Fig. 8). In the per-protocol analysis, active treatment decreased the rate by 60% (CI: 2 to 83%; $P = 0.03$). Further analysis demonstrated that active treatment mainly prevented Alzheimer's disease (Table 15).

The median MMSE score at randomization was 29 in both treatment groups. At the last available evaluation, systolic and diastolic blood pressures were 8.3 mm Hg and 3.8 mm Hg lower ($P < 0.001$) in the active treatment group, but on average the MMSE scores did not change in either group. However, in the placebo group the MMSE score decreased when systolic ($P = 0.001$) or diastolic ($P = 0.04$) blood pressure decreased. In the active

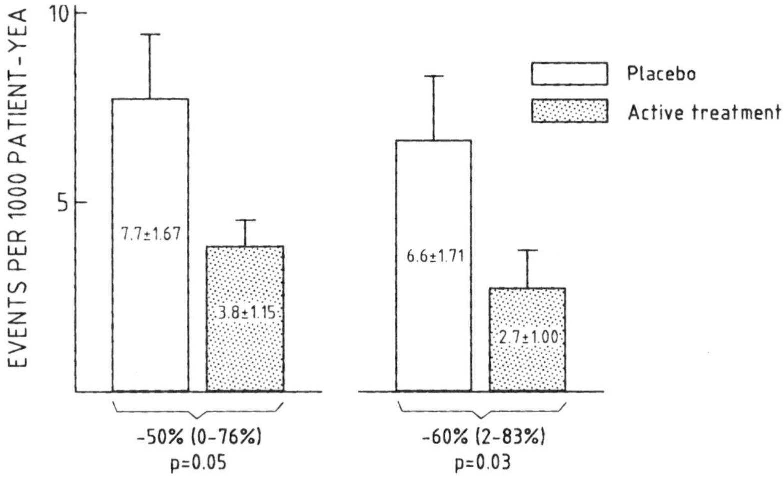

Fig. 8 Incidence of dementia by treatment group in the intention-to-treat and per-protocol analyses.

treatment group the MMSE scores remained unchanged ($P = 0.53$) or improved slightly ($P = 0.01$) with greater reductions in systolic or diastolic blood pressure. The between-group differences in these associations were significant for systolic ($P = 0.03$) and diastolic ($P = 0.002$) blood pressure.

The Syst-Eur findings suggest that in older people with isolated systolic hypertension, antihypertensive treatment may reduce the incidence of dementia. At the risk observed in the placebo group, treating 1000 hypertensive patients for 5 years could prevent 19 cases.

Table 15 Etiology of Dementia

Characteristic	Placebo	Active treatment	All patients
Intention-to-treat analysis			
Patient-years of follow-up	2737	2885	5622
All cases	21	11	32
Alzheimer's dementia	15	8	23
Mixed dementia	4	3	7
Vascular dementia	2	0	2
Per-protocol analysis			
Patient-years of follow-up	2260	2634	4894
All cases	15	7	22
Alzheimer's dementia	13	5	18
Mixed dementia	2	2	4
Vascular dementia	0	0	0

C. Prognostic Value of Conventional and Ambulatory Blood Pressure (45–47)

Within the framework of the Syst-Eur Trial, the Study on Ambulatory Blood Pressure Monitoring was set up to compare the prognostic accuracy of conventional and ambulatory blood pressure measurements (45–47). Follow-up of the placebo group also allowed the possibility of validating proposed diagnostic thresholds (48,49) for blood pressure monitoring in terms of morbidity and mortality. Of 198 Syst-Eur centers, 46 opted to enroll their patients.

Interim reports on the Study of Ambulatory Blood Pressure Monitoring showed: (a) that the daytime systolic blood pressure decreased by 2 to 3 mm Hg on long-term placebo treatment (50); (b) that in parallel-group trials or in clinical experiments focusing on the blood pressure course during the whole day, ambulatory blood pressure monitoring does not allow economizing on sample size (51); (c) and that it is possible to calculate the trough-to-peak ratio in parallel-group trials while fully accounting for placebo effects as well as interindividual variability (52).

In the main analysis of the Study on Ambulatory Blood Pressure Monitoring (47), 29 (3.5%) of 837 randomized patients with a 24-hour blood pressure recording at baseline were excluded because less than 80% of the required readings were available. Systolic and diastolic blood pressures were, on average, 21.9 mm Hg and 1.9 mm Hg higher ($P < 0.001$) on conventional than on daytime ambulatory measurement (Table 16). The corresponding mean ± 2 SD intervals ranged from −8.3 to +52.3 mm Hg and from −17.2 to +21.2 mm Hg, respectively. Awake and sleeping blood pressures were similar to daytime (from 10:00 AM to 8:00 PM) and nighttime (from midnight to 6:00 AM) blood pressures, respectively. The results of Cox regression were also comparable regardless of which of the two definitions of the diurnal high and low blood pressure spans was considered. Because short fixed-clocktime intervals (53) are easy to reproduce across studies, only the results for the daytime and the nighttime blood pressures were

Table 16 Conventional and Ambulatory Blood Pressures at Randomization in 808 Patients

	Systolic, mm Hg	Diastolic, mm Hg
Mean (SD) conventional* blood pressure in the sitting position	173.3 (10.8)	86.0 (5.8)
Mean (SD) ambulatory blood pressure		
24-hour	145.8 (15.6)	79.3 (8.9)
Daytime (10:00 AM–8:00 PM)	151.4 (16.2)	84.1 (9.8)
Nighttime (0–6:00 AM)	134.0 (18.6)	70.2 (10.1)
Nocturnal blood pressure fall†	17.4 (14.8)	13.8 (8.8)
Night-to-day blood pressure ratio‡	0.89 (0.09)	0.84 (0.10)
Awake	151.0 (15.8)	83.6 (9.4)
Sleeping	134.7 (18.1)	70.8 (9.9)

*Mean of six readings, i.e., two at each of three baseline visits, 1 month apart.
†Daytime minus nighttime blood pressure.
‡Dimensionless ratio of nighttime to daytime blood pressure.
Abbreviation: *SD*, standard deviation.

Table 17 Relative Hazard Rates* for Ambulatory Systolic Blood Pressure After Adjustment for the Conventional Systolic Blood Pressure and Various Entry Characteristics

	Mortality		Fatal and nonfatal endpoints combined		
	Total	Cardiovascular	Cardiovascular	Stroke	Cardiac
Placebo group (n = 393)					
24-hour pressure	1.19 (0.95–1.49)	1.29 (0.95–1.75)	1.27 (1.05–1.54)[b]	1.51 (1.06–2.15)[b]	1.14 (0.90–1.43)
Daytime pressure	1.14 (0.91–1.42)	1.25 (0.92–1.69)	1.20 (1.00–1.45)[b]	1.61 (1.14–2.28)[c]	1.06 (0.85–1.33)
Nighttime pressure	1.21 (1.00–1.47)[b]	1.39 (1.07–1.79)[b]	1.31 (1.12–1.53)[d]	1.25 (0.94–1.66)	1.22 (1.06–1.54)[b]
Active treatment (n = 415)					
24-hour pressure	0.95 (0.72–1.24)	0.89 (0.61–1.30)	1.05 (0.84–1.31)	1.15 (0.69–1.90)	1.05 (0.81–1.35)
Daytime pressure	0.81 (0.62–1.06)	0.86 (0.60–1.25)	0.94 (0.77–1.16)	0.82 (0.52–1.29)	0.97 (0.77–1.24)
Nighttime pressure	1.05 (0.86–1.27)	1.00 (0.77–1.30)	1.12 (0.95–1.32)	1.38 (0.96–2.00)	1.07 (0.89–1.29)
Both groups (n = 808)†					
24-hour pressure	1.09 (0.92–1.29)	1.11 (0.88–1.40)	1.17 (1.01–1.35)[b]	1.36 (1.04–1.79)[c]	1.11 (0.93–1.31)
Daytime pressure	0.98 (0.83–1.17)	1.07 (0.85–1.34)	1.08 (0.94–1.24)	1.25 (0.97–1.61)	1.03 (0.87–1.21)
Nighttime pressure	1.14 (1.00–1.30)[b]	1.18 (0.98–1.42)[a]	1.20 (1.08–1.35)[c]	1.31 (1.06–1.62)[b]	1.16 (1.02–1.33)[b]

*Relative hazard rates with 95% confidence interval between parentheses reflect the risk associated with a 10 mm Hg increase in systolic ambulatory blood pressure. Risk estimates were adjusted for sex, age, previous cardiovascular complications, smoking, residence in western Europe, and the conventional systolic blood pressure at entry; [a]indicates $P \leq 0.07$; [b]$P \leq 0.05$; [c]$P \leq 0.01$; and [d]$P \leq 0.001$.

†Also adjusted for active treatment.

reported. The mean (SD) within-subject coefficient of variation was significantly smaller for the nighttime than for the daytime blood pressure (8.7 [3.6]% vs 10.4 [3.3]%; $P < 0.001$).

With cumulative adjustments applied for sex, age, previous cardiovascular complications, smoking, and residence in western Europe (23), a higher systolic blood pressure at randomization predicted a worse prognosis, whereas the association between diastolic blood pressure and outcome was not significant. In the placebo group (n = 393), the 24-hour, daytime, and nighttime systolic ambulatory blood pressures predicted the incidence of cardiovascular complications even after further adjustment for the conventional blood pressure (Table 17). The nighttime systolic blood pressure behaved as a more accurate predictor of endpoints than the daytime level (except for stroke). The 24-hour level and the night-to-day ratio of systolic blood pressure were significantly and independently correlated with the incidence of all cardiovascular endpoints in the placebo group. The relative hazard rates associated with a 10 mm Hg increase in the 24-hour blood pressure and with a 10% higher night-to-day ratio were 1.23 (CI: 1.03–1.46; $P = 0.02$) and 1.41 (CI: 1.03–1.94; $P = 0.03$), respectively. In the placebo group, the cardiovascular risk conferred by a conventional systolic blood pressure of 160 mm Hg at randomization was similar to those associated with a 24-hour, daytime, or nighttime systolic blood pressure of 142 mm Hg (CI: 128–156 mm Hg), 145 mm Hg (CI: 126–164 mm Hg), or 132 mm Hg (CI: 120–145 mm Hg), respectively. In the active treatment group (n = 415), systolic blood pressure at randomization did not significantly predict cardiovascular risk, regardless of the technique of blood pressure measurement.

D. Pulse Pressure as Independent Cardiovascular Risk Factor (54)

Current guidelines for the management of hypertension rest almost completely on the measurement of systolic and diastolic blood pressure. However, the arterial blood pressure wave is more correctly described as consisting of a *pulsatile* (pulse pressure) and a *steady* (mean pressure) component. In a meta-analysis of the Syst-Eur (22) and Syst-China (55) trials and the former trial conducted by the European Working Party on High Blood Pressure in the Elderly (1), the independent roles of pulse pressure and mean pressure as determinants of cardiovascular prognosis in older hypertensive patients were further investigated (54).

The relative hazard rates associated with pulse pressure and mean pressure were calculated, using Cox regression with stratification for the three trials and with adjustments for sex, age, previous cardiovascular complications, smoking, and treatment group (54). A 10 mm Hg wider pulse pressure increased the risk of all major complications. After controlling for mean pressure and other covariates, the relative risks amounted to 15% for all-cause mortality (CI: 7 to 22%; $P < 0.001$), 22% for cardiovascular mortality (CI: 13 to 33%; $P < 0.001$), 17% for all cardiovascular endpoints (CI: 10 to 24%; $P < 0.001$), 17% for fatal and nonfatal stroke (CI:7 to 29%; $P < 0.001$), and 13% for coronary endpoints (CI: 2 to 24%; $P = 0.02$) (54). In a similar analysis, mean pressure predicted the incidence of cardiovascular complications but only after removal of pulse pressure as an explanatory variable from the model. Furthermore, the probability of a major cardiovascular endpoint increased with higher systolic blood pressure; at any given level of systolic blood pressure, it also rose with lower diastolic blood pressure, suggesting that indeed the wider pulse pressure was driving the risk of major complications (54).

IX. INTERPRETATION

Stepwise antihypertensive drug treatment in the Syst-Eur trial consisted of the dihydropyridine calcium-channel blocker nitrendipine, the converting-enzyme inhibitor enalapril and the thiazide diuretic hydrochlorothiazide. In elderly patients with isolated systolic hypertension, these drugs reduced the risk of stroke, the primary endpoint in the Syst-Eur trial, as well as the incidence of various other cardiovascular complications and dementia.

A. Syst-Eur, a Trial in Older Patients with Isolated Systolic Hypertension

The benefits of antihypertensive treatment in the Syst-Eur study were, in relative terms, similar to those in six other trials (1,2,4,56–58) in older patients with combined systolic and diastolic hypertension. Overall, in these studies, antihypertensive treatment reduced fatal stroke by 33% and cardiovascular mortality by 22% (59). In a subsequent quantitative review (60) that also included the SHEP trial (10) but not the small Japanese study by Kuramoto (57), these pooled estimates were also the same, that is, 33% and 22%.

The benefit of antihypertensive treatment is usually expressed in relative terms as the percentage reduction in the event rate compared with the control group. However, this quantity may be misleading, because in absolute terms the number of patient-years of treatment required to prevent one event varies proportionally with the underlying risk, as estimated from the event rate observed in the control group (60,61). Among nine intervention trials in the elderly (1,2,4,10,22,55–58), including the Syst-Eur trial (Fig. 9), the absolute benefit with regard to all strokes and cardiovascular mortality was small in the group of older (age 60 or older) patients enrolled in the Australian Trial in Mild Hypertension (4) and in the Medical Research Council Trial (58), and large in the Swedish Trial in Old Patients with Hypertension (56). Per 1000 patients treated for 5 years, the number of strokes or cardiovascular deaths prevented ranged from 10 (4,58) to 74 (56) and from 6 (4,58) to 67 (56), respectively. In the analysis by intention-to-treat, the Syst-Eur results with respect to the number of prevented strokes were in close agreement with those reported by the SHEP investigators (10). In relative terms, the percentage reduction in stroke incidence amounted to 42% and 36% (10), respectively, whereas in both trials nearly 1000 patients had to be treated for 5 years to prevent 30 strokes. For cardiovascular mortality, the relative benefit in the intention-to-treat analysis amounted to 27% and 20% (10), respectively, whereas 5000 patient-years of treatment prevented 18 and 10 (10) cardiovascular deaths.

Syst-Eur was the first outcome trial in hypertension that has recruited patients in eastern as well as western Europe. Of 8926 patients entered in the registers of screened patients, 52.6% were randomized. The Syst-Eur patients were recruited by population screening, at family practices (62), and at primary and secondary referral centers. On the other hand, the Syst-Eur trial included only 3.5% patients with previous myocardial infarction and 1.2% with a history of stroke. The exclusion of patients with major cardiovascular complications and the selection of individuals likely to comply with long-term follow-up and treatment are factors that must be taken into account when the Syst-Eur results are extrapolated. In the SHEP trial (10), 447,921 individuals were contacted, mainly by mass mailing and community screening. Of these, 11.6% met the initial criteria, 2.7% completed the baseline visit, and 1.1% (n = 4736) were randomized. In the SHEP trial, the maximal diastolic blood pressure at randomization was 5 mm Hg lower than in the

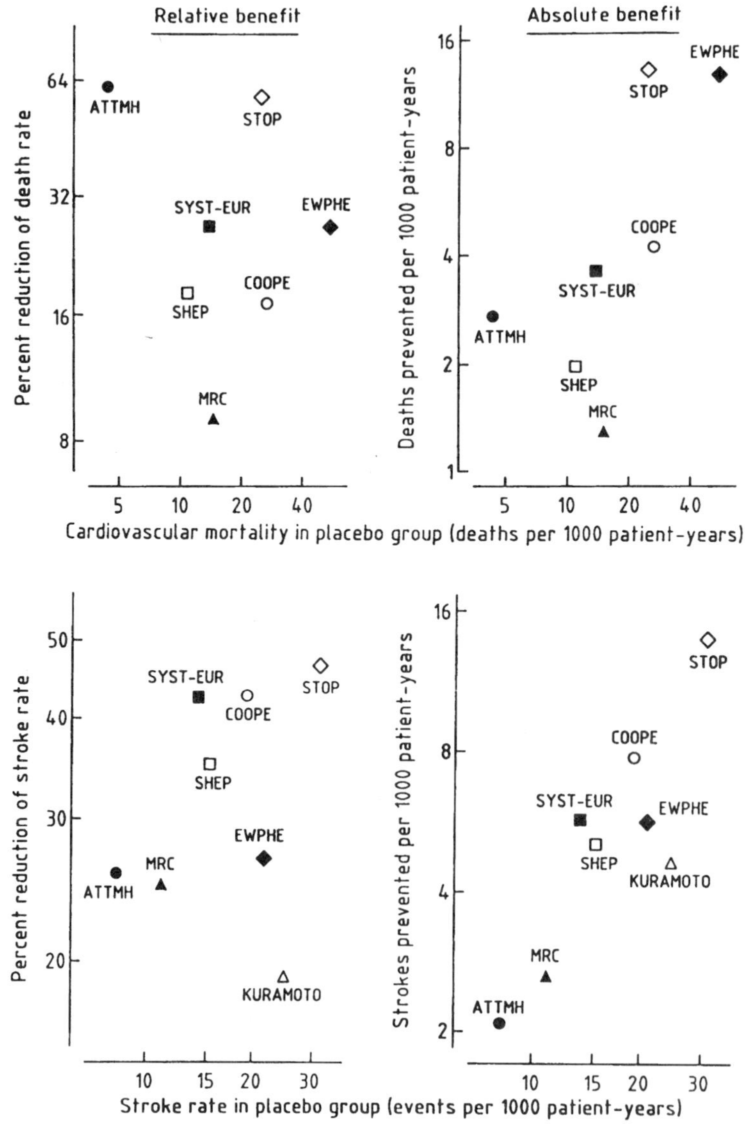

Fig. 9 Comparison of the relative (**left**) and absolute (**right**) benefits of antihypertensive drug treatment with regard to cardiovascular mortality (**top**) and fatal and nonfatal stroke (**bottom**) in the Systolic Hypertension in Europe Trial (Syst-Eur) and in older ($\geq$ 60 years) hypertensive patients enrolled in eight other intervention trials (Australian Therapeutic Trial in Mild Hypertension [ATTMH],[4] Coope and Warrender [COOPE],[2] European Working Party on High Blood Pressure in the Elderly Trial [EWPHE],[1] Kuramoto et al. [KURAMOTO],[57] Medical Research Council Trial [MRC],[58] Systolic Hypertension in the Elderly Program [SHEP],[10] Systolic Hypertension in China Trial [Syst-China],[55] and Swedish Trial in Older Patients with Hypertension [STOP][56]).

Syst-Eur study. In spite of these differences in recruitment and selection criteria, total and cardiovascular mortality in the placebo arms of the SHEP and Syst-Eur trials were approximately similar, that is, 23 versus 24 deaths per 1000 patient-years and 10 versus 13 deaths per 1000 patient-years.

The number of Syst-Eur patients initially (22) reported as lost to follow-up was substantially lower than, for instance, in the 176 general practices taking part in the Medical Research Council trial of mild hypertension (19%) (63). In the final Syst-Eur database (33), the proportion of patients lost to follow-up was similar to that in the Hypertension Optimal Treatment trial (2.6%), which stopped according to plan after 1100 events and after all patients had been followed for at least 3 years (64). The Syst-Eur experience confirms that in large multicenter trials terminating early, not all endpoints will be available when the main outcome results are published. Trialists should be encouraged to continue searching for unreported endpoints and to publish a final complete analysis. However, the update will not lead to different conclusions unless there was selective underreporting of events in one treatment group.

B. Syst-Eur and the Controversy on Calcium-Channel Blockers

Shortly after the first publication of the morbidity and mortality results of the Syst-Eur trial, the question arose whether the observed beneficial effects of active treatment could be ascribed to any of the drugs used in the trial. Further analyses suggested that the dihydropyridine calcium-channel blocker nitrendipine, independent of the other associated antihypertensive drugs, prevented cardiovascular complications in older patients with isolated systolic hypertension (27).

So-called ''post hoc'' analyses have inherent limitations, because they may not follow the lines of randomization. However, in the per-protocol analysis of all randomized patients, this problem was minimized. At 6 months, when most actively treated patients were still on monotherapy with nitrendipine or matching first-line placebo, the reduction in all cardiovascular endpoints was of the same order of magnitude as at 2 or 4 years of follow-up (Fig. 6). However, because no other antihypertensive drugs were compared to placebo, any difference between the two treatment groups may still have been the result of blood pressure reduction rather than to a drug-class effect.

To ascertain that the apparent benefit conferred by nitrendipine was not caused by selection bias in the control group, the 1327 patients remaining on monotherapy with active nitrendipine were matched by sex, age, previous cardiovascular complications, and systolic blood pressure at entry with an equal number of placebo patients, regardless of the type of placebos taken. In this analysis (Table 13), nitrendipine reduced cardiovascular mortality by 41%, all cardiovascular endpoints by 33%, and cardiac endpoints by 33%. In all randomized patients, the corresponding estimates of benefit in the per-protocol analysis (23) were 26% ($P = 0.13$), 32% ($P = 0.001$), and 26% ($P < 0.05$), respectively. Thus, the nearly one-third reduction of all cardiovascular endpoints in the subset of patients on monotherapy with nitrendipine is consistent with the overall benefit observed in all patients randomized to active treatment. This observation again suggests that cardiovascular prevention in the Syst-Eur trial may to a large extent be ascribed to calcium-channel blockade. The small number of patients on single treatment with enalapril made any search for specific effects of this drug impossible.

Three studies (55,65,66) investigated the effects of the dihydropyridine calcium-channel blockers in Chinese hypertensive patients but followed an unorthodox design

(66). The Cheng-Du nifedipine trial was a prospective placebo-controlled trial of 683 hypertensive patients (65). Over the 6 years of follow-up, the incidence of cardiovascular events decreased from 14.0% to 5.2% ($P = 0.05$). The Shanghai Trial of Nifedipine in the Elderly (STONE) was a single-blind trial, in which 1797 patients were alternatingly assigned to nifedipine (10 to 60 mg/day) or placebo with the possible addition in both treatment groups of active captopril (20 to 50 mg/day) or hydrochlorothiazide (25 mg/day) (66). Patients whose diastolic blood pressure exceeded 110 mm Hg were reallocated to nifedipine. A total of 165 patients were excluded from analysis, but all endpoints were blindly assessed. In an intention-to-treat analysis, total stroke incidence decreased by 57% (CI: −23 to −76%). In the nifedipine group, total mortality tended to decline by 45% (CI: −71 to 3%). No significant changes were observed in cardiovascular mortality (−26%; CI: −66 to 62%) or in the incidence of fatal and nonfatal myocardial infarction (−6%; CI: −87 to 566%) and cancer (−76%; CI: −95 to 13%) (66). The Systolic Hypertension in China (Syst-China) Trial was a placebo-controlled study in older (age 60 or older) Chinese patients with isolated systolic hypertension (55,67,68). The first-line antihypertensive agent in this study was also nitrendipine (10 to 40 mg/day) with the possible addition of captopril (12.5 to 50 mg/day) and hydrochlorothiazide (12.5 to 50 mg/day). At entry, the sitting blood pressure averaged 171 mm Hg systolic and 86 mm Hg diastolic, age averaged 66.5 years, and total serum cholesterol was 5.1 mmol/L. At 2 years of follow-up, the sitting systolic and diastolic blood pressures had fallen by 10.9 mm Hg and 1.9 mm Hg in the placebo group and by 20.0 mm Hg and 5.0 mm Hg in the active treatment group. The between-group differences were 9.1 mm Hg systolic (CI: 7.6 to 10.7 mm Hg) and 3.2 mm Hg diastolic (CI: 2.4 to 4.0 mm Hg). Active treatment reduced total stroke by 37% (CI: 14 to 53%; $P = 0.01$), all-cause mortality by 39% (CI: 16 to 57%; $P = 0.003$), cardiovascular mortality by 39% (CI: 4 to 61%, $P = 0.03$), stroke mortality by 58% (14 to 80%; $P = 0.02$), and all fatal and nonfatal cardiovascular endpoints by 37% (CI: 14 to 53%; $P = 0.004$) (55).

In 1995, a case-control study raised the possibility that calcium-channel blockers prescribed to patients with hypertension might increase the risk of myocardial infarction (19). In a quantitative review of 16 randomized secondary prevention trials, the use of short-acting nifedipine in patients with coronary heart disease was found to be associated with a 16% (CI: 1 to 33%) higher mortality (18). Furthermore, a prospective cohort study observed that the intake of verapamil and diltiazem, but not nifedipine, was correlated with a greater risk of gastrointestinal hemorrhage in hypertensive persons older than age 67 (16). Other findings in the same cohort suggested that treatment with calcium-channel blockers would be associated with a general increased risk of cancer (17,69).

These observational reports (16–19,69) left a large margin of uncertainty. With regard to myocardial infarction, confounding by indication could not be excluded. Furthermore, as suggested by one editorialist (70), the meta-analysis in patients with coronary heart disease hinged on the inclusion of the 2-week rather than the 6-month follow-up data of two reports (71,72) and included a group of patients with only mild coronary lesions (73). In sensitivity analyses, the increased risk also seemed to be confined to subjects taking at least 80 mg nifedipine per day (18). One report (17) associating the use of calcium-channel blockers with cancer was based on 47 exposed cases spread over a wide variety of cancer sites and only provided information on exposure to calcium-channel blockers at baseline. In the same cohort, patients taking calcium-channel blockers were more likely to be on treatment with warfarin (6.0% vs 2.6%; $P < 0.001$) or aspirin (37.3% vs 29.7%; $P < 0.001$) (17), which may have confounded the issue of gastrointestinal bleeding (16). A nested case-control analysis based on the information taken from the General Practice Research Database in the United Kingdom collected full information on exposure time but did not find an increased cancer risk in users of calcium-channel blockers or angiotensin converting-enzyme inhibitors relative to the patients on beta-blockers (74).

The first-line antihypertensive agent in the Syst-Eur trial was nitrendipine, a calcium-channel blocker of the dihydropyridine class with a terminal plasma half-life of 12 hours (9). The median duration of exposure in the active treatment group was 1.7 years (per-protocol analysis) (23). Compared with the placebo group, no changes occurred in noncardiovascular mortality and the incidence of cancer and bleeding. After termination of the trial on February 14, 1997, all Syst-Eur patients were offered the same treatment as those initially randomized to nitrendipine, enalapril, and hydrochlorothiazide. The Syst-Eur patients will remain in open follow-up to confirm the safety of dihydropyridines in the long-term management of isolated systolic hypertension (75).

C. Use of Calcium-Channel Blockers in Diabetic Patients

Recently, the controversy on the use of calcium-channel blockers found new life in a series of articles (32,76–79) and comments (80) suggesting that calcium-channel blockers, including second-generation dihydropyridines, such as amlodipine (76) or nisoldipine (32), might be harmful, particularly in hypertensive patients with diabetes mellitus. The Syst-Eur Trial is the first double-blind placebo-controlled outcome study that proved that antihypertensive treatment starting with a dihydropyridine calcium-channel blocker was particularly beneficial in diabetic patients (34,81). Cardiovascular benefit was observed as equal in the patients remaining on monotherapy with nitrendipine and in those progressing to combined treatment with nitrendipine plus enalapril, hydrochlorothiazide, or both (34,81).

The Syst-Eur findings in diabetic and nondiabetic patients were recently reinforced by a subgroup analysis of the placebo-controlled Syst-China Trial (68). Of 2394 Syst-China patients, 98 had diabetes (4.1%). On active treatment, the net placebo-subtracted differences in blood pressure after 2 years were −6.0/−4.7 mm Hg in the diabetic patients and −9.3/−3.1 mm Hg in the nondiabetics. With adjustment for possible confounders, active treatment decreased the relative risk in diabetic and nondiabetic patients as follows: −59% versus −36% for total mortality; −57% versus −33% for cardiovascular mortality; and −74% versus −34% for all cardiovascular endpoints. However, because of the small number of diabetic patients, the diabetes-by-treatment interaction terms were not statistically significant. Nevertheless, active treatment reduced the excess cardiovascular mortality and morbidity observed in the diabetic Syst-China patients to a nonsignificant level (68).

D. Prevention of Dementia

In older patients with isolated systolic hypertension, active treatment starting with the dihydropyridine calcium-channel blocker nitrendipine halved the rate of dementia from 7.7 to 3.8 cases per 1000 patient-years (36).

The primary hypothesis tested in the Syst-Eur project on cognitive function was that a reduction in blood pressure would protect against vascular dementia (35). In keeping with this hypothesis, the MMSE scores improved slightly with decreasing diastolic blood pressure in the active treatment group. The prevention of Alzheimer's disease was unexpected, although recent studies indicate that vascular factors, particularly hypertension, may play a role in the development of degenerative dementias as well as vascular dementia proper (82). On the other hand, the observation that antihypertensive treatment with a thiazide did not protect against cognitive impairment in the SHEP trial (10) argues against the prevention of dementia just by lowering the blood pressure. In vascular and degenerative dementias, the calcium-channel blocker nimodipine, compared with placebo, slightly improved the MMSE-scores (83). Thus, an additional or alternative explanation, albeit still unproven, could involve specific neuroprotection conferred by calcium-channel blockade (83–85). Indeed, the aging brain loses its ability to regulate intracellular calcium, leading to a cascade of cellular impairments and, ultimately, to cell death (84,85). In patients with Alzheimer's disease, beta-amyloid may raise the concentration of intraneuronal free calcium and through this very mechanism may sensitize the brain to neurotoxins, such as proinflammatory substances or pro-oxidants (85). The hypothesis of a possible central nervous action of nitrendipine is also supported by the observation that this drug crosses the blood-brain barrier and reduces the turnover of monoamine neurotransmitters (86), of which many are deficient in degenerative dementias (85). Nitrendipine-binding in the rat brain also occurs mainly at those sites that are primarily affected by Alzheimer's disease, such as the superficial cortex, thalamus, and hippocampus, and not in areas with low synaptic density (87).

The potential reduction by 50% of the incidence of dementias by antihypertensive drug treatment initiated with the dihydropyridine calcium-channel blocker nitrendipine may have important public health implications in view of the increasing longevity of populations worldwide. At the rate observed in the placebo group, treating 1000 hypertensive patients for 5 years could prevent 19 cases, a benefit that could even be larger in unselected higher risk groups. This beneficial outcome is in addition to the 53 major cardiovascular endpoints similarly prevented by the active drugs used in the Syst-Eur trial (22).

E. Ambulatory Blood Pressure as Cardiovascular Risk Factor

The Syst-Eur Trial was the first large-scale outcome trial in hypertension in which ambulatory blood pressure recordings were obtained in a substantial proportion of the randomized patients (45–47). In untreated older patients with isolated systolic hypertension, the ambulatory systolic blood pressure, over and above the conventional blood pressure, predicted cardiovascular risk. This was particularly manifest when the ambulatory systolic blood pressure was measured at night or when the whole-day, daytime, or nighttime systolic blood pressures exceeded 142 mm Hg, 145 mm Hg, or 132 mm Hg, respectively. Active treatment almost completely abolished the risk conferred by an increased ambulatory blood pressure at baseline. In the placebo group, the risk conferred by any level of conventional systolic blood pressure at entry declined by nearly one fifth for each 10 mm Hg increase in the white-coat effect (conventional minus daytime blood pressure). Introducing both the conventional and the ambulatory blood pressure as continuous variables in the same Cox regression model, avoided the use of arbitrary diagnostic thresholds to classify the patients into those with white-coat hypertension and those with sustained hypertension.

The hypothesis that nondipping would be associated with greater cardiovascular risk (88) is not generally accepted (89). Poor reproducibility of the dipping status (90) and the use of varying definitions for nondipping (91,92) sustain the controversy. To avoid arbitrary thresholds for the dipping status, the night-to-day blood pressure ratio was analyzed as a continuous variable (47). The hypothesis (88) of an inverse association between cardiovascular risk and the blood pressure fall at night was confirmed. Indeed, with adjustment for the 24-hour blood pressure and other risk factors (23), the cardiovascular risk in the placebo group increased by 41% for each 10% increment in the night-to-day ratio. In addition, in the placebo group and in all patients combined, the nighttime blood pressure behaved as a more consistent predictor of major endpoints than the daytime blood pressure. The influence of physical and psycho-emotional stress may weaken the predictive power of the daytime blood pressure, whereas the greater uniformity resulting from sleeping may help to demonstrate correlations with the nighttime blood pressure. The smaller within-subject coefficient of variation for the nighttime blood pressure than for the daytime blood pressure was in line with this hypothesis (47).

F. The Guidelines for Antihypertensive Drug Treatment Before and After Syst-Eur

In the early 1990s, the role of the newer classes of antihypertensive drugs in the pharmacological treatment of uncomplicated hypertension remained debated (28,93). According to the 1993 guidelines in the United States (94), diuretics and beta-blockers were the only classes of drugs that had been used in long-term controlled clinical trials and shown to reduce morbidity and mortality. They were, therefore, recommended as first-choice agents unless contraindicated or unacceptable, or unless there are special indications for other agents (94). In contrast, a joint committee of the World Health Organization and the International Society of Hypertension (95,96) was of the opinion that although most clinical trials tested diuretics, centrally acting drugs, vasodilators, or beta-blockers, often in combination, no evidence was available that the benefits would have been the result of any particular class of antihypertensive drugs rather than to the lowering of blood pressure per se. These experts recommended several drugs that may be prescribed as first-line treatment of mild sustained hypertension. They listed the drug classes in order of proven benefit on morbidity and mortality as (a) diuretics, (b) beta-blockers, and (c) converting-enzyme blockers, calcium-channel blockers, and alpha-adrenoceptor blocking drugs (95,96). Although both sets of guidelines (94,95) differed in their approach to designate the first-line antihypertensive agents, they were unanimous in recognizing the urgent need to evaluate the effectiveness of calcium-channel blockers and converting-enzyme inhibitors in reducing long-term morbidity and mortality in the treatment of hypertension.

The Syst-Eur trial provided evidence that the newer generations of antihypertensive drugs, particularly the long-acting dihydropyrides, improved prognosis in a large subset of the hypertensive population. In 1997, the Joint National Committee on Prevention, Detection, Evaluation and Treatment of Hypertension took the evidence provided by the Syst-Eur trial into account and revised the guidelines for treating older hypertensive patients (48). The committee recommended that in older patients with isolated systolic hypertension, diuretics remain preferred because they have significantly reduced multiple cardiovascular complications. In addition, the committee acknowledged that the Syst-Eur trial had shown a 42% reduction in fatal and nonfatal stroke over an average 2-year interval and that overall cardiovascular complications had been significantly reduced. The committee concluded that because nitrendipine is not available in the United States, other long-acting dihydropyridine calcium antagonists could be considered to be appropriate alternatives in older patients with systolic hypertension.

In agreement with earlier commentaries (97,98), it is likely that expert committees will further revise the current guidelines for the treatment of older hypertensive patients based on the Syst-Eur results in diabetes mellitus (34,99) and dementia (36). In addition, the observation that the ambulatory blood pressure is a significant predictor of outcome (47), over and above the conventional blood pressure, may lead to new guidelines for selecting patients with sustained hypertension as the most suitable candidates for antihypertensive treatment.

X. CONCLUSIONS

In summing-up the Syst-Eur trial, four conclusions emerge. First, this trial confirmed the SHEP findings (10) that antihypertensive treatment of older patients with isolated systolic hypertension prevents or postpones cerebrovascular and other cardiovascular complications (22,23). Second, the newer antihypertensive drug classes, exemplified by the calcium-channel blocker nitrendipine, with the possible addition of enalapril, are at least equipotent to conventional drugs and may well serve as substitutes for the prevention of cardiovascular complications (27,81). Third, long-acting dihydropyridine calcium-channel blockers may be particularly indicated in patients with isolated systolic hypertension who also have diabetes mellitus (34) or who are at risk of dementia (36). Finally, the circumstantial evidence (16–19,32,69,76–79) for potentially dangerous side effects of calcium-channel blockers has not been borne out when put to the more rigorous test of a double-blind placebo-controlled prospective trial with a median follow-up of 2 years.

ACKNOWLEDGMENTS

This chapter is dedicated to the memory of Prof. A. Amery, who died on November 2, 1994. The Syst-Eur trial was a concerted action of the BIOMED Research Program sponsored by the European Union. The trial was carried out in consultation with the World Health Organization, the International Society of Hypertension, the European Society of Hypertension, and the World Hypertension League. The trial was sponsored by Bayer A.G. (Wuppertal, Germany). The National Fund for Scientific Research (Brussels, Belgium) provided additional support. Study medication was donated by Bayer A.G. and Merck Sharpe and Dohme Inc. (West Point, PA, USA).

Clinical Investigators

Belgium: Guy Adriaens, MD; Bert Aertgeerts, MD; Clem Agten, MD; Robert André, MD; Jean-Marie Berthot, MD; Guy Beuken, MD; Fernand Bolly, MD; Wim Bos, MD; Etienne Bourdon, MD; Johan Buffels, MD; Erwin Buts, MD; Hilde Celis, MD (*Regional Coordinator*); Willem Ceyssens, MD; Jean Claus, MD; Denis Clement, MD; Koen Cornelli, MD; Paul De Cort, MD; Eddy De Graef, MD; Jean-François De Plaen, MD; Geert Decadt, MD; Eddy Dejaeger, MD; Luc Devriendt, MD; Frank Dewaele, MD; Edward Dierickx, MD; Hervé Dieu, MD; Marc Dobbeleir, MD; Michel Druart, MD; Herman Duprez, MD; Raymond Duyck, MD; Robert Fagard, MD; Frans Francis, MD; Marc Geeraert, MD; Phillippe Gilbert, MD; Michel Glibert-Walgraffe, MD; Jean Gremling, MD; Walter Holsters, MD; Jean-Bernard Lafontaine, MD; Benoit Langhoor, MD; Vera Leyssens, MD; Filip Libaut, MD; Pierre-Anne Lourtie, MD; Benny Maes, MD; Walter Onsea, MD; Walter Pelemans, MD; Henri Proost, MD; Jean-Paul Rijckaert, MD; Jan A. Staessen, MD; Chris Van Cauwenberge, MD; Hans Vandenabbeele, MD; André Vandenbroeck, MD; Stef

Vandervliet, MD; Roger Van Hoof, MD; Jan Van Lint, MD; Daniël Vantroyen, MD; Willy Vanverrewegen, MD; Paul Verhaert, MD; André Vlaeminck, MD.

Belorussia: Irina U. Korobko, MD; Irina V. Lazareva, MD; Maria M. Liventseva, MD; Tatjana A. Nechesova, MD; Georgy I. Sidorenko, MD.

Bulgaria: Rozmari P. Alahverdian, MD; Svesolav G. Andreev, MD; Eugeni D. Anev, MD; Malina N. Antova, MD; Vesselin G. Arabadjiev, MD; Boyan I. Asenov, MD; Valentina Baleva, MD; Anastas Batalov, MD; Sonia B. Beleva, MD; Radka M. Beltcheva, MD; Kolio M. Bianov, MD; Tzetana S. Bojanova, MD; Dimitar Z. Bozhinov, MD; Svetla T. Brayanova, MD; Maja P. Dabcheva, MD; Lilia M. Dentcheva, MD; Emil M. Dimitrov, MD; Lilia T. Dimitrova, MD; Todor I. Draganov, MD; Anna Elenkova, MD; Rumiana G. Eremieva, MD; Nicolai B. Ganov, MD; Svetoslav Z. Georgiev, MD; Vesselka I. Gergova , MD; Anton I. Gogov, MD; Eugeni G. Goshev, MD; Mladen Grigorov, MD; Vesselin S. Guidarsky, MD; Iasen G. Ianev, MD; Krassimira Jankulova, MD; Virjinia Jordanova, MD; Deljana K. Kamenova, MD; Rumiana Kermova, MD; Krastjo Kirilov, MD; Lidia Koeva, MD; Zoya Kuneva, MD; Gergana G Lazarova, MD; Emil Lilov, MD; Eli Lubenova, MD; Stefan I Mantov, MD; Temenuga Marinova, MD; Rossitsa P. Mateva, MD; Atanes K. Mihov, MD; Lilia Mitkova, MD; Choudomir Nachev, MD (*Regional Coordinator*): Luba Naidenova, MD; Natalia T. Nikolova, MD; Valeria N. Nikolova, MD; Svetla V. Obretenova, MD; Lilia S. Panteva, MD; Vasa Pasheva, MD; Anton P. Petkov, MD; Peter A. Petrov, MD; Anastas L. Popov, MD; Dimiter G. Popov, MD; Iulia K. Popova, MD; Theodora R. Poryasova, MD; Rada Prokopova, MD; Loida S. Radeva, MD; Rossitsa V. Radoeva, MD; Konstantin N. Ramshev, MD; Katja J. Raykova, MD; Peter B. Rusafov, MD; Boyan E. Shahov, MD (deceased); Zdravka Simeonova, MD; Vera Sirakova, MD; Albena T. Slavtcheva, MD; Diana S. Smilcova, MD; Panajot Solakov, MD; Anna Spasova, MD; Margarita Staneva, MD; Zlatinca M. Stereva, MD; Vassil Stoyanovsky, MD; Tsevtan Tchernev, MD; Snejana Tisheva, MD; Katja T. Todorova, MD; Maya Todorova, MD; Maria Tzekova, MD; Ivan N. Tzenov, MD; Vassel H. Vasilev, MD; Todorka N. Vasileva, MD; Ventrislav I. Veselinov, MD; Angel Volcov, MD; Kiril Yablanski, MD; Yoto T. Yotov, MD; Masusia A. Zaprianova, MD; Rozisa Zdravcova, MD; Zachezar Zozanov, MD.

Croatia: Nrfomkip Pivac, MD; Zvonk Rumboldt, MD.

Estonia: Tovio Laks, MD; Toomas Podar, MD; Uile Planken, MD.

Finland: Jari Airas, MD; Maija Alaluoto, MD; Riitta Antikainen, MD; Mikko V. Haapio, MD; Tapio Hakamäki, MD; Kari Halonen, MD; Matti Jääskivi, MD; Seppo Y. Junnila, MD; Ekki Karonen, MD; Paula Kivinen, MD; Paula S. Kohonen-Jalonen, MD; Pasi Kuusisto, MD; Aapo Lathonen, MD; Anneli Latva-Nevala, MD; Eero Lehmus, MD; Erkki Lehtomäki, MD; Raimo Puustinen, MD; Rita Ristolainen, MD; Eeva Ruotsalainen, MD; Cinzia Sarti, MD; Reijo Tilvis, MD; Jaakko Tuomilehto, MD (*Regional Coordinator*); Hannu Vanhanen, MD (*Associate Member of the Endpoint Committee*); Olavi Vänskä, MD; Hikka Viitanen, MD; Mirjami Viitaniemi, MD; Seija Vinni, MD; Hannu Wallinheimo, MD.

France: Philippe Archaud, MD; Jean-Marc Aupy, MD; Georges Baudassé, MD; Pierre Berger, MD; Antoine Berthelot, MD; Françis Bezot, MD; Benoît Bombecke, MD; Loic Boucher, MD; Jérôme Bousac, MD; Alain Boye, MD; Alain Campagne, MD; Jackie Castellani, MD; François Coisne, MD; Christian Copere, MD; Jean-Achille Cozic, MD; Eric De Sainte Lorette, MD; Alain Delelis-Fanien, MD; Bernard Diadema, MD; Gérard Donnarel, MD; Michèle Escande, MD; Gilles Etchegaray, MD; Hervé Feuiliette, MD; Yves-Michel Flores, MD; Françoise Forette, MD (*Regional Coordinator*); François Fouquet, MD; Gilles François, MD; Isabelie Gabilly, MD; Christian Gaillard, MD; Armelle Gentric, MD; Xavier Girerd, MD; Robert Gorlier, MD (deceased); Alexis Gracovetsky, MD; Michel Grégoire, MD; Ghislaine Henry, MD; Guy Herry, MD; Suzanne Houdry-Pavie, MD; Jean-Richard Israel, MD; Jean-Pierre Jacquemart, MD; Paul-Louis Jacquier, MD; Bruno La Salle, MD; Florence Latour, MD; Jean-Bernard Leblond, MD; Jean-Luc Lebrun, MD; Michel Masieri, MD; Gilles Merceay, MD; Charles-Henri Mercier, MD; Gilbert Meridjen, MD; Pierre Mours, MD; Alain Neveur, MD; Isabelle Périlliat, MD; Dominique Pineau-Valancienne, MD; Alain Pistre, MD; Louis-Marie Pommier, MD; André Ponsot, MD; Jean Pontonnier, MD; Hugues Pujade, MD; Elisabeth Quignard, MD; Didier Rabaud, MD; François Regnaut, MD; Jean-Pierre Ribat, MD; Joël Richard, MD; Claude Robin, MD; Philippe Romejko, MD; Michel Safard, MD; Raymond-Philippe Sarfati, MD; Alain Sarradon, MD; Nicole Savary, MD; Marie-Laure Seux, MD; Marie-Annick Terrienne, MD; Jean-Marc Vigne, MD; Marc Zecconi, MD; Georges Zerbé, MD.

Germany: Jutta Enderlein, MD; Hans-Dieter Faulhaber, MD; Claudia Heuel, MD; Stephan Matthias, MD; Eberhard Ritz, MD (*Regional Coordinator*); Gisela Schundau, MD; Uwe Zwettler, MD.

Greece: Aris D. Efstratopoulos, MD; Kyprionos Nikolaides, MD.

Ireland: Liza Bradley, MD; Danny Collins, MD; John Cox, MD; Joe Duggan, MD; Peter Dupont, MD; Doreen Fagan, MD; Pamela Lennox, MD; Brian Lucey, MD; Fáinsia Mee, RN; Catherine McElearny, MD; Eoin T. O'Brien, MD (*Regional Coordinator*); Kevin O'Malley, MD; Niall Power, MD; Rònan Ryan, MD; Michael Scully, MD.

Israel: Geoffrey Boner, MD; Custava Bott-Kanner, MD; Jose Fidel, MD; Adiv Goldhaber, MD; Eldad Kisch, MD; Irene Kruchin, MD; Alon Margalit, MD; Ilana Moran, MD; Gina Moshe, MD; Joseph Rosenfeld, MD (*Regional Coordinator*); Naftali Stern, MD; Chave Tabenkin, MD; Jack R. Viskoper, MD; Sarah Yodfat, MD; Yair Yodfat, MD; Chaim Yosephy, MD; Jose Zabludowski, MD; Serge Zerapha, MD.

Italy: Basem Abotel-Hag, MD; Ernesto Agostinacchio, MD; Aldrovandi Alessandro, MD; Michele Amoruso, MD; Francesco Bartolomucci, MD; Gratia Bergognoni, MD; Alfredo Bossini, MD; Vito Cagli, MD; Alberto Capra, MD; Mario Condorelli, MD; Mariarosa Del Torre, MD; Rosa Di Mise, MD; Claudio Diveroli, MD; Ernesta Dolce, MD; Monica Fastidio, MD; Roberto Fogari, MD; Evangelo Ivan, MD; Sattuada Lattuada, MD; Gastone Leonetti, MD (*Regional Coordinator*); Almado Libretti, MD; Fabio Lissoni, MD; Giuseppe Maiorano, MD; Giandomenico Malamani, MD; Massimo Merlo, MD; Francesco Minenna, MD; Pietro Nazarro, MD; Angela Palasciano, MD; Paolo Palatini, MD; Carlo Pasotti, MD; Riccardo Pieri, MD; Nazzaro Pietro, MD; Anna Pirrelli, MD; Alessandro Rappelli, MD; Elisabetta Roman, MD; Antonio Salvetti, MD; Michela Simi, MD; Laura Terzoli, MD; Franco Tettamanti, MD; Bruno Trimarco, MD; Alvaro Vaccarella, MD; Vito Vulpis, MD.

Lithuania: Marija R. Babarskiene, MD; Abromiskes Bickauskaite, MD; Jolanta Jasilionyte, MD; Juozas Paukstys, MD; Daiva Rastenyte, MD; Aldona Sereniene, MD.

The Netherlands: Willem H. Birkenhäger, MD (*Regional Coordinator*); Peter W. de Leeuw, MD; Willibrord H.L. Hoefnagels, MD; Arie T.J. Lavrijssen, MD; Arie H. Van den Meiracker, MD; Norbert F. Vogel, MD; Pieter H. Wassenberg, MD; Anton B. Wermenbol, MD; Anno Wester, MD; Arend J. Woittiez, MD.

Poland: Jacek Baszak, MD; Leszek Bieniaszewski, MD; Barbara Broniarczyk, MD; Danuta Czarnecka, MD; Urszula Czubeck, MD; Tomasz Grodzicki, MD; Barbara Gryglewska, MD; Urszula Iwicka, MD; Anna Jach, MD; Kalina Kawecka-Jaszcz, MD; Mariusz Kazmirowicz, MD; Marek Klocek, MD; Jozef Kocemba, MD (*Regional Coordinator*);

Barbara Krupa-Wojciechowska, MD; Marian Markiewicz, MD; Danuta Mroczek-Czernecka, MD; Edmund Nartowicz, MD; Wieslawa Piwowarska, MD; Krystyna Rachon, MD; Marek Rajzer, MD; Michal Tendera, MD.

Portugal: Rosa Afonso, MD; Teleforo B. Afonso, MD; Anabela Bitoque, MD; Anibal Caetano, MD; Almada Cardoso, MD; Manuel Carrageta, MD (*Regional Coordinator*); Helena Concalves, MD; Ana Costa, MD; Diniz Deolinda, MD; José Domingues, MD; Afredo Franco, MD; Gago Leiria, MD; Assuncao Martinez, MD; Armando Medeiros, MD; A. Moeda, MD; Ana Nunes, MD; Pedro Nunes, MD; Rogerio Nunes, MD; José Pascoal, MD; Salome Pereira, MD; Neves Rodrigues, MD; Gaime Segal, MD.

Romania: Speranta Babeanu, MD; Violeta Bogdaneanu, MD; State Doina, MD; Rozeta Draghici, MD; Diana Dumitrascu, MD; Dan L. Dumitrascu, MD; Lavinia Serban, MD.

Russian Federation: Olga Akimora, MD; Guramy G. Arabidze, MD (*Regional Coordinator*); Yuri B. Belousov, MD; Robert S. Bogachov, MD; Lada V. Budrina, MD; Tatjana A. Chlyabi, MD; Angela V. Demenova, MD; Olga V. Efremenkova, MD; Angelina E. Ershova, MD; Alla Y. Ivleva, MD; Tolyana B. Kasatova, MD; Victoriya Kirilyuk, MD; Janna D. Kobalava, MD; Irina A. Komisarenko, MD; Irina V. Kondratova, MD; Irina L. Konstantinova, MD; Alexander Kopelev, MD; Oleg A. Kozyrev, MD; Leonid B. Lazebnik, MD; Marina V. Leonova, MD; Veronika V. Lopykhova, MD; Irina P. Malaya, MD; Natalya V. Malysheva, MD; Olga M. Milyukova, MD; Sergey Moisseyev, MD; Valentin Moisseyev, MD; Sergey V. Nedogoda, MD; Taras M. Nesterenko, MD; Elena V. Oshchepkova, MD; Ludmila E. Salisheva, MD; Tatjana N. Sanina, MD; Inna M. Semenova, MD; Elena Senik, MD; Ekaterina Shkolnikova, MD; Madina M. Sidakova, MD; Boris A. Sidorenko, MD; Aleksei K. Starodoubtsev, MD; Gennady I. Storozhakov, MD; Marina V. Taranova, MD; Sergey Tereshchtenko, MD; Elena A. Toporova, MD; Galina A. Vereshchagina, MD; Sergey K. Zubkov, MD.

Slovakia: Zora Gérová, MD; Katha Jureckova, MD; Katha Sedlakova, MD.

Slovenia: Rok Accetto, MD; Bruno Bucic, MD; Jurij Dobovisek, MD; Primoz Dolenc, MD; Borut Kolsek, MD; Zdenko Lapanja, MD; Maja Mihelic-Brcic, MD; Jurij Petrin, MD; Olga Pirc-Cercek, MD; Ales Zemva, MD.

Spain: José Abellan, MD; Javier Aranda, MD; Manuel Arjona-Garcia, MD; Maria Barreda, MD; Gador Chamorro-Barrionuevo, MD; José Fernandez, MD; Blas Gill-Extremera, MD; Luis gonzalez-Gomez, MD; Pedro Aranda-Lara, MD; Antonia Maldonado-Martin, MD; Rafael Marin, MD; Josefina O. Martinez, MD; Fernando H. Meneguez, MD; Rex Molina, MD; José Mora-Macia, MD; Ernesto Lopez de Novales, MD; Joan Ocón-Pujadas, MD; José Ortega, MD; Alenta H. Pardell, MD; Fernanda Plaza, MD; Josep Redón, MD; José L. Rodicio, MD (*Regional Coordinator*); Luis M. Ruilope, MD; Leticia Soriano-Carrascosa, MD; Francisco F. Vega, MD.

United Kingdom: Peter Andrews, MD; Sally G. Armstrong, RN; Gareth D. Beevers, MD; Michèle Beevers, MD; P. Bruce-Jones, MD; Christopher J. Bulpitt, MD (*Regional Coordinator*); David Choat, MD; Wendy Crichton, RN; Peter Crome, MD; Christopher Davidson, MD; Colin T. Dollery, MD; Astrid E. Fletcher, PhD; Nicola Gainsborough, MD; Nandin D.P. Gunawardena, MD; Nigel Higson, MD; Stephen Jackson, MD; Christopher Kingswood, MD; David Kluth, MD; Dan Lee, MD; Peter J. Luce, MD; Ganesh Mankikar, MD; Anthony O'Brien, MD; Hugh O'Neal, MD; James C. Petrie, MD; Chakravarthi Rajkumar, MD; Andrew K. Scott, MD; Paul Sharpstone, MD; David I. Slovick, MD; Ian D. Starke, MD; Jean Timeyin, RN; Kenneth Tsang, MD; John Webster, MD; Peter Wilkinson, MD; Katia Witte, RN.

Committees and Coordination

Trial Coordinators: Robert Fagard, MD; Jan A. Staessen, MD.

Data Monitoring Committee: Christopher J. Bulpitt, MD; Astrid E. Fletcher, PhD; Jan A. Staessen, MD; Lutgarde Thijs, BSc.

Drug Committee: Hilde Celis, MD; Guy Demol, MD; Pierre Demol, MD; Robert Fagard, MD; Günther E. Hübner, MD; Jan A. Staessen, MD.

Endpoint Committee: Peter W. de Leeuw, MD; Robert Fagard, MD; Gastone Leonetti, MD; James C. Petrie, MD.

Ethics Committee: Willem H. Birkenhäger, MD; Colin T. Dollery, MD; Robert Fagard, MD.

Liaison Committee with the European Union: Willem H. Birkenhäger, MD; Fernando De Padua, MD; Colin T. Dollery, MD; Aris D. Efstratopoulos, MD; Robert Fagard, MD; Françoise Forette, MD; Detlev Ganten, MD; Eoin T. O'Brien, MD; Kevin O'Malley, MD; José L. Rodicio, MD; Jaakko Tuomilehto, MD; Charles van Ypersele, MD; Alberto Zanchetti, MD.

Publication Committee: Willem H. Birkenhäger, MD; Christopher J. Bulpitt, MD; Jan A. Staessen, MD; Alberto Zanchetti, MD.

Steering Committee: Guramy G. Arabidze, MD; Paul De Cort, MD; Robert Fagard, MD; Françoise Forette, MD; Kalina Kawecka-Jaszcz, MD; Gastone Leonetti, MD; Choudomir Nachev, MD; Eoin T. O'Brien, MD; José L. Rodico, MD; Joseph Rosenfeld, MD; Jaakko Tuomilehto, MD; John Webster, MD; Yair Yodfat, MD.

Coordinators of the Project on Ambulatory Blood Pressure Monitoring: Denis Clement, MD; Eoin T. O'Brien, MD; Giuseppe Mancia, MD; Gianfranco Parati, MD; Jan A. Staessen, MD; Lutgarde Thijs, BSc.

Coordinators of the Project on Vascular Dementia: Françoise Forette, MD; Thomas Strasser, MD.

Coordinators of the Project on Quality of Life: Christopher J. Bulpitt, MD; Astrid E. Fletcher, PhD.

Coordinators of General Practices: Hilde Celis, MD in collaboration with Jan Heyrman, MD; Gérard Stibbe, MD, and Michel Van den Haute, MD; Yair Yodfat, MD.

Coordinating Office: Nicole Auseloos; Hilde Celis, MD; Lut De Pauw, RN; Paul Drent, RN; Dimitri Emelianov, MD; Robert Fagard, MD; Heng Fan; J. Gasowski, MD; Tatjana Kutznetsova, MD; Viviane Mariën; Yvette Piccart; Jan A. Staessen, MD; Yvette Toremans; Lutgarde Thijs, BSc; Sven Vandenreycken; Roger Van Hoof, MD; Sylvia Van Hulle, RN; Jiguang Wang, MD (*Liaison with the Syst-China Trial Investigators*); Renilde Wolfs.

Regional Drug Dispatching Centers: Mariana Bontscheva, MD (Bulgaria); Carola Borsati, MD (Germany); Lesly Carmody, MD (United Kingdom); Efrat Caspi, MD; Daniel Koerner, MD (Israel); Sabine Coppens, MD (Belgium); Hans Eeltink, MD (the Netherlands); Mariangela Ferrari MD (Italy); Konsantin Gravilov, MD (Belorussia and the Russian Federation); Janko Hacundova, MD (Slovakia); Maija Kinnunen, MD (Estonia, Finland and Lithuania); Nada Lozey, MD (Slovenia); Antonio Nolasco, MD (Portugal); Janina Pawlowska, MD (Poland); Marc Pételaud, MD (France); Carmen Pinol, MD (Spain); George Sotiriadis, MD (Greece); Marija Stipic, MD (Croatia); Maya Thompson, MD (Ireland); Donia Verzea, MD (Romania); Jaroslava Vylitova, MD (Czech Republic).

REFERENCES

1. Amery A, Birkenhäger W, Brixko P, Bulpitt C, Clement D, Deruyttere M, de Schaepdryver A, Dollery C, Fagard R, Forette F, Forte J, Hamdy R, Henry JF, Joossens JV, Leonetti G, Lund-Johansen P, O'Malley K, Petrie J, Strasser T, Tuomilehto J, Williams B. Mortality and morbidity results from the European Working Party on High Blood Pressure in the Elderly trial. Lancet 1985; i:1349–1354.
2. Coope J, Warrender TS. Randomised trial of treatment of hypertension in elderly patients in primary care. Br Med J 1986; 293:1145–1151.
3. Hypertension Detection and Follow-up Program Cooperative Group. five-year findings of the Hypertension Detection and Follow-up Program. II. Mortality by race-sex and age. JAMA 1979; 242:2572–2577.
4. Management Committee. Treatment of mild hypertension in the elderly. A study initiated and administered by the National Heart Foundation of Australia. Med J Aust 1981; 2:398–402.
5. Kuramoto K, Matsushita S, Kuwajima I, Murakami M. Prospective study on the treatment of mild hypertension in the aged. Jpn Heart J 1981; 22:75–85.
6. Staessen J, Fagard R, Van Hoof R, Amery A. Mortality in various intervention trials in elderly hypertensive patients: a review. Eur Heart J 1988; 9:215–222.
7. Staessen J, Amery A, Fagard R. Editorial review. Isolated systolic hypertension in the elderly. J Hypertens 1990; 8:393–405.
8. Amery A, Birkenhäger W, Bulpitt CJ, Clement D, de Leeuw P, Dollery CT, Fagard R, Fletcher A, Forette F, Leonetti G, O'Brien ET, O'Malley K, Rodicio JL, Rosenfeld J, Staessen J, Strasser T, Terzoli L, Thijs L, Tuomilehto J, Webster J. Syst-Eur. A multicentre trial on the treatment of isolated systolic hypertension in the elderly: objectives, protocol, and organization. Aging Clin Exp Res 1991; 3:287–302.
9. Goa KL, Sorkin EM. Nitrendipine. A review of its pharmacodynamic and pharmacokinetic properties and therapeutic efficacy in the treatment of hypertension. Drugs 1987; 33:123–155.
10. SHEP Cooperative Research Group. Prevention of stroke by antihypertensive drug treatment in older persons with isolated systolic hypertension. Final results of the Systolic Hypertension in the Elderly Program (SHEP). JAMA 1991; 265:3255–3264.
11. Fletcher A, Spiegelhalter D, Staessen J, Thijs L, Bulpitt C. Implications for trials in progress of publication of positive results. Lancet 1993; 342:653–657.
12. Kaplan NM. Systolic Hypertension in the Elderly Program (SHEP) and Swedish Trial in Old Patients With Hypertension (STOP). The promises and the potential problems. Am J Hypertens 1992; 5:331–334.
13. Ménard J, Day M, Chatellier G, Laragh JH. Some lessons from Systolic Hypertension in the Elderly Program (SHEP). Am J Hypertens 1992; 5:325–330.
14. Staessen J, Fagard R, Amery A. Isolated systolic hypertension in the elderly: implications of SHEP for clinical practice and for the ongoing trials. J Hum Hypertens 1991; 5:469–474.
15. Staessen JA, Amery A, Birkenhäger W. Inverse association between baseline pressure and benefit from treatment in isolated systolic hypertension. Hypertension 1994; 23:269–270.
16. Pahor M, Guralnik JM, Furberg CD, Carbonin P, Havlik RJ. Risk of gastrointestinal haemorrhage with calcium antagonists in hypertensive persons over 67 years old. Lancet 1996; 347: 1061–1065.
17. Pahor M, Guralnik JM, Ferrucci L, Corti MC, Salive ME, Cerhan JR, Wallace RB, Havlik RJ. Calcium-channel blockade and incidence of cancer in aged populations. Lancet 1996; 348: 493–497.
18. Furberg CD, Psaty BM, Meyer JV. Nifedipine. Dose-related increase in mortality in patients with coronary heart disease. Circulation 1995; 92:1326–1331.

19. Psaty BM, Heckbert SR, Koepsell TD, Siscovick DS, Raghunathan TE, Weiss NS, Rosendaal FR, Lemaitre RN, Smith NL, Wahl PW, Wagner EH, Furberg CD. The risk of myocardial infarction associated with antihypertensive drug therapies. JAMA 1995; 274:620–625.
20. 41st World Medical Assembly. Declaration of Helsinki: recommendations guiding physicians in biomedical research involving human subjects. Bull Pan Am Health Organ 1990; 24:606–609.
21. *International Classification of Diseases. Manual of the International Statistical Classification of Diseases, Injuries, and Causes of Death. Based on the Recommendations of the Ninth Revision Conference, 1975, and Adopted by the Twenty-Ninth World Health Assembly.* Volume 1. Geneva, Switzerland: World Health Organization, 1977.
22. Staessen JA, Fagard R, Thijs L, Celis H, Arabidze GG, Birkenhäger WH, Bulpitt CJ, de Leeuw PW, Dollery CT, Fletcher AE, Forette F, Leonetti G, Nachev C, O'Brien ET, Rosenfeld J, Rodicio JL, Tuomilehto J, Zanchetti A, for the Systolic Hypertension in Europe (Syst-Eur) Trial Investigators. Randomised double-blind comparison of placebo and active treatment for older patients with isolated systolic hypertension [erratum published in Lancet 1997; 350: 1636]. Lancet 1997; 350:757–764.
23. Staessen JA, Fagard R, Thijs L, Celis H, Birkenhäger WH, Bulpitt CJ, de Leeuw PW, Fletcher AE, Babarskiene MR, Forette F, Kocemba J, Laks T, Leonetti G, Nachev C, Petrie JC, Tuomilehto J, Vanhanen H, Webster J, Yodfat Y, Zanchetti A, for the Systolic Hypertension in Europe (Syst-Eur) Trial Investigators. Subgroup and per-protocol analysis of the randomized European trial on isolated systolic hypertension in the elderly. Arch Intern Med 1998; 158: 1681–1691.
24. Cox DR. Regression models and life tables. J R Stat Soc B 1972; 34:187–220.
25. O'Brien PC, Fleming TR. A multiple testing procedure for clinical trials. Biometrics 1979; 35:549–556.
26. Report of a WHO Study Group. *Prevention of Diabetes Mellitus*. Geneva, Switzerland: World Health Organization, 1994.
27. Staessen JA, Thijs L, Fagard RH, Birkenhäger WH, Arabidze G, Babeanu S, Gil-Extremera B, Bulpitt CJ, Davidson C, de Leeuw P, Efstratopoulos AD, Fletcher AE, Fogari R, Jääskivi M, Kawecka-Jaszcz K, Nachev C, Petrie JC, Seux ML, Tuomilehto J, Webster J, for the Systolic Hypertension in Europe (Syst-Eur) Trial Investigators. Calcium channel blockade and cardiovascular prognosis in the European trial on isolated systolic hypertension. Hypertension 1998; 32:410–416.
28. Furberg CD, Psaty BM. Calcium antagonists: not appropriate as first line antihypertensive agents. Am J Hypertens 1996; 9:122–125.
29. Furberg CD, Psaty BM. JNC VI: timing is everything. Lancet 1997; 350:1413–1414.
30. Heckbert SR, Longstreth WT Jr, Psaty BM, Murros KE, Smith NL, Newman AB, Williamson JD, Bernick C, Furberg CD. The association of antihypertensive agents with MRI white matter findings and the Modified Mini-Mental State Examination in older adults. J Am Geriatr Soc 1997; 45:1423–1433.
31. Psaty BM, Furberg CD. Clinical implications of the World Health Organization—International Society of Hypertension statement on calcium antagonists. J Hypertens 1997; 15:1197–1200.
32. Estacio RO, Jeffers BW, Hiatt WR, Biggerstaff SL, Gifford N, Schrier RW. The effect of nisoldipine as compared with enalapril on cardiovascular outcomes in patients with non-insulin-dependent diabetes and hypertension. N Engl J Med 1998; 338:645–652.
33. Staessen JA, Thijs L, Birkenhäger WH, Bulpitt CJ, Fagard R, on behalf of the Syst-Eur Investigators. Update on the Systolic Hypertension in Europe (Syst-Eur) Trial. Hypertension 1999; 33:1476–1477.
34. Tuomilehto J, Rastenyte D, Birkenhäger WH, Thijs L, Antikainen R, Bulpitt CJ, Fletcher AE, Forette F, Goldhaber A, Palatini P, Sarti C, Fagard R, for the Systolic Hypertension in Europe (Syst-Eur) Trial Investigators. Effects of calcium-channel blockade in older patients with diabetes and systolic hypertension. N Engl J Med 1999; 340:677–684.

35. Forette F, Amery A, Staessen J, Strasser T, Thijs L, Beevers DG, Bert P, Clement D, Cox J, de Leeuw PW, De Plaen JF, Donnarel G, Escande M, Fagard R, Girerd X, Hickey A, Pandita-Gunawardena ND, Perilliat I, Ruilope M, Slovick D, Terzoli L, Varis R, Webster JR. Is prevention of vascular dementia possible? The Syst-Eur Vascular Dementia Project. Aging Clin Exp Res 1991; 3:373–382.
36. Forette F, Seux ML, Staessen JA, Thijs L, Birkenhäger WH, Babarskiene MR, Babeanu S, Bossini A, Gil-Extremera B, Girerd X, Laks T, Lilov E, Moisseyev V, Tuomilehto J, Vanhanen H, Webster B, Yodfat Y, Fagard R, on behalf of the Syst-Eur Investigators. Prevention of dementia in randomised double-blind placebo-controlled Systolic Hypertension in Europe (Syst-Eur) trial. Lancet 1998; 352:1347–1351.
37. Seux ML, Thijs L, Forette F, Staessen JA, Birkenhäger WH, Bulpitt CJ, Girerd X, Jääskivi M, Vanhanen H, Kivinen P, Yodfat Y, Vänskä O, Antikainen R, Laks T, Webster JR, Hakamäki T, Lehtomäki E, Lilov E, Grigirov M, Janculova K, Halonen K, Kohonen-Jalonen P, Kermova R, Nachev C, Tuomilehto J. Correlates of cognitive status of old patients with isolated systolic hypertension: the Syst-Eur Vascular Dementia Project. J Hypertens 1998; 16:963–969.
38. Folstein MF, Folstein SE, McHugh PR. ''Mini-Mental State.'' A practical method for grading the cognitive state of patients for the clinician. J Psychiat Res 1975; 12:189–198.
39. *Diagnostic and Statistical Manual of Mental Disorders*. Washington DC: American Psychiatric Association, 1987.
40. Letenneur L, Commenges RD, Dartigues JF, Barberger-Gateau P. Incidence of dementia and Alzheimer's disease in elderly community residents of south-western France. Int J Epidemiol 1994; 23:1256–1261.
41. Launer JL. Overview of incidence studies of dementia conducted in Europe. Neuroepidemiology 1992; 11 (suppl 1):2–13.
42. Ott A, Breteler MMB, van Harskamp F, Grobbee DE, Hofman A. The incidence of dementia in the Rotterdam study. In: Iqbal K, Winblad B, Nishimura T, Takeda K, Winieski H, eds. *Alzheimer's Disease, Biology, Diagnosis and Therapeutics*. New York: John Wiley and Sons Ltd., 1997; 1–10.
43. Loeb C, Gandolfo C. Diagnostic evaluation of degenerative and vascular dementia. Stroke 1983; 14:399–401.
44. Hachinski VC, Lliff LD, Zilkha E, Du Boulay GH, McAllister UL, Marshall J, Russel RWR, Symon L. Cerebral blood flow in dementia. Arch Neurol 1975; 32:632–637.
45. Staessen J, Amery A, Clement D, Cox J, De Cort P, Fagard R, Guo C, Marin R, O'Brien ET, O'Malley K, Mancia G, Parati G, Ravogli A, Thijs L, Webster J. Twenty-four hour blood pressure monitoring in the Syst-Eur trial. Aging Clin Exp Res 1992; 4:85–91.
46. Emelianov D, Thijs L, Staessen JA, Celis H, Clement D, Davidson C, Gasowski J, Gil-Extremera B, Fogari R, Jääskivi M, Lehtonen A, Nedogoda S, O'Brien E, Palatini P, Salvetti A, Vanhanen H, Webster J, Fagard R, on behalf of the Syst-Eur Investigators. Conventional and ambulatory blood pressure measurement in older patients with isolated systolic hypertension: baseline observations in the Syst-Eur trial. Blood Press Monit 1998; 3:173–180.
47. Staessen JA, Thijs L, Fagard R, O'Brien ET, Clement D, de Leeuw PW, Mancia G, Nachev C, Palatini P, Parate G, Tuomilheto J, Webster J, for the Systolic Hypertension in Europe Trial Investigators. Predicting cardiovascular risk using conventional vs ambulatory blood pressure in older patients with systolic hypertension. JAMA 1999; 282:539–546.
48. The Joint National Committee on Prevention Detection Evaluation and Treatment of High Blood Pressure. The sixth report of the Joint National Committee on Prevention, Detection, Evaluation, and Treatment of High Blood Pressure (JNC VI). Arch Intern Med 1997; 157: 2413–2446.
49. Staessen JA, O'Brien ET, Amery AK, Atkins N, Baumgart P, De Cort P, Degaute JP, Dolenc P, De Gaudemaris R, Enström I, Fagard R, Gosse P, Gourlay S, Hayashi H, Imai Y, James G, Kawasaki T, Kuschnir E, Kuwajima I, Lindholm L, Liu L, Macor F, Mancia G, McGrath B, Middeke M, Ming J, Omboni S, Otsuka K, Palatini P, Parati G, Pieper C, Verdecchia P,

Zachariah P, Zhang W. Ambulatory blood pressure in normotensive and hypertensive subjects: results from an international database. J Hypertens 1994; 12 (suppl 7):S1–S12.

50. Staessen JA, Thijs L, Bieniaszewski L, O'Brien ET, Palatini P, Davidson C, Dobovisek J, Jääskivi M, Laks T, Lehtonen A, Vanhanen H, Webster J, Fagard R, on behalf of the Systolic Hypertension in Europe (SYST-EUR) Trial Investigators. Ambulatory monitoring uncorrected for placebo overestimates long-term antihypertensive action. Hypertension 1996; 27:414–420.
51. Staessen JA, Thijs L, Mancia G, Parati G, O'Brien ET, on behalf of the Syst-Eur Investigators. Clinical trials with ambulatory blood pressure monitoring: fewer patients needed? Lancet 1994; 344:1552–1556.
52. Staessen JA, Thijs L, Bijttebier G, Clement D, O'Brien ET, Palatini P, Rodicio J, Rosenfeld J, Fagard R, on behalf of the Systolic Hypertension in Europe (SYST-EUR) Trial Investigators. Determining the trough-to-peak ratio in parallel-group trials. Hypertension 1997; 29:659–667.
53. Fagard R, Brguljan J, Thijs L, Staessen J. Prediction of the actual awake and asleep blood pressures by various methods of 24 h pressure analysis. J Hypertens 1996; 14:557–563.
54. Blacher J, Staessen JA, Girerd X, Gasowski J, Thijs L, Liu L, Wang JG, Fagard RH, Safar ME. Pulse pressure—not mean pressure—determines cardiovascular risk in older hypertensive patients. Arch Intern Med 2000; 160:1085–1089.
55. Liu L, Wang JG, Gong L, Liu G, Staessen JA, for the Systolic Hypertension in China (Syst-China) Collaborative Group. Comparison of active treatment and placebo for older patients with isolated systolic hypertension. J Hypertens 1998; 16:1823–1829.
56. Dahlöf B, Lindholm LH, Hansson L, Scherstén B, Ekbom T, Wester PO. Morbidity and mortality in the Swedish Trial in Old Patients with Hypertension (STOP-Hypertension). Lancet 1991; 338:1281–1285.
57. Kuramoto K, Mutsushita S, Kuwajima I. The pathogenetic role and treatment of elderly hypertension. Jpn Circ J 1981; 45:833–843.
58. MRC Working Party. Medical Research Council trial of treatment of hypertension in older adults: principal results. BMJ 1992; 304:405–412.
59. Thijs L, Fagard R, Lijnen P, Staessen J, Van Hoof R, Amery A. A meta-analysis of outcome trials in elderly hypertensives. J Hypertens 1992; 10:1103–1109.
60. Lever AF, Ramsay LE. Editorial review: treatment of hypertension in the elderly. J Hypertens 1995; 13:571–579.
61. Thijs L, Fagard R, Lijnen P, Staessen J, Van Hoof R, Amery A. Why is antihypertensive drug therapy needed in elderly patients with systolodiastolic hypertension? J Hypertens 1994; 12 (suppl 6):S25–S34.
62. Celis H, Yodfat Y, Thijs L, Clement D, Cozic J, De Cort P, Forette F, Grégoire M, Heyrman J, Stibbe G, Van den Haute M, Staessen J, Fagard R, on behalf of the Syst-Eur Investigators. Antihypertensive therapy in older patients with isolated systolic hypertension: the Syst-Eur experience in general practice. Fam Pract 1996; 13:138–143.
63. Medical Research Council Working Party. MRC trial of treatment of mild hypertension: principal results. BMJ 1985; 291:97–104.
64. Hansson L, Zanchetti A, Carruthers SG, Dahlöf B, Elmfeldt D, Julius S, Ménard J, Rahn KH, Wedel H, Westerling S, for the HOT Study Group. Effects of intensive blood pressure lowering and low-dose aspirin in patients with hypertension: principal results of the Hypertension Optimal Treatment (HOT) randomised trial. Lancet 1998; 351:1755–1762.
65. Hamet P, Gong L. Chinese contribution to trials on antihypertensive therapy. J Hypertens 1996; 14 (suppl 2):S123–S128.
66. Gong L, Zhang W, Zhu Y, Zhu J, 11 collaborating centres in the Shanghai area, Kong D, Pagé V, Ghadirian P, LeLorier J, Hamet P. Shanghai Trial of Nifedipine in the Elderly (STONE). J Hypertens 1996; 14:1237–1245.
67. Wang J, Liu G, Wang X, Zhang S, Sun M, Pan X, Jian M, Gong L, Thijs L, Staessen J, Fagard R, Liu L, on behalf of the Syst-China Investigators. Long-term blood pressure control in older

Chinese patients with isolated systolic hypertension: a progress report on the Syst-China trial. J Hum Hypertens 1996; 10:735–742.
68. Wang JG, Staessen JA, Gong L, Liu L, for the Systolic Hypertension in China (SYST-CHINA) collaborative group Chinese trial on isolated systolic hypertension in the elderly. Arch Intern Med 2000; 160:211–220.
69. Pahor M, Guralnik JM, Salive ME, Corti MC, Carbonin P, Havlik RJ. Do calcium channel blockers increase the risk of cancer? Am J Hypertens 1996; 9:695–699.
70. Opie LH, Messerli FH. Nifedipine and mortality. Grave defects in the dossier. Circulation 1995; 92:1068–1073.
71. Muller JE, Turi ZG, Pearle DL, Schneider JF, Serfas DH, Morrison J, Stone PH, Rude RE, Rosner B, Sobel BE, Tate C, Scheiner E, Roberts R, Hennekens CH, Braunwald E. Nifedipine and conventional therapy for unstable angina pectoris: a randomized double-blind comparison. Circulation 1984; 69:728–739.
72. Muller JE, Morrison J, Stone PH, Rude RE, Rosner B, Roberts R, Pearle DL, Turi ZG, Schneider JF, Serfas DH, Tate C, Scheiner E, Sobel BE, Hennekens CH, Braunwald E. Nifedipine therapy for patients with threatened and acute myocardial infarction: a randomized double-blind placebo-controlled comparison. Circulation 1984; 69:740–747.
73. Lichtlen PR, Hugenholtz PG, Rafflenbeul W, Hecker H, Jost S, Nikutta P, Deckers JW, on behalf of the INTACT Group Investigators. Retardation of coronary artery disease in humans by the calcium-channel blocker nifedipine: results of the INTACT Study (International Trial on Antiatherosclerotic Therapy). Cardiovasc Drugs Ther 1990; 4:1047–1068.
74. Jick H, Jick S, Derby LE, Vasilakis C, Myers MW, Meier CR. Calcium-channel blockers and risk of cancer. Lancet 1997; 349:525–528.
75. Gasowski J, Staessen JA, Celis H, Fagard RH, Thijs L, Birkenhäger WH, Bulpitt CJ, Fletcher AE, Arabidze GG, de Leeuw P, Dollery CT, Duggan J, Kawecka-Jaszcz K, Leonetti G, Nachev C, Safar M, Rodicio JL, Rosenfeld J, Seux ML, Tuomilehto J, Webster J, Yodfat Y, on behalf of the Systolic Hypertension in Europe Investigators. Systolic Hypertension in Europe (Syst-Eur) Trial Phase 2: objectives, protocol and initial progress. J Hum Hypertens 1999; 13:135–145.
76. Tatti P, Pahor M, Byington RB, Di Mauro P, Guarisco R, Strollo G, Strollo F. Outcome results of the Fosinopril versus Amlodipine Cardiovascular Events Randomized Trial (FACET) in patients with hypertension and NIDDM. Diabetes Care 1998; 21:597–603.
77. Alderman M, Madhavan S, Cohen H. Calcium antagonists and cardiovascular events in patients with hypertension and diabetes. Lancet 1998; 351:216–217.
78. Byington RP, Craven TE, Furberg CD, Pahor M. Isradipine, raised glycosylated haemoglobin, and risk of cardiovascular events. Lancet 1998; 350:1075–1076.
79. Pahor M, Kritchevsky SB, Zuccala G, Guralnik JM. Diabetes and risk of adverse events with calcium antagonists. Diabetes Care 1998; 21:193–194.
80. Pahor M, Psaty BM, Furberg CD. Treatment of hypertensive patients with diabetes. Lancet 1998; 351:689–690.
81. Staessen JA, Thijs L, Gasowski J, Celis H, Fagard RH, for the Systolic Hypertension in Europe (Syst-Eur) Trial Investigators. Treatment of isolated systolic hypertension in the elderly: further evidence from the Systolic Hypertension in Europe (Syst-Eur) Trial. Am J Cardiol 1998; 82:20R–22R.
82. Hofman A, Ott A, Breteler MMB, Bots M, Slooter AJC, van Harskamp F, van Duijn CN, Van Broeckhoven C, Grobbee DE. Atherosclerosis, apolipoprotein E, and prevalence of dementia and Alzheimer's disease in the Rotterdam Study. Lancet 1997; 349:151–154.
83. Morich FJ, Bieber F, Lewis JM, Kaiser L, Cutler NR, Escobar JI, Willmer J, Petersen RC, Reisberg B, the North American Nimodipine Study Group. Nimodipine in the treatment of probable Alzheimer's disease: result of two multicentre trials. Clin Drug Invest 1996; 11:185–195.
84. Thompson LT, Moyer JR Jr, Black J, Disterhoft JF. Cellular mechanisms for nimodipine's

reduction of aging related learning deficits. In: Meyer EM, Simpkins JW, Yamamoto J, Crews FT, eds. *Treatment of Dementias. A New Generation of Progress*. New York: Plenum Press, 1992:241–256.

85. Parneti L, Senin U, Mecocci P. Cognitive enhancement therapy for Alzheimer's disease. The way forward. Drugs 1997; 53:752–768.
86. Hong YL. The relationship between calcium antagonist-induced hypotension and central monoaminergic system in spontaneously hypertensive rats. Int J Clin Pharmacol Ther Toxicol 1987; 11:589–597.
87. Gould RJ, Murphy KMM, Snyder SH. Autoradiographic localization of calcium channel antagonist receptors in rat brain with [^{3}H]nitrendipine. Brain Res 1985; 330:217–223.
88. O'Brien E, Sheridan J, O'Malley K. Dippers and non-dippers. Lancet 1988; ii:397.
89. Fagard R, Staessen JA, Thijs L. The relationships between left ventricular mass and daytime and night-time blood pressures: a meta-analysis of comparative studies. J Hypertens 1995; 13:823–829.
90. Staessen J, Bulpitt CJ, O'Brien E, Cox J, Fagard R, Stanton A, Thijs L, Van Hulle S, Vyncke G, Amery A. The diurnal blood pressure profile. A population study. Am J Hypertens 1992; 5:386–392.
91. Verdecchia P, Porcellati C, Schillaci G, Borgioni C, Ciucci A, Battistelli M, Guerrieri M, Gatteschi C, Zampi I, Santucci A, Santucci C, Reboldi G. Ambulatory blood pressure. An independent predictor of prognosis in essential hypertension. Hypertension 1994; 24:793–801.
92. Staessen JA, Bieniaszewski L, O'Brien E, Gosse P, Hayashi H, Imai Y, Kawasaki T, Otsuka K, Palatini P, Thijs L, Fagard R, on behalf of the ''Ad Hoc'' Working Group. Nocturnal blood pressure fall on ambulatory monitoring in a large international database. Hypertension 1997; 29:30–39.
93. Swales JD. Pharmacological treatment of hypertension. Lancet 1994; 344:380–385.
94. The Joint National Committee on Detection Evaluation and Treatment of High Blood Pressure. The fifth report of the Joint National Committee on Detection, Evaluation, and Treatment of High Blood Pressure (JNC V). Arch Intern Med 1993; 153:154–183.
95. The Guidelines Subcommittee of the WHO/ISH Mild Hypertension Liaison Committee. 1993 guidelines for the management of mild hypertension. Memorandum from a World Health Organization/International Society of Hypertension Meeting. Hypertension 1993; 22:392–403.
96. Zanchetti A. Guidelines for the management of hypertension: the World Health Organization/International Society of Hypertension view. J Hypertens 1995; 13 (suppl 2):S119–S122.
97. Hansson L, Hedner T, Jern S. Break-through for calcium antagonists based on the Syst-Eur results. Blood Press 1998; 7:3–4.
98. Potter J. The SYST-EUR study—calcium channel blockers coming of age? J Hum Hypertens 1998; 11:619–620.
99. Birkenhäger WH, Staessen JA. Treatment of diabetic patients with hypertension. Current Hypertension Reports, 1999. In press.

15

Hypertension Optimal Treatment (HOT) Study

ALBERTO ZANCHETTI

Università di Milano, Ospedale Maggiore and Istituto Auxologico Italiano, Milan, Italy

LENNART HANSSON

University of Uppsala, Uppsala, Sweden

I. PRIOR HYPOTHESES

A. Cardiovascular Events in Treated Hypertensive Patients

A large number of randomized controlled trials have documented the benefit of lowering blood pressure with antihypertensive drugs, having shown a particularly striking reduction in fatal and nonfatal strokes and a less marked, although significant, reduction in coronary events (1). However, treated hypertensive patients are known to run a considerably higher risk of cardiovascular complications than matched normotensive subjects of the same age and sex. In the Dalby study, a significantly higher cardiovascular morbidity rate was found in most age groups when treated hypertensive patients in this southern Swedish community were compared with age and sex-matched normotensive individuals from the same community in a 3-year retrospective study (2). In the Dalby study, it was obvious that highly statistically significant reductions in arterial pressure had been obtained in the treated individuals. Despite this, blood pressure levels in the treated patients were still significantly higher than in the matched normotensive subjects (2). It is therefore not unlikely that the failure to ''normalize'' the risk in the treated patients may have been the result of the failure of ''normalizing'' their blood pressure.

A similar type of study in the Glasgow Blood Pressure Clinic investigated mortality in treated hypertensive patients (3). The mortality in almost 4000 patients with nonmalignant hypertension was compared with that of two control populations near Glasgow during a 6.5-year period. Somewhat disappointingly, the mortality in the treated hypertensive patients was found to be 2 to 5 times higher than in the normal populations (3).

Results of the kind shown in the Dalby and Glasgow studies, that is, higher cardiovascular morbidity and mortality in treated hypertensive patients than in matched normotensive subjects, could be explained by several different circumstances. It is obvious from the two studies that the level of blood pressure in the treated patients was higher than in the normotensive subjects and that benefits of treatment were greater in those in whom blood pressure had been reduced most. This suggests that insufficient lowering of the elevated blood pressure may have been an important explanation for the high morbidity and mortality found in the treated hypertensive patients.

It is also clear that substantial proportions of treated hypertensive patients do not reach goal blood pressure. This is not only shown by surveys of medical practices in various countries (4), but, as shown in Table 1, in controlled trials of antihypertensive therapy as well, where between one fifth and almost half of all treated patients failed to reach goal blood pressures.

B. The J-Shaped Curve Hypothesis

Even if the results of several intervention trials in hypertension suggest that blood pressure has been lowered insufficiently in many instances and that this could be one explanation for the suboptimal results of antihypertensive treatment, the opposite opinion also has been expressed, blood pressure lowered too vigorously could result in increased morbidity and mortality.

Theoretically, it must be assumed that the relationship between the level of blood pressure and the risk of any event, for instance of dying, must be J-shaped (5,6). In 1979, Stewart (7) claimed that in a retrospective analysis of 169 hypertensive patients, the risk of myocardial infarction was greater in patients in whom the diastolic blood pressure (fourth Korotkoff phase) was lowered to less than 90 mm Hg as compared with 100 to 109 mm Hg. In 1987 Cruickshank and coworkers published a retrospective analysis of

Table 1 Lack of Blood Pressure Control in Major Trials of Antihypertensive Treatment

Trial	Blood pressure goal	Patients not at goal (%)
HDFP (25)	DBP < 90 mm Hg	23–27
Australian (29)	DBP < 90 mm Hg	36
MRC-mild hypertension (26)	DBP < 90 mm Hg	23
EWPHE (43)	SBP/DBP < 160/90 mm Hg	25–32
IPPPSH (33)	DBP < 90 mm Hg	35
HAPPHY (44)	DBP < 95 mm Hg	23
SHEP (31)	SBP < 160 mm Hg or reduction ≥ 20 mm Hg	28–35
SystEur (30)	SBP < 150 mm Hg and reduction ≥ 20 mm Hg	56

Abbreviations: *HDFP*, Hypertension Detection and Follow-Up Program; *DBP*, diastolic blood pressure; *MRC*, Medical Research Council, *EWPHE*, European Working Party on High Blood Pressure in the Elderly; *SBP*, Systolic blood pressure; *IPPPSH*, The International Prospective Primary Prevention Study in Hypertensives; *HAPPHY*, Heart Attack Primary Prevention in Hypertension; *SHEP*, Systolic Hypertension in the Elderly Program; *SystEur*, Systolic Hypertension in Europe.

939 treated hypertensive patients in which they claimed that lowering the diastolic blood pressure to less than 85 to 90 mm Hg in patients with pre-existing ischemic heart disease was associated with an increase in fatal myocardial infarctions (8). Support for this view appeared to be provided by the study by Alderman et al., who followed 1765 previously untreated hypertensive patients during a 4.2-year observation period (9). They found that the 39 fatal and nonfatal myocardial infarctions that occurred in this study were significantly more common in patients with a small ($\leq$ 6 mm Hg) or a large ($\geq$ 18 mm Hg) fall in diastolic blood pressure, whereas patients with a reduction of diastolic blood pressure between 7 and 17 mm Hg had a significantly smaller risk (9). Some support for this view was also provided by the retrospective analysis by Samuelsson et al. (10).

Studies supportive of the J-shaped curve hypothesis have mostly been retrospective, often open, and commonly with too few events to reach significant conclusions (5,6). However, the real issue is not whether the relation between achieved blood pressure and cardiovascular events is J-shaped (as mentioned above, it must be), but whether there are additional benefits or risks in lowering blood pressure of patients with hypertension to fully normotensive levels, that is, between 70 mm Hg and 85 mm Hg diastolic blood pressure.

C. Effects of Antiaggregating Agents on Cardiovascular Events

Another possible approach to improving treatment benefits in patients with hypertension is to associate antihypertensive therapy with correction of their cardiovascular risk factors. Aggregation of platelets is an important mechanism for the development of thrombotic complications, such as occlusions of coronary or cerebral arteries, that lead to myocardial infarction or ischemic stroke. Therefore, many studies have explored the efficacy of antiplatelet drugs, principally acetylsalicylic acid (ASA, aspirin) in preventing recurrence of cardiovascular events in patients with a previous history of such events. In a meta-analysis of 25 trials with antiplatelet drugs involving 29,000 patients, cardiovascular mortality was reduced by 15% and the incidence of nonfatal cardiovascular events by 30% when ASA was administered (11). In more recent trials, low doses of ASA have been as effective as high doses in the secondary prevention of vascular events. Thus in the Swedish Aspirin Low dose Trial [SALT (12)], daily use of 75 mg ASA reduced the risk of stroke by 18% in patients with a previous history of transient ischemic attacks (TIA) or minor stroke.

Primary prevention trials with ASA have not shown uniform results. In the U.S. Physicians Health Study, which involved more than 22,000 male doctors, the risk of myocardial infarction was reduced by 44%, but this benefit was apparent only in participants aged 50 years or older (13). A similar trial in British doctors, however, did not show any significant effect of ASA on mortality, nonfatal stroke or myocardial infarction (14). No intervention studies with ASA have been done in patients with hypertension, possibly because the two major studies of primary prevention (13,14) have associated the use of aspirin with a small increase in the risk of cerebral hemorrhage, a risk that could be greater in hypertension.

II. PRIMARY AND SECONDARY OBJECTIVES OF THE HOT STUDY

The HOT study was designed to investigate the relationship between three different target diastolic blood pressures obtained with long-term antihypertensive treatment and cardiovascular mortality and morbidity. The three therapeutic goals were diastolic blood pres-

Table 2 Primary Objectives of the HOT study

1. To assess the relationship between major cardiovascular events (nonfatal myocardial infarction, nonfatal stroke, all cardiovascular deaths) and three target diastolic blood pressures (aimed at ≤ 90 mm Hg, ≤ 85 mm Hg and ≤ 80 mm Hg) during antihypertensive treatment (intention-to-treat analysis)
2. To assess the relationship between major cardiovascular events (nonfatal myocardial infarction, nonfatal stroke, all cardiovascular deaths) and diastolic blood pressure achieved during active antihypertensive therapy.
3. To assess if low-dose ASA in addition to antihypertensive therapy reduces major cardiovascular events (nonfatal myocardial infarction, nonfatal stroke, all cardiovascular deaths)

Abbreviations: *HOT*, Hypertension Optimal Treatment; *ASA*, acetylsalicylic acid.

sures of 90 mm Hg or less, 85 mm Hg or less, or 80 mm Hg or less. The study has also explored the possible benefits of adding a daily dose of 75 mg ASA, by comparing cardiovascular mortality and morbidity in patients receiving ASA or its placebo.

A. Primary Objectives

The primary objectives of the HOT study are detailed in Table 2. In brief, they were:

1. To assess the relationship between pooled major cardiovascular events and the target diastolic blood pressures of ≤ 80, ≤ 85, ≤ 90 mm Hg or the diastolic blood pressure achieved during antihypertensive treatment.
2. To determine whether the addition of a low dose of ASA to antihypertensive treatment reduces the incidence of pooled major cardiovascular events.

Table 3 Secondary Objectives of the HOT Study

1. To assess the relationship between target diastolic blood pressures and:
   a) fatal and nonfatal myocardial infarction
   b) fatal and nonfatal stroke
   c) cardiovascular mortality
   d) total mortality
   e) fatal congestive heart failure
   f) other fatal cardiovascular events
   g) impaired renal function (serum creatinine > 200 μmol/L)
   h) hospitalization (resulting from cardiovascular/noncardiovascular causes)
2. To assess if low-dose ASA added to antihypertensive treatment reduces:
   a) fatal and nonfatal myocardial infarction
   b) fatal and nonfatal stroke
   c) cardiovascular mortality
   d) total mortality
   e) fatal congestive heart failure
   f) other fatal cardiovascular events
   g) impaired renal function (serum creatinine > 200 μmol/L)
   h) hospitalization (resulting from cardiovascular/noncardiovascular causes)

Abbreviation: *ASA*, acetylsalicylic acid.

B. Secondary Objectives

Secondary analyses (Table 3) were planned to examine the relationship between target diastolic blood pressure and specific outcomes, such as total or cardiovascular mortality, fatal and nonfatal coronary heart disease or stroke, and hospitalization. The effects on these outcomes of adding a low dose of ASA to antihypertensive treatment were also assessed.

Other analyses were planned to investigate the influence of factors such as age, sex, previous history of myocardial infarction or stroke, diabetes mellitus, and smoking.

III. PROTOCOL OF THE STUDY (15)

A. Patients

Eligibility criteria are listed in Table 4.

B. Sample Size and Power Estimates

In the null hypothesis, it was assumed that the incidence of cardiovascular events would be linearly related to target diastolic blood pressures. A deviation from this linear relationship can be expressed as the distance of the incidence at 85 mm Hg to a line connecting the incidences at 80 mm Hg and 90 mm Hg. The sample size needed to detect a deviation depends on the expected incidence as well as the distance. Using the experience of the

Table 4 Eligibility Criteria for HOT Study Patients

Inclusion criteria
- Men and women
- Age between 50 and 80 years
- Essential hypertension
- Diastolic blood pressure $\geq$ 100 mm Hg or $\leq$ 115 mm Hg on two occasions, at least 1 week apart, after discontinuation of all antihypertensive medication (if any) at least 2 weeks before randomization.

Exclusion criteria
- Malignant hypertension
- Secondary hypertension
- Diastolic blood pressure $>$ 115 mm Hg
- Stroke or myocardial infarction within 12 months before randomization
- Decompensated congestive heart failure
- Other serious concomitant disease which, in the opinion of the investigator, could affect survival during the next 2–3 years
- Patients who, in the opinion of the investigator, required a β-blocker, ACE inhibitor, or diuretic for reasons other than hypertension
- Patients who, in the opinion of the investigator, required antiplatelet or anticoagulant treatment
- Insulin-treated diabetics
- Patients with known hypersensitivity to felodipine
- Patients with known contraindications to low-dose ASA

Abbreviations: *HOT*, Hypertension Optimal Treatment; *ACE*, angiotensin-converting enzyme; *ASA*, acetylsalicylic acid.

STOP-Hypertension study (16), it was assumed that a total of 18,000 patients followed up for 2.5 years would generate approximately 1100 major cardiovascular events (fatal and nonfatal), and that it would then be possible to detect an 18% deviation from the line by a two-sided test with a value of less than 0.05 and a power of 80%. The estimated sample size of 40,000 patient-years was also considered sufficient to reveal a 10% difference in cardiovascular event incidence rate between a placebo group and an ASA-treated group.

C. Statistical Analyses

In the analysis of trend and differences between target groups and the effects of ASA compared with placebo, a Cox proportional hazard model was used to calculate relative risk. In the analysis of the different events in relation to achieved blood pressure (mean since entry), a Poisson model was used. The logarithm of the hazard rate was modeled as a continuous function of mean blood pressure by connected linear and quadratic pieces of specified intervals. Time-dependent (updated) information was used for the covariates of current age, time from entry, and blood pressure from every 6 months. Two-tailed tests were used.

D. Randomization Procedures

A special coordinating center for the HOT study was set up at the Clinical Research Center (CRC) at the Östra Hospital in Göteborg, Sweden. Participating investigators worldwide were to submit by fax information on patients to be included in the study to the coordinating center. They were informed by return fax about the therapeutic goal to which the patient had been randomized. The following variables were taken into account when randomizing patients:

- Age
- Sex
- Previous myocardial infarction
- Other coronary heart disease
- Previous stroke
- Diabetes mellitus (treated with diet or drugs)
- Previous antihypertensive treatment
- Smoking

Before being enrolled, eligible patients were informed verbally and in writing about the purpose and conduct of the trial. Their informed consent was required.

Any ongoing antihypertensive medication was discontinued, and when the inclusion criteria (diastolic blood pressure $\geq$ 100 to $\leq$ 115 mm Hg) were met, the patients were randomized. At the randomization visit, three measurements of seated blood pressure were made and heart rate recorded after 5 minutes' rest.

E. Study Design

The study was a prospective, randomized, open trial with blinded clinical events evaluation (17) regarding the relationship between target blood pressure and cardiovascular mortality

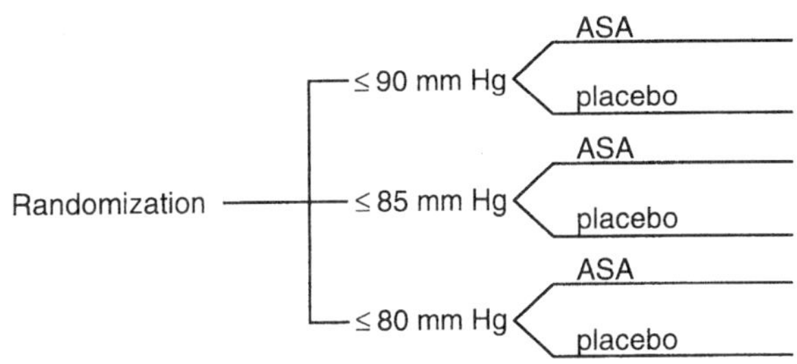

Fig. 1 HOT study design. (From Ref. 15.)

and morbidity; while regarding the effect of low-dose ASA, the study was randomized and double-blind. The study design is summarized in Figure 1.

After randomization, patients were again seen at 3 and 6 months and thereafter twice a year. A final visit was made within 1 month of the end of the study. At all visits, clinical information was collected and blood pressure was measured three times with the patients seated after 5 minutes of rest. An oscillometric semiautomatic device (Visomat OZ, D2, International, Hestia, Germany) was used. The apparatus was subjected to the tests of blood pressure measuring equipment proposed by the British Hypertension Society and was found to meet these criteria.

F. Treatment

In all patients, antihypertensive therapy was started with the long-acting calcium antagonist, felodipine, at a dose of 5 mg once a day. Additional therapy and dose increments in four further steps (Fig. 2) were prescribed to reach the randomized target blood pressure.

G. Definition of Endpoints

The primary endpoint (Table 5) was the rate of major cardiovascular events; secondary endpoints were fatal and nonfatal myocardial infarction, fatal and nonfatal stroke, cardiovascular mortality, and total mortality.

Major cardiovascular events were defined as all (fatal and nonfatal) myocardial infarctions, all (fatal and nonfatal) strokes, and all other cardiovascular deaths. Silent myocardial infarctions were documented by taking an electrocardiogram (ECG) at randomization and at the final visit.

A classification of all reported events was made by the independent clinical event committee based on all available information (hospital records, physician's records, death certificates, and necropsy reports). All events were classified without any knowledge of the actual medication or the treatment group to which the patients had been assigned. The approval rate of reported events by this committee was 76%.

If death occurred within 28 days of the onset of an event, that event was classified as fatal. If no obvious noncardiovascular cause of death was identified, the death was subsequently classified as cardiovascular. For the diagnosis of nonfatal myocardial infarction, at least two of the following criteria had to be fulfilled: central chest pain lasting for more than 15 minutes, transient elevation of enzymes indicating damage, or typical ECG changes. For the diagnosis of fatal myocardial infarction, the above criteria were required or the diagnosis was to be stated in hospital records or described in the necropsy report.

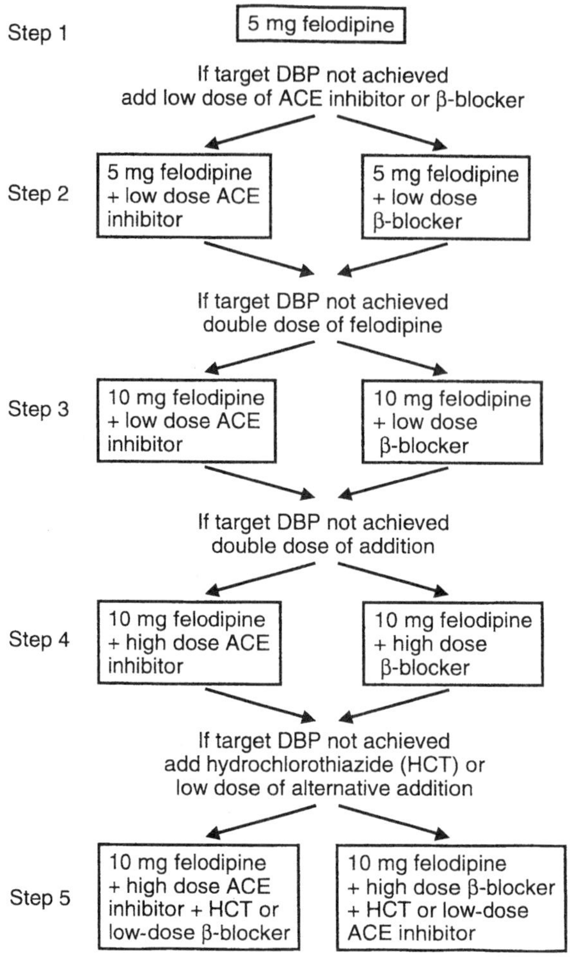

Fig. 2 Flow chart of treatment in the HOT study, showing the titration to target blood pressure. (From Ref. 15.)

Table 5 Primary and Secondary Endpoints in the HOT Study

Primary endpoint
- Rate of all major cardiovascular events (fatal and nonfatal myocardial infarction,* fatal and nonfatal stroke, all cardiovascular deaths)

Secondary endpoints
- Rate of all myocardial infarction (fatal and nonfatal)
- Rate of all myocardial infarction (fatal and nonfatal) including silent myocardial infarction
- Rate of all stroke (fatal and nonfatal)
- Rate of cardiovascular mortality
- Rate of total mortality

*Silent myocardial infarction was included among all myocardial infarctions according to the original protocol, but it was later decided to consider it separately as a secondary endpoint as time-dependent information could not be available for this event.

Abbreviation: *HOT*, Hypertension Optimal Treatment.

A 12-lead resting ECG was recorded at randomization and at the final visit. All ECGs were coded with the Minnesota code. The baseline ECGs were coded for signs of myocardial infarction (codes 1:1 or 1:2) as well as for signs of ischemia (codes 4:1-2 or 5:1-2). An ECG was recorded at randomization in 96% of all patients. A final ECG was recorded in 89% of all patients. The final ECGs were coded only for myocardial infarction (codes 1:1 and 1:2). In total, 54,911 codings were made. The final ECGs were compared with the baseline ECGs by two independent technicians. If discrepancies arose, the ECG committee members made the final classification. A finding of new Q or QS waves (codes 1:1 or 1:2), without clinical signs of myocardial infarction was defined as a silent myocardial infarction. Although the protocol listed silent myocardial infarctions among nonfatal infarction, it was subsequently decided to consider them separately, as time-dependent information could not be available for this type of event.

Diagnosis of a nonfatal stroke required unequivocal signs or symptoms of remaining neurological deficit, with a sudden onset and a duration of more than 24 h. Diagnosis of a fatal stroke also required the criteria given above. Alternatively, the diagnosis could be given in the hospital records or described in the necropsy report.

H. Study Organization

A total of 1904 investigators from 26 countries were involved in the study, mainly general practitioners and physicians at hospital outpatient clinics. The scientific aspects of the study were governed by the executive and steering committees. An independent clinical event committee evaluated all events (masked). Throughout the study, an independent safety committee had full access to all events (open). In each country, one or more monitors were in regular contact with the investigators to oversee the practical aspects of the study. An independent data audit committee visited randomly selected centers to audit the trial in accordance with the rules of the American Food and Drug Administration. Details on study organization are indicated in the Appendix.

IV. PRINCIPAL RESULTS (18)

A. Study Population

Overall, 19,193 patients from 26 countries, aged 50 to 80 years (mean 61.5 years), with hypertension and a diastolic blood pressure between 100 mm Hg and 115 mm Hg (mean 105 mm Hg) were randomly assigned a target blood pressure and acetylsalicylic acid or placebo. Because of the suspicion of incorrect inclusion or data handling at one center, 403 patients were excluded early in the trial. Patients were recruited from countries in Europe, North and South America, and Asia. The number of randomized patients by country is listed in Table 6. The average follow-up time was 3.8 years (range 3.3 to 4.9 years) and the total number of patient-years was 71,051. The first patient was enrolled in October 1992; randomization ended in April 1994; and the last day of follow-up was August 31, 1997 (19).

Patient characteristics by target group at randomization are shown in Table 7. Figure 3 summarizes the profile of the trial; 6264 patients were given the diastolic blood pressure target of 90 mm Hg or lower, 6264 a target of 85 mm Hg or lower, and 6262 a target of 80 mm Hg or lower. In addition, 9399 patients were randomly assigned acetylsalicylic acid and 9391 patients were assigned placebo.

Table 6 Number of Randomized Patients by Country/Area

Country/area	Number of randomized patients
Argentina	47
Austria	628
Belgium	755
Canada	838
Denmark	503
East Asia	205
Finland	373
France	1574
Germany	4674
Great Britain	131
Greece	335
Hungary	194
Israel	411
Italy	2702
Mexico	49
Norway	432
Spain	806
Sweden	492
Switzerland	797
The Netherlands	604
USA	2646

Table 7 Characteristics at Randomization

	Diastolic blood pressure target group		
	≤ 90 mm Hg (n = 6264)	≤ 85 mm Hg (n = 6264)	≤ 80 mm Hg (n = 6262)
Age (years)	61.5 (7.5)	61.5 (7.5)	61.5 (7.5)
Body mass index (kg, m^2)	28.4 (4.7)	28.5 (4.7)	28.4 (4.6)
Diastolic blood pressure (mm Hg)	105 (3.4)	105 (3.4)	105 (3.4)
Systolic blood pressure (mm Hg)	170 (14.4)	170 (14.0)	170 (14.1)
Serum creatinine (μmol/L)	89 (26)	89 (23)	89 (23)
Serum cholesterol (mmol/L)	6.0 (1.1)	6.1 (1.1)	6.1 (1.2)
Men/women (%)	53/47	53/47	53/47
Previous treatment (%)	52.3	52.7	52.6
Smokers (%)	15.9	15.8	15.9
Previous MI (%)	1.6	1.5	1.5
Other previous CHD (%)	5.9	6.0	5.9
Previous stroke (%)	1.2	1.2	1.2
Diabetes mellitus (%)	8.0	8.0	8.0

Data are mean (SD) or % of group.
Abbreviation: *MI*, myocardial infarction; *CHD*, coronary heart disease.

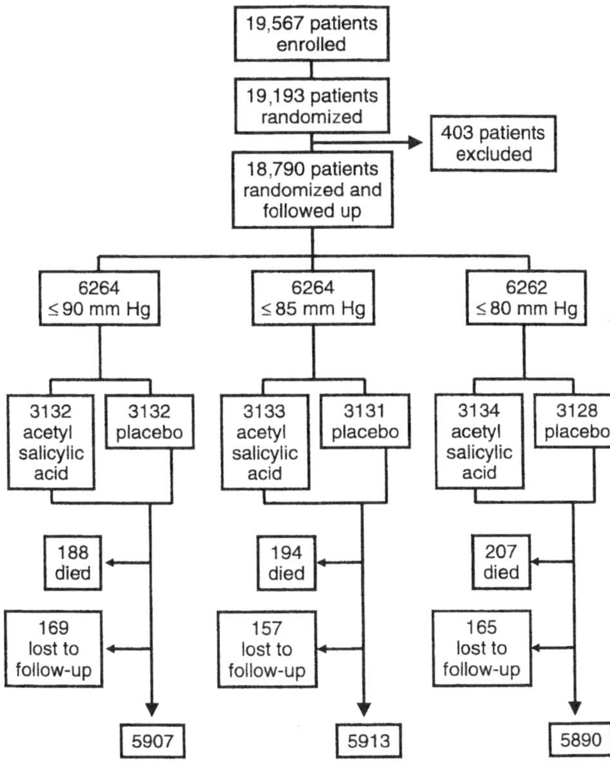

Fig. 3 HOT trial profile. (From Ref. 18.)

A total of 491 (2.6%) patients were lost to follow-up. Most were lost early in the study, for example, 130 patients did not return for any of the follow-up visits. The loss in terms of patient-years was 1269 (1.8%). The loss of patients in the three target groups was 169 from the 90 mm Hg or less target group, 157 from the 85 mm Hg or less target group, and 165 from the 80 mm Hg or less target group. Two hundred forty-five of those randomized to acetylsalicylic acid were lost; 246 were lost for the placebo group. The average age at randomization of those lost was 61.3 years and 61.5 years in those remaining in the study. Blood pressures of patients lost to follow-up and of those remaining in the study were identical at randomization. The age, sex distribution, previous morbidity, and previous antihypertensive treatment did not differ between those lost to follow-up and the remainder of the patients who form the basis for this report.

B. Treatment

Table 8 gives the percentages of patients taking the different antihypertensive agents at various times during the trial. At the end of the study, as many as 78% of patients were still taking felodipine, 41% received an angiotensin-converting enzyme (ACE) inhibitor, 28% a beta-blocker, and 22% a diuretic. Table 9 gives these data for diastolic blood pressure target group, and Figure 4 indicates the percentages of patients at the various treatment steps according to the diastolic blood pressure target to which they had been randomized. The proportion of subjects who remained in monotherapy (low-dose felodi-

Table 8 Percentages of Patients on Various Antihypertensive Agents at Various Times During the HOT Study

	3 m	6 m	24 m	36 m	Final
Felodipine	96	91	85	82	78
ACE inhibitor	30	36	40	41	41
Beta-blocker	19	23	27	28	28
Diuretics	6	10	18	20	22

Abbreviations: *HOT*, Hypertension Optimal Treatment; *ACE*, angiotensin-converting enzyme.

Table 9 Treatment at the End of the Study per Target Blood Pressure Group

	Diastolic blood pressure target group		
	≤ 90 mm Hg	≤ 85 mm Hg	≤ 80 mm Hg
Felodipine	77	78	79
ACE inhibitor	35	42	45
Beta-blocker	25	28	32
Diuretics	19	22	24

Abbreviation: *ACE*, angiotensin-converting enzyme.

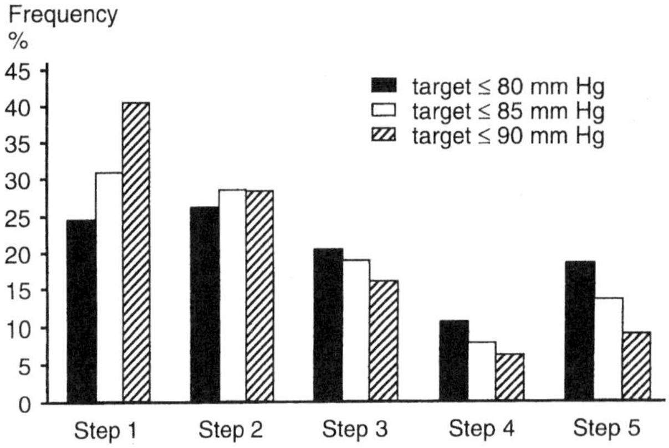

Fig. 4 Percentages of patients at the various treatment steps according to target blood pressure.

pine) was 40% in target group 90 mm Hg or lower and that decreased to 24% in subjects of target group 80 mm Hg or lower. The proportion of patients that progressed to higher steps of the treatment regimen obviously increased from target group 90 mm Hg or lower to target group 85 mm Hg or lower and to target group 80 mm Hg or lower, but even in the lowest target group as many as 80% of patients could continue a single- or two-drug regimen (steps 1, 2, 3, and 4).

Table 10 Achieved Blood Pressures and Heart Rate in Patients of the HOT Study: Mean (SD) of All Values from 6 Months After Randomization to the End of the Study

	Total	≤ 90 mm Hg	≤ 85 mm Hg	≤ 80 mm Hg
SBP (mm Hg)	141.6 (11.7)	143.7 (11.3)	141.4 (11.7)	139.7 (11.7)
DBP (mm Hg)	83.1 (5.3)	85.2 (5.1)	83.2 (4.8)	81.1 (5.3)
HR (beats/min)	74.9 (8.4)	75.5 (8.3)	75.0 (8.4)	74.2 (8.2)
ΔSBP (mm Hg)	−28.0 (13.4)	−26.2 (13.0)	−28.0 (13.2)	−29.9 (13.6)
ΔDBP (mm Hg)	−22.3 (5.8)	−20.3 (5.6)	−22.3 (5.4)	−24.3 (5.8)
ΔHR (beats/min)	−3.8 (9.4)	−3.2 (9.1)	−3.8 (9.4)	−4.4 (9.6)

Abbreviations: *SBP*, systolic blood pressure; *DBP*, diastolic blood pressure; *HR*, heart rate.

C. Effects on Blood Pressure

Compared with blood pressure at the time of randomization, average diastolic blood pressure was reduced by 20.3 mm Hg, 22.3 mm Hg, and 24.3 mm Hg and systolic blood pressure by 26.2 mm Hg, 28.0 mm Hg, and 29.9 mm Hg in the target groups 90 mm Hg or less, 85 mm Hg or less, and 80 mm Hg or less, respectively (Table 10). In the three target groups, the diastolic blood pressure was reduced from a mean of 105 mm Hg to a mean of 85.2 mm Hg, 83.2 mm Hg, and 81.1 mm Hg, respectively. The distribution curves of diastolic blood pressure for the three target groups are shown in Figure 5. A diastolic blood pressure greater than 90 mm Hg was found in 12% of the patients in the target group 90 mm Hg or less, 7% of the patients in target group 85 mm Hg or less, and in 6% of the patients randomized to the target group 80 mm Hg or less. On the whole, 91.5% of patients achieved a diastolic blood pressure of 90 mm Hg or less. Figure 6 indicates that the proportion of patients reaching the randomized target blood pressure increased gradually up to the 36-month visit. Also, systolic blood pressure continued to decrease until the end of the study (Fig. 7). There were no differences in achieved blood pressure between patients randomized to ASA or placebo (142.0/.83.2 mm Hg and 141.4/.82.9 mm Hg, respectively).

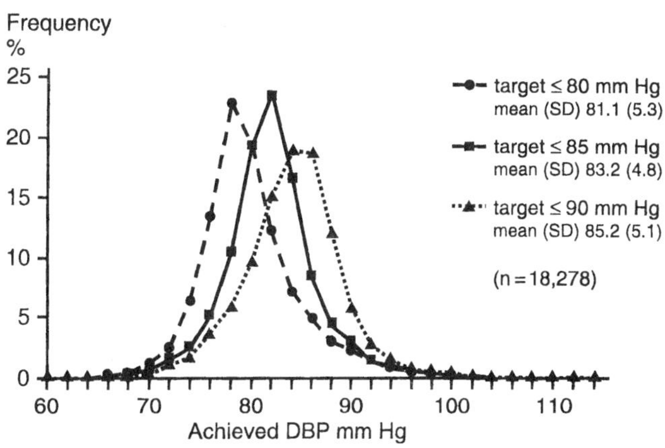

Fig. 5 Distribution of mean diastolic blood pressures, from 6 months' follow-up to the end of the HOT study. (From Ref. 18.)

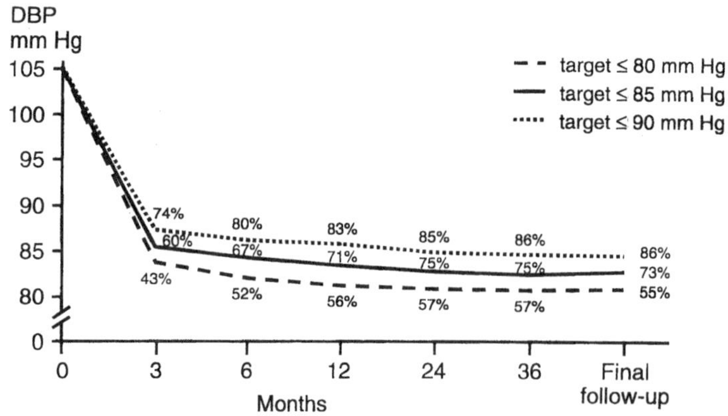

Fig. 6 Proportion (%) of patients reaching target diastolic blood pressure during the course of the HOT study.

Table 10 shows that heart rate slightly decreased in all three target groups without significant differences between groups. Table 11 indicates that treatment did not modify other risk factors for cardiovascular disease, such as serum cholesterol and serum creatinine.

D. Effects on Morbidity and Mortality

Cardiovascular morbidity and mortality in the three target blood pressure groups are indicated in Table 12. Because of the small blood pressure differences between groups, differences in event rates were rather small and only the trend for the rate of all myocardial infarction to be lower at a lower target blood pressure was of borderline significance: there was a 25% myocardial infarction reduction in the target group 85 mm Hg or less and a 28% reduction in the target group 80 mm Hg or less as compared with the target group 90 mm Hg or less.

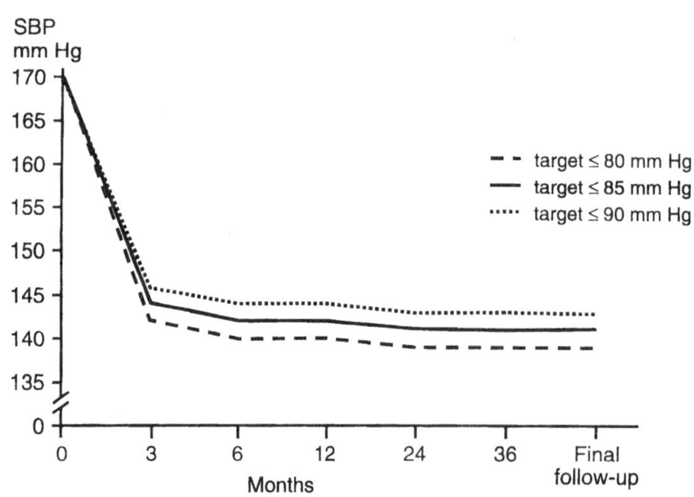

Fig. 7 Systolic blood pressure in the three target groups during the course of the HOT study.

Table 11 Serum Cholesterol and Serum Creatinine at Randomization and at Final Visit (means) in Patients of the Three Target Groups

	Diastolic blood pressure target group		
	Target ≤ 90	Target ≤ 85	Target ≤ 80
S-cholesterol mmol/L (mg/dl)			
Randomization	6.0 (233)	6.1 (235)	6.1 (234)
Final visit	5.9 (226)	5.9 (228)	5.9 (226)
S-creatinine μmol/L (mg/dl)			
Randomization	89 (1.0)	89 (1.0)	89 (1.0)
Final visit	90 (1.0)	89 (1.0)	90 (1.0)

Table 12 Events in Relation to Target Blood Pressure Groups (n = 6264, 6264, and 6262 in the Target Groups ≤ 90 mm Hg, ≤ 85 mm Hg, and ≤ 80 mm Hg, Respectively)

Events	No. of events	Events/1000 patient-years	*P*-value for trend	Comparison	Relative risk	95% confidence interval
Major cardiovascular events						
≤ 90 mm Hg	232	9.9		90 vs 85	0.99	0.83–1.19
≤ 85 mm Hg	234	10.0		85 vs 80	1.08	0.89–1.29
≤ 80 mm Hg	217	9.3	0.50	90 vs 80	1.07	0.89–1.28
Major cardiovascular events*						
≤ 90 mm Hg	274	11.7		90 vs 85	0.99	0.84–1.17
≤ 85 mm Hg	276	11.8		85 vs 80	1.05	0.88–1.24
≤ 80 mm Hg	263	11.3	0.66	90 vs 80	1.04	0.88–1.23
All myocardial infarction						
≤ 90 mm Hg	84	3.6		90 vs 85	1.32	0.95–1.82
≤ 85 mm Hg	64	2.7		85 vs 80	1.05	0.74–1.48
≤ 80 mm Hg	61	2.6	0.05	90 vs 80	1.37	0.99–1.91
All myocardial infarction*						
≤ 90 mm Hg	127	5.4		90 vs 85	1.19	0.92–1.54
≤ 85 mm Hg	107	4.6		85 vs 80	1.00	0.76–1.30
≤ 80 mm Hg	107	4.6	0.19	90 vs 80	1.19	0.92–1.53
All stroke						
≤ 90 mm Hg	94	4.0		90 vs 85	0.85	0.64–1.11
≤ 85 mm Hg	111	4.7		85 vs 80	1.24	0.94–1.64
≤ 80 mm Hg	89	3.8	0.74	90 vs 80	1.05	0.79–1.41
Cardiovascular mortality						
≤ 90 mm Hg	87	3.7		90 vs 85	0.97	0.72–1.30
≤ 85 mm Hg	90	3.8		85 vs 80	0.93	0.70–1.24
≤ 80 mm Hg	96	4.1	0.49	90 vs 80	0.90	0.68–1.21
Total mortality						
≤ 90 mm Hg	188	7.9		90 vs 85	0.97	0.79–1.19
≤ 85 mm Hg	194	8.2		85 vs 80	0.93	0.77–1.14
≤ 80 mm Hg	207	8.8	0.32	90 vs 80	0.91	0.74–1.10

*Silent myocardial infarction included.

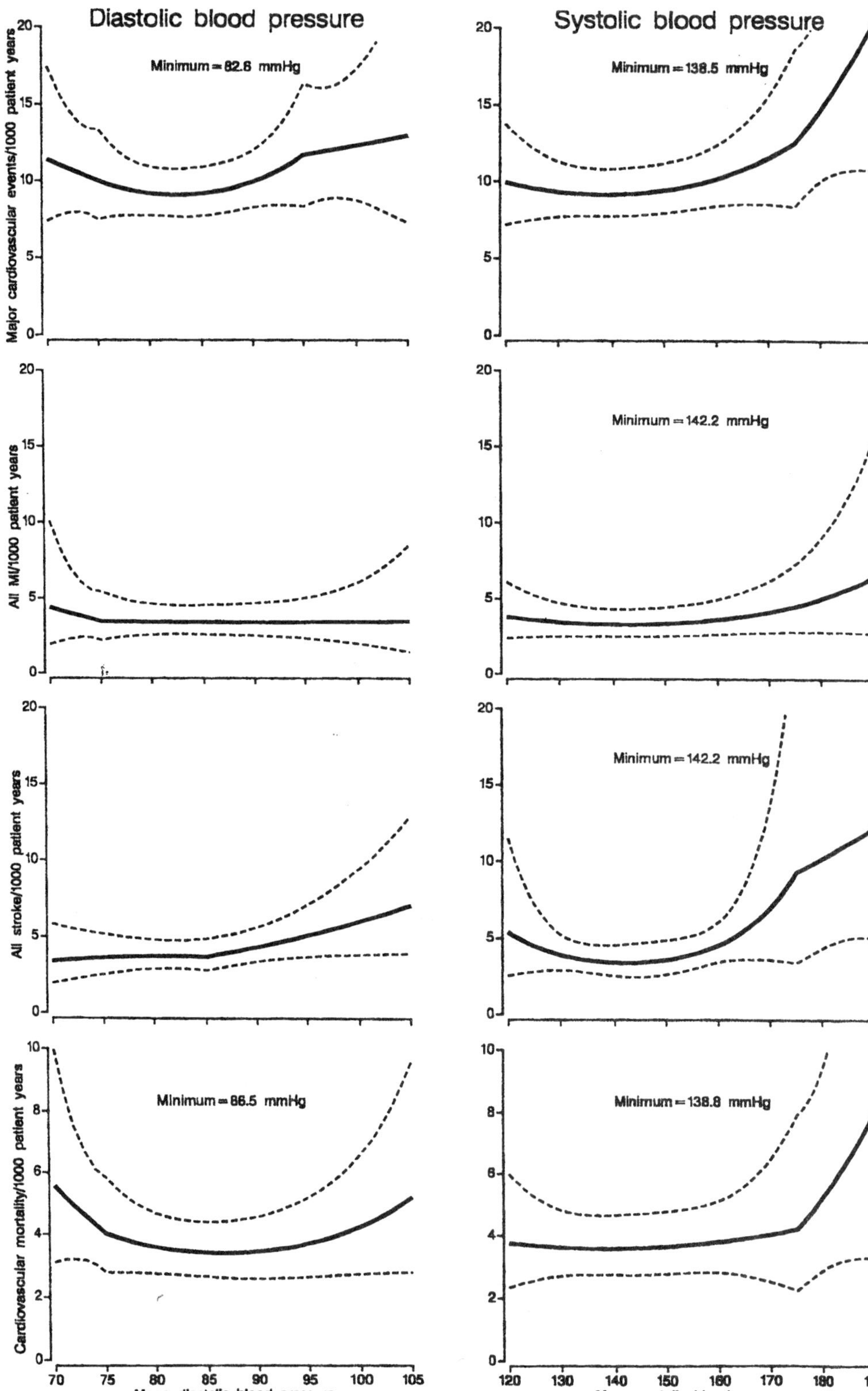

Fig. 8 Estimated incidence (95% confidence intervals) of cardiovascular events in relation to achieved mean diastolic and systolic blood pressure. The blood pressure at the lowest point of the curve is indicated (minimum). (From Ref. 18.)

E. Cardiovascular Event in Relation to Achieved Blood Pressure

The HOT study protocol had planned to analyze the incidence of cardiovascular endpoints in relation to achieved diastolic (and systolic) blood pressure as a powerful instrument to determine the optimal blood pressure level. Because blood pressure value separation between the three randomized groups was smaller than expected, this analysis was particularly informative. The results are illustrated in Figure 8.

Confidence intervals were narrowest in the diastolic blood pressure range of 75 to 95 mm Hg and in the systolic blood pressure range of 130 to 170 mm Hg, suggesting adequate precision of the estimated risk within these limits. For major cardiovascular events, the lowest point of risk was at a mean achieved diastolic blood pressure of 82.6 mm Hg and at a mean systolic blood pressure of 138.5 mm Hg. For all myocardial infarction, there was no definite minimum diastolic blood pressure, whereas the minimum risk was reached at a systolic blood pressure of 142.2 mm Hg. For all stroke, the lowest risk was below 80 mm Hg for diastolic and 142.2 mm Hg for systolic blood pressure. The lowest risk of cardiovascular mortality was at 86.5 mm Hg and 138.8 mm Hg for diastolic and systolic blood pressure, respectively.

Curves relating events to achieved blood pressure also give some indication of the number of events that could presumably be prevented in the study population by lowering blood pressure from the highest values present before randomization down to the minimum blood pressure. As illustrated in Figure 9, lowering of blood pressure from randomization

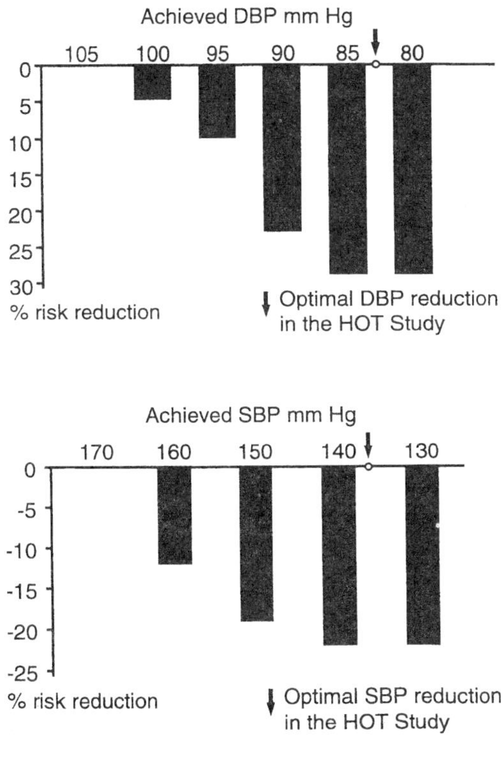

Fig. 9 Reduction of risk of a major cardiovascular event by reducing diastolic blood pressure (DBP, **upper panel**), and systolic blood pressure (SBP, **lower panel**) from randomization values to optimal values.

values down to the ''optimal'' values of between 80 and 85 mm Hg appeared to reduce major cardiovascular events by about 30%, and lowering systolic blood pressure to the optimal values of 135 to 140 mm Hg reduced major cardiovascular events by about 20%.

F. Effects of ASA on Cardiovascular Events

The rates of various types of cardiovascular events in patients randomized to either ASA or placebo is summarized in Table 13. Acetyl salicylic acid significantly ($P = 0.03$) reduced major cardiovascular events by 15%. The benefit of ASA was reduced to 9% when silent myocardial infarctions were included in the analysis. All myocardial infarction was 36% less frequent in the ASA group, a significant difference ($P = 0.002$). Inclusion of silent myocardial infarction reduced the benefit of ASA to 15%. There was no difference in stroke incidence between patients randomized to ASA or placebo. Cardiovascular mortality and total mortality were nonsignificantly lower by 5% ($P = 0.65$) and 7% ($P = 0.36$), respectively, in ASA-treated patients compared with patients receiving placebo. The effects of administering a small dose of ASA or placebo on major cardiovascular events, myocardial infarction, and stroke are also illustrated in Figure 10.

In the context of the study comparing ASA with its placebo, careful attention was paid to bleeding events (Table 14). Fatal bleeds (including cerebral) were equally common in the two groups, but nonfatal major bleeds were significantly more frequent among

Table 13 Events in Relation to Acetylsalicylic Acid (n = 9399) or Placebo (n = 9391)

Events	No. of events	Events/1000 patient-years	*P*-value	Relative risk	95% confidence interval
Major cardiovascular events					
ASA	315	8.9			
Placebo	368	10.5	0.03	0.85	0.73–0.99
Major cardiovascular events*					
ASA	388	11.1			
Placebo	425	12.2	0.17	0.91	0.79–1.04
All myocardial infarction					
ASA	82	2.3			
Placebo	127	3.6	0.002	0.64	0.49–0.85
All myocardial infarction*					
ASA	157	4.4			
Placebo	184	5.2	0.13	0.85	0.69–1.05
All stroke					
ASA	146	4.1			
Placebo	148	4.2	0.88	0.98	0.78–1.24
Cardiovascular mortality					
ASA	133	3.7			
Placebo	140	3.9	0.65	0.95	0.75–1.20
Total mortality					
ASA	284	8.0			
Placebo	305	8.6	0.36	0.93	0.79–1.09

*Silent myocardial infarction included.
Abbreviation: *ASA*, acetylsalicylic acid.

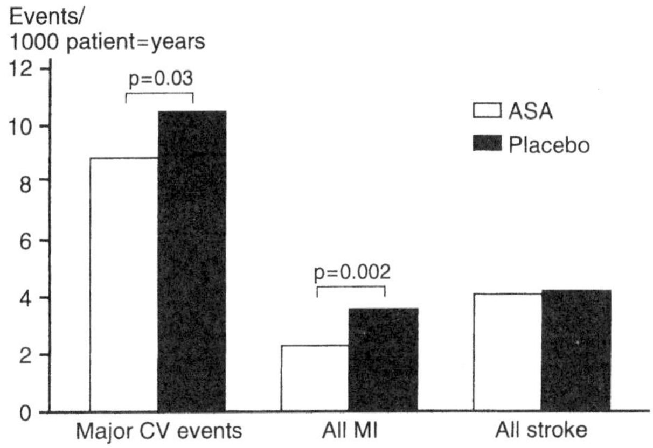

Fig. 10 Effects of acetylsalicylic acid (ASA) or placebo on major cardiovascular (CV) events, myocardial infarction (MI), and stroke.

Table 14 Bleeding Events Reported in ASA- and Placebo-Treated Patients

	ASA n = 9399	Placebo n = 9391
Fatal bleeds	7	8
Gastrointestinal	5	3
Cerebral	2	3
Other	—	2
Nonfatal major bleeds	129	70
Gastrointestinal	72	32
Cerebral	12	12
Nasal	22	12
Other	23	14
Minor bleeds	156	87
Gastrointestinal	30	18
Nasal	66	24
Purpura	45	25
Other	15	20

Abbreviation: *ASA*, acetylsalicylic acid.

patients receiving ASA than in those receiving placebo (risk ratio 1.8; $P < 0.001$); minor bleeds were also 1.8 times more frequent among patients who were taking ASA.

V. RESULTS IN SUBGROUPS OF PATIENTS

A. Diabetes Mellitus

Among the HOT patients, 1501 had a diagnosis of diabetes mellitus at baseline. Diabetes mellitus (18) was one of the variables taken into account for randomization, and therefore, diabetic patients were equally distributed between the three blood pressure target groups. As illustrated in Table 15, in diabetic patients a significant decline in the rate of major

Table 15 Events in Patients with Diabetes Mellitus at Baseline in Relation to Target Blood Pressure Groups (n = 501, 501, and 499 in the Target Groups ≤ 90 mm Hg, ≤ 85 mm Hg, and ≤ 80 mm Hg, Respectively)

Events	No. of events	Events/1000 patient-years	*P*-value for trend	Comparison	Relative risk	95% confidence interval
Major cardiovascular events						
≤ 90 mm Hg	45	24.4		90 vs 85	1.32	0.84–2.06
≤ 85 mm Hg	34	18.6		85 vs 80	1.56	0.91–2.67
≤ 80 mm Hg	22	11.9	0.005	90 vs 80	2.06	1.24–3.44
Major cardiovascular events*						
≤ 90 mm Hg	48	26.2		90 vs 85	1.13	0.75–1.71
≤ 85 mm Hg	42	23.3		85 vs 80	1.42	0.89–2.26
≤ 80 mm Hg	30	16.4	0.045	90 vs 80	1.60	1.02–2.53
All myocardial infarction						
≤ 90 mm Hg	14	7.5		90 vs 85	1.75	0.73–4.17
≤ 85 mm Hg	8	4.3		85 vs 80	1.14	0.41–3.15
≤ 80 mm Hg	7	3.7	0.11	90 vs 80	2.01	0.81–4.97
All myocardial infarction*						
≤ 90 mm Hg	18	9.7		90 vs 85	1.12	0.57–2.19
≤ 85 mm Hg	16	8.7		85 vs 80	1.07	0.53–2.16
≤ 80 mm Hg	15	8.1	0.61	90 vs 80	1.20	0.60–2.38
All stroke						
≤ 90 mm Hg	17	9.1		90 vs 85	1.30	0.63–2.67
≤ 85 mm Hg	13	7.0		85 vs 80	1.10	0.50–2.40
≤ 80 mm Hg	12	6.4	0.34	90 vs 80	1.43	0.68–2.99
Cardiovascular mortality						
≤ 90 mm Hg	21	11.1		90 vs 85	0.99	0.54–1.82
≤ 85 mm Hg	21	11.2		85 vs 80	3.0	1.29–7.13
≤ 80 mm Hg	7	3.7	0.016	90 vs 80	3.0	1.28–7.08
Total mortality						
≤ 90 mm Hg	30	15.9		90 vs 85	1.03	0.62–1.71
≤ 85 mm Hg	29	15.5		85 vs 80	1.72	0.95–3.14
≤ 80 mm Hg	17	9.0	0.068	90 vs 80	1.77	0.98–3.21

*Silent myocardial infarction included.

cardiovascular events was seen in relation to the target group (*P* for trend = 0.005). In the group randomized to 80 mm Hg or less, the risk of major cardiovascular events was halved compared with that of the target group 90 mm Hg or less. This change was attenuated but remained significant when silent myocardial infarctions were included. The approximate halving of the risk was also observed for all myocardial infarction, although it was not significant. All stroke also showed a declining rate with lower target blood pressure groups, with a risk reduction of about 30% in the 80 mm Hg or lower target group versus 90 mm Hg or lower target group. Cardiovascular mortality was also significantly lower in the 80 mm Hg or lower target group than in each of the other target groups.

B. Ischemic Heart Disease

Among the HOT patients, 3080 had ischemic heart disease (18) at baseline, as they had a history of previous myocardial infarction or other previous cardiac ischemic event, or a baseline ECG with Minnesota codes 1:1-2, 4:1-2, or 5:1-2. In these patients, as illustrated in Table 16, major cardiovascular events and all myocardial infarction declined nonsignificantly in relation to target groups. All stroke showed a significant reduction (*P* for trend = 0.046) with a 43% reduction in 80 mm Hg or lower target group compared with 90 mm Hg or lower target group. Cardiovascular mortality was not significantly affected.

C. Effects of Gender and Age

Fifty-three percent of the patients in the HOT study were men and 47% were women. The women were, on average, 1.5 years older and 10% (vs 21%) were smokers; otherwise, there were the expected gender-specific differences in demographic variables. Women had, on average, 4 mm Hg higher systolic blood pressure at the onset of the study, but there were only minimal differences at the end of the study in achieved blood pressure,

Table 16 Events in Patients with Ischemic Heart Disease at Baseline in Relation to Target Blood Pressure Groups (n = 1019, 1036, and 1025 in the Target Groups ≤ 90 mm Hg, ≤ 85 mm Hg, ≤ 80 mm Hg, Respectively)

Events	No. of events	Events/1000 patient-years	*P*-value for trend	Comparison	Relative risk	95% confidence interval
Major cardiovascular events						
≤ 90 mm Hg	77	20.7		90 vs 85	1.16	0.84–1.61
≤ 85 mm Hg	68	17.9		85 vs 80	1.08	0.76–1.52
≤ 80 mm Hg	62	16.6	0.20	90 vs 80	1.24	0.89–1.74
Major cardiovascular events*						
≤ 90 mm Hg	86	23.2		90 vs 85	1.08	0.80–1.47
≤ 85 mm Hg	81	21.5		85 vs 80	1.08	0.79–1.48
≤ 80 mm Hg	74	20.0	0.35	90 vs 80	1.16	0.85–1.58
All myocardial infarction						
≤ 90 mm Hg	25	6.6		90 vs 85	2.13	1.07–4.25
≤ 85 mm Hg	12	3.1		85 vs 80	0.62	0.30–1.27
≤ 80 mm Hg	19	5.0	0.33	90 vs 80	1.31	0.72–2.38
All myocardial infarction*						
≤ 90 mm Hg	35	9.3		90 vs 85	1.37	0.83–2.28
≤ 85 mm Hg	26	6.8		85 vs 80	0.82	0.49–1.38
≤ 80 mm Hg	31	8.3	0.63	90 vs 85	1.12	0.69–1.82
All stroke						
≤ 90 mm Hg	35	9.3		90 vs 85	1.18	0.73–1.93
≤ 85 mm Hg	30	7.9		85 vs 80	1.48	0.84–2.60
≤ 80 mm Hg	20	5.3	0.046	90 vs 80	1.75	1.01–3.04
Cardiovascular mortality						
≤ 90 mm Hg	28	7.3		90 vs 85	0.82	0.50–1.34
≤ 85 mm Hg	35	9.0		85 vs 80	0.98	0.62–1.57
≤ 80 mm Hg	35	9.2	0.37	90 vs 80	0.79	0.48–1.31
Total mortality						
≤ 90 mm Hg	54	14.1		90 vs 85	1.00	0.69–1.46
≤ 85 mm Hg	55	14.2		85 vs 80	0.95	0.65–1.37
≤ 80 mm Hg	57	15.0	0.75	90 vs 80	0.94	0.65–1.37

*Silent myocardial infarction included.

Table 17 Cardiovascular (CV) Events in Men (n = 9907) and Women (n = 8883) in the HOT Study

Variable		Events/1000 patient-years			
		Target group ≤ 90	Target group ≤ 85	Target group ≤ 80	*P*-value for trend
Major CV event	Men	11.3	12.8	11.8	0.70
	Women	8.3	6.9	6.5	0.11
MI	Men	4.1	4.1	3.4	0.38
	Women	3.0	1.2	1.7	0.034
Stroke	Men	4.5	5.1	4.4	0.9
	Women	3.4	4.3	3.1	0.73
CV mortality	Men	3.9	5.1	5.2	0.15
	Women	3.4	2.4	2.8	0.44
Total mortality	Men	9.1	10.2	11.0	0.14
	Women	6.6	5.9	6.3	0.78

Major events are CV death, myocardial infarction (MI), stroke.

as well as the percentage of patients on target, the percentage of patients still above 90 mm Hg, and the percentage of patients on the various titration steps between men and women (20,21). The principal results for the three randomized blood pressure target groups subdivided for men and women are shown in Table 17. Overall, the trend for a lower incidence of cardiovascular endpoints with a lower target blood pressure was more consistent in women; in particular, the trend for fewer myocardial infarctions achieved statistical significance in women ($P = 0.034$) but not in men.

Almost one third of the patients in the HOT study were aged 65 or older. There was an uneven gender distribution with 54% women and fewer smokers (11.7% vs 17.8%)

Table 18 Cardiovascular (CV) Events in Younger (< 65 years, n = 12,803) and Older (≥ 65 years, n = 6987) Patients in the HOT Study

Variable		Events/1000 patient-years			
		Target group ≤ 90	Target group ≤ 85	Target group ≤ 80	*P*-value for trend
Major CV event	Young	6.8	8.6	6.5	0.79
	Old	16.9	13.0	15.2	0.42
MI	Young	3.2	2.9	2.3	0.14
	Old	4.4	2.4	3.2	0.22
Stroke	Young	2.3	3.8	2.4	0.77
	Old	7.8	6.6	6.7	0.41
CV mortality	Young	1.9	2.9	2.2	0.52
	Old	7.6	5.7	8.0	0.81
Total mortality	Young	4.5	5.5	5.7	0.13
	Old	15.7	14.0	15.4	0.89

Major events are CV death, myocardial infarction (MI), stroke.

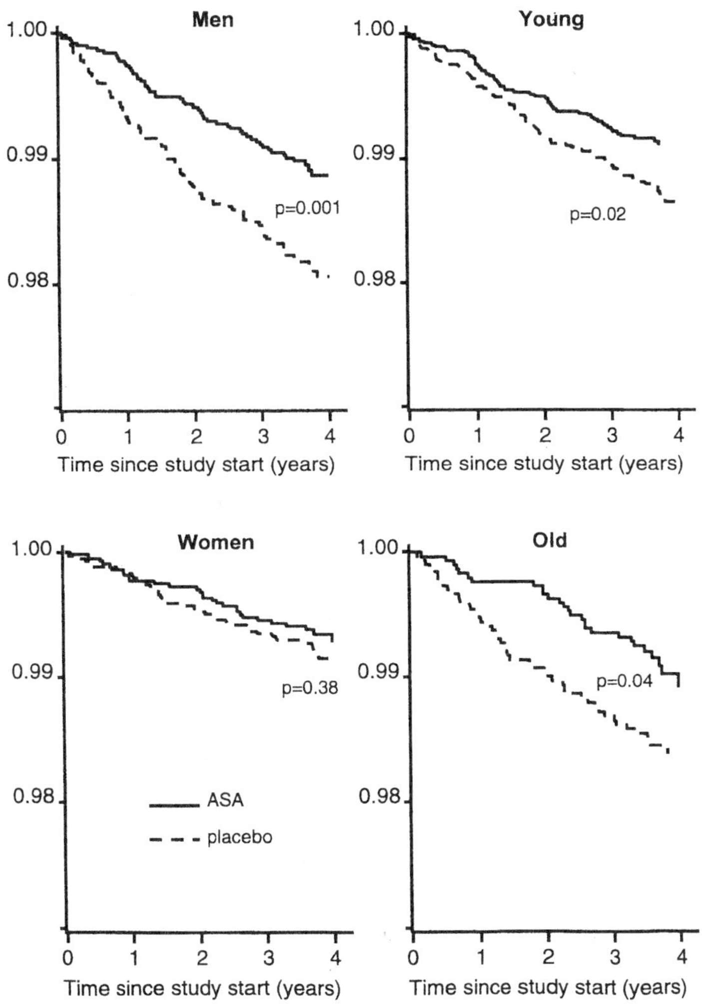

Fig. 11 Kaplan-Meier plots showing probability of follow-up without myocardial infarction in men, women, younger and older patients on ASA (*solid line*) compared with placebo (*dashed line*). (From Ref. 20.)

in the elderly group; otherwise, differences in demographic variables were as expected. Older patients had slightly higher systolic blood pressure and similar diastolic blood pressure as younger patients at baseline and tended to achieve 1 to 2 mm Hg lower diastolic blood pressure during treatment (20,21). There were trends toward fewer myocardial infarctions at lower target blood pressure in both younger and older subjects and trends toward fewer strokes at lower target blood pressure in older subjects, but none of these trends achieved statistical significance (Table 18).

D. Effects of ASA in Subgroups of Patients

The relative benefit of ASA on major cardiovascular events and all myocardial infarctions was about the same in the groups of patients with diabetes mellitus and with ischemic heart disease as in the whole HOT population (18). Aspirin lowered the incidence of myocardial infarction in men by 42% ($P = 0.001$), whereas the reduction in myocardial infarction was not significant in women. When subdividing into younger and older subjects, the effect of aspirin on major cardiovascular events was particularly marked (a 21% reduction) and statistically significant in the young ($P = 0.03$), whereas the reduction in myocardial infarction (by about one third) was significant in younger ($P = 0.02$) and older ($P = 0.04$) patients (20).

Figure 11 reports plots for survival without myocardial infarction and illustrates the significant effect of ASA in men and in both younger and older subjects. The effect appeared early after the onset of treatment and continued until the end of the trial.

VI. ADVERSE EFFECTS OF INTENSIVE ANTIHYPERTENSIVE TREATMENT AND QUALITY OF LIFE DURING THE HOT STUDY

A. Adverse Effects

The medication administered was well tolerated; the only reported adverse effects that exceeded 2% were dizziness, headache, leg edema, flushing, coughing—the latter three to a large extent attributable to the use of the calcium antagonist and ACE inhibitors (21,22). Table 19 indicates that peripheral edema, coughing, headache, and flushing were more prevalent in women (20) Peripheral edema, dizziness, and vertigo were more prevalent in older than younger patients, whereas the reverse occurred for coughing, flushing, and impotence (20). There was no significant increase in the incidence of adverse effects in the lowest target blood pressure group as compared with the others, although the rate of adverse effects was somewhat higher at the higher steps of the treatment regimen (Fig. 12) (22). It should also be remarked that the proportion of patients with reported adverse effects decreased gradually throughout the trial, from 16.9% at 3 months to 2.2% at the final visit (18).

B. Quality-of-Life Substudy

Nine hundred twenty-two hypertensive patients of the HOT study were included in a substudy that aimed to investigate the impact on quality of life of lowering the pressure and of intensified therapy (23). Seven hundred eighty-one patients completed both baseline

Table 19 Adverse Effects Reported Any Time During the Follow-Up (%) in Male and Female Patients in the HOT Study

Variable	Men (n = 9907)	Women (n = 8883)	*P*-value
Peripheral edema	11.4	17.0	< 0.001
Coughing	4.1	5.0	< 0.01
Headache	3.5	5.3	< 0.001
Flushing	2.1	4.3	< 0.001
Dizziness	2.7	2.9	n.s.
Impotence	2.7	—	
Fatigue	2.0	1.8	n.s.
Dyspepsia	1.4	1.6	n.s.
Abdominal pain	1.0	1.4	< 0.05

n.s. = not significant.

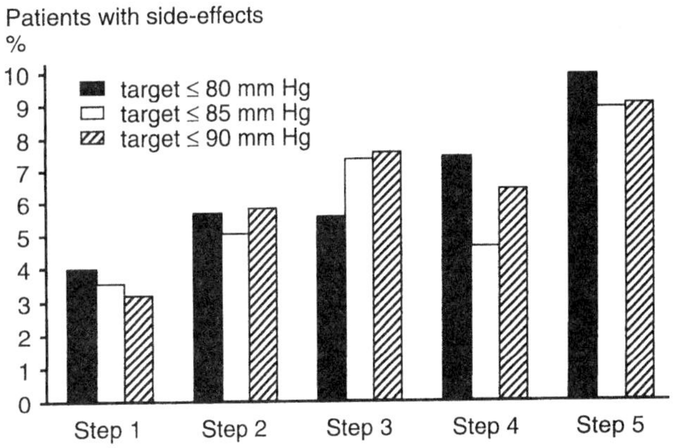

Fig. 12 Percentage of patients with side effects in the three target groups at 24 months in relation to dose titration step. (From Ref. 22.)

and follow-up questionnaires (intention-to-treat population), whereas 610 patients were included in a per-protocol analysis. Two self-administered validated questionnaires, the Psychological General Well-Being Index and the Subjective Symptoms Assessment Profile (SSA-P) were completed at baseline and after 6 months. As illustrated in Figure 13, the lower the diastolic blood pressure achieved, the greater the improvement in well-being ($P < 0.05$). The increase in well-being from baseline to 6 months was significant in target groups 80 mm Hg or less ($P < 0.01$) and 85 mm Hg or less ($P < 0.05$). The SSA-P domains' cardiac symptoms and dizziness improved in all groups, but the sex life score deteriorated in the 80 or less and 85 mm Hg or less groups in men. In all target groups, headaches were reduced ($P < 0.001$), whereas swollen ankles ($P < 0.001$) and dry cough

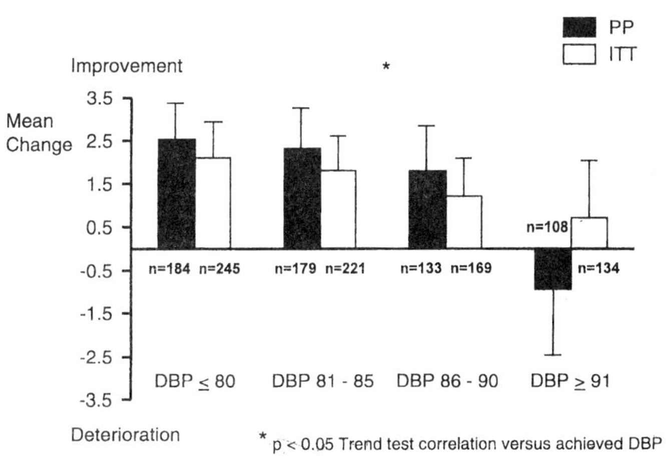

Fig. 13 The mean change (SEM) in the Psychological General Well-Being Index total scores from baseline to 6 months correlated to actual diastolic blood pressure achieved. Per protocol (PP) analysis included all patients that had evaluable data at baseline and at 6 months after entry; intention to treat (ITT) analysis also included patients who had violated inclusion or follow-up dates. Pitmans nonparametric permutation test: correlation was significant ($P < 0.05$) for PP analysis; $P = 0.11$ for ITT analysis. (From Ref. 23.)

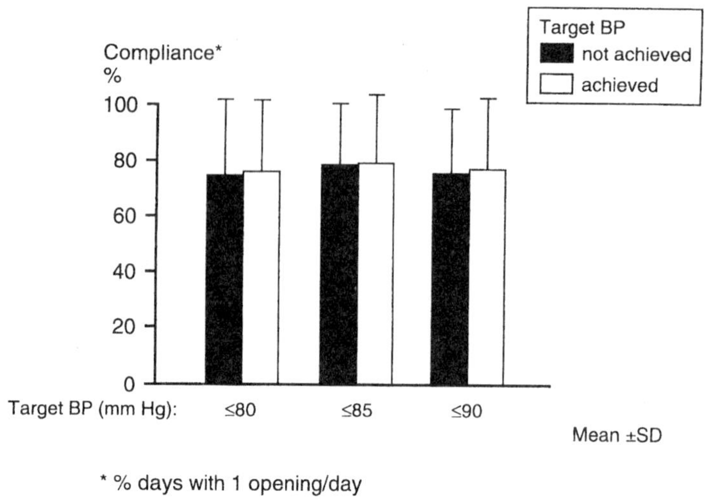

Fig. 14 Compliance to ASA in HOT study patients for target diastolic blood pressure group and according to achievement or lack of achievement of target blood pressure. (From Ref. 24.)

in the 80 mm Hg or less group ($P < 0.001$) increased. Although more intensive antihypertensive therapy is associated with a slight increase in subjective symptoms, it is nonetheless still associated with improvements in patients' well-being.

C. Compliance Substudy

Compliance to medication (24) in the HOT study was investigated in a subset of patients and evaluated as compliance to double-blind administration of aspirin or placebo in addition to antihypertensive treatment. Compliance was evaluated for 1 year in a subset (n = 530) of the study population (n = 18,790) by placing the medication in a container closed with an electronic cap that recorded precisely the time of each opening. The 1-year compliance rate (percentage of days with 1 opening/day) could be assessed in 501 patients. It averaged 78.3 ± 25% in aspirin-treated patients (n = 236, mean ±SD) as compared with 78.5 ± 25% in patients having received placebo (n = 265) and was not influenced by age, gender or country (Germany, Italy, Switzerland, United Kingdom). The compliance rate was also similar irrespective of the target blood pressure group and of whether the patients had reached their target blood pressure (Fig. 14), but it was significantly better during the first than the second 6-month monitoring period (84 ± 22% vs 72.3 ± 32%; n = 501). Thus, the high rate of compliance to aspirin or placebo observed in the HOT study suggests that the patients were highly motivated, which may account for the unusually good blood pressure control achieved in this trial during long-term antihypertensive treatment.

VII. DISCUSSION

A. Reasons Why the Study Was Done and Questions to be Answered

The large body of randomized trials of antihypertensive therapy demonstrated the benefits of lowering blood pressure (1), but none has approached the problem of how far blood pressure should be lowered. Even the Hypertension Detection and Follow-Up Program trial (25) was a comparison of more versus less frequent treatment of hypertension, rather than a comparison of different levels of achieved blood pressure. This uncertainty about the best level of blood pressure to be aimed at by treatment has been a main reason why physicians all over the world have been content to lower blood pressure by just a few mm Hg, extrapolating from trial meta-analyses that a 5 to 6 mm Hg reduction in diastolic blood pressure is enough to reduce stroke by about 40% (incorrectly ignoring that this reduction is the net difference from the placebo effect that can hardly be assessed in medical practice). The J-shaped curve concept (8) has been a further reason for doctors' concern about intensively treating hypertension. The HOT study, therefore, was planned not so much to disprove the J-shaped curve hypothesis (an unfalsifiable hypothesis, as obviously at 0 mm Hg blood pressure everyone would be dead) but rather to ascertain the level of diastolic blood pressure at which the treated hypertensive patient is at the lowest risk of cardiovascular events (15). Therefore, the first aim of the HOT study, as stated in the study protocol, was "to establish the optimal target blood pressure during antihypertensive treatment in order to reduce cardiovascular morbidity and mortality."

The second reason for which the HOT study was planned was to clarify the possible benefits of associating blood pressure lowering with antiplatelet therapy in hypertension and to ascertain whether a possible further reduction in the incidence of coronary events may be balanced by an increased risk of hemorrhagic stroke. Hence, the second aim of the HOT study, as indicated in the study protocol, was "to determine if the addition of low-dose ASA will further reduce cardiovascular morbidity and mortality."

B. Strengths and Weaknesses of the HOT Study

The design and conduct of the HOT study have several strengths: (a) the novelty of the two major objectives of the trial, namely, finding the optimal blood pressure to be aimed at and the possible benefits of associating intensive lowering of blood pressure with antiplatelet medication, objectives that had not been approached by any of the previous trials; (b) the large dimension of the study, with 19,193 patients randomized, of whom 18,790 followed up with a loss to follow-up of only 491 (2.6%) subjects (18). For comparison's sake, the largest trial of antihypertensive therapy previously completed, the Medical Research Council trial on mild hypertension (26), had randomized 17,354 patients with a loss of 19%; (c) the representativeness of the study that was conducted by 1904 investigators in 26 countries in Europe, North America, South America, and Asia; (d) the quality of the randomization procedure, that was computer generated and took into account a large number of relevant baseline variables, such as age, sex, previous antihypertensive therapy, smoking, previous myocardial infarction, other previous coronary heart disease, previous stroke, and diabetes mellitus (18,19); (e) the selection of patients with confirmed hypertension: in patients untreated at the enrolling visit, elevated blood pressure values had to be confirmed at two subsequent qualifying visits and averaged 171/106, 170/106, 169/105 mm Hg; in treated patients (52% of the total sample), withdrawal of treatment raised blood pressure from 161/99 mm Hg at enrolment to 169/105 and 170/106 mmHg at the two subsequent qualifying visits, thus ruling out inclusion of a substantial number of subjects with "white coat" hypertension (19); (f) both types of analyses that were used to relate events to blood pressure, namely, comparing event rates between different randomized target blood pressure groups of patients and relating event rates to achieved blood pressure, were indicated in the trial protocol (15). Likewise, separate analyses in diabetic patients or in subjects with previous ischemic heart disease concerned patients with characteristics included in the randomization procedure.

The HOT study also had weaknesses. (a) Diastolic blood pressure only was used as a target for treatment, and it may be objected that insufficient consideration was given to systolic blood pressure. However, when the protocol was designed in early 1991, no trials had yet demonstrated the value of lowering systolic blood pressure, and all available guidelines (27,28) insisted on using diastolic blood pressure as a guidance to treatment. Furthermore, using both systolic and diastolic blood pressure values as targets for randomized patients would have obviously complicated and perhaps endangered the conduct of the study. (b) The number of the events was smaller than initially calculated, as only 724 validated cardiovascular events in 683 patients occurred during an average follow-up of 3.8 years, whereas the expectation was for 1100 events during a follow-up of only 2.5 years (15). Event rates were obviously overestimated in the protocol, as calculations were based on the results of the STOP hypertension trial (16), which studied much older patients. Furthermore, as many as 24% of reported endpoints were rejected by the clinic event committee because of a lack of the criteria required by the protocol (18). It cannot be excluded that the rigorous criteria followed by the clinical events committee may have thus underassessed the real number of cardiovascular events. The attempt to increase the number of events by also considering ''silent'' myocardial infarctions (as indicated in the protocol) was made difficult by the unknown timing of a ''silent'' event that could only be diagnosed by the electrocardiogram done at the end of the trial; for all other events, their incidence was calculated by taking into account the time from randomization at which they occurred. Finally, the low incidence of events in the HOT trial patients may also be considered a strength rather than a weakness and taken as the consequence of the excellent blood pressure control achieved in virtually all patients (92%) of the study. (c) The major weakness of the HOT study is the small difference in diastolic (as well as systolic) blood pressure between the three target blood pressure groups to which the patients were randomized. Not only the average diastolic blood pressure differences between groups were of only 2 mm Hg instead of the expected 5 mm Hg, but, as evident from Figure 5, there was a large overlap of blood pressure values even in the groups randomized to 90 mm Hg or lower and to 80 mm Hg or lower (more than 50% of diastolic blood pressure values common to both groups). This markedly limited the power of the analysis per randomized target blood pressure group, which could show significant differences only for specific types of cardiovascular events (namely, all myocardial infarction) or for specific groups of patients (such as diabetics). More information has been derived from analyzing the relation of event rates with achieved blood pressure values. The continuous analysis was a very powerful mathematical model based on the average blood pressure of all 18,790 patients, that is, more than 105,000 standardized blood pressure measurements. However, a statistical analysis using achieved blood pressure may introduce weaknesses, compared with an analysis based on a randomized design. The potential source of error involving future information was avoided in our study by using a time-dependent model that was updated in its covariates. Because the model updated past mean of blood pressure, the time since randomization, and the age every 6 months, no future information was used in estimation of curves and confidence bands (18). Nevertheless, the estimated curves must be interpreted with caution, especially at the lowest and highest levels of blood pressure. At the extreme ends of the curves, patients with high risk because of coexisting disorders, such as malignancies and alcohol abuse, may accumulate. However, the possibility that patients with the lowest values of achieved blood pressure were those with the lowest values of baseline blood pressure (what may implicate a lower risk) is disproved

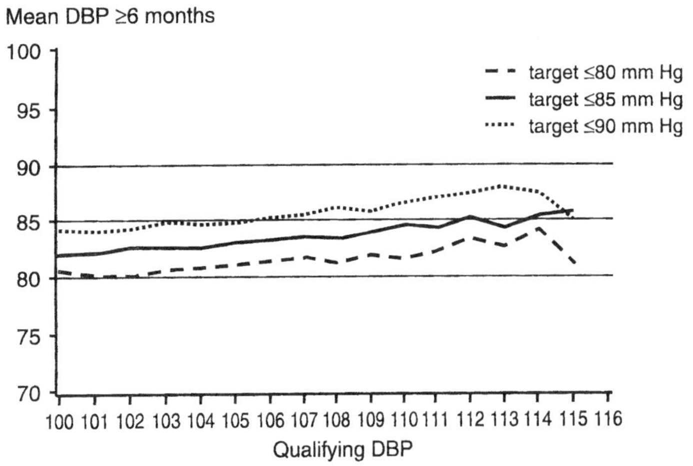

Fig. 15 Relation of achieved diastolic blood pressure (DBP) to qualifying DBP.

by the analysis summarized in Figure 15, showing that within each group of target blood pressure, baseline influenced achieved values by no more than 4 mm Hg. This was not the case for the extent of the blood pressure reduction, which was influenced more markedly (to a maximum of about 14 mm Hg) by baseline values (Fig 16). This suggested the opportunity of avoiding the correlation of cardiovascular endpoints with the extent of the blood pressure reduction induced by treatment.

C. Accomplishments

1. *Effectiveness of Intensive Antihypertensive Therapy in Significantly Lowering Blood Pressure*

An important accomplishment of the HOT study is the finding that substantial reductions in blood pressure can be achieved with a treatment regimen based on the long-acting

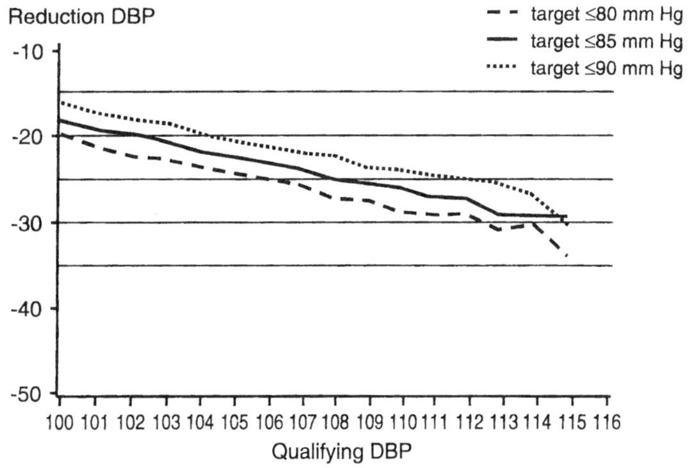

Fig. 16 Relation of reduction of diastolic blood pressure (DBP) to qualifying DBP.

calcium antagonist, felodipine, and with the frequent recourse to combination therapy. Even in patients who were receiving treatment before enrollment (52.6%), there was a striking further reduction in blood pressure with the treatment regimen used. The overall reductions in diastolic (20 to 24 mm Hg) and systolic blood pressure (26 to 30 mm Hg) are striking in comparison with those reported in the meta-analysis by Collins and colleagues (1) (5 to 6 mm Hg reduction in diastolic blood pressure and 9 to 10 mm Hg in systolic blood pressure). Admittedly, the blood pressure reductions observed in the HOT study are in relation to baseline values and not placebo subtracted, as was done in the meta-analysis of previous trials by Collins et al. (1). However, the reductions of both diastolic (22 mm Hg) and systolic blood pressures (28 mm Hg) obtained in the HOT study are definitely greater than those reported in the actively treated groups of most of the major trials included in that meta-analysis. For example, the reductions in diastolic blood pressure averaged 17 mm Hg in the Hypertension Detection and Follow-up Program (HDFP) (25), 12 mm Hg in the Australian and the MRC trials on mild hypertension (26,29), and even in the two major studies on isolated systolic hypertension, the SystEur (30) and the SHEP (31), the reductions in systolic blood pressure were slightly but definitely smaller (23 and 26 mm Hg) than in the HOT. It can be concluded, therefore, that the treatment regimen followed in the HOT study showed a greater effectiveness in lowering blood pressure, particularly diastolic blood pressure, than any previous study.

2. *Tolerability of Intensive Blood Pressure Lowering*

The medication administered in the HOT study was well tolerated. The only reported adverse effects that exceeded 2% were dizziness, headache, leg edema, flushing, and coughing, the latter three to a large extent attributable to the use of the calcium antagonist and ACE inhibitors. Furthermore, the substudy on patient well-being (23) showed an overall improvement as compared with baseline, and that this improvement was greater in the 80 mm Hg or lower target group than in the other target groups.

3. *Marked Reduction of Cardiovascular Events by Intensive Lowering of Blood Pressure*

The major cardiovascular event curves calculated from HOT study data suggest that from three to ten cardiovascular events can be prevented in every 1000 patients treated for 1 year by reducing blood pressure from baseline to the optimal blood pressure values of 80 to 85 mm Hg diastolic, and 130 to 140 mm Hg systolic. However, most of this benefit is achieved by lowering systolic blood pressure to about 140 mm Hg and diastolic blood pressure to about 90 mm Hg, and only a small additional benefit is obtained by reducing blood pressure any further. This conclusion agrees with a previous post hoc analysis of the MRC mild hypertension trial (32) that showed that the relation between on-treatment blood pressure and stroke flattens below systolic values of 135 to 140 mm Hg and diastolic values of 85 to 90 mm Hg, with no evidence of an increased incidence at lower values. Similar indications result from a post hoc analysis of the IPPPSH Study (33).

On the whole, the event rates in the HOT study were very low and definitely lower than the event rates in actively treated patients in the trial meta-analysis by Collins et al. (1) as revised by Collins and Peto (34). This is clearly shown in Table 20. It is unlikely that the baseline cardiovascular risk in HOT patients was lower than in previous trials meta-analyzed by Collins and Peto (34). In fact, the mean age of HOT patients was 5 years older than that of the patients of the meta-analysis; baseline systolic and diastolic blood pressures of HOT patients (170/105 mm Hg) were higher than in several of the

Table 20 Comparison of Event Rates (per 1000 patient-years) in the HOT Study and in Collins and Peto's Meta-Analysis of Previous Trials (33)

	HOT (mean age 61)	Previous trials* (mean age 56)
Total mortality	8.3	12.3
Cardiovascular mortality	3.8	6.5
All stroke	4.2	4.4
All myocardial infarction	3.0	7.8

*Actively treated patients.
Abbreviations: *HOT*, Hypertension Optimal Treatment.

major studies included in the meta-analysis [159/101 mm Hg in the HDFP (25), 158/100 in the Australian trial on mild hypertension (30), 156/98 in the MRC trial on mild hypertension (26)] and some of the previous trials (such as the Australian and the MRC trials (26,29) deliberately excluded patients with diabetes, previous myocardial infarction, stroke, and ischemic heart disease. Therefore, major difference of HOT from previous trials is in the percentage of actively treated patients that reached the target of 90 mm Hg or lower: this was 91.5% among HOT patients, whereas Table 1 shows that from 23% to 37% of patients in previous trials did not achieve this target. This is the most likely explanation of the particularly low rate of cardiovascular events in the HOT study. Alternatively, this low morbidity may be attributed to the prevalence of modern antihypertensive agents in the treatment regimen (78% of patients receiving felodipine and 41% an ACE inhibitor vs 28% receiving a β-blocker and 22% a diuretic).

4. *No J-Shaped Curve When Diastolic Blood Pressure Is Brought to "Normal" Values*

The HOT study has also shown that an additional lowering of blood pressure below minimum values does not produce a further reduction in events, but it is not harmful. There was no evidence of a J-shaped curve for the relation of major cardiovascular events, all myocardial infarction and all stroke with achieved blood pressure, at least in the ranges observed in our study (down to 70 mm Hg diastolic, and 120 mm Hg systolic). This was also true in the subgroup of more than 3000 patients with signs or history of ischemic heart disease at randomization.

We did find a slight, though nonsignificant, increase in cardiovascular deaths at the lowest level of blood pressure. As pointed out by Collins and Peto (34), because of the relatively short duration of trials of antihypertensive therapy, analyses of mortality are potentially unreliable and ''less informative than indirect assessment of that effect, based on analyses of the proportional effects of treatment on total stroke and on coronary events.'' Also, the slight increase in cardiovascular mortality was not caused by an increase in fatal myocardial infarctions or fatal strokes at the lowest achieved blood pressure.

There was also a small nonsignificant increase in total mortality with declining blood pressure, which was observed in the analysis of total mortality both in relation to target group and to achieved blood pressure. This increase was only partly accounted for by the increase in cardiovascular mortality. The small increment of total deaths in patients with the lowest blood pressures may be accounted for by the blood pressure lowering of poor health rather than by treatment.

5. Particularly Significant Benefits of Intensive Blood Pressure Lowering in Hypertensive Patients with Diabetes Mellitus

Intensive lowering of blood pressure produced such great benefits in the subgroup of patients with diabetes mellitus that these were clear and statistically significant even in the analysis by randomized target blood pressure groups, despite the small difference in blood pressure (18). Significant trends for greater event reduction at lower target diastolic blood pressure were found for major cardiovascular events and for cardiovascular mortality. Total mortality was also reduced with a *P* value (= 0.068) close to statistical significance. All myocardial infarctions were halved, but because of their small number, the reduction did not attain statistical significance. These results of the HOT study are consistent with those of the recent UK Prospective Diabetes Study (UKPDS) trial (35,36) demonstrating that a lower achieved blood pressure (144/82 mm Hg vs 154/87 mm Hg) was associated with significantly reduced risk of macrovascular and microvascular disease outcomes in diabetic patients.

6. Lower Myocardial Infarction Rate by Associating ASA to Antihypertensive Treatment

In a previous section of this chapter, it was mentioned that many controlled studies have proven the benefits of ASA in secondary prevention of myocardial infarction or of ischemic cerebrovascular disease (11), whereas only very few studies have investigated the effect of ASA in primary prevention of cardiovascular events, and with controversial effects (13,14). In particular, the effect of antiplatelet therapy has not been assessed in a prospective randomized trial of patients with hypertension. Indeed, hypertension has often been considered a contraindication to ASA because of the concern that possible benefits in the prevention of coronary events may be counterbalanced by an increased risk of cerebral bleeding.

The investigation of the effects of a small dose of ASA versus placebo in treated patients with hypertension, as we did in this study, provides very clear evidence of a substantial beneficial action of ASA on fatal and nonfatal acute myocardial infarctions, the incidence of which was reduced by as much as 36% (with the possibility of a benefit between 15% and 51%), and the prevention of 1.3 myocardial infarctions per 1000 patients treated for 1 year (and 2.5 myocardial infarctions per 1000 patient-years in subjects with diabetes mellitus) in addition to the benefit achieved by antihypertensive therapy. The relative benefit of ASA in patients with hypertension, as far as myocardial infarction is concerned, is similar to that observed in studies of patients with previous myocardial infarction or coronary disease (11). This benefit was achieved without any additional risk of strokes, which occurred at the same rates in patients with hypertension receiving ASA or placebo. Consequently, a significant benefit was also observed for major cardiovascular events, which were reduced by 15%. There was also a nonsignificant trend toward a lower cardiovascular mortality and total mortality in patients with hypertension who were receiving ASA. Inclusion of silent myocardial infarction among events limited the benefits of ASA, suggesting that silent myocardial infarctions may sometimes occur as a less severe event, from the prevention of an acute myocardial infarction. Although the number of fatal bleeds was similar in the ASA and placebo groups, the overall rate of major and minor bleeds (mainly gastrointestinal and nasal) was about 1.8 times higher in the ASA group.

Because of the importance of establishing the balance between the benefits for myocardial infarction and the risk of hemorrhage, we have carefully examined, in addition to the data from the HOT study, data from the recent Thrombosis Prevention Trial (TPT) of high-risk patients (37), from the two major primary prevention trials (13,14), and from a secondary prevention trial (the Swedish Aspirin Low Dose Trial, [SALT]) that used the same dose of the same ASA preparation given to the HOT patients (12). Admittedly, there are limitations in this approach, as all these studies were not very precise in the definition and verification of bleedings. Table 21 (38) shows the extreme variability of incidence of bleeds (expressed as bleeds per 1000 subject-years) and that, at any rate, the HOT is never the study with the highest bleed rate. ''All bleeds'' appears to be the least reliable variable (a range of values in the control groups between 4.62 in the HOT to 133.49 in the TPT). A narrower range is observed for all gastrointestinal bleeds, again with the lowest incidence in the HOT and the highest in the TPT. Only by restricting the analysis to major gastrointestinal bleeds did TPT show the lowest incidence (the highest one occurring in the SALT). Definition of a major gastrointestinal bleed is, however, much more restrictive in the TPT (''fatal and life-threatening, requiring transfusion or surgery'') and in the Physicians' Health Study (''fatal and requiring transfusion'') than in the HOT (''fatal, life-threatening, disabling, or requiring hospitalization'') and in the SALT and British Male Doctors' Study (''severe and requiring discontinuation'').

In conclusion, differences in bleed incidence between the various studies are most likely the result of differences in bleed reports and definitions and on the whole, in the hypertensive patients of the HOT study, aspirin was not associated with more bleedings than in other antiplatelet trials. However, the advantages of using ASA in hypertension have been shown in extremely well-treated patients with hypertension, such as those in our study, and do not necessarily extend to less well-treated patients with hypertension.

7. *Safety of Antihypertensive Treatment Based on Calcium Antagonists*

Although this was not the primary aim of the HOT study, its results provide important evidence in favor of the safety of an antihypertensive regimen based on calcium antagonists. All HOT patients were initiated on a low dose of felodipine and at the end of the study, 78% of them were still taking felodipine (in two-thirds of cases, in association with other antihypertensive agents). Although no comparative group with placebo or other antihypertensive drugs was included in the HOT study, the very low incidence of cardiovascular events observed in the course of the trial obviously indicates the safety of the therapeutic regimen used in the HOT. Together with the favorable results of controlled

Table 21 Bleeds in Five Cardiovascular Prevention Trials with Aspirin

	Subject years		Major GI		All GI		All bleeds	
Trial	A	P	A	P	A	P	A	P
HOT Study	35,716	35,686	2.16	1.04	3.0	1.54	8.18	4.62
Thrombosis Prevention Trial	8,105	8,071	0.75	0.25	18.38	13.13	143.86	113.49
Physicians Health Study	58,895	54,864	0.88	0.51	14.30	12.69	53.30	40.24
British Male Doctors' Study	18,820	9,470	3.67	—	—	—	—	—
SALT	1,724	1,568	5.22	2.55	6.38	2.55	28.42	14.03

Incidence of bleeds is expressed as bleeds/1000 subject-years. A: aspirin group; P: placebo group (no placebo in the British Male Doctors' Study control group). GI: gastrointestinal bleeds. Bleed rates are estimated from data given in or inferred from each paper.

Abbreviation: *SALT*, Swedish Aspirin Low-Dose Trial.

trials, such as the Syst-Eur (30), the Stone (39), and the Syst-China (40) that compared calcium antagonist-based treatment with placebo in elderly hypertensive patients, the HOT study results do not support the reservations raised by some authors against the use of calcium antagonists in the treatment of hypertension.

VIII. INFLUENCES EXERTED BY THE HOT STUDY RESULTS ON MEDICAL PRACTICE

It is too early to say how the principal results of the HOT study may influence medical practice, but they have certainly influenced several aspects of the 1999 WHO/ISH guidelines (41) that often cite information provided by this study. The following are the major clinical applications of HOT study evidence.

A. The Possibility of Lowering Blood Pressure to Goal

In the HOT study patients, the goal of 90 mm Hg diastolic blood pressure was achieved in 91.5%, an accomplishment that was not obtained in any of the previous trials of antihypertensive therapy. Choosing a target of 85 or 80 mm Hg and below, rather than 90 or below, may have helped to obtain a more generalized control of diastolic blood pressure, as in the target groups 85 or 80 mm Hg or less only 7% and, respectively, 6% of patients failed to achieve the level of 90 mm Hg, whereas 12% of patients in the target group 90 mm Hg or lower failed to achieve this target. As explained in a previous section of this chapter, the HOT study only used diastolic blood pressure as an objective of treatment, and we cannot say whether reaching a systolic blood pressure target of 140 mm Hg or lower would be equally successful.

B. Broad Use of Combination Therapy in Antihypertensive Management

The 1999 WHO/ISH guidelines (41) mention that the HOT study has demonstrated that combination therapy was necessary in about 70% of patients to achieve target blood pressure. It is appropriate to underline that target blood pressure could be achieved in almost two thirds of HOT patients by either low-dose monotherapy (with the calcium antagonist felodipine) or low-dose combination of two agents (usually, a low dose of felodipine with a low dose of either an ACE inhibitor or a beta blocker). Therefore, the HOT study shows that, in the greatest proportion of hypertensive patients, blood pressure can be controlled to a satisfactory degree without having to prescribe too many compounds or too large doses.

C. Good Tolerability of Antihypertensive Therapy

Intensive lowering of blood pressure by drugs, as progressively combined in the HOT study, was very well tolerated by patients, and the substudy on well being has shown that the lower the target or the achieved blood pressure, the better the quality of life of the patients (23). This refutes the common belief that antihypertensive drugs worsen quality of life.

D. No Increased Risk in "Normalizing" Blood Pressure

The principal results of the HOT study demonstrated the benefits of lowering blood pressure in patients with hypertension to about 140 mm Hg systolic and 85 mm Hg diastolic or lower. Efforts to lower blood pressure further, down to fully "normal" or "optimal" values of 120 mm Hg systolic and 70 mm Hg diastolic, give little further benefit but do not cause additional risk. This was also true in the patients with baseline history or signs of ischemic heart disease, that is, the group of patients for whom the concept of the J-shaped curve was developed (8). Obviously, this does not rule out that a J-shaped curve exists, and indeed it is likely to exist, but if the point of inflexion is below 120/70 mm Hg, this means there is no risk in "normalizing" blood pressure.

E. Importance of Intensive Blood Pressure Lowering in Diabetic Hypertensives

The HOT study, having involved the largest number of diabetic hypertensives as compared with any other intervention trial, is a very important piece of evidence in favor of the recommendation to lower blood pressure to normal or optimal values in diabetic patients. This is recognized in the WHO/ISH guidelines (41). As treatment in the HOT study was based on a calcium antagonist, the study indicates that calcium antagonists can be used to lower blood pressure in diabetic patients. This conclusion is supported by a substudy of diabetic patients in the Syst-Eur trial (42).

F. Benefits of Associating Antihypertensive Therapy with Antiplatelet Agents

The WHO/ISH guidelines (41) recognize that "in view of the results of the HOT study, it is reasonable to recommend the use of low-dose aspirin in hypertensive patients whose blood pressure has been rigorously controlled, who are at high risk of coronary heart disease and are not particularly at risk of bleeding from the gastrointestinal tract or from other sites." Analyses of the HOT data by gender (20) suggests that men may derive more significant benefits from addition of aspirin to antihypertensive therapy.

APPENDIX

Study Organization

Executive committee—L Hansson (Sweden) and A Zanchetti (Italy; chairmen), SG Carruthers (Canada), KH Rahn (Germany), S Julius (USA), J Ménard (France), H Wedel (Sweden; statistician), B Dahlöf (Sweden; secretary), D Elmfeldt (Sweden; nonvoting), S Westerling (Sweden; nonvoting).

Steering committee—DL Clement (Belgium), F Fyhrquist (Finland), B-G Hansson (Sweden), H Ibsen (Denmark), KA Jamerson (USA), SE Kjeldsen (Norway), R Kolloch (Germany), P Larochelle (Canada), G Leonetti (Italy), G McInnes (UK), J-M Mallion (France), T Rosenthal (Israel), LM Ruilope (Spain), F Skrabal (Austria), P Toutouzas (Greece), B Waeber (Switzerland), H Wesseling (The Netherlands), J-R Zhu (People's Republic of China).

National coordinators—R Sanchez (Argentina), E Kekes (Hungary).

Independent safety committee—JD Swales (UK), S Pocock (UK), JL Rodicio (Spain).

Independent clinical event committee—L Rydén (Sweden), C Dal Palù (Italy), H Holzgreve (Germany).

Independent data audit committee—LH Lindholm (Sweden), JK McKenzie (Canada).

Additional studies committee—T Hedner (Sweden), G Mancia (Italy), D Elmfeldt (Sweden).

ECG committee—S Jern (Sweden), J Wikstrand (Sweden).

HOT study coordinating group—J Allgen (Sweden), B Virdborg (Sweden), I Warnold (Sweden), S Westerling (Sweden).

Data handling and statistics group—A Hagelin (Sweden), P Lilja (Sweden), J Lindquist (Sweden), A Odén (Sweden), N-G Pehrsson (Sweden), H Wedel (Sweden).

ACKNOWLEDGMENTS

The principal sponsor of the HOT Study was Astra AB, Sweden, now AstraZeneca. Local sponsors were Astra Merck Inc, USA; TEVA, Israel; and Hoechst, Argentina. We thank the 1904 participating investigators and coworkers and all those who acted as monitors in the participating countries for their dedicated work. We also acknowledge the skillful and meticulous administrative work of A Holmner and S Lilja at the Hot study coordinating center.

REFERENCES

1. Collins R, Peto R, MacMahon S, Hebert P, Fiebach NH, Eberlein KA, Godwin J, Qizilbash N, Taylor JO, Hennekens CH. Blood pressure, stroke, and coronary heart disease. Part 2, Short-term reductions in blood pressure: overview of randomised drug trials in their epidemiological context. Lancet 1990; 335:827–838.
2. Lindholm L, Ejlertsson G, Scherstén B. High risk of cerebrocardiovascular morbidity in well treated male hypertensives: a retrospective study of 40–59 year old hypertensives in a Swedish primary care district. Acta Med Scand 1984; 216:251–259.
3. Isles CG, Walker LM, Beevers GD, Brown I, Cameron HL, Clarke J, Hawthorne V, Hole D, Lever AF, Robertson JW. Mortality in patients of the Glasgow Blood Pressure Clinic. J Hypertens 1986; 4:141–156.
4. Zanchetti A. Contribution of fixed low-dose combinations to initial therapy in hypertension. Eur Heart J 1999; 1(Suppl L):L5–L9.
5. Hansson L. How far should blood pressure be lowered? What is the role of the J-curve? Am J Hypertens 1990; 3:726–729.
6. Zanchetti A. To what level should blood pressure be brought by antihypertensive treatment? High Blood Pressure 1992; 1:197–200.
7. Stewart IM. Relation of reduction in pressure to first myocardial infarction in patients receiving treatment for severe hypertension. Lancet 1979; 1:861–865.
8. Cruickshank JM, Thorn JM, Zacharias FJ. Benefits and potential harm of lowering high blood pressure. Lancet 1987; 1:581–584.
9. Alderman MH, Ooi WL, Madhavan S, Cohen H. Treatment-induced blood pressure reduction and the risk of myocardial infarction. JAMA 1989; 262:920–924.
10. Samuelsson O, Wilhelmsen L, Andersson OK, Pennert K, Berglund G. Cardiovascular morbidity in relation to change in blood pressure and serum cholesterol levels in treated hypertension: results from the Primary Prevention Trial in Göteborg, Sweden. JAMA 1987; 258:1768–1776.
11. Antiplatelet Trialists' Collaborative overview of randomised trials of antiplatelet therapy, 1: prevention of death, myocardial infarction and stroke by prolonged antiplatelet therapy in various categories of patients. BMJ 1994; 308:81–106.
12. The SALT Collaboration Group. Swedish Aspirin Low-dose Trial (SALT) of 75 mg aspirin

as secondary prophylaxis after cerebrovascular ischaemic events. Lancet 1991; 338:1345–1349.

13. Hennekens CH, Buring JE, Sandercock P, Collins R, Peto R. Aspirin and other antiplatelet agents in the secondary and primary prevention of cardiovascular disease. Circulation 1989; 80:749–756.
14. Peto R, Gray R, Collins R, Wheattey K, Hennekens C, Jamrozik K, Warlow C, Hafner B, Thompson E, Norton S. Randomised trial of prophylactic daily aspirin in British male doctors. BMJ 1988; 296:313–316.
15. Hansson L, Zanchetti A, for the HOT Study Group. The Hypertension Optimal Treatment Study (the HOT Study) Blood Pressure 1993; 2:62–68.
16. Dahlöf B, Lindholm L, Hansson L, Scherstèn B, Ekbom T, Wester PO. Morbidity and mortality in the Swedish trial in old patients with hypertension (STOP-Hypertension). Lancet 1991; 338:1281–1285.
17. Hansson L, Hedner T, Dahlöf B. Prospective Randomized Open Blinded End-point (PROBE) Study a novel design for intervention trials. Blood Pressure 1992; 1:113–119.
18. Hansson L, Zanchetti A, Carruthers SG, Dahlof B, Elmfeldt D, Menard J, Rahn KH, Wedel H, Westerling S, for the HOT Study Group. Effects of intensive blood pressure lowering and low dose aspirin in patients with hypertension: principal results of the Hypertension Optimal Treatment (HOT) randomised trial. Lancet 1998; 351:1755–1762.
19. Hansson L, Zanchetti A, for the HOT Study Group. The Hypertension Optimal Treatment (HOT) Study. Patient characteristics, randomization, risk profiles, and early blood pressure results. Blood Pressure 1994; 3:322–327.
20. Kjeldsen SE, Kolloch RE, Leonetti G, Mallion JM, Zanchetti A, Hansson L, for the HOT Study Group. Influence of gender and age on preventing cardiovascular disease by antihypertensive treatment and acetylsalicylic acid. The HOT Study. J Hypertens 2000; 18:629–642.
21. Hansson L, Zanchetti A, for the HOT Study Group. The Hypertension Optimal Treatment (HOT) Study: 12-month data on blood pressure and tolerability, with special reference to age and gender. Blood Pressure 1995; 4:313–319.
22. Hansson L, Zanchetti A, for the HOT Study Group. The Hypertension Optimal Treatment (HOT) Study: 24-month data on blood pressure and tolerability. Blood Pressure 1997; 6:313–317.
23. Wiklund I, Halling K, Rydèn-Bergsten T, Fletcher A, on behalf of the HOT Study Group. Does lowering the blood pressure improve the mood? Quality-of-life results from the Hypertension Optimal Treatment (HOT) Study. Blood Pressure 1997; 6:357–364.
24. Waeber B, Leonetti G, Kolloch R, McInnes GT, for the HOT Study Group. Compliance with aspirin or placebo in the Hypertension Optimal Treatment (HOT) Study. J Hypertens 1999; 17:1041–1045. In publication.
25. Hypertension Detection and Follow up Program Cooperative Group. Five-year findings of the Hypertension Detection and Follow-up Program. I. Reduction in mortality of persons with high blood pressure, including mild hypertension. JAMA 1979; 242:2562–2571.
26. Medical Research Council Working Party. MRC trial of treatment of mild hypertension: principal results. BMJ 1985; 291:97–104.
27. Joint National Committee: 1988 Report of the Joint National Committee on detection, evaluation and treatment of high blood pressure. Arch Intern Med 1988; 148:1023–1038.
28. Guidelines Sub-Committee. 1989 Guidelines for the management of mild hypertension: memorandum from a World Health Organization-International Society of Hypertension meeting. J Hypertens 1989; 7:689–693.
29. Management Committee. The Australian Therapeutic Trial in Mild Hypertension. Lancet 1980; i:1261–1267.
30. Staessen JA, Fagard R, Thijs L, Celis H, Arabidze GG, Birkenhäger WH, Bulpitt CJ, de Leeuw PW, Dollery CT, Fletcher AE, Forette F, Leonetti G, Nachev C, O'Brien ET, Rosenfeld J, Rodicon JL, Tuomilehto J, Zanchetti A, for the Systolic Hypertension in Europe (Syst-Eur)

Trial Investigators. Randomised double-blind comparison of placebo and active treatment for older patients with isolated systolic hypertension. Lancet 1997; 350:757–764.
31. SHEP Cooperative Research Group. Prevention of stroke by antihypertensive drug treatment in older persons with isolated systolic hypertension, final results of the Systolic Hypertension in the Elderly Program (SHEP). JAMA 1991; 1265:3255–3264.
32. Medical Research Council Working Party on Mild to Moderate Hypertension. The MRC Mild Hypertension Trial: some subgroup results. In: Strasser T, Ganten D, eds. Mild Hypertension: From Drug Trials to Practice. New York: Raven Press, 1987; 9–20.
33. The IPPPSH Collaborative Group. Cardiovascular risk and factors in a randomised trial of treatment based on the beta-blocker oxprenolol. The International Prospective Primary Prevention Study in Hypertensives (IPPPSH). J Hypertens 1985; 36:379–392.
34. Collins R, Peto R. Antihypertensive drug therapy: effects on stroke and coronary heart disease. In: Swales JD, ed. Textbook of Hypertension. Oxford: Blackwell Scientific Publications, 1994: 1156–1164.
35. UK Prospective Diabetes Study Group. Tight blood pressure control and risk of macrovascular and microvascular complications in type 2 diabetes: UKPDS 38. BMJ 1998; 317:703–713.
36. UK Prospective Diabetes Study Group. Efficacy of atenolol and captopril in reducing risk of macrovascular and microvascular complications in type 2 diabetes: UKPDS 39. BMJ 1998; 317:713–720.
37. Medical Research Council General Practice Research Framework. Thrombosis Prevention Trial: randomized trial of low-intensity oral anticoagulation with warfarin and low dose aspirin in the primary prevention of ischemic heart disease in men at increased risk. Lancet 1998; 351:233–241.
38. Zanchetti A, Hansson L, on behalf of the HOT Executive Committee. Risk of major gastrointestinal bleeding with aspirin. Reply. Lancet 1999; 353:149–150.
39. Gong L, Zhang W, Zhu Y, Kong D, Page V, Ghadirian P, LeLorier J, Hamet P, Shanghai trial of nifedipine in the elderly (STONE). J Hypertens 1996; 14:1237–1245.
40. Liu L, Wang JG, Gong L, Liu G, Staessen JA, for the Systolic Hypertension in China (Syst-China) Collaborative Group. Comparison of active treatment and placebo for older Chinese patients with isolated systolic hypertension. J Hypertens 1998; 16:1823–1829.
41. Guidelines Subcommittee. 1999 World Health Organization—International Society of Hypertension Guidelines for the Management of Hypertension. J Hypertens 1999; 17:151–183.
42. Tuomilehto J, Rastenyte D, Birkenhäger WH, Thijs L, Antikainen R, Bulpitt CJ, Fletcher AE, Forette F, Goldhaber A, Palatini P, Sasti C, Fagard R, for the Systolic Hypertension in Europe Trial Investigators. Effects of calcium-channel blockade in older patients with diabetes and systolic hypertension. N Engl J Med 1999; 340:677–684.
43. Amery A, Birkenhäger W, Brixko P, Bulpitt C, Clement D, Delaruyttere M, De Schaepdryuer A, Dollery C, Fagard R, Forette F. Mortality and morbidity results from the European Working Party on High Blood Pressure in the Elderly Trial. Lancet 1985; i:1350–1354.
44. Wilhelmsen L, Berglund G, Fitzsimons D, Holzgreve H, Hosie J, Pennert K, Tuomilehto J, Wedel H, on behalf of the Heart Attack Primary Prevention in Hypertension Trial Research Group. Beta-blockers versus diuretics in hypertensive men: main results from the HAPPHY trial. J Hypertens 1987; 5:561–572.

16

Beta-Blocker Heart Attack Trial

ROBERT P. BYINGTON

Wake Forest University School of Medicine
Winston-Salem, North Carolina

I. BACKGROUND

The availability of proven therapies to reduce the clinical consequences of atherosclerotic disease has accelerated remarkably over the last 25 years. In the nonacute setting, major trials were still being conducted in the 1970s to test whether risk factor reduction would reduce the occurrence of clinical atherosclerotic events. For example, major trials, such as the Hypertension Detection and Follow-Up Program (1,2), tested whether antihypertensive therapy of hypertensive patients would reduce the occurrence of cerebrovascular events. Similarly, other major trials, such as the Coronary Primary Prevention Trial (3,4), were being conducted to test whether lipid-lowering therapy of high-risk patients would reduce the occurrence of cardiovascular events.

In the acute setting, within the last quarter-century the treatment of myocardial infarction (MI) has progressed greatly beyond simple bed rest, the alleviation of symptomatic pain, and the possible administration of one of the early antiarrhythmics. Of particular concern to clinicians, epidemiologists, and other public health authorities was the occurrence of sudden death. Without warning, individuals with undetected atherosclerotic disease or undetected (and mostly untreated) risk factors were dying before they even reached a hospital. No treatment was available to prevent this, either in the primary or secondary setting.

A conference was sponsored in 1976 by the United States National Heart and Lung Institute (now the National Heart, Lung, and Blood Institute, or NHLBI) to discuss potential agents to be used in either a primary or secondary prevention setting to reduce the incidence of sudden death (5). After reviewing what was then known about the epidemiology of sudden death and the mechanisms thought to be involved in the evolution of a clinical event, the conference participants considered therapeutic agents that might be useful in suppressing arrhythmias or limiting ischemia. Because it was recognized that a trial with an events outcome could easily require a large sample size followed up for many years, the conference participants also considered which populations might have an event rate that would make a sudden death trial both logistically and economically feasible. Ultimately, a recommendation was given to the NHLBI that a beta-adrenergic blocking agent (or beta-blocker) should be tested in patients who recently survived an acute MI. Such an agent was selected for recommendation because it could block the sympathetic nervous activity thought to be important in the pathophysiology of sudden death and, in animal models, beta-blockers could limit the size of an infarct and decrease myocardial ischemia (6,7). Also, and most importantly, there was evidence from five small trials to suggest that such an agent would be efficacious in reducing events (8–15).

Based on that recommendation, the Beta-Blocker Heart Attack Trial (BHAT) was initiated by the NHLBI in 1977. The particular beta-blocker selected, propranolol, was the only one then available for use in the United States. To reduce the possibility of outcome ascertainment bias, all-cause mortality, rather than sudden death was to be used as the primary outcome measure.

Before the trial, propranolol, a nonselective beta-blocker without sympathomimetic activity, was being used clinically to relieve angina pectoris and reduce ventricular arrhythmias. It was also a documented antihypertensive. By the mid-1970s, using preliminary data from other investigations, propranolol was even being advertised in some markets as being able to reduce the incidence of a first MI among hypertensives, compared with other antihypertensives (16).

This chapter reviews the design and primary results of that trial and focuses on the subgroup of participants who had a self-reported history of hypertension.

II. DESIGN AND CONDUCT OF THE BETA-BLOCKER HEART ATTACK TRIAL

A. Trial Design

The protocol-specified objectives and subgroup hypotheses for the BHAT are listed in Table 1. The primary objective was to test whether the chronic administration of the beta-blocker, propranolol hydrochloride, given to 3837 acute MI patients, would reduce the incidence of all-cause mortality over a 2- to 4-year period (17). It was designed as a randomized, placebo-controlled, double-masked, multicenter clinical trial. Protocol-specified secondary objectives included testing whether propranolol would reduce the incidence of coronary heart disease (CHD) mortality, sudden cardiac mortality (death within 1 hour of the onset of symptoms), and the combination of fatal CHD plus definite nonfatal recurrent MI (total ''coronary incidence''). Other outcomes of interest included the incidence or recurrence of anginal events, heart failure, stroke, and coronary artery bypass graft surgery (CABG). The description of the sample size calculations is provided below.

Recruitment for the trial began in June 1978 and ended in October 1980. Patients were recruited and followed up in 31 centers with 134 participating hospitals across the United States and Canada. (Appendix A lists the investigators and institutions participating in BHAT and Appendix B describes the BHAT Steering Committee and its subcommittees.) Follow-up ended in October 1981, 8 months ahead of the scheduled termination, because data accumulated to that point provided compelling evidence that propranolol

Table 1 BHAT Objectives and Subgroup Hypotheses as Specified in the Protocol

A. Primary objective	To determine whether the regular administration of propranolol to patients who have had at least one documented myocardial infarction would result in a significant reduction in mortality from any cause over the follow-up period.
B. Secondary objectives	1. To evaluate the effect of the regular administration of propranolol on: a. the incidence of coronary heart disease mortality b. the incidence of sudden cardiac death, defined as death within 1 hour of the onset of symptoms c. the combined incidence of nonfatal myocardial infarction plus coronary heart disease mortality 2. To evaluate the possible side effects of propranolol with chronic use 3. To evaluate the possible mechanisms of action of propranolol if it is successful in reducing mortality and morbidity 4. To evaluate the natural history of coronary heart disease in the placebo group population
C. Subgroup hypotheses to be tested	Propranolol is effective in reducing sudden cardiac death: 1. in patients with a prior myocardial infarction who have ventricular arrhythmias at baseline 2. in patients with a prior anterior myocardial infarction

Abbreviation: *BHAT*, Beta-Blocker Heart Attack Trial.

was effective in reducing all-cause mortality (18). The BHAT participants were followed up for a minimum of 12 and a maximum of 40 months; the average length of follow-up was 25 months.

Men and women, age 30 through 69, who had been hospitalized for 5 to 21 days for an MI (documented by specific symptoms, enzyme changes, and electrocardiographic evidence) were potentially eligible for the trial. The major inclusion and exclusion criteria are listed in Table 2. Patients with obvious indications or contraindications for a beta-blocker were not eligible for the trial. Blood pressure parameters were considered: patients were ineligible if they exhibited uncontrolled hypertension or pulmonary hypertension with right ventricular failure or if they had symptomatic hypotension.

Over the more than 2-year recruitment period, approximately 16,400 age-eligible patients with the BHAT definition of an MI who had survived at least 5 days were screened by the BHAT investigators. It was from these patients that the trial enrolled the 3837 participants (23% of the 16,400). Of the 77% who were not enrolled, screenees were judged ineligible because of contraindications to propranolol (18%), use or anticipated use of propranolol (18%), trial design/conduct issues (for example, living too far from a clinic, having a concomitant life-threatening illness, or having had cardiac surgery, 26%), or because consent could not be obtained (15%).

Before randomization, eligible participants went through a baseline interview and examination process (Table 3). Demographic and medical history data were collected (including pre- and in-hospitalization histories), as well as history data regarding medication use. The BHAT physician, after reviewing the patient's history and conducting the physical examination, recorded an opinion regarding whether the patient had a history of angina

Table 2 BHAT Inclusion and Exclusion Criteria

Inclusion criteria
Men and women
Aged 30 to 69 years at time of myocardial infarction
Admitted to coronary care unit
Having had a confirmed, BHAT-defined myocardial infarction
Gives informed consent
Randomized 5 to 21 days after infarction
Exclusion criteria
Contraindication to propranolol use (e.g., heart rate <50 beats/minute)
Indication for beta-blocker use (e.g., severe angina or hypertension uncontrolled by diuretic)
History of adverse reaction to a beta-blocker
Hypertension uncontrolled by therapy (≥190 mm Hg systolic or ≥110 mm Hg diastolic)
Pulmonary hypertension with right ventricular failure
Symptomatic hypotension
Cardiogenic shock
"Brittle" insulin-dependent diabetes
History of severe congestive heart failure
Heart failure within 3 days before last possible date for randomization
History of severe asthma as an adult
Women capable of becoming pregnant
Concomitant condition making it unlikely that patient would survive follow-up (e.g., cancer)

Abbreviation: *BHAT*, Beta-Blocker Heart Attack Trial.

and heart failure. The Rose Questionnaire (19) was used separately to identify angina. A resting electrocardiogram, a chest x-ray, urinalysis, and serum cholesterol determination were obtained as part of the physical examination. A 24-hour ambulatory Holter monitor was conducted in 3266 (85%) of the randomized participants.

While still in the hospital, eligible patients were randomized to receive propranolol (1916 patients) or matching placebo (1921 patients). Blinded study medication began immediately after randomization. The initial dose of propranolol was 20 mg, which was increased to 40 mg every 8 hours if no adverse reactions were noted. Blood was drawn after a minimum of six 40-mg doses and 8 hours after the last dose. Serum propranolol levels were measured at a central laboratory and the measurements reported to the coordinating center. If the serum propranolol level was less than 20 ng/mL, then the coordinating center instructed the clinical center to increase the study medication dosage at the 1-month visit to 80 mg three times a day (or 240 mg/day). If the level was 20 ng/mL or greater, then the clinical center was instructed to increase the dosage to 60 mg three times a day (or 180 mg/day). To keep the clinical center blinded to the true treatment group assignment of each participant, the clinics were also instructed to "increase" the "dose" for patients randomized to the placebo group.

These dosage levels were to be maintained through-out the follow-up period unless a reduction was clinically warranted (for example, because of a perceived side effect). At the end of the recruitment period, 82% of the 3837 randomized participants had been assigned to the 180 mg/day dosage and 18% to the 240 mg/day dosage. These proportions were equal between the treatment groups at baseline (20). At the 6-month follow-up visit, the mean propranolol level among the propranolol patients assigned to the 180 mg/day

Table 3 BHAT Procedures by Visit

Visit	Interview	Physical examination	Electrocardiogram*	24-hour Holter*	Chest X-ray†	Determination of serum propranolol level*	Hematocrit, WBC count, urinalysis†	Potassium*	Cholesterol, SGOT, creatinine*
Baseline	X	X	X	X	X	X	X	X	X
1 mo‡	X	X							
1.5 mo	X	X		X§		X		X	
3 mo	X	X							
6 mo	X	X				X			
9 mo	X	X							
12 mo	X	X	X		X	X	X	X	X
15 mo	X	X							
18 mo	X	X				X			
21 mo	X	X							
24 mo	X	X	X			X	X	X	X
27 mo	X	X							
30 mo	X	X				X			
33 mo	X	X							
36 mo	X	X	X			X	X	X	X
39 mo	X	X							
42 mo	X	X				X			

*Analyzed centrally.
†Analyzed locally at clinical center.
‡Specific purposes of this visit are to assess overall health status, adherence, possible side effects, and to increase drug dosage (see text).
§Performed in a subset of participants.
Abbreviations: *BHAT*, Beta-Blocker Heart Attack Trial; *WBC*, white blood cell; SGOT, serum glutamate oxaloacetate transaminase.

dose was 73 ng/mL, which was only slightly higher than the mean 67 ng/mL level among the propranolol patients assigned to the 240 mg/day dose (personal notes by the author, 1982).

The first follow-up clinic visits occurred 4, 6, and 12 weeks after randomization (Table 3). All subsequent visits occurred every 3 months for the duration of the trial. In addition to the dispensation of study medication, these follow-up visits were designed to monitor and record adherence to study medications, perceived side effects, current health status (including use of non-study medications), and the occurrence of prespecified clinical events. Good compliance to all aspects of the protocol was constantly stressed. The annual postrandomization visits were more elaborate, with the collection of laboratory data and the performance of a resting electrocardiogram.

Mortal events were blindly classified by a mortality classification subcommittee of the steering committee. Any information concerning the death (death certificates, hospital records, witness/family interview materials) was obtained and used in the committee's deliberations (21). At the end of the trial, vital status could not be ascertained on only 11 participants.

A detailed algorithm was developed to classify the recurrent nonfatal MIs (22). Like the entry criteria for the qualifying infarction, the classification algorithm for the recurrent infarctions used specific and documented symptom, enzyme, and electrocardiographic evidence. Unlike the criteria for qualifying infarction, the electrocardiographic evidence now required evidence of an evolving event (such as development of a new Q-wave). Using standardized data collected by the clinics, a nonfatal event subcommittee was able to classify the infarction event as definite, probable, or other (that is, not able to meet the BHAT definition of a recurrent MI).

The incidences or recurrences of heart failure or stroke were monitored by the clinics, and computer algorithms using data collected by the clinics to classify the events as definite or probable (22) were used. The incidence or recurrence of angina was determined by a positive Rose Questionnaire (19,22).

B. Definition of Hypertension and Prevalence of Hypertension at Baseline in BHAT

As noted in the above description and in the entry criteria listed in Table 2, being hypertensive per se was neither a specific entry requirement nor a specific entry exclusion criterion (unless severe and untreated). At baseline, there was no attempt to identify specifically and without error which patients were "hypertensive" and which were not. Using the responses from various baseline questions and physical examination findings, however, a number of definitions were constructed during the course of the trial, including definitions that simply identified which patients had higher blood pressure levels (although it was recognized that acute infarction patients would have temporarily lower pressures).

Two definitions were used most often during trial monitoring. The first was a positive response to the baseline interview question "Prior to this hospitalization, were you ever told that you had high blood pressure or hypertension?" Using this definition, 1565 BHAT participants had a history of hypertension (40.8% prevalence). The second definition was an extension of the first. A positive response to the first question began a second set of questions on whether the hypertension was treated with drugs. This second definition thus had three levels to it: a history of treated hypertension (1128 participants, 29.4%

prevalence), a history of untreated hypertension (437 participants, 11.4% prevalence), and no history of hypertension (2272 participants).

The hypertension-specific analyses presented in this chapter will usually use the first definition, the self-reported history of hypertension without regard to treatment. For ease of presentation, BHAT participants will be categorized as ''hypertensive'' or ''nonhypertensive,''although it is recognized that there may be some misclassification. As will be described below, this definition does, however, identify people at increased risk of experiencing an event during follow-up.

C. *Sample Size Calculation for the BHAT*

The original targeted sample size for the trial was 4020 randomized participants (17). This assumed an average of 3 years of follow-up, a two-sided alpha of 0.05, and 90% power. Using data from observational studies of patients with an acute MI, the 3-year mortality in the placebo group was assumed to be 18%. Using data from the earlier, smaller trials of beta-blockers (8–15), it was assumed that a beta-blocker could reduce that mortality rate by 28% to a 3-year rate of 12.96%. Taken together, the 3-year absolute difference in the mortality rates between the two treatment groups was thus estimated to be about 5% (=18% − 13%). When incorporated into a standard sample-size formula, these assumptions initially indicated that approximately 2150 participants would be needed to answer the question of whether a beta-blocker could reduce all-cause mortality in patients who had recently experienced an MI (1075 randomized to each treatment group).

However, it was also recognized that some of the patients randomized to the propranolol group would, over the course of follow-up, stop taking their study medication (that is, drop out of the active treatment group). It was also recognized that some patients randomized to placebo would begin taking an open-labeled beta-blocker (or drop into active treatment). Based on data from observational studies, the 3-year drop-out rate from the propranolol group was assumed to be 26%, and the 3-year drop-in rate for the placebo participants was assumed to be 21%. If a beta-blocker really did reduce mortality (as assumed), these crossovers would have the effect of lowering the 3-year mortality rate in the placebo group to 17.46% and increasing the mortality rate in the propranolol group to 13.75%. A revised 3-year absolute difference in the mortality rates between the two treatment groups was now estimated to be a smaller, tighter 3.7%. Because all analyses were to follow the intention-to-treat principle, these new estimates of the expected mortality rates were used in a final sample-size estimation procedure, providing the investigators with the final, and much larger, required targeted sample size of 4020.

D. BHAT Analyses Presented in This Chapter

The BHAT results presented in this chapter were previously reported in published BHAT papers found in the author's records and notes from the trial (from his time at the BHAT coordinating center), or were newly calculated using data supplied to the author by the sponsor of the trial, the National Heart, Lung, and Blood Institute.

Prevalence ratios of categorical and means of continuous characteristics were estimated at baseline. Simple rates were also estimated for follow-up events occurring over the average 25 months of follow-up. Life-table estimates were made for all-cause mortality and coronary incidence (defined as the first occurrence of a definite nonfatal reinfarction

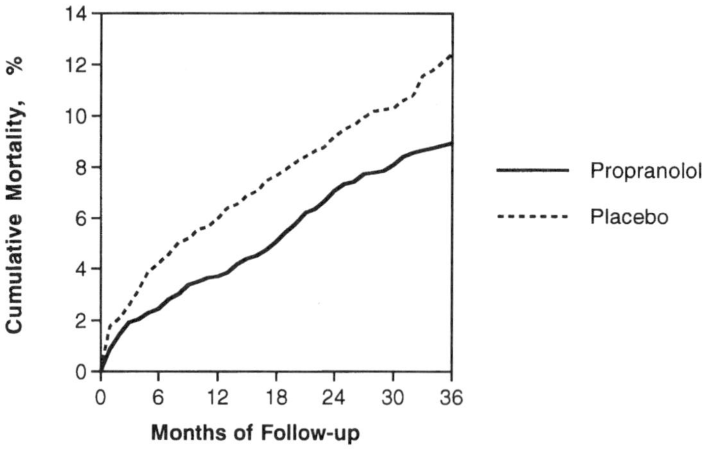

Fig. 1 Lifetable cumulative mortality curves for Beta-Blocker Heart Attack Trial (BHAT) participants. (From Ref. 21.)

or a fatal atherosclerotic event). Statistical differences between hypertensives and nonhypertensives were estimated using standard procedures to test for significance (23). Tests of "treatment X hypertensive status" interactions were conducted using the Mantel-Haenszel procedure (24). All analyses were conducted following the intention-to-treat principle.

It should be remembered that BHAT had one primary protocol-specified outcome measure and three secondary protocol-specified outcome measures. In the two original papers describing the results of the trial (21,22), the BHAT investigators appropriately only presented *P*-values for these measures because of the issues involved with multiple statistical testing. For ease of presentation, this chapter will not follow that original practice. All statistical tests (and the many resultant *P*-values) presented in this chapter, other

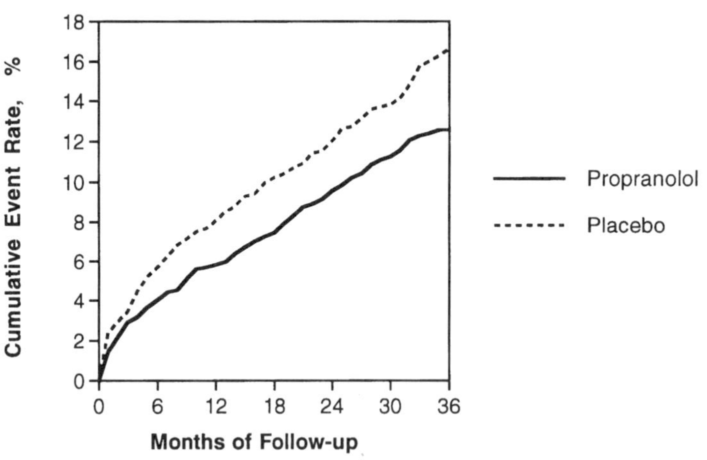

Fig. 2 Lifetable cumulative coronary incidence event curves for Beta-Blocker Heart Attack Trial (BHAT) Participants. Coronary incidence: first occurrence of a definite nonfatal reinfarction or a fatal atherosclerotic event. (From Ref. 22.)

than the four protocol-specified tests, should be viewed as post hoc hypotheses. The additional, unadjusted *P*-values are provided to the reader as simple guides for judging possible significance. A nominal *P*-value of 0.05 or less is used as a marker for highlighting a difference between groups.

III. BASELINE CHARACTERISTICS OF THE ENTIRE BHAT COHORT, AND BASELINE COMPARISON OF PARTICIPANTS WITH AND WITHOUT A HISTORY OF HYPERTENSION

Table 4 describes the baseline characteristics of the 3837 randomized patients participating in the trial. As noted above, 40.8% of the participants had a self-reported history of hypertension; 29.4% had a history of treatment for hypertension.

The overall mean age was 55.3 years; ages ranged from 30 to 69 years. Approximately 15% of the participant were female and 9% were black. Over 80% were current or former smokers, and the mean serum cholesterol value was 213 mg/dL. The mean body mass index was 26.4 kg/m^2. Fifteen percent had had a prior MI and about 10% had a history of heart failure (9%) or diabetes (12%). Angina was measured both as the BHAT physician's opinion (37%) and as a positive response to the Rose Questionnaire (12%). This difference in the anginal measures has been described previously (25).

Over one third (36%) of the randomized participants had electrocardiographic evidence of an anterior infarction. Nine percent had an infarction that did not fulfill the strict BHAT definition of a qualifying MI (non-BHAT MI). Because this classification was determined after randomization, these patients remained in the trial as full participants (although the mortality results were examined separately in this subgroup (21)). Because of the manner in which these data were collected, it was not possible to identify the location of the infarct in participants with a non-BHAT MI.

Table 4 Baseline Description of BHAT Participants, and Comparison of Those With and Without a History of Hypertension Before Hospitalization

	Entire BHAT population (n = 3837)	History of hypertension* (n = 1565)	No history of hypertension (n = 2272)	*P*-value of difference
Mean age, yr	55.3	56.1	54.8	**<0.001**
Male, %	84.3	79.8	87.4	**<0.001**
Black, %	8.7	12.3	6.2	**<0.001**
White, %	88.9	85.0	91.6	
Mean systolic BP, mm Hg	112.0	115.3	109.7	**<0.001**
Mean diastolic BP, mm Hg	74.4	74.6	70.9	**<0.001**
Mean heart rate, beats/minute	75.9	76.9	75.4	**<0.001**
Mean serum cholesterol, meq/l	213.3	214.6	212.3	0.12
Mean weight, kg				
Men	80.2	82.2	78.7	**<0.001**
Women	67.0	68.5	65.1	**0.002**
Mean body mass index, mean kg/m^2	26.4	27.0	25.9	**<0.001**
Cigarette smoking status, %				
Current	57.2	50.4	62.0	**<0.001**
Former	25.8	28.1	24.1	
Never	17.0	21.5	13.9	

Table 4 Continued

	Entire BHAT population (n = 3837)	History of hypertension* (n = 1565)	No history of hypertension (n = 2272)	*P*-value of difference
Medical history, %				
Prior MI	14.8	16.4	13.7	**0.02**
Angina (physician's opinion from exam)	36.7	41.2	33.7	**<0.001**
Angina (by Rose Questionnaire)	11.5	14.6	9.4	**<0.001**
Heart failure	9.3	10.8	8.2	**0.007**
Diabetes	11.6	16.6	8.1	**<0.001**
Use of a beta-blocker, just before MI	7.1	12.5	3.4	**<0.001**
In-hospital events occurring before randomization, %				
Atrial fibrillation	6.3	7.0	5.8	0.13
Congestive heart failure	14.7	16.6	13.4	**0.006**
Ventricular tachycardia	23.2	23.2	23.3	0.92
Medications used at time of randomization, %				
Antiarrhythmic	17.3	16.8	17.6	0.52
Anticoagulant	14.5	14.8	14.4	0.73
Antiplatetet	6.9	6.5	7.2	0.40
Diuretic	17.1	27.5	9.9	**<0.001**
Vasodilator	36.2	39.0	34.3	**0.003**
Digitalis	12.8	14.5	11.6	**0.009**
Insulin	3.5	3.9	3.2	0.23
Oral hypoglycemic	2.0	2.7	1.6	**0.02**
Location of BHAT MI, %				
Anterior only	26.8	25.1	27.9	0.52
Anterior and inferior	9.6	10.4	9.1	
Inferior only	32.0	32.8	31.5	
Subendocardial	22.8	23.0	22.6	
Non-BHAT MI	8.9	8.8	9.0	
Abnormalities noted on resting ECG, %				
Q-QS waves	67.7	67.2	68.0	0.62
ST depression	26.4	30.6	23.4	**<0.001**
ST elevation	13.4	13.8	13.1	0.55
T-wave abnormalities	65.5	65.0	65.9	0.59
Ventricular conduction defects	9.0	9.2	8.9	**0.70**
Atrioventricular conduction defects	3.7	4.4	3.3	**0.09**
Cardiomegaly on chest X-ray†, %	36.0	41.5	32.3	**<0.001**
Mean # VPBs/hour on 24-hour Holter‡	13.3	14.1	12.8	0.64
Presence of multiform VPBs on 24-hour Holter‡	32.1	34.4	30.5	**0.02**

*Self-reported positive response to baseline interview question: Prior to this hospitalization, were you ever told by a doctor that you had high blood pressure or hypertension?

†X-ray obtained on 3266 of 3837 randomized participants (85%).

‡24-hour ambulatory Holter obtained on 3290 of 3837 randomized participants (86%).

Notes: %, percent; #, number; *BP*, blood pressure; *MI*, myocardial infarction; *VPB*, ventricular premature beats. P-values ≤ 0.05 are in **bold**.

More than two thirds (68%) of the participants had Q-QS waves on the baseline resting electrocardiogram and about 25% had an ST-segment depression. During the hospitalization for this event, 6% of the participants had experienced atrial fibrillation, 23% ventricular tachycardia, and 15% heart failure (not severe enough to prevent randomization into the trial). Just prior to the MI, 7% of the participants were taking a beta-blocker. At the time of randomization, 36% of the participants were taking a vasodilator, 17% a diuretic, 17% an antiarrhythmic, 15% an anticoagulant, and 13% digitalis. Thirty-six percent had evidence of cardiomegaly on the chest X-ray and 32% had multiform ventricular premature beats (VPBs) on the 24-hour ambulatory Holter. The mean number of VPBs per hour was 13.3.

The mean number of days between the day of admission for the MI and randomization was 10.0 days (range 5 to 21). Overall, there was excellent comparability between the baseline characteristics of those participants assigned to the propranolol group and those assigned to the placebo group (17,21).

Table 4 also compares the baseline characteristics of 1565 self-reported hypertensive versus 2272 nonhypertensive BHAT participants. The two groups of participants differed on most of the characteristics described in this table (with P-values of 0.05 or less). Hypertensive patients were slightly older (mean 56 vs. 55 years) and had larger proportions of women (20% vs. 13%) and blacks (12% vs. 6%). Hypertensives also had higher mean blood pressures (115/75 vs. 110/71) and higher mean body mass indices (27 vs. 26 kg/m^2). Larger proportions of hypertensives had histories of prior MI (16 vs. 14%), angina (41 vs 37% for physician-defined angina and 15 vs 9% for Rose Questionnaire angina), heart failure (11 vs 8%), and diabetes (17 vs 8%). Just prior to the MI, 13% of the hypertensives and 3% of the nonhypertensives were taking a known beta-blocker.

Except for the occurrence of heart failure, hypertensives and nonhypertensives had almost equivalent rates of in hospital complications: 17% of the hypertensives experienced heart failure during hospitalization compared with 13% of the nonhypertensives. The resting electrocardiographic parameters were also nearly identical, with the exception of ST-segment depression: hypertensives had a higher prevalence than nonhypertensives (31% vs. 23%).

IV. OVERALL EVENT OUTCOME RESULTS IN BHAT

A. Effect of Propranolol on All-Cause Mortality

Table 5 summarizes the major fatal and nonfatal outcome results for the trial. The primary BHAT outcome measure was all-cause mortality. After an average follow-up period of 25 months, 138 patients in the propranolol group died (3.5%/year) compared with 188 in the placebo group (4.7%). This 26% reduction in the primary trial outcome attributable to propranolol use is depicted in Figure 1 and was highly statistically significant ($P = 0.004$). Even after adjusting for baseline characteristics that were differentially distributed between the two treatment groups and for those characteristics that were known to be predictive of mortality in post-MI patients, the treatment group difference remained (21).

Interpreting the curves presented in Figure 1, the BHAT investigators noted in the original paper (21) that the beneficial effect of propranolol began very soon after randomization and was greatest during the first 1½ years after MI, although the curves remained parallel for the duration of follow-up. This latter observation suggested continued benefit

Table 5 Fatal and Nonfatal Events by Treatment Group (Mean 25 Month Follow-Up Period)

	Propranolol (n = 1916)		Placebo (n = 1921)		Percent relative reduction in risk	Absolute risk reduction 100 pts/yr	*P*-value of absolute reduction
	Events		Events				
	Number	Rate/100/yr	Number	Rate/100/yr			
All-cause mortality	138	3.5	188	4.7	26	−1.2	0.004
Cardiovascular death	127	3.2	171	4.3	26	−1.1	0.009
Atherosclerotic death	119	3.0	164	4.1	27	−1.1	0.006
Atherosclerotic sudden death (<1 hour)	64	1.6	89	2.2	28	−0.6	0.04
Recurrent definite nonfatal MI	85	2.1	101	2.5	16	−0.4	0.24
Coronary incidence*	192	4.8	249	6.2	23	−1.4	0.004
Definite heart failure	129	3.2	128	3.2	−1	0.0	0.93
Rose Questionnaire angina	747	18.7	733	18.3	−2	0.4	0.60
Definite stroke	29	0.7	30	0.7	3	0.0	0.90
Bypass surgery	174	4.4	202	5.0	14	−0.7	0.14

*Coronary incidence: first occurrence of a definite nonfatal reinfarction or a fatal atherosclerotic event.
Abbreviation: *MI*, myocardial infarction.

up through 40 months. The authors also noted the consistency of the positive results between BHAT and the recently completed long-term trial of timolol (26) and short-term trial of metoprolol (27). In both of these trials, a beta-blocker given after MI was associated with a reduction in total mortality.

Accordingly, and in the absence of data beyond 40 months, the original BHAT investigators recommended that propranolol be used for at least 3-years in postinfarction patients who do not have a contraindication to beta-blockade.

B. Effect of Propranolol on Other Fatal Events

The other fatal outcome measures are also presented in Table 5 and in each case, propranolol was associated with a reduction in deaths. Cardiovascular deaths were reduced by 26% (3.2%/year vs. 4.3%, $P = 0.009$), atherosclerotic deaths were reduced by 27% (3.0% vs. 4.1%, $P = 0.006$), and atherosclerotic sudden deaths (specifically, deaths within 1 hour of symptoms) were reduced by 28% (1.6% vs. 2.2%, P = 0.04). The last two outcomes were protocol-specified secondary outcome measures in the trial.

The complementary causes of death were reported in the original results paper (21). The treatment group differences in nonsudden atherosclerotic deaths, other cardiovascular deaths, and all noncardiovascular deaths were never statistically significant. These results suggested that the reduction in all-cause mortality was mediated through the beneficial effects of propranolol on the cardiovascular system.

C. Effect of Propranolol on Nonfatal Events

The lower portion of Table 5 presents the effects of propranolol on other trial outcome measures. Eighty-five participants in the propranolol group experienced a recurrent definite nonfatal MI, compared with 101 in the placebo group. Although the propranolol group rate was 16% lower, the difference between the treatment groups did not reach statistical significance ($P = 0.24$). Twelve participants had multiple infarcts during follow-up, five in the propranolol group and seven in the placebo (22). Of the 85 propranolol participants who had had a recurrent MI, 12 (14.1%) subsequently died; of the 101 placebo participants who had had a recurrent event, 17 (16.8%) subsequently died (22).

When the nonfatal MIs were combined with the atherosclerotic deaths (''coronary incidence''), there was a 23% statistically significant reduction in events (4.8%/year propranolol vs 6.2% placebo). This latter outcome measure, depicted in Figure 2, was also a protocol-specified secondary outcome measure. Similar to what was noted in Figure 1 for all-cause mortality, the coronary incidence event curves in Figure 2 began to separate immediately after randomization.

The fear of causing or exacerbating existing heart failure was a concern during the development of the trial protocol. For that reason, patients with severe heart failure or failure within 3 days of the last possible day of randomization were ineligible for randomization. During the trial, 257 participants experienced a definite heart failure episode, equally divided between the two treatment groups [129 events in the propranolol group and 128 in the placebo group, $P = 0.93$ (Table 5)]. When these events were stratified by prior history of heart failure (including failure before the BHAT MI or heart failure during hospitalization for the MI), there was a slight tendency for there to be more events in the propranolol group among those with a pre-BHAT history (22). Among the 345 propranolol patients with a history of heart failure, 14.8% experienced a recurrence; among the 365 placebo patients with a prior history, 12.6% experienced a recurrence. The rates of incident heart failure among patients without a history were lower and more equivalent: 5.0% of the propranolol participants and 5.3% of the placebo participants experienced incident heart failure during the BHAT follow-up period (22).

Detailed analyses of the BHAT heart failure data revealed that the effect of propranolol on heart failure was especially pronounced in the short term among those with a prior history (28). Among propranolol patients without a history of heart failure, 1.3% experienced heart failure during the first 30 days after randomization; among placebo patients without a history, a comparable 1.1% experienced heart failure during the first 30 days; and among placebo patients with a history, the 30-day rate of recurrence was only slightly higher at 1.6%. However, among propranolol patients with a history of heart failure, 4.3% (1 of every 25 treated), experienced an episode of recurrent heart failure during the first 30 days of treatment. After this initial period, however, the rate of heart failure was equivalent for all groups (28).

Table 5 also describes the effect of propranolol on the occurrence of Rose Questionnaire angina, definite stroke, and CABG surgery. For each of these outcomes, there was no statistically significant reduction in the rates that could be attributable to the beta-blocker. This was an unexpected result for angina (18.7%/year propranolol vs. 18.3%/year placebo) because propranolol was marketed as an antianginal agent. This lack of an effect was also noted when the data were stratified by baseline history of angina (22). Possible explanations for this incongruity are that the Rose Questionnaire does not measure pain severity well and anginal frequency should have been taken into account.

D. Subgroup Findings of the Overall Results

The overall mortality and morbidity results from the trial have been stratified by many subgroup characteristics and presented in detail in many BHAT papers. The clear beneficial effects of propranolol were evident in almost all subgroups. Specifically, all-cause mortality was reduced by the beta-blocker in the young and old (21,29), women and men (21,30), in patients with and without severe ventricular arrhythmias (31,32), and in patients with and without a complicated BHAT infarction (21,33). Similarly, coronary incidence was reduced by the beta-blocker in the young and old and in patients with and without a complicated MI (22).

E. Overall Safety Issues in BHAT

In addition to the prespecified clinical outcome measures of interest in the trial, the trial investigators collected information regarding possible or perceived side effects. During the follow-up visit interviews, participants were questioned about specific events often thought to be related to beta-blocker therapy, such as blacking out, tiredness, frequent nightmares, or a decrease in sexual activity. If a participant had to stop the blinded BHAT medication, or if the assigned protocol dose had to be reduced, the specific reason for this was recorded.

Table 6 presents the treatment group proportions of BHAT participants reporting specific complaints at anytime during follow-up. The following complaints were reported to be more common among the propranolol participants (21): tiredness (66.9% propranolol vs. 62.3% placebo, $P = 0.003$), bronchospasm (31.2% vs. 27.1%, $P = 0.005$), cold hands or feet (10.1 vs. 7.7%, $P = 0.01$), and diarrhea (5.5% vs. 3.6%, $P = 0.007$). Although there was a treatment group difference in the average 25-month incidence of tiredness (a commonly heard complaint for propranolol use in general practice), it is noted that the

Table 6 Percent of BHAT Participants with Complaints at Any Time During Follow-Up

Complaint	Propranolol (n = 1916)	Placebo (n = 1921)	Percent relative difference in risk	Absolute risk difference/ 100 pts	*P*-value of absolute difference
Tiredness	66.9	62.3	6.8%	4.6	0.003
Bronchospasm	31.2	27.1	13.3%	4.1	0.005
Nightmares	39.7	36.9	7.1%	2.8	0.08
Cold hands, feet	10.1	7.7	23.7%	2.4	0.01
Insomnia	21.1	18.8	10.8%	2.3	0.08
Faintness	28.6	26.6	7.1%	2.0	0.17
Diarrhea	5.5	3.6	33.5%	1.8	0.007
Hallucinations	5.9	4.5	23.1%	1.4	0.06
Shortness of breath	66.8	65.5	1.9%	1.3	0.39
Nausea	6.0	4.8	19.9%	1.2	0.11
Reduced sexual activity	43.2	42.0	2.7%	1.2	0.46
Abdominal pain	5.7	4.8	16.2%	0.9	0.20
Depression	40.7	39.8	2.3%	0.9	0.56
Burning hands, feet	8.4	7.5	10.3%	0.9	0.33
Blurred vision	7.5	6.7	10.8%	0.8	0.33
Hair loss	1.2	0.7	43.4%	0.5	0.10
Eye dryness	0.6	0.5	8.6%	0.0	0.83
Flushing	1.4	1.5	−4.2%	−0.1	0.87
Constipation	3.0	3.3	−7.6%	−0.2	0.68
Dry mouth	2.3	2.6	−12.0%	−0.3	0.58
Rash, itching	4.8	5.1	−6.3%	−0.3	0.67
Blacking out	9.1	10.4	−14.1%	−1.3	0.18
Rapid heart beat	10.8	15.1	−40.2%	−4.3	0.001

Sorted by "Absolute Risk Difference." Complaints at head of list are associated with use of propranolol.
Abbreviation: *BHAT*, Beta-Blocker Heart Attack Trial.

absolute difference in the rates was 4.6%, or about 2.3% per year. More than 60% of the placebo patients had experienced tiredness. This is an example of a "side effect" that, although truly related to treatment, is only so to a small degree. Ninety-five percent of the propranolol patients experienced tiredness, not because of propranolol, but because they were sick individuals.

It was also noted that other complaints usually associated with propranolol use (depression and nightmares) were equally distributed between the placebo and propranolol groups (21).

With respect to having a change in BHAT medication because of a perceived side effect, the following reasons were more commonly given among the propranolol participants (21): reduced sexual activity (0.2% propranolol vs. 0.0% placebo, $P < 0.05$), gastrointestinal problems (1.0% vs. 0.3%, $P < 0.01$), and hypotension (1.2% vs. 0.3%, $P < 0.005$). Although associated with the use of propranolol, each of these reasons had a very low incidence.

The overall conclusion of these findings was that propranolol use was safe in this group of patients who had no contraindication to beta-blockade.

V. EFFECT OF PROPRANOLOL TREATMENT ON CLINICAL EVENTS AMONG HYPERTENSIVES IN THE BHAT

A. Effect of Baseline Hypertension Status on Clinical Events in the BHAT Placebo Group

Before an attempt was made to determine the effect of propranolol on clinical events among BHAT participants with and without a history of hypertension, the rates of these events were examined by hypertensive status in the placebo group. The objective of this exercise was to determine whether either of the self-reported definitions of hypertension history used by the trial did well (or better) in predicting events among patients not exposed to propranolol.

Figure 3 presents the rates of fatal and nonfatal events, stratified by a history of treatment for hypertension, history of untreated hypertension, and no history of hypertension. For each outcome measure, the rate is noted to be lowest among those patients without a history of hypertension. For all-cause mortality, atherosclerotic mortality, and coronary incidence, the rates were highest among treated hypertensives and were almost equal for untreated hypertensives and nonhypertensives. For sudden death (death within 1 hour), there was a stepped-reduction in death with treated hypertensives having the highest rate and untreated hypertensives having an intermediate rate. For heart failure, the rates were equivalent between the two hypertension groups. For stroke, untreated hypertensives had the highest rate.

Because the nonhypertensives consistently had the lower rates, and given the inconsistent patterns among treated and untreated hypertensives, the two hypertensive groups were next grouped together for analysis. This is presented in Table 7, where the effect of simply having a self-reported history of hypertension is noted to be predictive of clinical events (placebo group only). For each of the events, hypertensives had a higher rate,

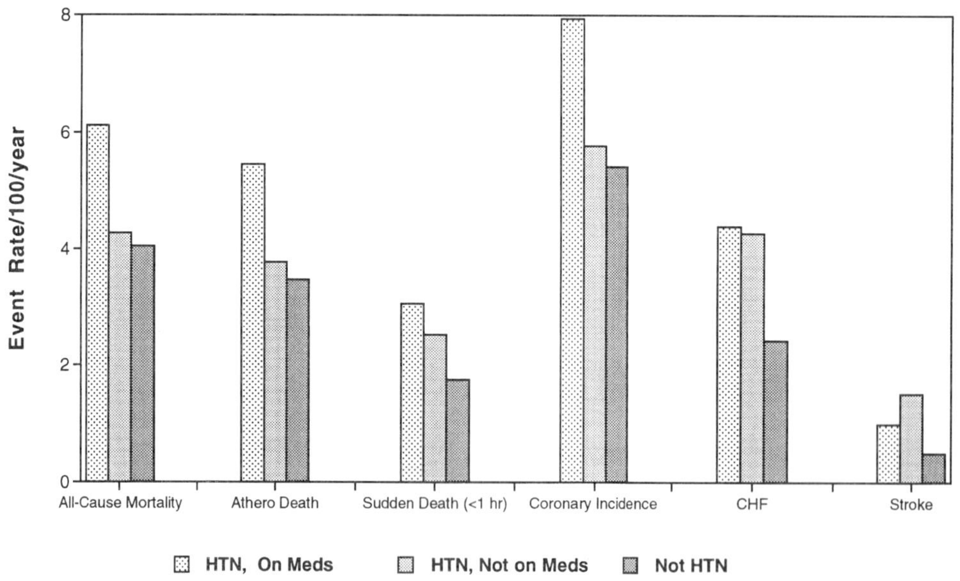

Fig. 3 Events in the Beta-Blocker Heart Attack Trial (BHAT) placebo group by self-reported hypertensive status. Athero: atherosclerotic; HTN: self-reported history of hypertension before BHAT MI; coronary incidence: first occurrence of a definite nonfatal reinfarction or a fatal atherosclerotic event.

Table 7 Fatal and Nonfatal Events in the BHAT Placebo Group by History of Hypertension (Mean 25-Month Follow-Up Period)

	History of hypertension (n = 771)		No history of hypertension (n = 1250)				
	Events		Events		Relative risk	Absolute risk 100 pts/yr	*P*-value of absolute difference
	Number	Rate/100/yr	Number	Rate/100/yr			
All-cause mortality	91	5.7	97	4.0	1.40	1.6	0.02
Cardiovascular death	84	5.2	87	3.6	1.44	1.6	0.01
Atherosclerotic death	81	5.0	83	3.5	1.46	1.6	0.01
Atherosclerotic sudden death (<1 hour)	47	2.9	42	1.8	1.67	1.2	0.01
Recurrent definite nonfatal MI	47	2.9	54	2.3	1.30	0.7	0.18
Coronary incidence*	119	7.4	130	5.4	1.37	2.0	0.008
Definite heart failure	70	4.4	58	2.4	1.80	1.9	0.001
Rose Questionnaire angina	315	19.6	418	17.4	1.12	2.2	0.05
Definite stroke	18	1.1	12	0.5	2.24	0.6	0.03
Bypass surgery	84	5.2	118	4.9	1.06	0.3	0.66

Notes: History of hypertension: self-report of history of hypertension before hospitalization for BHAT infarction.
*Coronary incidence: first occurrence of a definite nonfatal reinfarction or a fatal atherosclerotic event.
Abbreviations: *BHAT*, Beta-Blocker Heart Attack Trial; *MI*, myocardial infarction.

Table 8 Deaths by Treatment Group and History of Hypertension (Mean 25-Month Follow-Up Period)

	Propranolol			Placebo			Percent relative reduction in risk	Absolute risk reduction 100 pts/yr	P-value of absolute reduction	Interaction P-value
	Deaths		Tot number in group	Deaths		Tot number in group				
	Number	Rate/100/yr		Number	Rate/100/yr					
All-cause mortality										
Hx of HTN	69	4.2	794	91	5.7	771	26	−1.5	0.04	0.94
No Hx of HTN	69	3.0	1122	97	4.0	1150	27	−1.1	0.04	
Overall:	138	3.5	1916	188	4.7	1921	26	−1.2	0.004	
Cardiovascular death										
Hx of HTN	63	3.8	794	84	5.2	771	27	−1.4	0.04	0.83
No Hx of HTN	64	2.7	1122	87	3.6	1150	25	−0.9	0.08	
Overall:	127	3.2	1916	171	4.3	1921	26	−1.1	0.009	
Atherosclerotic death										
Hx of HTN	57	3.4	794	81	5.0	771	32	−1.6	0.02	0.60
No Hx of HTN	62	2.7	1122	83	3.5	1150	23	−0.8	0.10	
Overall:	119	3.0	1916	164	4.1	1921	27	−1.1	0.006	
Atherosclerotic sudden death (<1 hour)										
Hx of HTN	30	1.8	794	47	2.9	771	38	−1.1	0.03	0.36
No Hx of HTN	34	1.5	1122	42	1.8	1150	17	−0.3	0.41	
Overall:	64	1.6	1916	89	2.2	1921	28	−0.6	0.04	

Notes: History of hypertension (Hx of HTN): self-report of history of hypertension before hospitalization for BHAT infarction.

reaching statistical significance for all but two categories, recurrent definite nonfatal MI ($P = 0.18$) and bypass surgery ($P = 0.66$). Over the average 25 months of follow-up, hypertensives died at a rate 40% higher than nonhypertensives (5.7%/year vs. 4.0%, $P = 0.02$) and had a rate of sudden death that was 67% higher (2.9%/year vs. 1.8%, $P = 0.01$). Hypertensives also had higher rates of heart failure (4.4%/year vs. 2.4%, $P = 0.001$), Rose Questionnaire angina (19.6%/year vs. 17.4%, $P = 0.05$), and (although the rates were low) stroke (1.1%/year vs. 0.5%, $P = 0.03$).

B. Effect of Propranolol on Fatal and Nonfatal Clinical Events in Post-MI Patients With and Without a History of Hypertension

The treatment group-specific fatal and nonfatal event rates in Table 5 were next stratified by hypertensive status. The analyses of the fatal events are presented in Table 8. For each outcome measure, an average 26% relative reduction in mortality attributable to propranolol is noted for patients with and without the self-reported history of hypertension. Also for each outcome, the treatment group differences among hypertensives are nominally statistically significant; for the nonhypertensives, only the treatment group differences for all-cause mortality and cardiovascular death reached statistical significance, because the absolute reductions in risk were smaller. However, the outcome-specific *treatment X hypertensive status* interaction *P*-values did not provide evidence that hypertensives benefited more or less from treatment with propranolol. Because hypertensives were at a higher risk of death, the absolute reductions in risk were always greater for the hypertensives. This indicates that on a population level, more deaths would be averted among treated post-MI hypertensives than among treated nonhypertensives.

The effects of propranolol on all-cause mortality (the BHAT primary outcome measure) among hypertensives and nonhypertensives were examined in detail. Although the overall death rates were higher among the hypertensives (Table 7), both hypertensives and nonhypertensives experienced similar relative reductions in deaths (26% to 27%). This is graphically depicted in Figure 4, where it is noted that the group with the highest

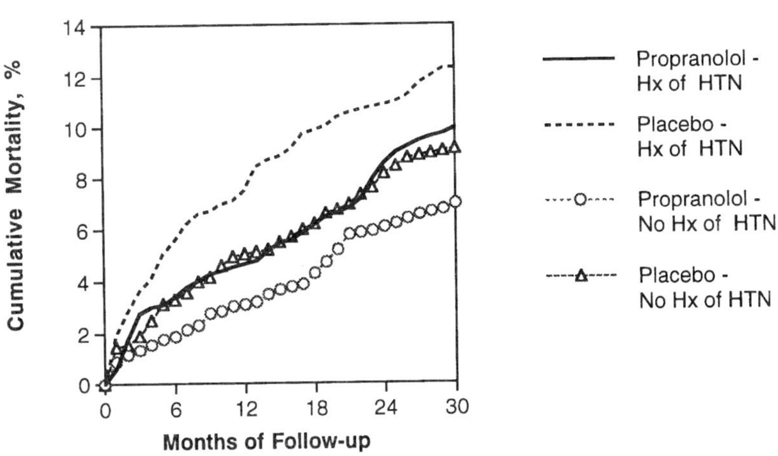

Fig. 4 Lifetable cumulative mortality curves by treatment group and history of hypertension. Hx of HTN: history of hypertension. *Note*: Graph ends at 30 months of follow-up because of instability in rates beyond this point.

Table 9 Other Events Occurring During Follow-up By Treatment Group and History of Hypertension (Mean 25-Month Follow-Up Period)

	Propranolol			Placebo						
	Events			Events						
	Number	Rate/100/yr	Tot number in group	Number	Rate/100/yr	Tot number in group	Percent relative reduction in risk	Absolute risk reduction 100 pts/yr	*P*-value of absolute reduction	Interaction *P*-value
Recurrent definite nonfatal MI										
Hx of HTN	34	2.1	794	47	2.9	771	30	−0.9	0.11	0.27
No Hx of HTN	51	2.2	1122	54	2.3	1150	3	−0.1	0.87	
Overall:	85	2.1	1916	101	2.5	1921	16	−0.4	0.24	
Coronary incidence*										
Hx of HTN	84	5.1	794	119	7.4	771	31	−2.3	0.004	0.22
No Hx of HTN	108	4.6	1122	130	5.4	1150	15	−0.8	0.19	
Overall:	192	4.8	1916	249	6.2	1921	23	−1.4	0.004	
Definite heart failure										
Hx of HTN	58	3.5	794	70	4.4	771	20	−0.9	0.20	0.07
No Hx of HTN	71	3.0	1122	58	2.4	1150	−25	0.6	0.19	
Overall:	129	3.2	1916	128	3.2	1921	−1	0.0	0.93	
Definite stroke										
Hx of HTN	22	1.3	794	18	1.1	771	−19	0.2	0.58	0.23
No Hx of HTN	7	0.3	1122	12	0.5	1150	40	−0.2	0.24	
Overall:	29	0.7	1916	30	0.7	1921	3	0.0	0.90	
Rose Questionnaire angina										
Hx of HTN	324	19.6	794	315	19.6	771	0	0.0	0.98	0.65
No Hx of HTN	423	18.1	1122	418	17.4	1150	−4	0.6	0.50	
Overall:	747	18.7	1916	733	18.3	1921	−2	0.4	0.60	
Bypass surgery										
Hx of HTN	68	4.1	794	84	5.2	771	21	−1.1	0.12	0.43
No Hx of HTN	106	4.5	1122	118	4.9	1150	8	−0.4	0.52	
Overall:	174	4.4	1916	202	5.0	1921	14	−0.7	0.14	

Notes: History of hypertension (Hx of HTN): self-report of history of hypertension before hospitalization for BHAT infarction.
*Coronary incidence: first occurrence of a definite nonfatal reinfarction or a fatal atherosclerotic event.
Abbreviation: *MI*, myocardial infarction; *BHAT*, Beta-Blocker Heart Attack Trial.

mortality included hypertensive patients not taking propranolol; the group with the lowest mortality included nonhypertensive patients taking propranolol. In between, the mortality rate for hypertensive propranolol patients was almost always equivalent to the rate for nonhypertensive patients not taking propranolol; that is, the deleterious effect of hypertension was removed for patients taking propranolol.

Table 9 describes the effects of propranolol on the nonfatal outcome measures, stratified by hypertensive status. For each event type, except heart failure and stroke, the effect of treatment on the outcome was not greatly different for hypertensives or nonhypertensives. As was noted overall in Table 5, propranolol patients experienced relatively large reductions in fatal/nonfatal coronary incidence and smaller reductions in recurrent nonfatal MIs and bypass surgery; there was no effect of propranolol on Rose Questionnaire angina.

Figure 5 presents the treatment group-specific lifetable curves for coronary incidence stratified by hypertension status. Here, and supported to some extent by the point estimates in Table 9 (although not by the nonsignificant interaction *P*-value), propranolol might have had more of an effect in reducing total coronary events among hypertensives (31% reduction versus a 15% reduction among nonhypertensives, Table 9). Mirroring what was noted in Figure 4 for all-cause mortality, the group with the highest coronary event rate in Figure 5 included hypertensive patients not taking propranolol; the group with the lowest event rate included nonhypertensive patients taking propranolol. In between again, but now only slightly higher than the lowest group, the event rates for hypertensive propranolol patients and nonhypertensive placebo patients were almost always equivalent.

For heart failure, there is a suggestion that only hypertensives experienced a reduction in events because of propranolol; nonhypertensives may actually experience slightly more failure events. For this outcome, the interaction *P*-value of 0.07 almost reaches nominal significance. However, given the number of post hoc statistical tests performed and given that this observation has not been noted in other trials, this suggestion of harm may be considered a statistical fluke.

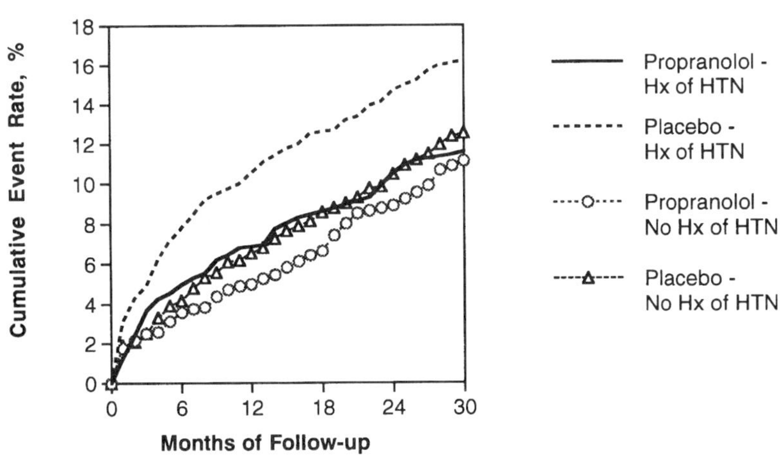

Fig. 5 Lifetable cumulative coronary incidence event curves by treatment group and history of hypertension. Coronary incidence: first occurrence of a definite nonfatal reinfarction or a fatal atherosclerotic event; Hx of HTN: history of hypertension. *Note*: Graph ends at 30 months of follow-up because of instability in rates beyond this point.

VI. EFFECT OF PROPRANOLOL ON OTHER BLOOD PRESSURE CHARACTERISTICS

A. Effect of Propranolol on Blood Pressure Levels in Post-MI Patients With and Without a History of Hypertension

At baseline, the mean in-hospital blood pressures of BHAT patients randomized to propranolol and placebo were 112/73 and 112/72 mm Hg, respectively ($P = 0.22$). As these survivors of an MI became removed in time from the data of their BHAT MI, their blood pressures increased, with the placebo patients increasing to a slightly higher mean pressure (Fig. 6). At the first annual visit, the mean blood pressures for the propranolol and placebo patients were 127/80 and 130/81, respectively ($P < 0.001$). This was a 15 mm Hg (13.4%) increase in systolic blood pressure (SBP) and a smaller 7 mm Hg (9.9%) increase in diastolic blood pressure (DBP) among the propranolol participants. Among the placebo participants, the absolute and relative increases were greater: there was an 18 mm Hg (16.0%) increase in SBP and a 9 mm Hg (11.9%) increase in DBP.

The mean blood pressures were not that different at the second annual visit. At this visit, the minimum blood pressures were 80 and 90 mm Hg systolic and 50 and 40 mm Hg diastolic for the propranolol and placebo patients, respectively.

As might be expected, the patterns were similar, although shifted, for the patients with and without a self-reported history of hypertension (Fig. 7). The BHAT participants with a history of hypertension had higher mean blood pressures at baseline (as also noted in Table 4). As time progressed, and although they started at a higher blood pressure to begin with, hypertensive patients experienced greater absolute and relative increases in blood pressure in both treatment groups, although to a lesser extent among patients assigned to propranolol.

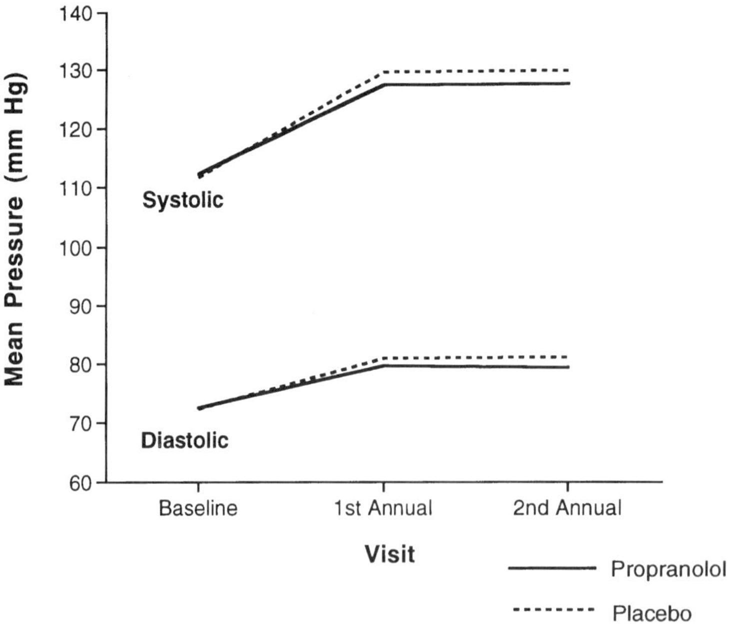

Fig. 6 Differences in mean blood pressure levels by treatment group and time. $P < 0.001$ at both annual follow-up visits.

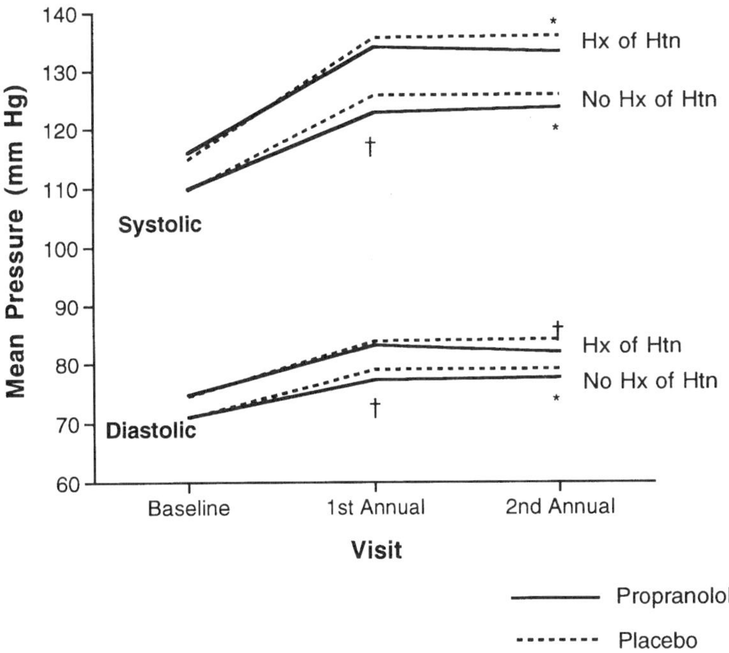

Fig. 7 Differences in mean blood pressure levels by treatment group, history of hypertension, and time. Hx of HTN: baseline self-reported history of hypertension. $^*P \leq 0.05$; $^\dagger P \leq 0.01$.

Specifically, the mean inhospital baseline blood pressures for the hypertensive propranolol and placebo patients were 116/75 and 115/75 mm Hg, respectively. At the first annual visit, the pressures had increased to 134/83 and 136/84 mm Hg, respectively, treatment group differences that were not statistically significant. This was an 18 mm Hg (18.2%) increase in SBP and a 9 mm Hg (11.4%) increase in DBP among the propranolol hypertensives. Among the placebo hypertensives, the absolute and relative increases were greater still: there was a 21 mm Hg (18.2%) increase in SBP and a 9 mm Hg (12.6%) increase in DBP.

Among nonhypertensive patients, the mean baseline blood pressure for both propranolol and placebo patients was 110/71 mm Hg. At the first annual visit, the pressures had increased to 123/77 and 126/79 mm Hg, respectively, treatment group differences that were highly statistically significant ($P < 0.001$). This was a 13 mm Hg (11.8%) increase in SBP and a 6 mm Hg (8.9%) increase in DBP among the propranolol hypertensives. Among the placebo hypertensives, the absolute and relative increases were greater: there was a 16 mm Hg (14.7%) increase in SBP and an 8 mm Hg (11.4%) increase in DBP.

B. Effect of Propranolol on Use of Open-Labeled Antihypertensives in Post-MI Patients With and Without a History of Hypertension

Figure 8 describes the use of open-labeled antihypertensive medications by treatment group over time. As noted above, 29.4% of the BHAT participants had reported taking an antihypertensive medication before the BHAT MI. This was evenly distributed between the two treatment groups (28.6% propranolol, 30.2% placebo, $P = 0.28$). At the time of

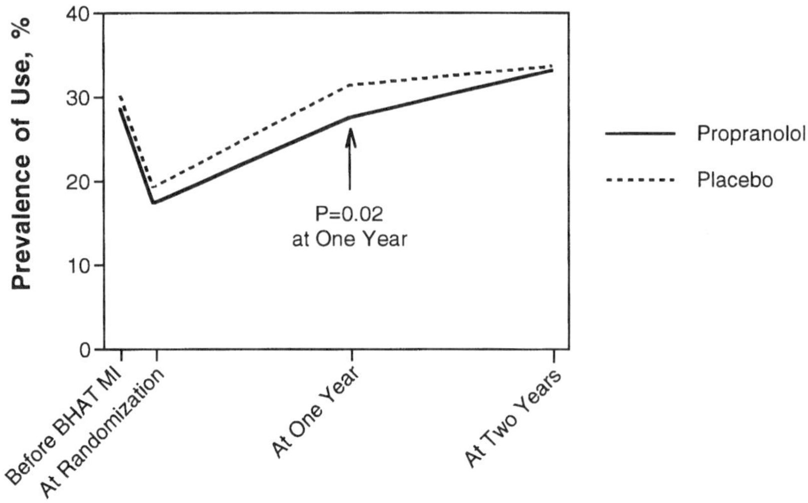

Fig. 8 Use of open-labeled antihypertensive medications by treatment group over time.

randomization, however, these prevalences had dropped (17.4% propranolol, 19.3% placebo, $P = 0.32$). Using these randomization prevalences as a new starting point, the use of open-labeled antihypertensive medication increased from baseline to the first annual visit, by 59% for the propranolol patients and 63% for the placebo patients. At this visit, at which time there had been great increases in mean blood pressure levels from baseline (Fig. 6), there was now a statistically significant difference between the treatment groups in the use of open-labeled antihypertensives: 27.6% propranolol versus 31.4% placebo ($P = 0.02$). However, between the first and second annual visits, the prevalence of antihypertensive use increased in the placebo group to 33.7%, whereas the prevalence in the propranolol group increased to an almost identical 33.2% ($P = 0.84$, for the difference in prevalences). It is noted that the postrandomization prevalence estimates of about 30% are only slightly higher than the preinfarction prevalence estimates of 29%.

C. Adherence to Trial Medication: Hypotension as a Reason for Noncompliance

During the operational life of the BHAT, the trial investigators continually monitored adherence to all aspects of the protocol. Of particular concern was adherence to study medications. The goals were to keep BHAT participants on their assigned, blinded medications and off open-labeled beta-blockers. If a perceived side effect was clinically judged to be related to the medication, the clinic physician had the option of taking a participant completely off the medication or simply reducing the dose to a level below the assigned protocol dose. The specific reasons why a drug was completely withdrawn or why a dose was lowered were recorded and also monitored. A major a priori concern of the BHAT investigators was that some propranolol participants may become hypotensive. For this reason, ''hypotension'' was monitored as one of the reasons for noncompliance.

During the course of the trial, 48% of the propranolol patients and 52% of the placebo patients had completely stopped their trial medications at least once ($P = 0.04$). Forty-seven percent of the propranolol patients and 36% of the placebo patients had had

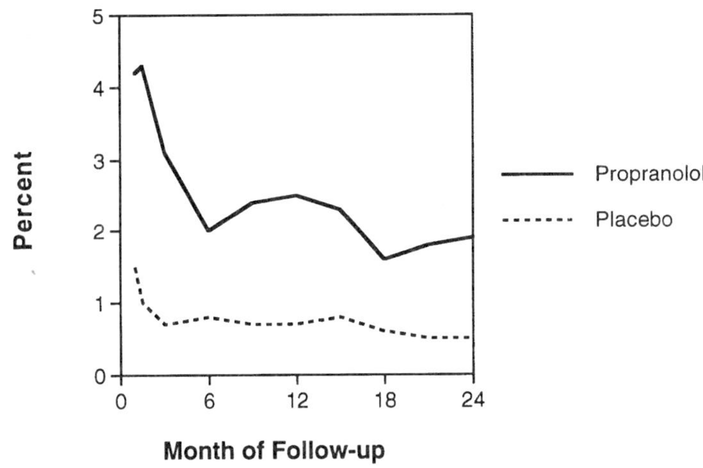

Fig. 9 Proportion of Beta-Blocker Heart Attack Trial (BHAT) participants not compliant with blinded trial medication because of hypotension by treatment group and time after randomization. (Noncompliance: completely off trial medication or on less than full protocol dose.)

their assigned trial dosage level reduced at least once ($P \leq 0.001$). Because there was overlap in these two measures of compliance, a more global measure was ''being off medication or not being at protocol dose.'' For this measure, 66% of the propranolol patients and 61% of the placebo patients were not compliant at least once ($P \leq 0.001$).

The BHAT participants fell in and out of this characterization of noncompliance as clinic personnel worked with them to improve compliance. This is indicated by visit-specific data. For example, at the final clinic visit for the trial, the prevalences of noncompliance (that is being off medication or not being at protocol dose) were 13% for the propranolol patients and 6% for the placebo patients (values much lower than 66% and 61%).

Figure 9 presents the treatment group and follow-up specific prevalences of being noncompliant because of hypotension. (Data were not available to stratify these results by history of hypertension.) Although the propranolol participants always had more noncompliance participants because of hypotension ($P \leq 0.001$), the proportions were always very small: at the second annual visit (24 months), 1.9% of the propranolol patients were noncompliant because of hypotension compared with 0.7% of the placebo patients. This 1.2% difference indicates that for every 100 patients treated with propranolol, only about 1% might develop hypotension severe enough to warrant a change in dosage.

VII. GENERALIZATION OF THE OVERALL BHAT RESULTS

A major issue for any clinical trial is how generalizable the trial results are. This is a function of the trial inclusion and exclusion criteria. As noted above and in Table 2, many of the exclusions were related to the patient having a contraindication to propranolol. It is unlikely that these patients would be given a beta-blocker, and obviously, the trial results cannot be extrapolated to them. These patients comprised about 18% of all age-eligible patients who survived 5 days. Many other exclusions were related to the strong likelihood that the patient would be given a beta-blocker. Given the consistency of the reported beneficial effects of propranolol in the previously reported subgroup analyses (21,29–33) and in the analyses of hypertensives presented in this chapter, there is no reason to believe that these patients would not benefit from beta-blocker therapy. These patients also comprised 18% of the age-eligible 5-day survivors of an acute MI. Finally, most of the remaining exclusion criteria concerned design and conduct issues, and again, there is no reason to believe that these patients would not benefit from beta-blocker therapy.

Thus, the BHAT results strongly suggest that up to three fourths of 30- to 69-year-old post-MI patients who had survived at least 5 days and who had no contraindication to beta-blockade could benefit from therapy.

VIII. IMPACT OF THE BHAT

The BHAT did not occur in a vacuum. It and the other contemporary beta-blocker trials (25,26) were landmark clinical trials that demonstrated that the risk of mortality and coronary events could be reduced in post-MI patients if given soon after a heart attack. The major strength of the study, built on its solid design and well-managed conduct, was its unequivocal findings: propranolol, when begun within 3 weeks of a heart attack, could safely and easily reduce the 3-year incidence of all-cause mortality, atherosclerotic mortality, sudden death, and the 3-year incidence of fatal and nonfatal coronary events. This benefit was seen in almost all examined subgroups, including hypertensives. These were major findings and were reported, not only in the medical literature, but on the major network news stations in the United States.

When designing a trial, decisions are made on how to conduct it in a standardized fashion. Each decision made diminishes the opportunities of obtaining answers to other questions. Thus, limitations for the trial are those that were built into the trial design. The BHAT was not designed to address the question of whether beta-blockade reduces events if treatment were begun months after the MI. Similarly, BHAT was not designed to address the question of whether post-MI patients should continue a beta-blocker for more than 3 years.

Unfortunately, news of this great benefit has not been widely applied. Although the BHAT results were first reported in 1981 (34) and, although the results suggested that up to three fourths of post-MI patients could benefit from treatment, secondary prevention trials of post-MI coronary patients begun much later still had large proportions of participants not on a beta-blocker. For example, the baseline use of beta-blocker therapy was only 36% among the post-MI patients in the Survival and Ventricular Enlargement (SAVE) trial (begun in 1987) (35), 40% among the post-MI patients in the Cholesterol and Recurrent Events (CARE) trial (begun in 1989) (36), 57% among the post-MI patients in the Scandinavian Simvastatin Survival Study (4S) trial (begun in 1987) (37), 47% among the coronary patients in the Long-Term Intervention with Pravastatin in Ischaemic Disease (LIPID) trial (begun in 1989) (38), 63% among the coronary patients in the Prospective Randomized Evaluation of the Vascular Effects of Norvasc Trial (PREVENT) (begun in 1992) (39), and 33% among the women with coronary disease in the Heart and Estrogen/progestin Replacement Study (HERS) (begun in 1993) (40).

To many, the concept of evidence-based medicine seems so self evident that it can be ignored. However, when very large proportions of coronary patients are not given beta-blockade, it is a demonstration that evidence-based medicine is not being practiced. As might be expected, this underutilization of appropriate therapy is not random. A 1999 report suggests that physicians who work on randomized control trials were more likely to use beta-blockers appropriately, compared with physicians in routine clinical practice

(41). The authors of that report also note that the 1990 American College of Cardiology/ American Heart Association national guidelines for the early management of postinfarction patients (42) did not result in an increase in the prevalence of appropriate beta-blocker use. In contrast, another 1999 report presented evidence that intense local guidelines and physician re-education could result in an increase in beta-blocker use (43).

No evidence presented over the last 17 years has diminished the 1982 conclusion of the BHAT investigators: ''Based on the BHAT results, in conjunction with those of studies reported previously, the investigators recommend the use of propranolol for at least three years in patients with no contraindications to beta-blockade who have had a recent MI'' (21).

ACKNOWLEDGMENTS

This chapter uses data supplied by the NHLBI, NIH, and DHHS. The views expressed in this chapter are those of the author and do not necessarily reflect the views of the NHLBI.

APPENDIX A: INSTITUTIONS PARTICIPATING IN BHAT: PRINCIPAL INVESTIGATORS AND CO-INVESTIGATORS

A. Clinical Centers

Baylor College of Medicine; Houston, Texas
Craig M. Pratt, M.D., Principal investigator
John Farmer, M.D.
William Fennell, M.D.
Richard R. Miller, M.D.
James B. Young, M.D.
Boston University School of Medicine; Boston, Massachusetts
Pantel S. Vokonas, M.D., Principal investigator
Bruce Abramowitz, M.D.
Brown University Affiliated Hospitals; Providence, Rhode Island
Robert J. Capone, M.D., Principal investigator
Abdul Khan, M.D.
Richard S. Shulman, M.D.
Emory University; Atlanta, Georgia
Robert C. Schlant, M.D., Principal investigator
Daniel Arensberg, M.D.
Evanston Hospital; Evanston, Illinois
Gary N. Wilner, M.D., Principal investigator
William Barnhart, M.D.
Cary Berkowitz, M.D.
Edward Winslow, M.D.
Geisinger Medical Center; Danville, Pennsylvania
Charles A. Laubach, M.D., Principal investigator
John H. Chapman, M.D.
Greater Baltimore Medical Center; Baltimore Maryland
Thaddeus E. Prout, M.D., Principal investigator
James H. Biddison, M.D.
Luis F. Gonzales, M.D.

James C. Ricely, M.D.
Robert Peters, M.D.
Henry Ford Hospital; Detroit, Michigan
Gerald M. Breneman, M.D., Principal investigator
Remingio Garcia, M.D.
Tennyson Lee, M.D.
Kaiser Foundation Hospital; Portland Oregon
John A. Grover, M.D., Principal investigator
Merwyn Greenlick, Ph.D.
John B. Wild, M.D.
Lankenau Hospital; Philadelphia, Pennsylvania
William L. Holmes, Ph.D., Principal investigator
Leonard S. Dreifus, M.D.
Long Island Jewish-Hillside Medical Center; New Hyde Park, New York
Kul D. Chadda, M.D., Principal investigator
Robert H. Kramer, M.D.
Robert I. Hamby, M.D.
Morris Jampol, M.D.
Stephen Rabinowitz, M.D.
Paul Samuel, M.D.
Steven Zeldis, M.D.
Maimonides Medical Center; Brooklyn, New York
Edgar Lichstein, M.D., Principal investigator
Alvin Greengart, M.D.
Gerald Hollander, M.D.
Michael Sanders, M.D.
Prem Gupta, M.D.
Medical College of South Carolina; Charleston, South Carolina
Peter C. Gazes, M.D., Principal investigator
William H. Barnwell, II, M.D.
Medical College of Virginia; Richmond, Virginia
David W. Richardson, M.D., Principal investigator
Zubair UI Hassan, M.D.
A. Jarrell Raper, M.D.
Donald Romhilt, M.D.
William K. Smith, M.D.
Miami Heart Institute; Miami, Florida
Frank L. Canosa, M.D., Principal investigator
Jeff Raines, Ph.D.
Montreal Heart Institute; Montreal, Quebec, Canada
Pierre A. Théroux, M.D., Principal investigator
David D. Waters, M.D.
Mt. Sinai Hospital; Minneapolis, Minnesota
Phillip J. Ranheim, M.D., Principal investigator
Reuben Berman, M.D.
Marvin Segal, M.D.
Hans Bauer, M.D.
William D. Kimber, M.D.

Northwestern University Medical School; Chicago, Illinois
Olga M. Haring, M.D., Principal investigator
David Berkson, M.D.
Gustave Bermudez, M.D.
Richard Davison, M.D.
Overlook Hospital; Summit, New Jersey
John J. Gregory, M.D., Principal investigator
Donald Brock, M.D.
Joel Cannilla, M.D.
John Farry, M.D.
Kenneth Jacobson, M.D.
R. Gregory Sachs, M.D.
Martin J. Sheehy, M.D.
Pacific Health Research Institute; Honolulu, Hawaii
J. Judson McNamara, M.D., Principal investigator
John J. Cogan, M.D.
Samuel C. Gresham, M.D.
Providence Medical Center; Portland, Oregon
Gordon L. Maurice, M.D., Principal investigator
Frank D. McBarron, M.D.
James H. Mackay, M.D.
Rush-Presbyterian-St. Lukes Medical Center; Chicago, Illinois
James A. Schoenberger, M.D., Principal investigator
Joseph V. Messer, M.D.
Gilberto S. Neri, Jr., M.D.
Rutgers Medical School Raritan Valley Hospital; New Brunswick, New Jersey
Peter T. Kuo, M.D., Principal investigator
Paul Jennings, M.D.
John B. Kostis, M.D.
Norman Reitman, M.D.
Salt Lake Clinic Research Foundation; Salt Lake City, Utah/Ogden Research Center; Ogden, Utah
Allan H. Barker, M.D., Principal investigator (Salt Lake City)
C. Basil Williams, M.D., Principal investigator (Ogden)
Kenneth A. Crockett, M.D.
Michael J. Preece, M.D.
Ernest Wilkinson, M.D.
G. Thomas Blanch, M.D.
State University of New York at Buffalo; Buffalo, New York
Robert M. Kohn, M.D., Principal investigator
Dennis Dubois, M.D.
Philip D. Morey, M.D.
Douglas L. Roberts, M.D.
Joseph Wanka, M.D.
University of California, Davis; Davis, California
Nemat O. Borhani, M.D., Principal investigator
Thomas Evans, M.D.
Allen Frankel, M.D.

University of California, San Francisco; San Francisco, California
Mary Anne Warnowicz, D.O., Principal investigator
Robert W. Peters, M.D.
Randolph Byrd, M.D.
Edward S. Kersh, M.D.
University of Rochester School of Medicine; Rochester, New York
Paul N. Yu, M.D., Principal investigator
Theodore Biddle, M.D.
William Henion, M.D.
P. K. Mathew, M.D.
Alvani Santos, M.D.
University of Southern California, Los Angeles; Los Angeles, California
L. Julian Haywood, M.D., Principal investigator
Maria De Guzman, M.D.
Veterans Administration Hospital; Little Rock, Arkansas
Marvin L. Murphy, M.D., Principal investigator
Moshen Sakhaii, M.D.
Neil De Soyza, M.D.
Veterans Administration Hospital; West Roxbury, Massachusetts
Kevin M. McIntyre, M.D., Principal investigator
Edward Gillie, M.D.
Kenneth LaBresh, M.D.
William Neill, M.D.
Alfred F. Parisi, M.D.
G.V.R. K. Sharma, M.D.
William E. Strauss, M.D.

B. Coordinating Center

University of Texas School of Public Health; Houston, Texas
C. Morton Hawkins, Sc.D., Principal investigator
Rose Lee Bell, M.P.H., Ph.D.
Robert P. Byington, M.P.H., Ph.D.
Darwin R. Lalbarthe, M.D., Ph.D.
J. David Curb, M.D.
Robert J. Hardy, Ph.D.
Ronald B. Harrist, Ph.D.

C. Resting ECG Reading Center

University of Minnesota; Minneapolis, Minnesota
Richard S. Crow, M.D., Principal investigator
Henry Blackburn, M.D.
Ronald Prineas, M.D.

D. Ambulatory ECG Reading Center

Anthropometrics Heart Clinic; Haddonfield, New Jersey
Joel Morganroth, M.D., Principal investigator
Leonard Dreifus, M.D.
John Kastor, M.D.

E. Central Laboratory

Bio-Science Laboratories; Van Nuys, California
Frank Ibbott, Ph.D., Principal investigator

F. Drug Distribution Center
Department of Health and Human Services
United States Public Health Service, Perry Point, Maryland

G. National Heart, Lung, and Blood Institute (Sponsor)
Bethesda, Maryland
- Curt Furberg, M.D., Project officer
- Lawrence M. Friedman, M.D.
- David L. DeMets, Ph.D.
- William T. Friedewald, M.D.
- Eugene Passamani, M.D.

H. Policy/Data Monitoring Board
- John Naugton, M.D., Chairman
- Paul L. Canner, Ph.D.
- Lawrence J. Cohen, M.D.
- Max Halperin, Ph.D.
- Lois Pratt, Ph.D.
- Burton Sobel, M.D.
- Harold Strauss, M.D.
- William T. Friedewald, M.D. (Ex Officio) (nonvoting)

APPENDIX B: THE BHAT STEERING COMMITTEE AND ITS SUBCOMMITTEES

A. BHAT Steering Committee
Charge: To provide overall scientific direction for the trial at the operational level. Specific functions included: to advise and assist all study units on and with all operational matters; to monitor the performance of the individual clinical centers with respect to patient recruitment and adherence; to monitor the quality of the performance of the clinical centers and the central units; to review all proposed ancillary studies; to keep the trial investigators informed about the progress of the trial; to report major problems to the policy/data monitoring board.

Permanent members
- Sidney Goldstein, M.D., Chairman
- Nemat O. Borhani, M.D.
- Richard S. Crow, M.D.
- Curt Furberg, M.D.
- C. Morton Hawkins, Sc.D.
- Frank Ibbott, Ph.D.
- Joel Morganroth, M.D.
- Thaddeus E. Prout, M.D.

B. Subcommittees of the BHAT Steering Committee
Adherence subcommittee—monitored patient adherence and reviewed methods for maintaining good adherence to study treatment protocol and medication.
- Kevin M. McIntyre, M.D., Chairman
- Rose Lee Bell, M.P.H.
- Lawrence M. Friedman, M.D.
- William L. Holmes, Ph.D.
- Frank D. McBarron, M.D.

Pantel S. Vokonas, M.D.
C. Basil Williams, M.D.

Bibliography subcommittee—created and maintained a current bibliography on propranolol and other beta-blocking agents pertinent to the BHAT.

L. Julian Haywood, M.D., Chairman
Curt Furberg, M.D.
Olga M. Haring, M.D.
Paul Jennings, M.D.
Darwin R. Labarthe, M.D., Ph.D.
J. J. McNamara, M.D.
Phillip J. Ranheim, M.D.
Douglas L. Roberts, M.D.

Editorial review subcommittee—reviewed and recommended approval or disapproval of every scientific paper using unpublished BHAT data (including ancillary study data) as well as every paper using published BHAT data that purports to represent official BHAT views or policy. This applied to papers prepared for publication or oral presentation. Also reviewed proposed ancillary studies to ensure that patient safety and BHAT design and scientific integrity were not compromised. Suggested special studies that might be conducted at one or several centers on an ancillary basis.

James A. Schoenberger, M.D., Chairman
James K. Alexander, M.D.
Nemat O. Borhani, M.D.
Curt Furberg, M.D.
Sidney Goldstein, M.D.
Merwyn Greenlick, Ph.D.
C. Morton Hawkins, Sc.D.
Jeff Raines, Ph.D.
Richard S. Shulman, M.D.

Holter monitoring advisory subcommittee—advised the ECG centers and the steering committee on questions relating to methodology and analysis of Holter recordings.

Edgar Lichstein, M.D. Chairman
Theodore Biddle, M.D.
Robert P. Byington, M.P.H., Ph.D.
Robert J. Capone, M.D.
Richard S. Crow, M.D.
Neil de Soyza, M.D.
John J. Gregory, M.D.
Ronald B. Harrist, Ph.D.
John B. Kostis, M.D.
Joel Morganroth, M.D.
Craig Pratt, M.D.
William Ruberman, M.D.

Mortality classification subcommittee—reviewed in a blinded fashion all information concerning cause and circumstance of death of BHAT patients and coded this information for each decedent.

Gary N. Wilner, M.D., Chairman
Daniel Arensberg, M.D.
Allen H. Barker, M.D.

Robert P. Byington, M.P.H., Ph.D.
Lawrence M. Friedman, M.D.
Charles A. Laubach, Jr., M.D.
Robert W. Peters, M.D.
Donald W. Romhilt, M.D.

Natural history subcommittee—suggested appropriate natural history analyses based on placebo group data. Initiated publications and presentations based on these analyses.

Thaddeus E. Prout, M.D., Chairman
William H. Barnwell, II, M.D.
Gerald M. Breneman, M.D.
Robert P. Byington, M.P.H., Ph.D.
Lawrence M. Friedman, M.D.
Darwin R. Labarthe, M.D., Ph.D.
James H. Mackay, M.D.
Marvin L. Murphy, M.D.
Ronald Prineas, M.D.
William Ruberman, M.D.

Nonfatal events subcommittee—classified, in a blinded and standardized fashion, specific nonfatal events. Its primary function was to review and classify information concerning nonfatal myocardial infarctions.

Paul N. Yu, M.D., Chairman
Robert P. Byington, M.P.H., Ph.D.
Kul D. Chadda, M.D.
Richard S. Crow, M.D.
J. David Curb, M.D.
John A. Grover, M.D.
Eugene Passamani, M.D.
Ronald Prineas, M.D.
Norman Reitman, M.D.
G.V.R.K. Sharman, M.D.

Quality control subcommittee—monitored the performance of the clinical centers and the central units. Blinded data were not reviewed by this subcommittee.

Curt Furberg, M.D., Chairman
Rose Lee Bell, M.P.H.
Richard S. Crow, M.D.
Ronald B. Harrist, Ph.D.
Frank Ibbott, Ph.D.
Robert M. Kohn, M.D.
David W. Richardson, M.D.

REFERENCES

1. Hypertension Detection and Follow-Up Program Cooperative Group. Five-year findings of the Hypertension Detection and Follow-Up Program. I. Reduction in mortality of persons with high blood pressure, including mild hypertension. JAMA 1979; 242:2562–2571.
2. Hypertension Detection and Follow-Up Program Cooperative Group. Five-year findings of the Hypertension Detection and Follow-Up Program. II. Mortality by race-sex and age. JAMA 1979; 242:2572–2577.

3. Lipid Research Clinics Program. The Lipid Research Clinics Coronary Primary Prevention Trial results. I. Reduction in incidence of coronary heart disease. JAMA 1984; 251:351–364.
4. Lipid Research Clinics Program. The Lipid Research Clinics Coronary Primary Prevention Trial results. II. The relationship of reduction in incidence of coronary heart disease to cholesterol lowering. JAMA 1984; 251:365–374.
5. Workshop on Chronic Antiarrhythmic Therapy and the Prevention of Sudden Death: Summary Report. Cardiac Diseases Branch, National Heart, Lung, and Blood Institute. Bethesda, Maryland: National Institutes of Health, 1976.
6. Maroko PR, Kjekshus JK, Sobel BE, Watanabe T, Covell JW, Ross J Jr, Braunwald E. Factors influencing infarct size following coronary occlusions. Circulation 1971; 43:67–82.
7. Reimer KA, Rasmussen MM, Jennings RB. Reduction by propranolol of myocardial necrosis following temporary coronary artery occlusion in dogs. Circ Res 1973; 33:353–363.
8. Reynolds JL, Whitlock RML. Effects of β-adrenergic receptor blocker in myocardial infarction treated for one year from onset. Br Heart J 1972; 34:252–259.
9. Wilhelmsson C, Vedin JA, Wilhelmsen L, Tibblin G, Werkö L. Reduction of sudden deaths after myocardial infarction by treatment with alprenolol: preliminary results. Lancet 1974; 2: 1157–1160.
10. Vedin A, Wilhelmsson C, Werkö L. Chronic alprenolol treatment of patients with acute myocardial infarction after discharge from hospital: effects on mortality and morbidity. Acta Med Scand 1975; 575(suppl):1–56.
11. Ahlmark G, Saetre H, Korsgren M. Reduction of sudden deaths after myocardial infarction. Lancet 1974; 2:1563.
12. Ahlmark G, Saetre J. Long-term treatment with β-blockers after myocardial infarction. Eur J Clin Pharmacol 1976; 10:77–83.
13. Barber JM, Boyle DM, Chaturvedi NC, Singh N, Walsh MJ. Practolol in acute myocardial infarction. Acta Med Scand 1975; 587(suppl):213–219.
14. Multicentre International Study. Improvement in prognosis of myocardial infarction by long-term beta-adrenoceptor blockade using practolol. BMJ 1975; 3:735–740.
15. Multicentre International Study. Reduction in mortality after myocardial infarction with long-term β-adrenergic blockade using practolol. BMJ 1977; 2:419–421.
16. Inderal (propranolol) advertisement in United Kingdom. J R Coll Phys 1976; 11:33–34.
17. Beta-Blocker Heart Attack Trial Research Group (monograph prepared by Robert P. Byington). Beta-Blocker Heart Attack Trial: Design, methods and baseline results. Cont Clin Trials 1984; 5:382–437.
18. DeMets DL, Hardy RJ, Friedman LM, Lan KKG. Statistical aspects of early termination in the Beta-Blocker Heart Attack Trial. Cont Clin Trials 1984; 5:362–372.
19. Rose GA. The diagnosis of ischaemic heart pain and intermittent claudication in field surveys. Bull WHO 1962; 27:645–658.
20. Walle T, Byington RP, Furberg CD, McIntyre K, Vokonas P. Biologic determinants of propranolol disposition: results from 1308 patients in the Beta-Blocker Heart Attack Trial. Clin Pharm Ther 1985; 38:509–518.
21. Beta-Blocker Heart Attack Trial Research Group. A randomized trial of propranolol in patients with acute myocardial infarction. I. Mortality results. JAMA 1982; 247:1707–1714.
22. Beta-Blocker Heart Attack Trial Research Group. A randomized trial of propranolol in patients with acute myocardial infarction. II. Morbidity results. JAMA 1983; 250:2814–2819.
23. GW Snedecor, WG Cochran. Statistical Methods, 7th ed. Ames, IA: The Iowa State University Press, 1980.
24. Mantel N, Haenszel W. Statistical aspects of the analysis of data from retrospective studies of disease. J Natl Cancer Inst 1959; 22:719–748.
25. Friedman LM, Byington RP, and the Beta-Blocker Heart Attack Trial Research Group. Assessment of angina pectoris after myocardial infarction: comparison of ''Rose Questionnaire''

with physician judgment in the Beta-Blocker Heart Attack Trial. Am J Epidemiol 1985; 121: 555–562.
26. Norwegian Multicenter Study Group. Timolol-induced reduction in mortality and reinfarction in patients surviving acute myocardial infarction. N Engl J Med 1981; 304:801–807.
27. Hjalmarson A, Herlitz J, Malék I, Rydén L, Vedin A, Waldenström A, Wedel H, Elmfeldt D, Holmburg S, Nyberg G, Swedberg K, Waagstein F, Waldenström J, Wilhelmsen L, Wilhelmsson C. Effect on mortality of metoprolol in acute myocardial infarction: a double-blind randomised trial. Lancet 1981; 2:823–827.
28. Chadda K, Goldstein S, Byington R, Curb JD. Effect of propranolol after acute myocardial infarction in patients with congestive heart failure. Circulation 1986; 73:503–510.
29. Hawkins CM, Richardson DW, Vokonas PS, for the Beta-Blocker Heart Attack Trial Research Group. Effect of propranolol in reducing mortality in older myocardial infarction patients—The Beta-Blocker Heart Attack Trial experience. Circulation 1983; 67(suppl I):I-94–I-97.
30. Furberg CD, Friedman LM, MacMahon SW. Women as participants in trials of the primary and secondary prevention of cardiovascular disease-Part II. Secondary prevention—The Beta-Blocker Heart Attack Trial and the Aspirin Myocardial Infarction Study. In: Eaker ED, Packard B, Wenger NK, Clarkson TB, Tyroler HA, eds. Coronary Heart Disease in Women Proceedings of an NIH Workshop. New York: Haymarket Dogma, Inc., 1987.
31. Beta-Blocker Heart Attack Trial Research Group (prepared by Friedman LM, Byington RP, Capone RJ, Furberg CD, Goldstein S, Lichstein E). Effect of propranolol in patients with myocardial infarction and ventricular arrhythmia. J Am Coll Cardiol 1986; 7:1–8.
32. Kostis JB, Wilson AC, Sanders MR, and Byington RP, for the BHAT Study Group. Prognostic significance of ventricular ectopic activity in survivors of acute myocardial infarction who receive propranolol. Am J Cardiol 1988; 61:975–978.
33. Furberg CD, Hawkins CM, Lichstein E, for the Beta-Blocker Heart Attack Trial Study Group. Effect of propranolol in post-infarction patients with mechanical or electrical complications. Circulation 1984; 69:761–765.
34. Beta-Blocker Heart Attack Study Group. The Beta-Blocker Heart Attack Trial. JAMA 1981; 246:2073–2074.
35. Pfeffer MA, Braunwald E, Moye LA, Basta L, Brown EJ, Cuddy TE, Davis BR, Geltman EM, Goldman S, Flaker GC, Klein M, Lamas GA, Packer M, Rouleau J, Rouleau JL, Rutherford J, Wertheimer JH, Hawkins CM, on behalf of the SAVE Investigators. Effect of captopril on mortality and morbidity in patients with left ventricular dysfunction after myocardial infarction. N Engl J Med 1992; 327:669–677.
36. Sacks FM, Pfeffer MA, Moye LA, Rouleau JL, Rutherford JD, Cole TG, Brown L, Warnica JW, Arnold JMO, Wun C-C, Davis BR, Braunwald E, for the Cholesterol and Recurrent Events Trial Investigators. The effect of pravastatin on coronary events after myocardial infarction in patients with average cholesterol levels. N Engl J Med 1996; 335:1001–1009.
37. Scandinavian Simvastatin Survival Study Group. Randomised trial of cholesterol lowering in 4444 patients with coronary heart disease: the Scandinavian Simvastatin Survival Study (4S). Lancet 1994; 344:1383–1389.
38. The Long-Term Intervention with Pravastatin in Ischaemic Disease (LIPID) Study Group. Prevention of cardiovascular events and death with pravastatin in patients with coronary heart disease and a broad range of initial cholesterol levels. N Engl J Med 1998; 339:1349–1257.
39. Byington RP, Miller ME, Herrington D, Riley W, Pitt B, Furberg CD, Hunninghake DB, Mancini GBJ, for the PREVENT Investigators. Rationale, design, and baseline characteristics of the Prospective Randomized Evaluation of the Vascular Effects of Norvasc Trial (PREVENT). Am J Cardiol 1997; 80:1087–1090.
40. Hulley S, Grady D, Bush T, Furberg C, Herrington D, Riggs B, Vittinghoff, for the Heart and Estrogen/progestin Replacement Study (HERS) Research Group. Randomized trial of estrogen plus progestin for secondary prevention of coronary heart disease in postmenopausal women. JAMA 1998; 280:605–613.

41. Kitzer JR, Cannon CP, McCabe CH, Mueller HS, Schweiger MJ, Davis VG, Perritt R, Antman EM, for the TIMI Investigators. Trends in the use of pharmacotherapies for acute myocardial infarction among physicans who design and/or implement randomized trials versus physicians in routine clinical practice—the MILIS-TIME experience. Am Heart J 1999; 137:79–92.
42. ACC/AHA Task Force. Guidelines for the early management of patients with acute myocardial infarction: a report of the American College of Cardiology/American Heart Association Task Force on Assessment of Diagnostic and Therapeutic Cardiovascular Procedures (Subcommittee to Develop Guidelines for the Early Management of Patients with Acute Myocardial Infarction). J Am Coll Cardiol 1990; 16:249–292.
43. Sarasin FP, Maschiangel M-L, Schaller M-D, Héliot C, Mischler S, Gaspoz J-M. Successful implementation of guidelines for encouraging the use of beta-blockers in patients after acute myocardial infarction. Am J Med 1999; 106:499–505.

17

Effect of Enalapril on Morbid and Mortal Events Among SOLVD Participants with Hypertension

JOHN B. KOSTIS and MICHAEL C. RUDDY

University of Medicine and Dentistry of New Jersey–Robert Wood Johnson Medical School, New Brunswick, New Jersey

I. INTRODUCTION

Unlike most of the other clinical trials described in this volume, the Studies of Left Ventricular Dysfunction (SOLVD) were not designed as a study in hypertensives but addressed the effect of the angiotensin-converting enzyme (ACE) inhibitor, enalapril, in patients with systolic left ventricular dysfunction with or without heart failure. SOLVD trial is included in this book because approximately 2000 patients had hypertension as well as left ventricular dysfunction. A statistically and clinically significant reduction in ischemic events, heart failure hospitalization, and total mortality was seen in the hypertensive subset as well as in SOLVD as a whole.

II. RATIONALE OF SOLVD

The study was designed in the mid-80s when there was no proof that pharmacological intervention could alter the long-term survival of patients with left ventricular dysfunction and heart failure (1). Short-term studies of ACE inhibitors had shown hemodynamic and symptomatic benefits in patients with heart failure, but there was no conclusive evidence of a mortality benefit with these agents. SOLVD was one of several clinical trials designed to assess the effects of ACE inhibitors on mortality in these patients. One of these, CONSENSUS (Cooperative North Scandinavian Enalapril Survival Study), was designed to evaluate the effect on mortality of the addition of the ACE inhibitor, enalapril, to digitalis and diuretic therapy in patients with severe New York Heart Association [(NYHA) class IV] heart failure. The VHeFT (Veterans Administration Vasodilator Heart Failure Trial) focused on the effect of prazosin and of the combination of isosorbide dinitrate and hydralazine on mortality of patients with less severe (NYHA class II and II) heart failure who were also taking digoxin and diuretics.

CONSENSUS was interrupted by the data safety monitoring board after 253 patients were randomized because of a statistically significant 27% decrease in mortality in the enalapril treatment group (2). In this trial fewer than 200 patients were followed up for more than 6 months and only about 100 for more than 1 year. In VHeFT, patients randomized to the hydralazine or isosorbide dinitrate combination, but not those randomized to prazosin, had a lower mortality than placebo (3). Thus, during the design and conduct of SOLVD, available data suggested a benefit of vasodilator therapy on survival of patients with heart failure. However, confirmation was needed, especially when long-term therapy was considered for mildly symptomatic or asymptomatic patients (1).

III. THE DESIGN OF SOLVD

The SOLVD trial was designed in 1984 and 1985 and initiated in 1986 to evaluate the effects of the ACE inhibitor, enalapril, on long-term mortality and morbidity in patients with systolic left ventricular dysfunction with or without symptomatic heart failure. In the middle to late 80s, it was not known whether pharmacological therapy could improve long-term survival of patients with left ventricular systolic dysfunction and heart failure. When SOLVD was designed and initiated (1984–1986), data indicated favorable hemodynamic effects of ACE inhibitors, and small studies suggested a trend toward lower mortality. The SOLVD trial was designed to evaluate the effect of enalapril on mortality in a broad spectrum of patients with left ventricular dysfunction with and without heart failure (1). The primary objective of SOLVD was to answer the following question: can long-term survival be improved by taking enalapril:

1. in patients with left ventricular dysfunction (resting ejection fraction ≤ 0.35) and no history of overt heart failure (for the prevention trial), and
2. in patients with left ventricular dysfunction (resting ejection fraction ≤ 0.35 with a history of overt heart failure (for the treatment trial).

A secondary analysis was the effect of treatment on survival in all participants in the study (treatment and prevention trials combined). In addition, the treatment was assessed in five subgroups: (1) tertiles of plasma sodium; (2) patients using versus those not using a vasodilator at baseline; (3) tertiles of baseline ejection fraction; (4) etiology (coronary artery, hypertensive heart disease, and other); and (5) by NYHA functional classification (this was added after the results of CONSENSUS became known). The protocol neither stipulated nor precluded the administration of antihypertensive therapy. Patients with uncontrolled hypertension, defined as systolic blood pressure > 140 mm Hg AND diastolic blood pressure > 95 mm Hg, were excluded. Information on the duration of hypertension is not available. In SOLVD, some patients were taking pharmacologic agents with antihypertensive properties such as diuretics (43%), β-blockers (18%), and calcium channel antagonists (33%). However, the reason for the administration of these agents was not known but could be the presence of either hypertension or heart failure (diuretics), coronary artery disease (β-blockers, calcium channel antagonists), or other indications for these drugs. Analysis of the effect of enalapril compared with placebo in patients with hypertension was not a prespecified analysis in SOLVD. The analysis of the hypertensive subset of SOLVD was prompted by the high number of patients with hypertension as defined in Joint National Committee (JNC)-V and JNC-VI, who were randomized in SOLVD (4,5). Recruitment in SOLVD started in June 1986 and ended in May 1990 (March 1989 for the treatment trial). In addition to the primary and secondary hypotheses addressed in SOLVD, seven substudies were carried out to investigate the effect of treatment on a variety of outcomes that might mediate the effect of enalapril treatment in the two trials, elucidate the mechanisms of action of enalapril, and answer mechanistic questions.

Inclusion criteria of SOLVD were two: age between 21 and 80 years, inclusive, and left ventricular ejection fraction < 0.35 measured by radionuclide angiography, left ventricular contrast angiography or two-dimensional echocardiography within 3 months of the day of consent. Exclusion criteria were noncardiac diseases likely to limit survival, certain cardiac conditions other than primary myocardial dysfunction, intolerance to enalapril, and a substantial likelihood of nonadherence to the assigned medication (Table 1) (1). Randomization was stratified by trial (treatment or prevention) and hospital.

To evaluate patient adherence and tolerability of ACE inhibition, a 2- to 7-day prerandomization drug challenge period was instituted (4). During this period, patients eligible for randomization were given enalapril, 2.5 mg twice per day, were contacted by telephone regarding adverse effects a day later, and then seen 2 to 7 days after starting to receive medication. At this visit (first visit after starting enalapril), heart rate and blood pressure were measured, adverse effects were recorded, and blood was drawn for complete blood count, electrolytes, and creatinine. The patients were given placebo for 14 to 17 days (mean 15 days) and then returned to the clinical center for randomization. At randomization, enalapril or matching placebo was started at 2.5 mg twice daily and titrated in succeeding visits as tolerated to a maximum of 10 mg twice daily (Table 2). After randomization, visits were scheduled at 2 weeks, 6 weeks, 4 months, and then every 4 months until the end of the study. Changes in clinical condition and functional status, the use of nonstudy drugs, hospitalizations, and adherence to the study drug were noted at each follow-up visit. Measurements of electrolytes, blood urea nitrogen, creatinine, and complete blood count were obtained at specified intervals during follow-up. Adverse effects was ascertained by questioning the participants at follow-up visits and by inquiring about the reasons for withdrawing or changing the dose of the study drug. All randomized patients were retained in the analyses that were performed by the intention-to-treat approach.

The SOLVD trial was carried out in 23 clinical centers (total of 92 hospitals) in the United States (20) Canada (2), and Belgium (1). The coordinating center, the project office in the Clinical Trials Branch of the National Heart, Lung, and Blood Institute, and the Drug and Distribution Center rounded out the structure of SOLVD. The steering committee was composed of the principal investigators of the clinical centers and coordinating center and the project officer. The Data and Safety Monitoring Board, appointed by the director of the National Heart, Lung, and Blood Institute, reviewed the protocol and periodically monitored the study for outcomes, toxicity, and safety (1).

A. Sample Size

Sample size was calculated using a model based on the normal approximation to the binomial distribution with adjustment for lack of adherence and the following assump-

Table 1 Inclusion and Exclusion Criteria of SOLVD

Inclusion criteria
Age 21 to 80 years, inclusive.
Left ventricular ejection fraction—6.35.
Exclusion criteria
Medical history of intolerance to enalapril.
Prospective participant already receiving an ACE inhibitor and unable to discontinue.
Myocardial infarction in the last 30 days.
Hemodynamically significant primary valvular or outflow tract obstruction (e.g., mitral valvular stenosis, asymmetric septal hypertrophy, or malfunctioning prosthetic valve).
Constrictive pericarditis.
Complex congenital heart disease.
Syncopal episodes presumed to be result of life-threatening arrhythmias. (Asymptomatic cardiac arrhythmia including ventricular tachycardia is not an exclusion criterion.)
Any prospective participant in whom cardiac surgery, including transplantation, is likely in the near future (e.g., participant's name is on cardiac transplant list). In particular, if a potential participant is likely to need CABG surgery in the immediate future, he or she should be excluded but can be reassessed for eligibility after surgery.
Unstable angina pectoris (defined as angina at rest) or severe stable angina (more than an average of two attacks/day) despite treatment.
Uncontrolled hypertension at the time of randomization. (Uncontrolled blood pressure is defined as systolic blood pressure $>$ 140 mm Hg AND diastolic blood pressure $>$ 95 mm Hg.)
Cor pulmonale (right ventricular failure secondary to pulmonary disease).
Advanced pulmonary disease ($FEV_1/FVC = \leq 50$, peak expiratory flow rate $<$ 200 ml/s, FVC $<$ 60% of predicted).
Major neurologic diseases that could lead to early death (i.e., Alzheimer's disease, advanced Parkinson's disease).
Cerebrovascular disease (e.g., significant carotid artery stenosis) that could potentially be complicated or rendered unstable by administration of an ACE inhibitor. (Prospective participants who may be at increased risk for stoke should their blood pressure decrease excessively. The mere presence of a carotid bruit need not in itself exclude participants.)
Collagen vascular disease other than rheumatoid arthritis (i.e., systemic lupus erythematosus, polyarteritis nodosa, scleroderma).
Suspected significant renal artery stenosis.
Renal failure (i.e., creatinine $>$ 2.5 mg/dl or dialysis patients).
Malignancies, except for surgically cured skin cancer, carcinoma in-situ, or 5 years free of disease after the diagnosis of solid tumors.
Requirement for immunosuppressive therapy. (The use of steroids for non–life-threatening diseases such as arthritis is not an exclusion.)
Active myocarditis.
Significant primary liver disease.
Likelihood of a prospective participant being nonadherent because of chronic alcoholism, lack of a fixed address, drug addiction, etc.
Other life-threatening disease or prospective participant who is not realistically expected to be discharged alive from the hospital.
Pregnant woman or woman of child-bearing potential who is not protected from pregnancy by any method.
Prospective participant who is simultaneously receiving other investigational drug protocols (other than for compassionate use).
Failure to give consent.

Abbreviations: *SOLVD*, Studies of Left Ventricular Dysfunction; *ACE*, angiotensin-converting enzyme; *CABG*, coronary artery bypass grafting; FEV_1, forced expiratory volume; FVC, forced vital capacity.
(From Ref. 1.)

Table 2

Eligibility established: EF $\leq$ 0.30 etc.
Prerandomization run-in: enalapril 2.5 mg b.i.d.
2–7 days (median 6 days)
Exclusion of patients with noncompliance or side effects
Prerandomization placebo phase and placebo
14–17 days
Exclusion of unstable and noncompliant patients
RANDOMIZATION
(enalapril or placebo)
2.5 or 5 mg b.i.d. at physician judgment
2 weeks
5 mg or 10 mg b.i.d.
Follow-up visits
Physicians encouraged to maintain patients at 10 mg b.i.d. or as tolerated

Abbreviation: *EF*, ejection fraction.

Table 3 Outcomes Measures in the SOLVD Trial

Treatment trial	Prevention trial	Combined trials (ischemic events)
Deaths	Death	Myocardial infarction
Deaths or hospitalizations for CHF	All causes	Fatal
Cardiovascular deaths	Cardiovascular causes	Nonfatal
Cardiac	Cardiac	Either
Arrhythmia without worsening CHF	Arrhythmia without worsening CHF	Hospitalization for angina
Heart failure or arrhythmia with CHF	Progressive heart failure (pump failure or arrhythmias with CHF)	MI or hospitalization for angina
MI	Myocardial infarction	Cardiac deaths or nonfatal MI
Other	Other	Cardiac death, nonfatal MI, or hospitalization for angina
Stroke	Stroke	All deaths, nonfatal MI or hospitalization for angina
Other vascular or unknown	Other vascular cause of unknown	
Noncardiovascular deaths	Noncardiovascular causes	
	Development of CHF	
	Development of CHF and anti-CHF therapy	
	First hospitalization for CHF	
	Multiple hospitalizations for CHF	
	Death or development of CHF	
	Death or hospitalization for CHF	

Abbreviations: *SOLVD*, Studies of Left Ventricular Dysfunction; *CHF*, Congestive heart failure; *MI*, myocardial infarction.

tions: (1) a one-sided significance level of 0.025; (2) power of 90%; (3) a 3-year mortality of 32% in the control group in the treatment trial; (4) average follow-up of 3.0 years; (5) a 3-year mortality of 17% in the control group in the Prevention Trial; (6) a 25% reduction in mortality given 100% adherence with treatment; (7) a 3-year adherence proportion of 80% in the treatment trial and 85% in the prevention trial; and (8) that nonadherers revert to event rates of the other treatment group. Using these assumptions, a sample size of 2100 was calculated for the treatment trial and 4000 for the prevention trial. The sample size was then adjusted upward to avoid underpowering the study if the above assumptions did not hold true (for example, lower event rates or poorer adherence) to 2500 for the treatment trial and 4600 for the prevention trial. The power of the combined study (the treatment and prevention trials; 7100 patients, together) was 90% to detect a 13% reduction in mortality (1).

IV. MAJOR FINDINGS OF SOLVD

During the open-label prerandomization drug challenge phase, enalapril, 2.5 mg twice per day, was given on an outpatient basis for 7 days (mean 6.1, range 2 to 7, and median 7) to 7487 patients. Four hundred forty-four (5.93%) patients reported side effects, including symptoms attributed to hypotension (in 166 patients [2.2%]). Of the patients who reported side effects, 77.9% agreed to continue their participation in the study with a 50-50 chance of receiving enalapril. Ninety-eight (1.3%) of 7487 patients were not willing to continue because of side effects (0.5% because of symptoms attributed to hypotension). Thus, outpatient initiation of enalapril therapy was well tolerated by patients in SOLVD (4).

In the treatment trial, 1284 patients were randomized to placebo and 1285 to enalapril (approximately 90% in NYHA class II and III) (5). During an average follow-up of 41.4 months, there were 510 deaths in the placebo group (39.7%) and 452 in the enalapril group (35.2%) (relative risk reduction 16%, 95% confidence interval [CI]) 5% to 26% $P = 0.0036$, Tables 3 and 4). The largest mortality reduction was in deaths attributed to progressive heart failure with no significant change on arrhythmic death. In addition, the rate of hospitalization for worsening heart failure was higher in the placebo group (736) than in the enalapril group (613; 26% risk reduction, 95% CI 18% to 34% $P < 0.0001$).

In the prevention trial, patients were randomly assigned to receive either placebo (n = 2117) or enalapril (n = 2111) for an average follow-up of 37.4 months (6). Three hundred thirty-four deaths occurred in the placebo group and 313 in the enalapril group (relative risk reduction 8%, 95% CI 8% [an increase of 8%] to 21%, $P = 0.30$, Table 5). The combined endpoint of death and development of heart failure occurred less frequently in the enalapril group (630 events) than in the placebo group (818 events, relative risk reduction, 29%, 95% CI 21% to 36%, $P < 0.001$). Four hundred thirty-four patients died or were hospitalized for heart failure in the enalapril group versus 518 in the placebo group (relative risk reduction 20%, 95% CI 9% to 30%, $P < 0.001$).

In both the treatment (127 vs. 158, $P < 0.02$) and prevention trials (161 vs. 204, $P < 0.01$) as well as the combined trial (288 vs. 362, relative risk reduction 23%, 95% CI 11% to 34%; $P < 0.001$), fewer patients developed myocardial infarction in the enalapril group than the placebo group (Table 6) (7). Unstable angina requiring hospitalization developed in 499 in the enalapril group compared with 595 in the placebo group (risk reduction 20%, 95% CI 9% to 29%, $P < 0.001$). There were fewer cardiac deaths (615) in the enalapril group compared with placebo (711, $P < 0.003$). The combined endpoint of death, myocardial infarction, and unstable angina was reduced by enalapril (20% risk reduction, 95% CI 14% to 26%, $P = 0.001$).

Table 4 Effect of Treatment on Mortality and Hospitalization for Congestive Heart Failure, and Proportion of Patients Taking Angiotensin-Converting-Enzyme Inhibitors After Various Periods in the SOLVD Treatment Trial*

Months of follow-up	Mortality			Death or hospitalization for heart failure			Proportion taking inhibitors†	
	Placebo	Enalapril	Risk reduction (95% CI)	Placebo	Enalapril	Risk reduction (95% CI)	Placebo	Enalapril
	Number		Percent	Number		Percent	Percent	
3	69	47	33 (2–53)	164	92	46 (30–57)	6	91
6	126	91	29 (8–46)	259	150	45 (33–55)	10	88
12	201	159	23 (5–37)	401	262	40 (30–48)	12	86
24	344	277	23 (10–34)	559	434	30 (21–38)	20	83
36	450	396	16 (4–27)	680	555	28 (19–35)	23	82
48	504	443	17 (5–27)	731	607	27 (18–34)	30	83
Overall	510	452	16 (5–26)	736	613	26 (18–34)	—	—
	$Z = 2.69$; $P = 0.0036$			$Z = 5.65$; $P < 0.0001$				

*The 95% confidence intervals (CI) correspond to a two-sided P value of < 0.05 or a one-sided P value of < 0.025. Risk reductions were calculated by the log-rank test from the data available at each specific time.

†Values shown for 3 and 6 months were based on data obtained after the visits at 4 and 8 months, respectively.

The inhibitors were angiotensin-converting-enzyme inhibitors.

Abbreviation: *SOLVD*, Studies of Left Ventricular Dysfunction.

Table 5 Deaths, Causes of Death, Development of Heart Failure, and Hospitalization for Heart Failure, According to Treatment Group in the SOLVD Prevention Trial

Cause of death or type of event	Placebo (n = 2117)	Enalapril (n = 2111)	Reduction in risk (95% CI)*	Z score	*P* value†
	No. (%)		%		
Death‡					
All causes	334 (15.8)	313 (14.8)	8 (−8 to 21)	1.02	0.30
Cardiovascular causes	298 (14.1)	265 (12.6)	12 (−3 to 26)	1.57	0.12
Cardiac	271 (12.8)	238 (11.3)	13 (−3 to 27)	1.63	0.10
Arrhythmia without worsening CHF	105 (5.0)	98 (4.6)	7 (−22 to 30)	0.54	NS
Progressive heart failure (pump failure or arrhythmia with CHF)	106 (5.0)	85 (4.0)	21 (−5 to 41)	1.64	0.10
Myocardial infarction	52 (2.5)	46 (2.2)	14 (−28 to 42)	0.74	ND
Other	8 (0.4)	9 (0.4)	—	—	ND
Stroke	13 (0.6)	10 (0.5)	—	—	ND
Other vascular cause or unknown	14 (0.7)	17 (0.8)	—	—	ND
Noncardiovascular causes	36 (.7)	48 (2.3)	—	—	ND
Morbidity and combined outcomes					
Development of CHF	640 (30.2)	438 (20.7)	37 (28 to 44)	7.47	< 0.001
Development of CHF and anti-CHF therapy	477 (22.5)	293 (13.9)	43 (33 to 50)	7.59	< 0.001
First hospitalization for CHF	273 (12.9)	184 (8.7)	36 (22 to 46)	4.65	< 0.001
Multiple hospitalizations for CHF	102 (4.8)	58 (2.7)	44 (23 to 59)	3.61	< 0.001
Death or development of CHF	818 (38.6)	630 (29.8)	29 (21 to 36)	6.55	< 0.001
Death or hospitalization for CHF	518 (24.5)	434 (20.6)	20 (9 to 30)	3.46	< 0.001

*By the log-rank test. CI denotes confidence interval. A negative number indicates an increase in risk.
†NS denotes not significant and ND not done (i.e., no statistical test was performed).
‡After August 31, 1991, but before the final follow-up visits, there were eight additional deaths in the placebo group and four in the enalapril group. Therefore, the total numbers of deaths were 342 in the placebo group and 317 in the enalapril group (risk reduction, 9% $Z = 1.23$; $P = 0.22$). The corresponding numbers for mortality from cardiovascular causes were 304 and 269 (risk reduction, 13%; 95% confidence interval, −2 to 26; $Z = 1.71$; $P = 0.09$).
Abbreviations: *SOLVD*, Studies of Left Ventricular Dysfunction; *CHF*, congestive heart failure.
(From Ref. 6.)

Table 6 Effect of Enalapril on Development of Myocardial Infarction, Hospitalization for Worsening Angina, and Cardiac and Total Mortality in the Combined SOLVD Trials

Outcome	No. of events (%) Placebo	No. of events (%) Enalapril	Risk reduction (%) (95% CI)	Z score	*P*
Treatment trial					
Myocardial infarction					
Fatal	91 (1.7)	69 (5.4)	27 (1, 46)	1.99	0.04
Nonfatal	83 (6.5)	66 (5.1)	23 (−6, 44)	1.58	0.11
Either	158 (12.3)	127 (9.9)	23 (2, 39)	2.17	0.02
Hospitalization for angina*	240 (18.7)	187 (14.6)	27 (12, 40)	3.29	0.001
MI or hospitalization for angina	350 (27.3)	282 (21.9)	25 (12, 36)	3.63	0.001
Cardiac deaths or nonfatal MI	505 (39.3)	429 (33.4)	19 (8, 29)	3.21	0.001
Cardiac death, nonfatal MI, or hospitalization for angina	659 (51.3)	547 (42.6)	23 (14, 32)	4.63	0.0001
All deaths, nonfatal MI or hospitalization for angina	700 (54.5)	592 (46.1)	22 (13, 30)	4.51	0.0001
Prevention trial					
Myocardial infarction					
Fatal	66 (3.1)	70 (3.3)	−4 (−45, 26)	−0.21	0.83
Nonfatal	147 (6.9)	103 (4.9)	32 (13, 47)	3.06	0.001
Either	204 (9.1)	161 (7.6)	24 (6, 38)	2.59	0.01
Hospitalization for angina*	355 (16.8)	312 (14.8)	14 (0, 26)	1.99	0.05
MI or hospitalization for angina	509 (24.0)	425 (20.1)	20 (9, 29)	3.35	0.001
Cardiac deaths or nonfatal MI	413 (19.5)	329 (15.6)	23 (11, 33)	3.49	0.001
Cardiac death, nonfatal MI, or hospitalization for angina	691 (32.6)	570 (27.0)	21 (12, 29)	4.13	0.0001
All deaths, nonfatal MI or hospitalization for angina	722 (34.1)	613 (29.0)	19 (9, 27)	3.37	0.0001
Combined trials					
Myocardial infarction					
Fatal	157 (4.6)	139 (4.1)	14 (−8, 32)	1.32	0.19
Nonfatal	230 (6.8)	169 (5.0)	29 (13, 41)	3.39	0.001
Either	362 (10.6)	288 (8.5)	23 (11, 34)	3.38	0.001
Hospitalization for angina*	595 (17.5)	499 (14.7)	20 (9, 29)	3.61	0.001
MI or hospitalization for angina	859 (25.3)	707 (20.8)	22 (14, 29)	4.89	0.0001
Cardiac deaths or nonfatal MI	918 (27.0)	758 (22.3)	21 (13, 28)	4.72	0.0001
Cardiac death, nonfatal MI, or hospitalization for angina	1350 (39.7)	1117 (32.9)	22 (16, 28)	6.20	0.0001
All deaths, nonfatal MI or hospitalization for angina	1422 (41.8)	1205 (35.5)	20 (14, 26)	5.82	0.0001

*Data for hospitalization for angina include both primary and secondary discharge diagnosis. Numbers of patients hospitalized with a primary diagnosis of worsening angina are: prevention trial (329 placebo, 296 enalapril, Z = 1.61), treatment trial (204 placebo, 166 enalapril, Z = 2.55) and combined trials (533 placebo, 462 enalapril, Z = 2.84).

Abbreviations: *SOLVD*, Studies of Left Ventricular Dysfunction; *MI*, myocardial infarction.

(From Ref. 7.)

Enalapril was well tolerated in SOLVD. However, hypotension, azotemia, cough, fatigue, and other side effects caused discontinuation of therapy in a significant minority of patients (8). During an average of 40 months of follow-up, side effects were reported by 28.1% of patients randomized to enalapril and by 16.0% of those randomized to placebo ($P < 0.0001$). Enalapril use was associated with a higher rate of symptoms related to hypotension [14.8% vs 7.1% of the placebo group, $P < 0.0001$ (Table 7)]. Additionally,

Table 7 Side Effects Reported During Follow-Up in the Placebo and Enalapril Groups of SOLVD

	Placebo					Enalapril			
	SE (no.)	SE (%)	DISC (no.)	DISC (%)	DISC if SE Present %	SE (%)	SE (%)	DISC (%)	DISC if SE present (%)
Hypotension	242	7.1	95	2.8	39.3	500	14.8	5.4	36.2
Taste	28	0.8	10	0.3	35.7	32	0.9	0.5	50.0
Skin rash	48	1.4	40	1.2	83.3	56	1.7	1.3	78.6
Azotemia	55	1.6	29	0.9	52.7	128	3.8	2.1	55.5
Fatigue	120	3.5	65	1.9	54.2	196	5.8	2.8	48.5
GI	70	2.1	40	1.2	57.1	98	2.9	1.7	57.1
Angioedema	4	0.1	4	0.1	100.0	12	0.4	0.3	83.3
Cough	67	2.0	47	1.4	70.1	169	5.0	3.3	66.9
Vision	12	0.4	5	0.1	41.7	24	0.7	0.3	41.7
Hyperkalemia	14	0.4	2	0.1	14.3	41	1.2	0.7	56.2
Impotence	19	0.6	7	0.2	36.8	22	0.7	0.5	81.8
Leukopenia	6	0.2	3	0.1	50.0	13	0.4	0.3	76.9
Proteinuria	16	0.5	9	0.3	56.3	6	0.2	0.1	50.0
Other	95	2.8	58	1.7	61.1	114	3.4	1.8	54.4
Any SE	542	16.0	291	8.6	53.7	949	28.1	15.2	54.1
Patients (no.)	3387					3382			

Abbreviations: *SOLVD*, Studies of Left Ventricular Dysfunction; *SE*, side effect; *DISC*, discontinued blinded treatment because of side effect; *GI*, gastrointestinal; *Hypotension*, symptoms attributed to hypotension. (From Ref. 4.)

the following were reported more frequently in the enalapril group: azotemia (3.8% vs. 1.6%, $P < 0.0001$), cough (5.0% vs. 2.0%, $P = 0.0001$), fatigue (5.8% vs. 3.5%, $P < 0.0001$), hyperkalemia (1.2% vs. 0.4%, $P = 0.0002$), and angioedema (0.4% vs. 0.1%, $P < 0.05$). Blinded therapy was discontinued because of side effects in 15.2% of the enalapril group versus 8.6% in the placebo group ($P < 0.0001$).

V. CHARACTERISTICS OF THE HYPERTENSIVE SUBSET OF SOLVD

Of the 6797 patients who were randomized into SOLVD, 2652 gave a history of hypertension at randomization. One thousand five hundred eight patients had systolic blood pressure (SBP) of 140 mm Hg or higher and 985 patients had diastolic blood pressure (DBP) 90 mm Hg or higher at randomization. In the retrospective analysis of the SOLVD database, the hypertensive population of SOLVD was defined in three alternative ways, using three overlapping subsets (history of hypertension, SBP $\geq$ 140 mm Hg, and DBP $\geq$ 90 mm Hg). The fact that similar results were observed in analyzing all three subsets strengthens the conclusions of the analysis. The three subgroups overlapped; some patients had both high SBP and high DBP, and some with history of hypertension also had SBP of 140 mm Hg or higher or DBP of 90 mm Hg or higher, whereas others did not (Table 8). Five hundred seventy-six patients had elevation of both systolic and diastolic blood pressure (285 randomized to placebo and 291 randomized to enalapril). Separate analysis of this subset was not performed because of its smaller size and the large overlap (58%) with the subset with elevated diastolic blood pressure (9,10).

Table 8 Number of SOLVD Participants with High Blood Pressure at Baseline Who Were Randomized to Placebo and Enalapril

	SBP ≥ 140 mm Hg			DBP ≥ 90 mm Hg		
Trial	Placebo	Enalapril	Total	Placebo	Enalapril	Total
Prevention	482	440	922	319	316	635
Treatment	279	307	586	162	188	350
Combined	761	747	1508	481	504	985

Abbreviations: *SOLVD*, Studies of Left Ventricular Dysfunction; *SBP*, systolic blood pressure; *DBP*, diastolic blood pressure.
(From Ref. 10.)

Table 9 Baseline Characteristics in SOLVD Participants with High Blood Pressure at Baseline-Combined Trials

	Baseline DBP ≥ 90 mm Hg				Baseline SBP ≥ 140 mm Hg			
	Placebo		Enalapril		Placebo		Enalapril	
	N	%	N	%	N	%	N	%
Age (Yrs)								
20–29	19	4.0	18	3.6	7	0.9	10	1.3
40–49	74	15.4	72	14.3	46	6.0	53	7.1
50–59	158	32.8	167	33.1	183	24.1	186	24.9
60–69	173	36.0	196	38.9	366	48.2	340	45.6
70–80	57	11.8	51	10.1	158	20.8	157	21.0
Male	423	87.9	438	86.9	643	84.5	610	87.1
Female	58	12.1	66	13.1	118	15.5	137	18.3
Race								
Black	80	16.6	88	17.5	91	12.0	111	14.9
White	389	80.9	407	81.1	659	86.6	622	83.5
Other	12	2.5	7	1.4	11	1.4	12	1.6
No prior MI	167	34.7	151	30.0	270	35.5	226	30.3
Prior MI	314	65.3	352	70.0	491	64.5	519	69.7
No prior angina	325	67.7	342	67.9	503	66.2	497	66.5
Prior angina	155	32.3	162	32.1	257	33.8	250	33.5
No prior CABG	362	75.3	385	76.4	564	74.1	543	72.7
Prior CABG	119	24.7	119	23.6	197	25.9	204	27.3
Etiology								
Ischemic HD	342	71.1	362	72.0	563	74.0	555	74.5
Unknown/idiopathic	74	15.4	72	14.3	120	15.8	108	14.5
Other	65	13.5	69	13.7	78	10.2	82	11.0
NYHA class I	213	44.3	245	48.6	344	45.2	331	44.3
Class II	213	44.3	205	40.7	335	44.0	322	43.1
Class III	52	10.8	52	10.3	79	10.4	91	12.2
Class IV	3	0.6	2	0.4	3	0.4	3	0.4
Age (yrs)	481	58.1	504	58.3	760	62.7	746	62.4
EF	481	27.0	504	27.3	761	27.7	747	28.2
SBP (mm Hg)	481	141.9	504	141.5	761	148.8	747	148.9
DBP (mm Hg)	481	92.9	504	92.8	761	84.5	747	84.7

Abbreviations: *SOLVD*, Studies in left Ventricular Dysfunction; *DBP*, diastolic blood pressure; *SBP*, systolic blood pressure; *MI*, myocardial infarction; *CABG*, coronary artery bypass graft; *HD*, heart disease; *NYHA*, New York Heart Association; *EF*, ejection fraction.
(From Ref. 10.)

The placebo and enalapril groups of the hypertension subsets of SOLVD were balanced with respect to baseline characteristics as shown in Table 9. Among the 26 comparisons shown, only one statistically significant difference was seen between the enalapril and placebo groups: among patients with high systolic blood pressure at baseline, prior myocardial infarction was significantly more frequent in the enalapril group (P = .034).

In this post hoc subgroup analysis of the hypertensive subset of SOLVD, crude event rates were calculated as the percentage of patients experiencing the event. Relative risks were computed using a Cox regression analysis, with treatment group as the only independent variable. Homogeneity of treatment effects between hypertensive and nonhypertensive subgroups was tested by examining the interaction between treatment group and hypertension in the Cox regression model.

A. Effect on Blood Pressure

During follow-up, enalapril was associated with lower SBP and DBP. The average difference in blood pressure between the placebo and enalapril groups was 6/4 mm Hg. Blood pressure at baseline, at year 1, and at year 2 of follow-up is shown in Table 10 (10). All differences between enalapril and placebo were statistically significant with $P < .01$ with two exceptions: in the subgroup with high SBP and high DBP at year 1, the difference in DBP was significant with $P = .04$. At year 2, the differences in both DBP and SBP were not statistically significant (small N).

B. Effect on Morbid and Mortal Events

In the SOLVD hypertensive subset, the relative risk for a cardiac event or death was consistently in favor of enalapril for all endpoints considered. The SOLVD study was not powered to detect differences within these small hypertension subgroups. However, either a statistically significant benefit or a favorable trend for risk reduction was seen in all hypertensive subgroups examined (Table 11). For the combined trials, therapy with enalapril was associated with an 18% reduction in the relative risk of death (95% CI: 2% to 32%, $P = 0.03$) and lower crude mortality rate from 26.1% for placebo to 21.5% (difference 4.6%, 95% CI; 18.3 to 0.9) (Fig. 1). The number needed to treat (NNT) to prevent one death during the trial was 21.8. The relative risk reduction of mortality in the treatment trial was 24% (95% CI: 3% to 41%, $P = 0.03$) and in the prevention trial 17% (95% CI: −9% to 37%, $P = 0.18$). As a result of the lower mortality rates, the average follow-up time during the combined trials was 0.11 years longer (95% CI: 0.00 to 0.20 years) for patients receiving enalapril. Adjusting survival time for NYHA class had little effect on the reported findings (Table 10) (11). The magnitudes of the treatment effects were similar in the hypertensive and nonhypertensive subgroups (Table 9). There were no statistically significant interactions between treatment group and hypertensive status, implying that enalapril has similar effects regardless of hypertensive and normotensive patients with left ventricular dysfunction.

The effects on congestive heart failure hospitalization on the combined ischemic event of cardiac mortality, myocardial infarction, and unstable angina were statistically significant in the individual analyses of each trial and each blood pressure subset studied (Table 11). Thus, the rate of hospitalization for congestive heart failure was lower in the enalapril group than the placebo group among patients with history of hypertension (35% lower), among those with elevated DBP at baseline (43% lower), or high SBP at baseline (33% lower). The effect of enalapril on lowering the rate of hospitalization for congestive

Table 10 Mean Change in Blood Pressure in the SOLVD Combined Trials

	Year 1							
	Placebo				Enalapril			
Group	N	Pre	Post	Change	N	Pre	Post	Change
Changes in systolic blood pressure								
SBP normal, DBP normal	2040	117.8	122.5	4.7	2077	118.0	117.1	−0.9
SBP normal, DBP high	165	128.9	130.3	1.4	190	127.9	124.5	−3.4
SBP high, DBP normal	390	147.2	139.3	−7.8	393	147.1	132.6	−14.5
SBP high, DBP high	235	150.8	140.8	−10.0	242	151.2	136.1	−15.0
Changes in diastolic blood pressure								
SBP normal, DBP normal	2040	74.2	76.2	2.0	2077	74.3	72.9	−1.5
SBP normal, DBP high	165	92.1	84.8	−7.3	190	91.6	81.2	−10.3
SBP high, DBP normal	390	79.4	78.8	−0.6	393	79.5	75.8	−3.7
SBP high, DBP high	235	93.3	85.4	−7.9	242	93.5	83.3	−10.2

	Year 1				Year 2			
	Placebo				Enalapril			
Group	N	Pre	Post	Change	N	Pre	Post	Change
Changes in systolic blood pressure								
SBP normal, DBP normal	1562	117.9	123.1	5.2	1614	117.9	117.6	−0.3
SBP normal, DBP high	123	129.1	127.7	−1.4	150	128.1	121.5	−6.6
SBP high, DBP normal	286	147.0	140.4	−6.6	310	147.0	131.1	−15.9
SBP high, DBP high	176	150.1	138.0	−12.1	195	150.7	136.4	−14.3
Changes in diastolic blood pressure								
SBP normal, DBP normal	1562	74.3	75.6	1.4	1614	74.4	72.8	−1.6
SBP normal, DBP high	123	92.1	83.0	−9.1	150	91.9	77.8	−14.1
SBP high, DBP normal	286	79.5	78.1	−1.4	310	79.6	74.8	−4.8
SBP high, DBP high	176	93.5	82.4	−11.0	195	93.5	81.5	−11.9

Abbreviations: *SOLVD*; Studies of Left Ventricular Dysfunction; *Change*, change in blood pressure; *SBP*, systolic blood pressure; *DBP*, diastolic blood pressure.
(From Ref. 10.)

Table 11 Mortality, Myocardial Infarction, Unstable Angina, Stroke, and Hospitalization for Congestive Heart Failure in SOLVD Patients with and Without History of Hypertension and in Those with Elevated Systolic or Diastolic Blood Pressure at Baseline

	No H/O HT				H/O HT			
	EN	PL	RR	P	EN	PL	RR	P
N	2068	2077			1328	1324		
Total mortality	20.6	24.1	0.866	.006	24.8	25.8	0.927	.323
CHF	16.7	24.1	0.647	<.001	20.6	28.3	0.664	<.001
Stroke	3.0	3.8	0.775	.132	5.4	5.4	0.979	.898
MI	8.3	11.0	0.729	.002	8.7	10.0	0.836	.159
Angina	13.5	17.3	0.743	<.001	16.5	17.7	0.900	.263
Combined endpoint	30.4	38.5	0.744	<.001	34.2	39.4	0.825	.003
	DBP ≥ 90				SBP ≥ 140			
	EN	PL	RR	P	EN	PL	RR	P
N	504	481			747	761		
Total mortality	19.6	23.7	0.791	.088	23.4	27.3	0.841	.091
CHF	16.5	26.0	0.574	<.001	19.5	27.7	0.647	<.001
Stroke	5.2	6.4	0.755	.289	5.0	6.8	0.707	.105
MI	8.9	9.6	0.889	.575	9.5	11.6	0.806	.176
Angina	15.9	15.2	0.872	.42	14.3	16.0	0.867	.280
Combined endpoint	29.0	36.0	0.762	.015	30.8	38.8	0.766	.002

Abbreviations: *SOLVD*, Studies of Left Vertricular Dysfunction; *H/O HT*, history of hypertension; *SBP*, systolic blood pressure at baseline; *CHF*, hospitalization for heart failure; *MI*, acute myocardial infarction; *No H/O HT*, no history of hypertension; *PL*, crude rate in the placebo group; *RR*, relative risk based on a life-table analysis (note that 100 (1-RR) is the percent risk reduction associated with enalapril therapy); *combined endpoint*, myocardial infarction, unstable angina, cardiac mortality; *DBP*, diastolic blood pressure at baseline; *stroke*, development of stroke; *angina*, hospitalization for angina; *EN*, crude rate in the enalapril group.

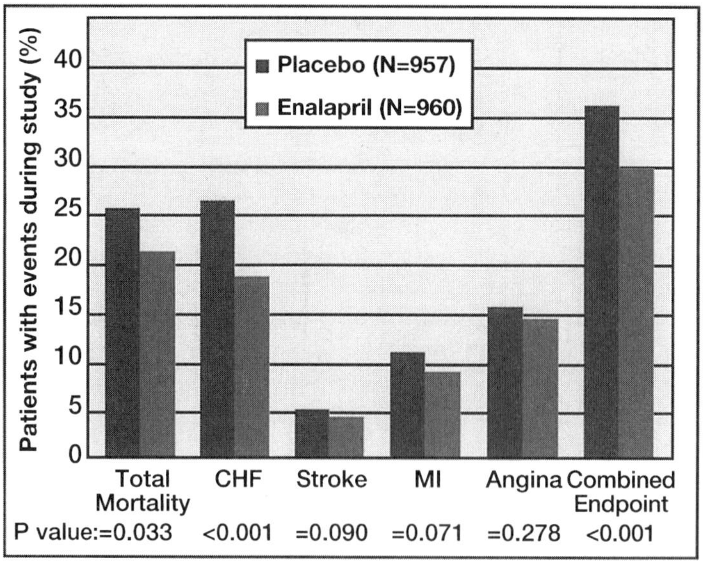

Fig. 1 Enalapril reduced the risk of all major cardiovascular clinical events in the Studies of Left Ventricular Dysfunction (SOLVD) and also reduced total mortality. (From Ref. 9.)

heart failure was more pronounced in patients who were receiving β-blockers during follow-up than those who were not taking these agents (relative risk 0.403 vs. 0.696, P = .037 for lack of homogeneity). This effect was also more pronounced in patients who did not receive diuretics compared with those who received diuretics during follow-up (relative risk 0.489 vs. 0.721, P = .038 for lack of homogeneity). These findings may reflect a lesser degree of illness severity in patients receiving β-blockers not receiving diuretics.

The relationship of the blood pressure during treatment (i.e., at 6 weeks after baseline) to events in the total cohort showed that patients with low systolic (≤ 100 mm Hg) or low diastolic (≤ 60 mm Hg) blood pressure at 6 weeks were more likely to be hospitalized during follow-up, although at each BP stratum, congestive heart failure hospitalization was less likely in the enalapril group compared with the placebo group. Also, a beneficial effect or trend of enalapril on morbidity and mortality was observed when the relationship of events to the change in blood pressure between baseline and at 6 weeks follow-up was considered.

VI. THE ECONOMIC IMPACT OF THERAPY WITH ENALAPRIL IN SOLVD PATIENTS WITH HYPERTENSION

In recent years, emphasis has been placed on cost of treating hypertension. In the SOLVD hypertensive subset, the risk imposed by the coexistence of hypertension and systolic left ventricular dysfunction justifies the use of ACE inhibitors on both clinical and economic grounds. This is described briefly in the following cost and benefit considerations (11). In this analysis, hospital costs were estimated by multiplying the Diagnostic Related Group weight for each hospitalization type with the average federal reimbursement rate that excluded adjustments by the Health Care Financing Administration for capital expenditures, free care, and medical education. Physician fees were estimated using relative value units (RVU) from the Medicare Fee Schedule and the average Federal reimbursement per RVU. Deaths occurring outside the hospital were assigned a cost of \$1,000, cost of ambulatory care was set at \$436, and the cost of enalapril was based on the Federal supply schedule price list. A \$2.50 per month dispensing fee was added. The cost per year of life saved and the cost per quality-adjusted year of life saved were estimated using a 5% annual discount rate for both costs and effects (11).

In the combined analysis of the trial events, therapy with enalapril was associated with a statistically significant 37% reduction in the number of hospitalizations. For all types of hospitalizations, there were 32 fewer hospitalizations per 100 patients receiving enalapril (95% CI: 11.8 to 52.2, NNT = 3.1 patients). The savings from the reduction in hospitalization costs (\$2,650 per patient for the duration of the study) were higher than the cost of enalapril and the extra ambulatory care expense because of the lower mortality with enalapril. As a result, the clinical benefits of treatment with the ACE inhibitor were associated with cost savings (\$1,560 per patient for the duration of the study) rather than expenses (Table 12). In the treatment trial, patients randomized to enalapril had a cost reduction of \$3,198 per patient (95% Cl, \$657 to \$5,739). In the prevention trial, the average cost savings per patient on enalapril were \$744 (95% Cl: cost reduction of \$2,011 to cost increase of \$523 per patient). The cost analysis for patients with asymptomatic and undiagnosed left ventricular dysfunction (similar to patients in the prevention trial) may be somewhat less because of the lower frequency of outpatient visits in this group. Also, the cost of the (left ventricular dysfunction) screen (MUGA, echo, cath, etc.) is not included in the model.

Table 12 Mortality and Years of Follow-Up by NYHA Class During the Period of Observation in SOLVD Patients with Hypertension at Baseline with 95% Confidence Intervals for the Difference

	Enalapril	Placebo	Difference E–P	95% Cl
Combined analysis*				
Deaths during trial (%)	21.5	26.1	−4.6	(−8.3, −0.9)
Years of follow-up†				
NYHA class I	1.32	1.12	0.21	
NYHA class II	1.27	1.30	−0.03	
NYHA class III	0.26	0.33	−0.07	
NYHA class IV	0.02	0.02	0.00	
Total years	2.87	2.76	0.11	(0.00, 0.20)
Quality adjusted yrs.	1.87	1.78	0.09	(0.02, 0.16)
Treatment trial	(n = 376)	(n = 336)		
Deaths during trial (%)	31.6	39.3	−7.6	(−14.7, −0.6)
Years of follow-up†				
NYHA class I	0.49	0.33	0.16	
NYHA class II	1.72	1.64	0.08	
NYHA class III	0.59	0.66	−0.07	
NYHA class IV	0.04	0.04	0.00	
Total years	2.84	2.68	0.17	(0.00, 0.34)
Quality adjusted yrs.	1.74	1.62	.13	(0.02, 0.23)
Prevention trial	(n = 584)	(n = 621)		
Deaths during trial (%)	15.6	18.4	−2.8	(−7.0, 1.5)
Years of follow-up*				
NYHA class I	1.82	1.59	0.23	
NYHA class II	1.00	1.09	−0.09	
NYHA class III	0.06	0.13	−0.07	
NYHA class IV	0.01	0.00	0.00	
Total years	2.88	2.81	0.07	(−0.07, 0.21)
Quality adjusted yrs.	1.94	1.87	0.07	(−0.02, 0.160)

*Due to different numbers of patients between treatment groups within the two trials, combined results were based on a weighted average of the treatment (37.1%) and prevention (62.9%) trial results.
†Statistically significant trend toward better NYHA classes with enalapril ($P < .01$).
Abbreviations: *SOLVD*, Studies of Left Ventricular Dysfunction; *CI*, confidence interval; *NYHA*, New York Heart Association.
(From Ref. 11.)

A. Lifetime Projection

For lifetime projections, a state transition model was used to estimate survival in each of the four NYHA classes and to assess quality-adjusted survival. Quality-adjusted survival was estimated based on the predicted survival time in each NYHA class weighted by the set of quality adjustment factors. Patients receiving enalapril were projected to live an average of 2.14 years longer than those randomized to receive placebo (95% CI: 0.05 to 4.21 years). In addition, this gain in life expectancy occurred mainly while patients were in a better health state (NYHA classes I and II). Unlike the period of observation during the trial, the beneficial impact of enalapril on survival was projected to be greater in the prevention trial (2.72 years) than in the treatment trial (1.15 years). As seen in the trial analysis for the combined group, patients receiving enalapril were projected to save an average of $1,456 during their lifetime (95% Cl; cost increase of $9,243 to cost reduction of $12,527 per patient). These savings accrued from patients enrolled in the treatment trial ($7,884 reduction per patient; 95% Cl: cost reduction of $16,180 to cost increase $622). In the prevention trial, patients receiving enalapril were projected to experience a net cost of $2,342 compared with placebo (95% Cl: cost reduction of $14,429 to cost increase of $18,397) corresponding to a cost per life year saved of $1,816 ($2,342/1.29).

The exact mechanism of the beneficial effect of ACE inhibitors in improving the clinical outcomes of patients with left systolic left ventricular dysfunction is not known. Converting enzyme inhibition results in a multitude of effects related to decreased production of angiotensin-II as well as increased bradykinin and prostaglandin effects. Lowering blood pressure may contribute to the benefit and this effect may be more pronounced in hypertensive patients.

VII. STRENGTHS AND WEAKNESSES OF THE ANALYSIS OF THE HYPERTENSIVE SUBSET OF SOLVD

This analysis suggests that the beneficial effects of enalapril in preventing mortal and morbid events demonstrated in SOLVD are also present and have similar magnitude in patients with hypertension and left ventricular dysfunction. Similar observations may be made in other clinical trials on patients with left ventricular dysfunction using ACE inhibitors. Although subset analysis in patients with a history of hypertension was not presented, 43% of the patients who participated in the Survival and Ventricular Enlargement Trial (SAVE) had a history of hypertension, and in the Acute Infarction Ramipril Efficacy (AIRE) study, a benefit of ACE inhibition was present in 28% of patients who had a history of hypertension requiring therapy (12,13). In these trials, as well in SOLVD, ACE inhibitor therapy was not given for the treatment of hypertension, and doses were not a adjusted to achieve a predetermined blood pressure level. Also, SOLVD was not powered to detect differences between the normotensive and hypertensive subgroups.

Additional limitations of this study include the fact that it is a retrospective subset analysis rather than a prespecified analysis, that the assessment of economic outcomes was done after the end of the study, and that there is no comparison to another antihypertensive agent. Although open label use of ACE inhibitors was allowed in the trial, this was not incorporated into the economic analysis. In addition, it was assumed that the underlying processes related to hazards for death and hospitalization present during the trial (as measured in our survival analysis and equations predicting the hospitalization rate) would continue unchanged after discontinuation of the trial.

On the other hand, the additional blood pressure drop of approximately 6/4 mm Hg compared with placebo may have been an important contributor to the overall benefit of enalapril in SOLVD. In addition, the analysis presented here, combined with findings of SAVE and AIRE, implies that ACE inhibitors are effective in lowering the chance of mortal and morbid events in patients with hypertension and systolic left ventricular dysfunction. Because left ventricular dysfunction carries a worse prognosis than that of mild or moderate hypertension, treatment of the former condition should take priority when the two conditions coexist. The coexistence of hypertension with left ventricular dysfunction does not appear to limit the powerfully beneficial effects of ACE inhibitor therapy on clinical outcome.

VIII. IMPACT OF SOLVD

The impact of SOLVD, combined with the effect of similar trials with ACE inhibitors (CONSENSUS, SAVE, AIRE, TRACE), on clinical practice has been enormous. Although not all patients with left ventricular dysfunction who are candidates for ACE inhibition receive such therapy, the majority receive one of these agents (14,15). It appears that cardiologists are more likely to prescribe ACE inhibitors and to use a higher (more appropriate) dose than generalists (14). In addition, ACE inhibition has been incorporated in the AHCPR guidelines for heart failure (16). The JNC-VI has classified the presence of heart failure in hypertensive patients as an indication for the use of ACE inhibitors. This was at least in part based on SOLVD and supported by JNC-VI (17).

REFERENCES

1. The SOLVD Investigators. Studies of Left Ventricular Dysfunction (SOLVD)—Rationale, design and methods: two trials that evaluate the effect of enalapril in patients with reduced ejection fraction. Am J Cardiol 1990; 66:315–322.
2. The CONSENSUS Trial Study Group. Effects of enalapril on mortality in severe heart failure: results of the Cooperative North Scandinavian Enalapril Study (CONSENSUS). N Engl J Med 1987; 316:429–435.
3. Cohn JN, Archibald DG, Ziesche S, Franciosa JA, Harston WE, Tristani FE, Dunkman WB, Jacobs W, Francis GS, Flohr KH et al. Effect of vasodilator on mortality in chronic congestive heart failure. Results of a Veterans Administration Cooperative Study. N Engl J Med 1986; 314(24):1547–1552.
4. Kostis JB, Shelton BJ, Yusuf S, Weiss MB, Capone RJ, Pepine CJ, Gosselin G, Delahaye F, Probstfield JL, Cahill L, Dutton D. Tolerability of enalapril initiation by patients with left ventricular dysfunction: results of the medication challenge phase of Studies of Left Ventricular Dysfunction (SOLVD). Am Heart J 1994; 128(2):358–364.
5. The SOLVD Investigators. Effect of enalapril on survival in patients with reduced left ventricular ejection fractions and congestive heart failure. N Engl J Med 1991; 325:293–302.
6. The SOLVD Investigators. Effect of enalapril on mortality and the development of heart failure in asymptomatic patients with reduced left ventricular ejection fractions. N Engl J Med 1992; 327:685–691.
7. Yusuf S, Pepine W, Garces C, Pouleur H, Salem D, Kostis J, Benedict C, Rousseau M, Bourassa M, Pitt B. Effect of enalapril on myocardial infarction and unstable angina in patients with low ejection fractions. Lancet 1992; 340(8829):1173–1178.
8. Kostis JB, Shelton B, Gosselin G, Goulet C, Hood WB Jr, Kohn RM, Kubo SH, Schron E, Weiss MB, Willis PW III, Young JB, Probstfield J, for the SOLVD Investigators. Adverse effects of enalapril in the Studies of Left Ventricular Dysfunction (SOLVD). Am Heart J 1996; 131:350–355.
9. Kostis JB. The effect of enalapril on mortal and morbid events in patients with hypertension and left ventricular dysfunction. Am J Hypertens 1995; 8:909–914.
10. Kostis JB. Response to letters to the editor. Am J Hypertens 1996; 9(6):615–619.
11. Cook JR, Glick H, Gerth W, Kinosian B, Kostis JB. The cost and cardioprotective effects of enalapril in hypertensive patients with left ventricular dysfunction. Am J Hypertens 1998; 11(12):1433–1441.
12. Pfeffer MA, Braunwald E, Moye LA, et al. Effect of captopril on mortality and morbidity in patients with left ventricular dysfunction after myocardial infarction. N Engl J Med 1992; 327: 669–677.
13. The Acute Infarction Ramipril Efficacy (AIRE) Study Investigators: effect of ramipril on mor-

tality and morbidity of survivors of acute myocardial infarction with clinical evidence of heart failure. Lancet 1993; 342:821–828.
14. Stafford RS, Saglam D, Blumenthal D. National patterns of angiotensin-converting enzyme inhibitor use in congestive heart failure. Arch Intern Med 1997; 157(21):2460–2464.
15. Philbin EF, Andreaou C, Rocco TA, Lynch LJ, Baker SL. Patterns of angiotensin-converting enzyme inhibitor use in congestive heart failure in two community hospitals. Am J Cardiol 1996; 77(10):832–838.
16. Chodoff P, Bischof RO, Nash DB, Laine C. The AHCRP guidelines on heart failure: comparison of a family medicine and an internal medicine practice with the guidelines and an educational intervention to modify behavior. Clin Perform Qual Health Care 1996; 4(4):179–185.
17. Joint National Committee. The fifth report of the Joint National Committee on detection, evaluation, and treatment of high blood pressure (JNC V). Arch Intern Med 1993; 153:154–183.

18

Captopril in Type I Diabetic Nephropathy

EDMUND J. LEWIS

Rush-Presbyterian-St. Luke's Medical Center, Chicago, Illinois

Hypothesis. To determine whether the angiotensin II enzyme inhibitor, captopril, protects renal function in the patient with type I diabetes mellitus and overt nephropathy by an intrarenal mechanism that is independent of the systemic antihypertensive effect of this drug.

Primary Objectives.

1. To determine the time to doubling of the baseline serum creatinine to a value of at least 2 mg/dl
2. To determine the time to the combined endpoints of death, dialysis, or renal transplantation

Secondary Objectives. To determine the course of renal function as measured by:

1. Serum creatinine
2. Twenty-four hour creatinine clearance
3. Urine protein excretion

Study Design. The Collaborative Study Group trial of captopril in diabetic nephropathy was a randomized, double-blind, placebo-controlled trial of 409 subjects (age 18 to 49 years) with type I diabetes mellitus (Table 1) (1). Patients had to have had onset of diabetes mellitus before age 30 and a duration of diabetes of at least 7 years. To establish the diagnosis of diabetic nephropathy, patients were required to have a 24-hour urine protein excretion of 500 mg/day or higher and the presence of diabetic retinopathy. If patients did not have diabetic retinopathy, they were required to have proteinuria of 500 mg/day or higher and a renal biopsy diagnosis of diabetic nephropathy. The upper limit

Table 1 Captopril in Diabetic Nephropathy: Methods

Study design:	Randomized, double-blind, placebo-controlled
Study population:	409 patients with IDDM with onset before age 30 and ≥ 7 years' duration
Study entry:	24-hour urinary protein excretion ≥ 500 mg/24 h, creatinine < 2.5 mg/dl, and diabetic retinopathy or biopsy-proven nephropathy
Medication:	Captopril 25 mg tid or matching placebo + Conventional antihypertensive therapy as needed for blood pressure control (<140/90 mm Hg)
Patient follow-up:	1.8 to 4.8 years; median, 3 years

Abbreviation: *IDDM*, insulin-dependent diabetes mellitus.
Source: Ref. 1.

of baseline serum creatinine was 2.5 mg/dl (Table 1). Exclusion criteria included the assessment that either angiotensin-converting enzyme (ACE) inhibitor therapy or calcium channel blocker therapy was required for the patient's management. Calcium channel blocker use was prohibited during the trial (Table 2). Eligible patients were randomized to receive captopril, 25 mg three times a day, or matching placebo. In addition, antihypertensive medications other than ACE inhibitors or calcium channel blockers were required therapy in a stepped-care approach to both treatment groups using diuretics, beta-blockers, central alpha-adrenergic blockers, and peripheral vasodilators to control the blood pressure to 140 mm Hg or lower systolic and 90 mm Hg or lower diastolic pressure (Table 3). The patient who was above these blood pressure goals at any visit during the course of

Table 2 Captopril in Diabetic Nephropathy: Key Exclusion Criteria

Clinical requirement for ACE inhibitors or calcium channel blockers
Contraindications to captopril
Serum potassium ≥ 6.0 mEq/L
WBC < 2500/μL
Bilateral renal artery stenosis
Hypersensitivity reactions to captopril
Pregnancy or lactation

Abbreviation: *ACE*, angiotensin-converting enzyme.
Source: Ref. 1.

Table 3 Captopril in Diabetic Nephropathy: Goals of Blood Pressure Treatment

Seated DBP < 90 mm Hg
Seated SBP
<140 mm Hg
If baseline ≥ 150 mm Hg, decreases at least 10 mm Hg
Maximum SBP of 160 mm Hg
Patients had to achieve blood pressure goal to continue study medication

Abbreviations: *DBP*, diastolic blood pressure; *SBP*, systolic blood pressure.
Source: Ref. 1.

the study had to add other blood pressure medication to bring the values below these goals. The blood pressure of record was the seated office measurement. Patients were followed up for a minimum of 1.8 years.

Sample Size Determination. For purposes of sample size determination, we assumed that the proteinuric diabetics would be recruited at a uniform rate over a 2-year interval and that half the patients would receive captopril and half placebo. All patients would be followed up for an additional 2 years after the close of recruitment. Therefore, the average follow-up of these patients would be 3 years with a range of follow-up of 2 to 4 years. The outcome used for sample size determination would be the time to a 50% loss in glomerular filtration rate (GFR) from baseline as measured by doubling of baseline serum creatinine. This outcome was chosen because it was considered clinically relevant and it would be of sufficient sensitivity to detect a therapeutic effect. For sample size evaluation, some distributional assumptions were made. It was assumed that the time to a 50% loss in initial GFR would follow an exponential distribution with hazard rate λ. Therefore, the expected treatment-specific cumulative incidence of a 50% loss in initial GFR at time t would be $CI(t) = 1 - e^{-\lambda t}$ (2).

Little published data were available that described the cumulative proportion of proteinuric type I diabetic patients whose GFR would decline by 50% or more as a function of time. The investigators in this study, based on their clinical experience, had indicated that it was reasonable to expect that 50% of such patients would show at least a 50% loss in initial GFR within 2 years of follow-up. This assumption is also supported by data from Viberti, who showed that proteinuric diabetics with a median initial GFR of 60 ml/minute/1.73 m^2 had an average decline of 29.8 ml/minute/24 months (3). This constituted an average reduction in GFR of 50% in 2 years, which corresponded to an exponential hazard rate of $\lambda = 0.35$.

Sample size determination in a clinical trial requires the specification of a difference between the treatment groups considered to be of clinical interest. The clinical investigators in this study consider a one third or more reduction in the hazard rate for proteinuric diabetics treated with placebo ($\lambda_c = 0.35$) to be of clinical interest (i.e., $\lambda_e = 0.23$ for those treated with captopril). If the time to a 50% loss in initial GFR among captopril-treated proteinuric diabetics followed an exponential distribution with a hazard rate of $\lambda_e = 0.23$ or less, then the study sample size should have sufficient statistical power to detect this treatment difference $(\lambda_c - \lambda_e) = (0.35 - 0.23) = (1/3)\,(0.35) = 0.12$ (2).

The method of sample size determination for a test of a difference between treatment-specific exponential distributions for the case of a limited recruitment period and administrative censoring was based on the asymptotic normality of the maximum likelihood estimator of λ as described by Lachin (4). This method had been shown to approximate the power function of the distribution free log-rank test for the difference between two survival distributions. The total sample size required to assure 90% power (1-β) of detecting a difference in hazard rates of $\lambda_c - \lambda_e = 0.12$ or more was calculated to be $n = 351$. The total sample size of $n = 351$ was based on a level of significance of 5% (α, one-tailed) with equal-sized treatment groups (4).

The total sample size of 351 was based on the assumption of no losses to follow-up. The sample size was extended to allow for losses to follow-up (1). In this study, it was believed unlikely that the losses to follow-up in both groups combined would exceed 15%. Therefore, an adjusted total sample size of $n_L = 400$ in the presence of 15% losses to follow-up was approximately equivalent to an effective sample size of $n = 350$ with no losses to follow-up. It was decided that the total sample size objective would be 400

Table 4 Captopril in Diabetic Nephropathy: Selected Baseline Characteristics*

Characteristic	Placebo (n = 202)	Captopril (n = 207)
Age (yr)	34 ± 8	35 ± 7
Male (%)	54	52
Race: white (%)	87	91
black (%)	10	5
Duration of diabetes (yr)	22 ± 7	22 ± 7
Hypertensive (%)	76	75
Seated MAP (mm Hg)	104 ± 13	102 ± 12
Serum creatinine (mg/dl)	1.3 ± 0.4	1.3 ± 0.5
24-hour urinary protein excretion (g/day)	3 ± 2.6	2.5 ± 2.5†
24-hour creatinine clearance (ml/min)	79 ± 35	84 ± 46

*Plus-minus values are mean ± standard deviation.
†Statistically significant.
Abbreviation: *MAP*, mean arterial pressure.
Source: Ref. 1.

patients recruited at the rate of 200 per year over 2 years. Each patient would be followed up for at least 2 years resulting in an average follow-up of 3 years.

The actual power of the study to detect a difference in the treatment-specific hazard rates was based on a sample size of losses that a total sample size of 400 patients, in the presence of 15% losses to follow-up, afforded a high probability (power ≥ 85%) of detecting a one third or more reduction in the hazard rate for captopril-treated patients.

The study was conducted in 30 centers in the United States and Canada. Patient enrollment started in December 1987 and ended in September 1990. Patient follow-up was completed in September 1992.

Baseline characteristics were similar for patients randomized to captopril or placebo (Table 4) (1). The only significant difference was that patients assigned to placebo had a slightly higher 24-hour urine protein excretion than those assigned to captopril. The mean age for both groups was approximately 34 years, and a little over half the patients were male. Almost 90% of the patients were white. The patients had diabetes for an average of 22 years. Approximately 75% of the patients were hypertensive at the start of the study. The seated mean arterial pressure for all patients entered into the study was 102 to 104 mm Hg.

I. RESULTS

Doubling of Serum Creatinine. During the trial, 68 patients doubled their baseline serum creatinine, 25 (12%) in the captopril group and 43 (21%) in the placebo group (Fig. 1). Captopril significantly reduced the risk of doubling of serum creatinine by 51.1% ($P = 0.004$) compared with placebo. Using iothalamate clearances, the doubling of serum creatinine event was documented as an event indicating halving of the baseline GFR. In fact, the median decrease in iothalamate clearance at the time of a doubling of serum creatinine was −60%.

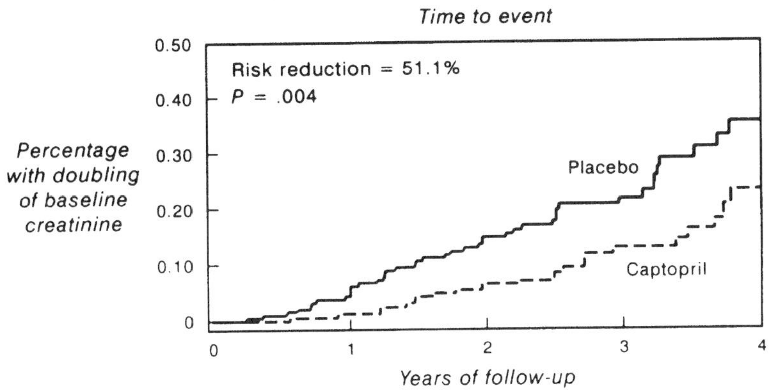

Fig. 1 Doubling of serum creatinine. (Data from Ref. 1.)

End-Stage Renal Disease or Death. At the end of the trial, 65 patients developed end-stage renal disease or died: 23 (11%) in the captopril group and 42 (21%) in the placebo group. Captopril significantly reduced the risk of death, dialysis, or renal transplantation by 50.5% ($P = 0.006$) compared with the placebo group (Fig. 2).

Blood Pressure Control During the Study. The magnitude of blood pressure lowering in the captopril and placebo groups was comparable throughout the study (Fig. 3). The median seated systolic blood pressure ranged from 128 to 134 mm Hg for the captopril group and from 129 to 136 mm Hg for the placebo group. At most quarterly follow-up intervals, the difference was no more than 2 mm Hg. The median seated diastolic pressure ranged from 77 to 82 mm Hg for the captopril group and from 80 to 84 mm Hg for the placebo group. At most quarterly follow-up visits, the difference was less than 4 mm Hg.

The mean ± (SD) arterial pressure, averaged over all follow-up visits, was 96 ± 8 mm Hg in the captopril group and 100 ± 8 mm Hg in the placebo group. Decrease in baseline mean arterial pressure in the 155 patients in the captopril group who had pre-

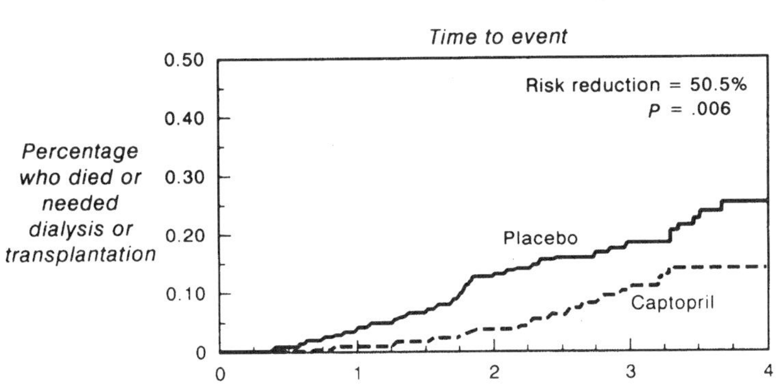

Fig. 2 End-stage renal disease (ESRD) or death. (Data from Ref. 1.)

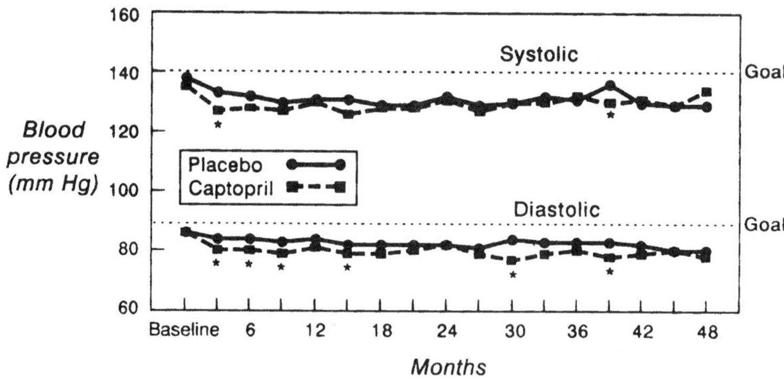

Fig. 3 Median seated systolic and diastolic blood pressures. $^*P < 0.05$, captopril vs placebo. (Data from Ref. 1.)

existing hypertension averaged 7 ± 11 mm Hg and it averaged 5 ± 11 mm Hg in the 153 patients with pre-existing hypertension in the placebo group. This difference in blood pressure control was not significant ($P = 0.16$). Among patients who were not hypertensive before entry into the trial (52 in the captopril group and 49 in the placebo group), the difference in the control of mean arterial pressure was more pronounced, averaging 5 mm Hg through the follow-up period ($P \leq 0.001$). Thus, the overall difference in blood pressure control between the two groups is explained by the antihypertensive effect of captopril as compared with placebo in patients defined as nonhypertensive. In fact, relatively few patients in this latter category reached study endpoints (Table 5). The significant results of the study were, in fact, determined by the results in those patients defined as hypertensive at the beginning of the study (Table 5). Blood pressure control was similar in the captopril and placebo groups for these hypertensive patients. Thus, when the effect of mean arterial blood pressure on doubling of serum creatinine, end-stage renal disease, or mortality were evaluated using a time-dependent analysis, the estimated risk reduction of doubling of serum creatinine associated with captopril therapy was not significantly altered by adjusting for mean arterial pressure (7) (Table 5). Similarly, the reduction of end-stage renal disease or mortality in the captopril group was not significantly changed. The beneficial effects of captopril could not be explained by the small differences in blood pressure control between the groups (Fig. 4).

Table 5 Effect of Baseline Blood Pressure on Time to Doubling of Baseline Serum Creatinine

	Number of Patients		
Baseline blood pressure	Captopril (n = 207)	Placebo (n = 202)	% Reduction in risk
Hypertensive	22/155	36/153	47.7*
Normotensive	3/52	7/49	58.2

*Statistically significant.
Source: Ref. 1.

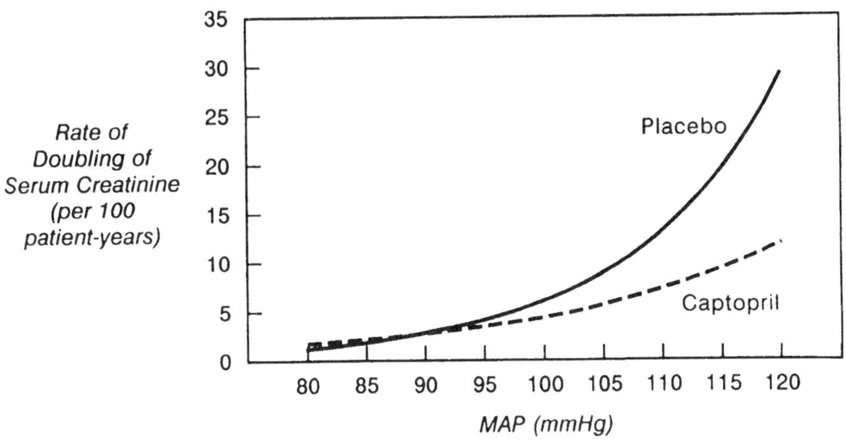

Fig. 4 Relationship between blood pressure and doubling of serum creatinine.

II. THE IMPACT OF BLOOD PRESSURE CONTROL ON OUTCOME

During the course of the study, many patients tended to have an increase in blood pressure above goal during the 3-month intervals between study visits. The patients were then required to receive more intensive antihypertensive therapy to be brought back to goal. In fact, only four patients had to leave the study because of an inability to reach blood pressure goal: one in the captopril group and three in the placebo group. Examination of the relationship between the highest blood pressure recorded during the study and the likelihood of doubling of serum creatinine was carried out using a gamma-Poisson analysis (Fig. 4). This analysis revealed that patients in the captopril group who experienced a rise of blood pressure during the study were nevertheless protected when compared with patients with a similar increase in blood pressure in the placebo group. At a mean arterial pressure of 120 mm Hg, patients in the placebo group were three times as likely to reach the doubling of serum creatinine endpoint compared with those in the captopril group. According to this analysis, patients whose blood pressure was well controlled below 95 mm Hg throughout the study had similar doubling of serum creatinine rates in both groups. This finding is most likely explained by the limited follow-up among these normotensive patients whose diabetic nephropathy was progressing slowly. A much longer follow-up period would have been required to demonstrate renal protection using doubling of serum creatinine as the endpoint criterion for these latter patients. Renal protection in this group using stabilization or diminution of proteinuria as the criterion for renal protection has been described in other studies (see below).

III. THE EFFECT OF BASELINE SERUM CREATININE ON RISK REDUCTION OF END-STAGE RENAL DISEASE OR MORTALITY

The effect of the initial serum creatinine on the risk reduction of the endpoints of doubling of serum creatinine, end-stage renal disease, or mortality was assessed over a wide range of baseline serum creatinine values. At a baseline serum creatinine of 2.25 mg/dl, the risk reduction for either doubling of serum creatinine or end-stage renal disease or mortality was diminished by 75% (Fig. 5). At lower serum creatinine levels, the risk reduction were

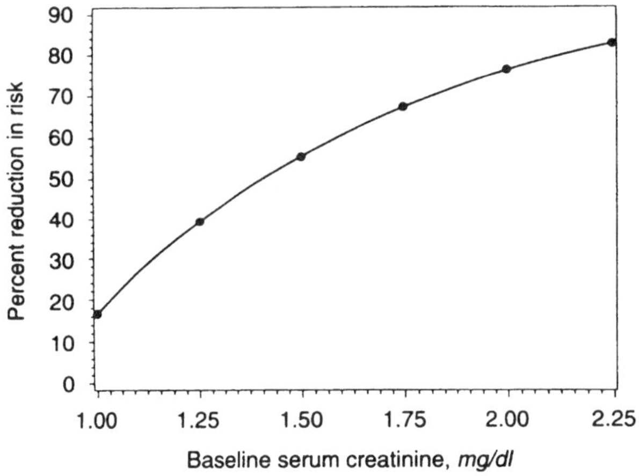

Fig. 5 Time to doubling of serum creatinine percent reduction in risk with captopril as a function of baseline serum creatinine.

proportionately lower. This did not indicate variation in the degree of renal protection relative to the degree of renal failure at baseline. Rather, it was an indicator of the fact that patients with higher baseline serum creatinine levels, and therefore lower baseline GFRs, had to lose fewer ml/min of GFR to reach the endpoints of either doubling of serum creatinine or end-stage renal disease. Obviously, a patient entering the study with a serum creatinine of 2.25 and a GFR of 40 ml/min would have to lose only 20 ml/min of GFR to double serum creatinine. On the other hand, a patient entering the study with a serum creatinine of 1.25 mg/dl and a GFR of 100 ml/min would have to lose 50 ml/min of GFR during the same 3-year period to double serum creatinine.

IV. THE EFFECT OF PRE-EXISTING HYPERTENSION ON TIME TO DOUBLING OF BASELINE SERUM CREATININE

The effect of pre-existing hypertension on doubling of baseline serum creatinine was assessed (Table 6). Captopril was associated with a 47.7% reduction in the risk of doubling

Table 6 Risk Reduction with Captopril: Adjustment for MAP During the Trial

	Doubling of serum creatinine	ESRD or all-cause mortality
Unadjusted		
Risk reduction	51.1%	50.5%
P value	.004	.006
Adjusted for MAP		
Risk reduction	43.3%	45.9%
P value	.025	.019

Abbreviations: *MAP*; mean arterial pressure; *ESRD*, end-stage renal disease.
Source: Ref. 1.

Table 7 Overall Percentage Use of Concomitant Antihypertensive Medications*

	Captopril (n = 207)	Placebo (n = 202)
Baseline	60%	58%
1 Year	58%	70%
2 Years	67%	77%
3 Years	67%	84%
4 Years	70%	92%

*Percentage of patients remaining in study at each time point.
Source: Ref. 1.

of serum creatinine in the hypertensive patients and a 58.2% reduction risk in the normotensive patient. Thus, the beneficial effect of captopril was independent of the prior existence of hypertension. However, it should be noted that there were 58 doubling of serum creatinine events in those with pre-existing hypertension (22 in the captopril group and 36 in the placebo group), compared with only 10 doubling of serum creatinine events in those who were defined as not having pre-existing hypertension (three in the captopril group and seven in the placebo group) (Table 5).

V. CONCOMITANT ANTIHYPERTENSIVE MEDICATIONS (TABLE 7)

At baseline, 58% of the patients in the placebo group and 60% of those in the captopril group were already receiving antihypertensive medication. Sixty-four percent of the hypertensive patients in the placebo group were receiving diuretic agents at baseline, and this value ranged from 79% to 93% during the study. By comparison, 62% of the hypertensive patients in the captopril group were receiving diuretics at baseline, and this value ranged from 74% to 87% during the study. At no quarterly interval was the difference between groups statistically significant except at month 24 ($P = 0.033$). Fifteen percent of the hypertensive patients in the placebo group were receiving beta-adrenergic antagonists at baseline and 34% to 46% were receiving them during the study, whereas 11% of the hypertensive patients in the captopril group were receiving these drugs at baseline and 15% to 53% were receiving them during the study. The difference between the groups was significant only during the first 12 months of the study. There was no significant difference in the use of other agents, including labetalol, clonidine, methyldopa, prazosin, hydralazine, guanabenz, terazosin, and minoxidil. Overall, little difference was found in the use of antihypertensive agents between the two groups of patients.

VI. THE EFFECT OF PROTEINURIA AT BASELINE ON DOUBLING OF SERUM CREATININE

As noted above (Table 1), there was a small imbalance in the baseline proteinuria between the two groups. The effect of this difference on the doubling of serum creatinine, end-stage renal disease or mortality, using a time-dependent analysis, revealed that the risk reduction for the primary endpoints was not significantly changed (Table 8).

Table 8 Risk Reduction with Captopril: Adjustment for Baseline Urinary Protein Excretion

	Doubling of serum creatinine	ESRD or all-cause mortality
Unadjusted		
Risk reduction	51.1%	50.5%
P value	.004	.006
Adjusted for proteinuria		
Risk reduction	46.8%	49.2%
P value	.016	.012

Abbreviation: *ESRD*, end-stage renal disease.
Source: Ref. 1.

VII. RATE OF INCREASE IN SERUM CREATININE

The effect of treatment on renal function, using serum creatinine as a measure, revealed a mean rate of increase in serum creatinine with an average follow-up period of 2.7 years per patient of 0.25 ± 0.76 (SD) mg/dl per year for the captopril-treated patients and 0.47 ± 0.85 mg/dl per year for placebo-treated patients ($P = 0.004$). This represents a 53% decrease in the rate of increase of serum creatinine in mg/dl/yr among those patients receiving captopril. With respect to the percent decline in creatinine clearance per year, patients in the captopril group had a decrease of 11 ± 21 ml/min/yr, compared with 17 ± 20 ml/min/yr ($P = 0.027$). This represents a 64% decrease in the decline in creatinine clearance per year among those patients receiving captopril. Therefore, the renal protective effects of captopril that have been reflected in the risk reduction of doubling of serum creatinine or end-stage renal disease or death in this time-to-event analysis study are not simply reflected among those patients who were losing renal function rapidly enough to reach the primary endpoints. The renal protective effects of captopril were seen in the entire patient population under study as reflected by the alteration in rate of change of renal function using creatinine parameters.

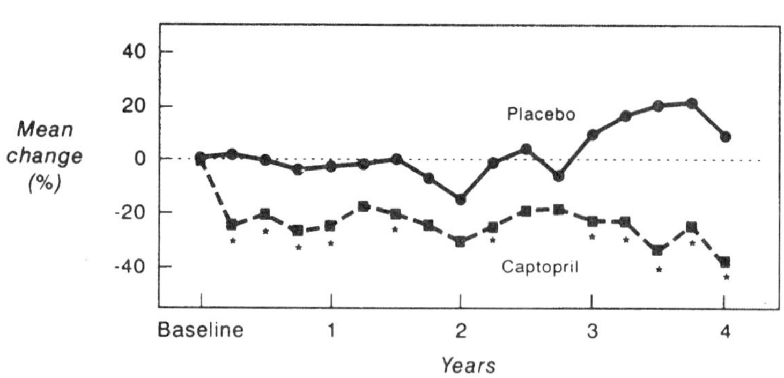

Fig. 6 Percentage change from baseline in urinary protein excretion in patients who did not reach the stop point—geometric mean change in percent. *$P \leq 0.05$, captopril vs placebo. (Data from Ref. 1.)

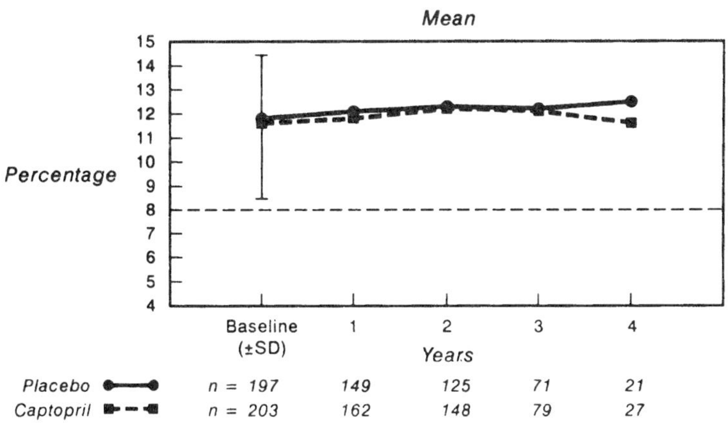

Fig. 7 Total glycosylated hemoglobin—approximately one third higher than HbA_{IC}. (Data from Ref. 1.)

VIII. PERCENT CHANGE FROM BASELINE AND URINE PROTEIN EXCRETION

Measurement of the median 24-hour urine protein excretion revealed that urine protein was decreased in the captopril-treated group by the 3-month visit. The decrease from baseline in the captopril-treated group was significantly greater than the change from baseline in the placebo-treated patients at all succeeding time points (Fig. 6).

IX. GLUCOSE CONTROL AND DIET

Total glycosylated hemoglobin levels were equal in the two groups throughout the trial. Dietary protein intake calculated from urine urea excretion was also equal in the two groups (Figs. 7 and 8).

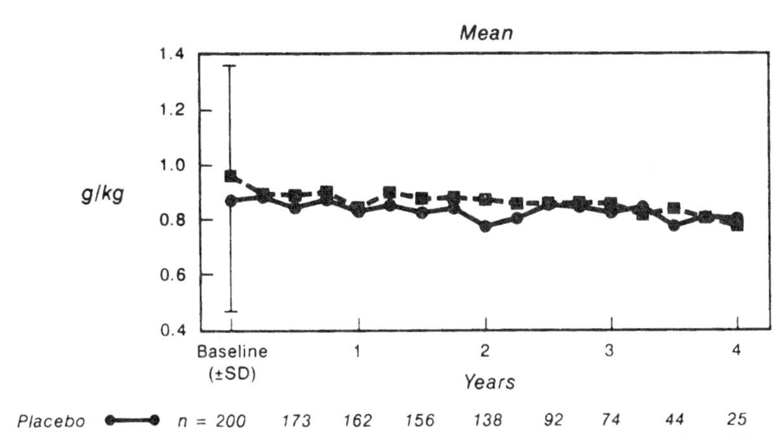

Fig. 8 Estimated dietary protein intake. (Data from Ref. 1.)

Table 9 "Captopril-Specific" Side Effects Leading to Discontinuation of Study Medication

Event	Captopril (n = 207)	Placebo (n = 202)
Hyperkalemia*	6 (2.9%)	0
Dizziness	5 (2.4%)	2 (1.0%)
Hypotension	3 (1.4%)	1 (0.5%)
Orthostatic hypotension	3 (1.4%)	0
Taste disturbance	2 (1.0%)	1 (0.5%)
Neutropenia	1 (0.5%)	2 (1.0%)
Cough	1 (0.5%)	0
Rash	1 (0.5%)	0

*P = .03.
Source: Ref. 1.

X. ADVERSE EVENTS

At the time of the last study visit, 84% (128/153) of the surviving captopril-treated patients who had not reached primary endpoints were still taking the coded medication compared with 91% (110/121) patients who were taking coded medication in the placebo group. Few adverse events were reported in either the placebo- or captopril-treated groups (Table 9). There were no significant differences between the groups in adverse effects or intercurrent illness. As would be expected with an ACE inhibitor, some episodes of hyperkalemia occurred. Hyperkalemia, defined as a serum potassium level above 6 mEq/L was recorded in only six patients (2.9%). This unexpectedly low event rate for hyperkalemia may be explained by the extensive use of diuretics during the study. None of the 207 patients treated with captopril developed acute renal failure.

XI. DISCUSSION

In conclusion, this study revealed that the long-term administration of the angiotensin II converting enzyme inhibitor, captopril, to patients with type I diabetes mellitus with nephropathy: (1) significantly reduced the progression of renal disease; (2) significantly reduced the need for dialysis or renal transplantation and improved survival; and (3) provided a renal protective benefit that was independent of the systemic antihypertensive effects of this drug, as the dramatic differences achieving the endpoints could not be explained by blood pressure control alone. These results were obtained in the context of a highly acceptable safety profile during the course of the study. As a result of this study, the Food and Drug Administration approved this drug as renoprotective in patients with overt type I diabetic nephropathy, declaring this to be a new specific indication that was independent of the use of the drug as an antihypertensive agent. Captopril remains the only drug approved by the Food and Drug Administration as "renoprotective." However, this therapeutic effect appears to be applicable to the class of ACE inhibitors as a whole and not to the specific agent itself. The renoprotective benefit of captopril during this trial was demonstrated in the primary time-to-event analyses (Figs. 1, 2). The secondary analyses relative to the effect of the agent on the rate of change of creatinine parameters

Table 10 Captopril in Diabetic Nephropathy: Sequential Measurements of Renal Function

	Captopril	Placebo	*P*-value
Mean rate of increase in serum creatinine (mg/dl/year)	0.2 ± 0.8	0.5 ± 0.8	$P = .004$
Mean % decline in creatinine clearance/year	11 ± 21	17 ± 20	$P = .03$

Source: Ref. 1.

(Table 10), and the gamma-Poisson analysis (Fig. 4) also revealed captopril to be renoprotective, even among patients who had episodes of elevated blood pressure during the study.

The rationale for carrying out this study was based on a body of evidence derived from studies of the pathogenesis of glomerular injury in experimental animals rendered diabetic (5–7). Angiotensin II converting enzyme inhibition prevented the progressive glomerular damage that occurs in animals with experimental diabetes mellitus to develop proteinuria and glomerulosclerosis. In addition, several small clinical studies had been undertaken, the results of which supported the notion that therapy with an angiotensin II converting enzyme inhibitor preserved renal function, particularly with respect to a decrease in the amount of proteinuria among treated patients (8–11). These previous studies, all done in smaller cohorts of patients, either examined different endpoints such as decreased proteinuria or microalbuminuria and were confounded by significantly lower mean arterial pressures in the ACE inhibitor-treated groups. Marre et al. (12) reported the benefit of ACE inhibition in normotensive patients, but their study was limited by a small sample size and a significant decrease in mean arterial pressure in the group receiving ACE inhibitors. Kasiske et al. (13) demonstrated by meta-analysis that ACE inhibition was more likely to diminish proteinuria in patients with diabetic nephropathy than were other antihypertensive agents, thus implying a direct renal protection by these agents. However, this was the first study of a large cohort of patients in which the beneficial effects of captopril on preserving renal function were shown to be independent of the effect of lowering the systemic blood pressure. The confirmation that the renoprotective effect of ACE inhibition was independent of the blood pressure-lowering mechanism was crucial, as it had been well documented that blood pressure control by itself could slow the rate of loss of renal function in diabetic nephropathy (14–18).

The path from basic scientific and experimental animal observations to the demonstration of a clinical therapeutic effect is rarely a straight line from point A to point B. More often there are an interrupted series of meandering steps that can involve chance, unexpected insightful observations, the practical application of established scientific evidence, the heroic development of a novel new hypothesis, and the successful testing of a hypothesis in animals under rigidly controlled experimental circumstances, all of which may come together and provide a rationale for further scientific evaluation in a controlled clinical therapeutic trial. The earliest observations that ultimately led to the development of ACE inhibitors and their application to human disease began in research laboratories where investigators pursued studies that they could not have believed would ultimately have a dramatic impact in the field of diabetic nephropathy. One must first consider the beginnings of the development of the first ACE inhibitor. This concept originated with the study of a component of the venom of the Brazilian pit viper, *Bothrops jararaca*, which was responsible for the painful and hypotensive sequelae of snake bite (19). The study of the factor in the snake venom that might cause a lowering of blood pressure ultimately led to the isolation of teprotide, a substance inhibitory to the kininase II family of enzymes, which includes the angiotensin II converting enzyme. Teprotide is a nonapeptide. Ondetti and Cushman (20) created three-dimensional models of the enzyme, which led them to an understanding of the likely complementary three-dimensional structure of the receptor site that was believed to exist on the angiotensin II converting enzyme. What followed was a brilliant approach to the development of a small molecule believed to be capable of reacting with the active site of the enzyme and serving as a competitive inhibitor to angiotensin II. The substituted proline compound designed by these chemists turned out to be captopril.

The study of the hemodynamic mechanism that could account for the progressive nature of glomerular injury suffered by rodents who had experienced no direct glomerular insult but had been subjected to renal ablation surgery, ultimately led Brenner and his colleagues (5–7) to apply their understandings of glomerular hemodynamics to the treatment of the glomerular alterations in the experimental diabetic state. These investigators developed techniques that allowed them to directly measure intraluminal pressure within the afferent and efferent arterioles of the renal glomerulus, as well as the glomerular capillary loops. As a result of these studies, it was noted that the diabetic state is associated with an increase in the intraluminal pressure of glomerular capillaries, which could be accounted for on the basis of an increase in the tone of the efferent artery draining the renal glomerulus, thus causing increased resistance to the drainage of blood from this capillary structure (Fig. 9). The increased efferent arterial tone appeared to be under the control of the renin-angiotensin system and blockade of the constrictive effects of angiotensin II relieved the efferent arteriolar vasoconstriction of the diabetic state and diminished glomerular capillary pressure. The hypothesis was generated that glomerular injury in the diabetic state could be explained by barotrauma caused by increased intracapillary pressure. The use of angiotensin II converting enzyme inhibition was shown to diminish glomerular capillary pressures and glomerular capillary injury in the experimental diabetic state in the rat. These seminal experiments and the application of this physiological information to the understanding of the potential treatment of diabetic nephropathy provided a remarkable model for the understanding of the nature of glomerular injury in type I diabetes mellitus and served as the rationale for the clinical trial. Of course, there was no certainty that the results obtained in diabetic rats would be duplicated in patients with

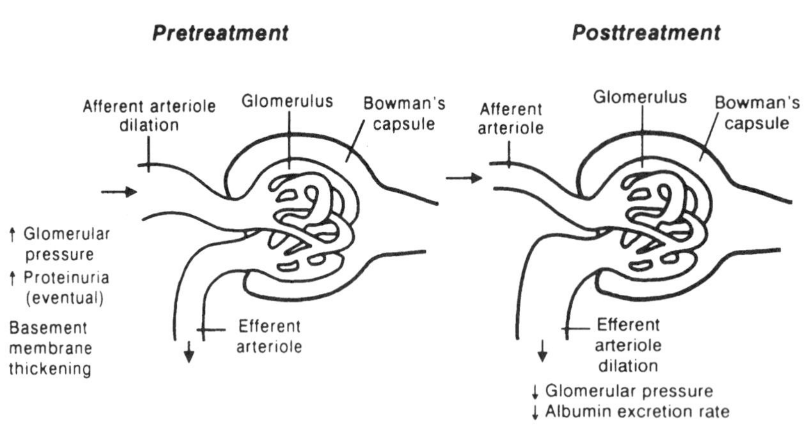

Fig. 9 Intrarenal effects of angiotensin-converting enzyme inhibitors—rat model of diabetes. (From Ref. 7.)

diabetic nephropathy. In a similar situation, an equally strong rationale for the use of low-protein diets in patients with chronic renal disease was based on strong evidence that low-protein diets had a beneficial effect on the abnormal hemodynamics that developed in animals with progressive renal disease (21). Small clinical trials indicated a beneficial impact of a low-protein diet in some patients (22–24). Unfortunately, the proposed beneficial effects were not confirmed in a large clinical trial (25). The latter experience underscores the importance of valid clinical trials, even in situations where a well-reasoned hypothesis and strong experimental animal results are convincing.

Results of this trial support the proposal that angiotensin II converting enzyme inhibition can beneficially influence the altered glomerular hemodynamics in patients with diabetes, thus achieving renal protection. Although the removal of the tonic constrictor effect of angiotensin II on efferent arterioles, hence lowering glomerular intracapillary pressure, would explain the reason why the administration of captopril dramatically preserves renal function, there are other possible explanations for the beneficial intrarenal actions of this agent. It is conceivable that ACE inhibitors may interfere with trophic properties of angiotensin II that promote cellular and glomerular hypertrophy or diminish the accumulation of mesangial matrix (26). Angiotensin II is capable of stimulating release of the cytokine transforming growth factor (TGF)-beta that can stimulate the production of connective tissue elements (27–31). Angiotensin-converting enzyme inhibition might therefore interfere with this scarring process. In addition, ACE inhibitors are known to decrease urine protein excretion in patients with diabetes and other glomerulopathies, as has been demonstrated in this and other studies (1, 32). This decrease in proteinuria may itself be associated with a decrease in the rate of progression of kidney damage. The transit of large amounts of filtered protein may be toxic to both glomerular and tubulointerstitial structures (32–34). Thus the possibility cannot be ruled out that amelioration of proteinuria might be pathogenetically relevant in the captopril-treated patients in our study.

It is well recognized that many advances in clinical management of chronic diseases actually result in an increased cost to the health care system. This is because the amount of money spent for health care in most long-term situations is directly proportional to the lifespan of the patient. The effect of captopril therapy in patients with diabetic nephropathy is an unusual example of a therapeutic success leading to a projected decrease in the overall expenditure of health care dollars for this patient population (35). The reason for this optimistic cost-effective projection resides in the fact that patients with overt diabetic nephropathy who receive captopril and have careful blood pressure control have a significant extension of life without the requirement of dialysis or transplantation when compared with patients who have blood pressure control alone. This therapy therefore significantly defers the substantial health care costs of the end-stage renal disease program, which currently costs about $50,000 per year for each patient requiring dialysis. In addition, many patients can have their life expectancy extended to the point where mortality, usually from cardiovascular causes, occurs before there is ever a need for renal replacement therapy. Hence, in those patients, the cost of dialysis and transplantation is avoided entirely. In more recent studies, we have demonstrated that careful blood pressure control to a mean arterial pressure of 100 mm Hg or less using ACE inhibition may be associated with stabilization and even regression of nephropathy in the type I diabetic patient (36). A formal economic analysis performed by the Arthur D. Little Corporation revealed that the captopril study had the potential of an aggregate health care cost savings of $475,000,000 per year within 10 years of the publication of the study and a cumulative health care savings cost of $2.4 billion over this 10-year period. Even if these predictions are optimistic, there is little doubt that captopril can prolong life and save money in patients with type I diabetic nephropathy because of its remarkable positive therapeutic effects and because the alternative outcome of end-stage renal disease is so expensive. Although one may quibble about the total amount of money that will be saved in a finite period, it is clear that the savings gained by avoiding even 1 year of dialysis in a single patient will buy more than a lifetime supply of captopril.

To summarize, the remarkable risk reductions with respect to renal endpoints exhibited during the course of this study and attributable to captopril changed the standard of care for patients with type I diabetic nephropathy. The purpose of the study was to determine whether captopril was renoprotective, which required equal blood pressure control in the captopril and placebo groups. We were able to conclude that renoprotection was indeed an independent effect of therapy with this agent.

A few comments might be in order with respect to the way things might have been done, knowing what we know now. Clearly, the claim of renoprotection required equal control of the blood pressure in both groups. A difference in blood pressure control could always raise the question of whether the known beneficial effects of blood pressure lowering in diabetic nephropathy could explain the results. Although the actual difference in mean arterial pressure between the two groups was small throughout the trial, the inclusion of patients who were normotensive at the beginning of the trial confused some observers. As expected, captopril lowered the blood pressure in these normotensive patients, whereas placebo did not. In retrospect, if patients with type I diabetic nephropathy who were normotensive had been excluded from the trial, no significant difference would have occurred in systemic arterial pressure between the two groups and some confusion could have been avoided. Further, if the entry criteria for the study had required some elevation of the baseline serum creatinine, those with a relatively high entry GFR would have been excluded. As these patients were unlikely to halve their GFR during the 3-year mean follow-up of the trial, they could not contribute to the results in a time-to-event analysis. That having been said, it must be noted that these comments are made in retrospect; each limitation in the entry criteria for a clinical trial narrows the window for attainment of the required sample size. An ideal clinical protocol may end up being too restrictive to allow the successful recruitment of the required sample size and the proper conduct of a clinical trial. Fortunately, the time-to-event analysis used in this study and the dramatic effect of the therapeutic agent negated any possible weakness that might have been accounted for by the inclusion of patients who had less severe renal disease.

A final point should be made regarding the primary event chosen for our analysis. As previously noted, at the time of the design of this study, very little information in the literature addressed the rate of loss of renal function to be expected in a large population of patients with type I diabetic nephropathy. It was decided that during the course of an average follow-up of 3 years that halving of the initial GFR would be a significant event. Within the range of serum creatinine that was anticipated in the entry criteria for the study, it was reasoned that a halving of the GFR would cause a doubling of the baseline serum creatinine. The use of the serum creatinine as an endpoint in the study, rather than the determination of serial GFR determinations significantly decreased the cost of the study, always a consideration in clinical trials. In addition, the ease of obtaining a blood sample for creatinine allowed us to collect more observational points during the course of the study than would the cumbersome clearance technique. The reasoning regarding the accuracy of doubling of serum creatinine as an endpoint was supported by the finding that both creatinine clearance and iothalamate clearance decreased by approximately 60% at the time the event was recorded. The median time from the recording of a doubling of serum creatinine to end-stage renal disease, defined as the initiation of dialysis therapy or the attainment of a serum creatinine of 6 mg/dl or more was 9.3 months. This short interval between doubling of serum creatinine and end-stage renal disease accounts for the similar results in the two time-to-event analyses used in this study. In many respects, our introduction of the use of "doubling of the serum creatinine" as an endpoint has become a current standard for large clinical trials in the field of nephrology. It is an example of how a simple and inexpensive, although accurate and reproducible, method can become preferred technology in this complex world.

REFERENCES

1. Lewis EJ, Hunsicker LG, Bain RP, Rohde RD, for the Collaborative Study Group. A clinical trial of an angiotensin converting enzyme inhibitor in the nephropathy of insulin-dependent diabetes mellitus. N Engl J Med 1993; 329(20):1456–1462.
2. Bain R, Rohde R, Hunsicker LG, McGill J, Kobrin S, Lewis EJ, for the Collaborative Study Group. A controlled clinical trial of angiotensin-converting enzyme inhibition in type I diabetic nephropathy: Study design and patient characteristics. J Am Soc Nephrol 1992; 3(1):S97–S103.
3. Viberti GC, Bilous RW, Mackintosh D, Keen H. Monitoring glomerular function in diabetic nephropathy: a prospective study. Am J Med 1983; 74:256–264.
4. Lachin JM. Introduction to sample size determination and power analysis for clinical trials. Controlled Clin Trials 1981; 2:93–113.
5. Zatz R, Meyer TW, Rennke HG, Brenner BW. Predominance of hemodynamic rather than metabolic factors in the pathogenesis of diabetic glomerulopathy. Proc Natl Acad Sci U S A 1985; 82:5963–5967.
6. Zatz R, Dunn BR, Meyer TW, Anderson S, Rennke HG, Brenner BM. Prevention of diabetic glomerulopathy by pharmacologic amelioration of glomerular capillary hypertension. J Clin Invest 1986; 77:1925–1930.
7. Anderson S, Rennke HG, Garcia DL, Brenner BM. Short and long term effects of antihypertensive therapy in the diabetic rat. Kidney Int 1989; 36:526–536.
8. Björck S, Nyberg G, Mulec H, Granerus G, Herlitz H, Aurell M. Beneficial effects of angiotensin converting enzyme inhibition of renal function in patients with diabetic nephropathy. BMJ 1986; 293:471–474.
9. Hommel E, Parving H-H, Mathiesen E, Edsberg B, Damkjaer Nielsen M, Giese J. Effect of captopril on kidney function in insulin-dependent diabetic patients with nephropathy. BMJ 1986; 293:467–470.
10. Björck S, Mulec H, Johnsen SA, Nyberg G, Aurell M. Contrasting effects of enalapril and metoprolol on proteinuria in diabetic nephropathy. BMJ 1990; 300:904–907.
11. Parving H-H, Hommel E, Smidt UM. Protection of kidney function and decrease in albuminuria by captopril in insulin dependent diabetics with nephropathy. BMJ 1988; 297:1086–1091.
12. Marre M, Leblanc H, Suarez L, Guyanne TT, Menard J, Passa P. Converting enzyme inhibition and kidney function in normotensive diabetic patients with persistent microalbuminuria. BMJ 1987; 294:1448–1542.
13. Kasiske BL, Kalil RSN, Ma JZ, Liao M, Keane WF. Effect of antihypertensive therapy on the kidney in patients with diabetes: a meta-regression analysis. Ann Intern Med 1993; 118: 129–138.
14. Mogensen CE. Progression of nephropathy in long-term diabetics with proteinuria and effect of initial anti-hypertensive treatment. Scand J Clin Lab Invest 1976; 36:383–388.
15. Christlieb AB, Warram JH, Krolewski AS, Busick EJ, Ganda OP, Asmol AC, Soeldner S, Bradley RF. Hypertension: the major risk factor in juvenile-onset insulin dependent diabetics. Diabetes 1981; 30(suppl 2):90–96.

16. Mogensen CE. Long-term antihypertensive treatment inhibiting progression of diabetic nephropathy. BMJ 1982; 285:685–688.
17. Parving H-H, Andersen AR, Smidt UM, Svendsen PA. Early aggressive antihypertensive treatment reduces rate of decline in kidney function in diabetic nephropathy. Lancet 1983; i:1175–1179.
18. Parving H-H, Andersen AR, Hommel E, Smidt U. Effects of long-term antihypertensive treatment on kidney function in diabetic nephropathy. Hypertension 1985; 7:suppl II:II-114–II-117.
19. Ondetti MA, Rubin B, Cushman DW. Design of specific inhibition of angiotensin converting enzyme: new class of orally active antihypertensive agents. Science 1977; 196:441–444.
20. Ondetti MA, Williams NJ, Sabo EF, Cheung HS, Cushman DW. Angiotensin converting enzyme inhibitors from the venom of *Bothrops jaracaca*; isolation, elucidation of structure and synthesis. Biochemistry 1971; 10:3033–3039.
21. Brenner BM, Meyer TW, Hostetter TH. Dietary protein intake and the progressive nature of kidney disease: the role of hemodynamically-mediated glomerular injury in the pathogenesis of progressive glomerular sclerosis in aging, renal ablation and intrinsic renal disease. N Engl J Med 1982; 307:652–659.
22. Mitch WE. The influence of the diet on the progression of renal insufficiency. Ann Rev Med 1984; 35:249–264.
23. Walser M. Ketoacids in the treatment of uremia. Clin Nephrol 1975; 3:180–186.
24. Walser M. Progression of chronic renal failure in man. Kidney Int 1990; 37:1195–1210.
25. Klahr S, Levey AS, Beck GJ, Caggiula AW, Hunsicker L, Kusek JW, Striker G, for the Modification of Diet in Renal Disease Study Group. The effects of dietary protein restriction and blood-pressure control on the progression of chronic renal disease. Modification of Diet in Renal Disease Study Group. N Engl J Med 1994; 330:877–884.
26. Berk BC, Vekshtein V, Gordon HM, Tsuda T. Angiotensin II-stimulated protein synthesis in cultured vascular smooth muscle cells. Hypertension 1989; 13:305–314.
27. Ziyadeh FN. The extracellular matrix in diabetic nephropathy. Am J Kidney Dis 1993; 22: 736–744.
28. Yamamoto T, Nakamura T, Noble NA, Ruoslahti E, Border WA. Expression of transforming growth factor β is elevated in human and experimental diabetic nephropathy. Proc Natl Acad Sci U S A 1993; 90:1814–1818.
29. Sharma K, Guo I, Jin Y, Ericksen M, Ziyadeh FN. Anti-TGF-β antibody attenuates renal hypertrophy and matrix expansion in diabetic mice. J Am Soc Nephrol 1994; 5:972–978.
30. van Det NF, Tamsma JT, van den Born J, Berden JHM, Daha MR, Löwik CWGM, van der Woude FJ, Verhagen NAM. Differential effects of angiotensin II and transforming growth factor β on the production of heparin sulfate proteoglycan by mesangial cells in vitro. J Am Soc Nephrol 1996; 7:1015–1023.
31. Wolf G, Ziyadeh FN. The role of angiotensin II in diabetic nephropathy: emphasis on nonhemodynamic mechanisms. Am J Kidney Dis 1997; 29:153–163.
32. Gruppo Italiano di Studi Epidemiologici in Nefrologia (GISEN). Randomized placebo-controlled trial of effect of ramipril in decline in glomerular filtration rate and risk of terminal renal failure in proteinuric non-diabetic nephropathy. Lancet 1997; 349:1847–1863.
33. Remuzzi A, Puntorieri S, Battaglia C, Bertani T, Remuzzi G. Angiotensin converting enzyme inhibition ameliorates glomerular filtration of macromolecules and water and lessens glomerular injury in the rat. J Clin Invest 1990; 85:541–549.
34. Ruggenenti P, Remuzzi G. The renoprotective action of angiotensin-converting enzyme inhibitors in diabetes. Exp Nephrol 1996; 4(supp 1):53–60.
35. Rodby RA, Firth LM, Lewis EJ, and the Collaborative Study Group. An economic analysis of captopril in the treatment of diabetic nephropathy. Diabetes Care 1996; 19:1051–1060.
36. Lewis JB, Berl T, Bain RP, Lewis EJ, and the Collaborative Study Group. Effect of intensive blood pressure control on the course of type 1 diabetic nephropathy. Am J Kidney Dis 1999; 34:809–817.

19

Attenuation of Ventricular Enlargement: The SAVE Study

LEMUEL A. MOYÉ and MARC A. PFEFFER

University of Texas School of Public Health, Houston, Texas

I. INTRODUCTION

The development of ACE inhibitor therapy for use in the post-myocardial infarction (MI) setting ranks among the primary contributions to cardiovascular medicine in the 1990s. This treatment for post-myocardial ventricular enlargement developed from both the early observations of the natural history of postinfarction clinical outcomes and the painstaking evaluation of treatment to ameliorate left ventricular (LV) dysfunction.

Before the theoretical benefit of angiotensin-converting enzyme (ACE) therapy in the postinfarction setting could become reality, the demands of a skeptical medical community had to be satisfied. The standards by which new medical interventions are judged have consistently risen. By the 1980s, cardiologists and regulatory agencies required a demonstration of safety and efficacy through disciplined research methods strong enough to satisfy epidemiological causality tenets while broad enough to include major demographic subgroups and important comorbidity subsets. The mechanism of ACE inhibitor action had to be clear, and the therapy benefits had to be consistent within a spectrum of endpoints tightly linked to the natural history of left ventricular dysfunction. The only research methodology available to satisfactorily address these issues was a prospectively designed, double-blind, placebo-controlled clinical trial.

However, the design and execution of such a study promised to be complicated and difficult. Well-defined exclusion criteria designed to provide the clearest view of therapy benefit could potentially obstruct successful patient identification for the trial. In addition, the availability of new medications to extend survival in the postinfarction setting would continue to exert downward pressure on clinical event rates, jeopardizing any ability to detect meaningful event rate differences attributable to ACE inhibitor therapy.

The Survival and Ventricular Enlargement (SAVE) trial was the original study designed to address the impact of ACE inhibitor therapy on survival in patients with LV dysfunction post-MI. Echocardiographic data were prospectively incorporated into the study to further test whether the mechanism by which captopril produced improved survival was through an attenuation of LV remodeling.

II. BACKGROUND AND PATHOPHYSIOLOGY OF HEART FAILURE

The survivors of MI are at increased risk for subsequent cardiovascular events, heart failure, recurrent MI, and death. This risk is a complex function of the severity of myocardial dysfunction, the severity of underlying coronary artery disease, the arrhythmia profile, the presence of concomitant disease, and age. The degree of LV dysfunction is often assessed by global ejection fraction, which is perhaps the most important determinant of risk factor stratifications. All of these factors interact as determinants of clinical outcomes following MI (1–3).

Postinfarction LV enlargement has been the subject of study for 2 decades. The process of ventricular enlargement can be detected in the early phases after MI (by the echocardiogram) as infarct expansion, a process characterized by elongation and thinning of the infarct-containing ventricular segment (4,5). Patients manifesting this process are at a greater risk for the development of aneurysms, heart failure, and fatal events. However, patients demonstrating early infarct expansion are also at risk for progressive and global ventricular enlargement (6,7). Early animal and preliminary clinical studies demonstrated that the ventricular dilation that occurs after MI was related to the extent of myocardial damage (8), and that this enlargement, once present, would continue the destructive cycle of progressive dilation, leading to further increases in systolic and diastolic wall stress, which in turn provides an environment for LV enlargement and dysfunction (9).

This pathophysiological construct provided the basis for the initial animal studies in which the ACE inhibitor, captopril, was administered to rats after experimental infarctions. This research program demonstrated the attenuation of this progressive increase in ventricular chamber size. When continued for up to 1 year, ACE inhibition both diminished the tendency to LV enlargement and prolonged the survival of animals with experimental infarction (10). It was shown that this reduction in LV volume enlargement was a consequence of both reduced filling pressure (distension) and actual structural remodeling. These initial studies confirmed that, for comparable degrees of histologically determined infarct size, this chronic administration of an ACE inhibitor was associated with smaller ventricular volumes and improved survival in the animal model.

Applicability of these animal studies to patients was supported by small mechanistic experiments specifically designed to determine if ACE inhibitor therapy in patients would favorably alter the process of ventricular enlargement following MI (11,12). However, because the specific endpoint of each of these trials was ventricular size, these trials were not designed with sufficient statistical power to identify this potential effect on clinical events. Given the importance of ventricular enlargement and function on overall prognosis after MI, a hypothesis that ACE inhibition therapy would be effective in improving survival, reducing LV dysfunction, and reducing cardiovascular morbidity in myocardial infarct survivors with LV dysfunction was constructed.

III. DESIGN OF SAVE

The SAVE trial was designed to (a) determine whether the use of an ACE inhibitor could favorably alter clinical outcomes in patients with LV dysfunction, and to (b) establish the mechanistic support for the concept of using an ACE inhibitor to prevent further deterioration in ventricular performance.

A. The Role of Randomization in Clinical Trials, and Its Implementation in SAVE

Randomization is the hallmark of modern experiments. An adaptation that appeared in the 20th century, it has had a major impact on the development of clinical research programs. When nonexperimentalists speak of random events, they often mean events that occur in chaos, without order, or predictability. On the contrary, random mechanisms in clinical experiments are carefully considered and methodically implemented. Generally, in clinical trials, there are two levels of randomization. The first is the random selection of subjects from the population, and the second is the random allocation of the experimental intervention. Each of these two levels of randomization has a different goal and follows a different procedure. In general, clinical experiments must incorporate both levels of randomization.

1. Random Selection of the Population at Large

In SAVE, the ability to generalize conclusions from those patients chosen in the sample to the larger population of patients with LV dysfunction was critical. The methodologic mechanism on which this generalization rests is the random selection of subjects from the population at large. This procedure requires that every subject in the population have the same constant probability of being included in the experimental sample. The strength of this simple random sampling approach is that, because the sample is representative of the population at large, findings in the sample can be generalized to the population at large. The SAVE investigators worked to randomize patients from major medical centers in the United States and Canada. The SAVE trial was conducted in 45 centers, reflecting the inclusion of patients from 114 hospitals across the United States and Canada. The trial randomized men and women, ages 21 to 79, who recently sustained an MI with resultant LV ejection fractions less than or equal to 40%. Inclusion and exclusion criteria are as listed in Table 1, chosen to obtain a sample of patients accurately reflecting the post-MI population with LV dysfunction. However, despite this effort, the random selection of subjects from the population in large, randomized clinical trials in the United States, such as SAVE, is not guaranteed. This widespread recruitment effort is an attempt to be as inclusive as possible, and its result is an approximation of a random selection mechanism.

2. Random Allocation of Therapy

Once the sample of patients from the general population was chosen, the manner of allocating captopril therapy must be determined. Unlike in an observational program, experimental programs incorporate the use of an intervention whose implementation is under the complete control of the investigator. The SAVE trial was designed as a prospective experiment, with the use of captopril strictly controlled by the experimental protocol. The investigators used this control by agreeing that patients would receive captopril according to the dictates of random therapy allocation.

Table 1 SAVE Major Inclusion and Exclusion Criteria

Inclusions
Men and women between ages 21 to 79
Confirmed acute myocardial infarction between 3 and 16 days preceding randomization
Radionuclide ejection fraction of 40% or less
Exclusions
Women of childbearing potential unless contraception is used
Patients with contraindication to captopril
Patients with congestive heart failure despite treatment with digitalis and diuretics
Any patient with:
Serum creatinine > 2.5 mg/dl
Malignancy thought to reduce survival or require radiation therapy
Hypertension requiring vasodilator therapy at the time of screening
Severe valvular heart disease likely to require a surgical procedure
Other conditions thought to limit survival
Psychological disorder making the patient unsuitable for a clinical trial
Participation in another investigational drug trial
Clinical ischemia with no corrective procedure prior to this scheduled randomization
Ischemia or hypertension after the test dose of captopril before randomization
Unwilling to consent

Abbreviation: *SAVE*, Survival and Ventricular Enlargement.

This is the second level of randomization in clinical trials and its use is critical for the clearest attribution of effect. Accordingly, the decision for each patient's therapy group assignment was not based on a characteristic of the patient that would blur the attribution of effect, but on a random mechanism. If the only difference between patients who receive the active medication and those who receive control or placebo therapy is the therapy itself, then differences in the outcome measure can be ascribed to the therapy. Alternatively, the absence of randomization quickly dilutes the ability of investigators to successfully ascribe effects seen in the experiment to the intervention itself. In SAVE, patients were randomized to placebo therapy or active therapy, which consisted of 50 mg of captopril t.i.d (Table 2). Both active and placebo therapy were placed on top of the standard regimen for LV dysfunction, including the use of digitalis, diuretics, and nitrate therapy. The use of this background therapy provided the optimum environment in which the additional benefit captopril provided could be assessed.

3. *Sample Size Computation*

The goal of the SAVE trial was to assess whether treatment with captopril would improve survival without significant deterioration of LV performance of patients who have recovered from an acute MI (13). The prospectively specified primary study endpoint was total mortality. However, an experiment designed to determine a 20% reduction in total mortality from a cumulative placebo mortality rate of 20% with a type I error rate of 0.05 (two-

Table 2 Drug Treatment Protocol

Placebo group—standard therapy for left ventricular dysfunction + placebo
Active group—standard therapy for left ventricular dysfunction + 50 mg captopril t.i.d.

sided) and a power of 90% would require 3868 patients. Consideration of the likely event of patients who change their assigned therapy would increase the sample size to more than 4000 patients, a sample size goal too ambitious to attain. Therefore, although interest remained in the total mortality outcome, emphasis was placed on a combined measure of mortality and morbidity. This new endpoint counted death plus survival with a major reduction in radionuclide ventricular LV ejection fraction (RVG-EF) from baseline of at least nine absolute percentage points.

The change in RVG-EF was chosen as a component of this endpoint of SAVE because it was anticipated to occur infrequently but, when present, was deemed to be of major clinical significance. Before any final RVG-EF examinations were obtained, an exploratory analysis was undertaken of the baseline RVG-EF studies to determine the variability of the RVG-EF measurement. The reproducibility of the RVG-EF was obtained by determining the standard deviation of the 200 baseline RVG-EFs obtained from SAVE clinical centers. This measurement suggested that a change of nine percentage points in the RVG-EF observed in the SAVE participants would signify a biological, clinically relevant decrease in RVG-EF in the population. In addition, observations of repeat RVG-EF determinations confirmed that patients with ejection fraction deteriorations $\geq 9\%$ were experiencing an increased risk of death, making this magnitude of deterioration clinically relevant. Thus, the occurrence of this uncommon RVG-EF event, which was evidence of significant deterioration in LV function, was likely to be of clinical importance with a longer duration of patient follow-up. After review of this interim data but before any RVG-EFs were obtained at the study's end, the decision was made to set the minimum change in RVG-EF as a deterioration of ≥ 9 units for the component of the primary endpoint in a patient surviving to the end of the trial. A goal of 2220 randomized participants was accepted as the recruitment goal for SAVE. This number was based on the following assumptions as to the size of the sample:

1. The primary end point is either death from any cause or survival, a ≥ 9 unit reduction, or both in ejection fraction as determined by RVG-EF.
2. The average follow-up time for patients in the study is 3.5 years.
3. The efficacy, uncorrected for patients who change therapy group, is 25%.
4. The cumulative mortality rate for the SAVE placebo group is 20%.
5. The overall percentage of surviving patients experiencing a reduction (in ejection fraction) of more than 9 units is 9% in the placebo group.
6. The projected yearly dropout rate for patients who are initially assigned to active therapy but in whom the active medication is discontinued is 17% the first year, 9% the second year, and 7% the third year.
7. The projected yearly drop-in rate for patients who are initially assigned to placebo therapy but go on active open-label therapy is 9% for the first year, 7% for the second year, and 5% for the third year.
8. In a two-tailed test of significance, the maximum type I error is 0.05, and the power for statistical test on the primary endpoint of SAVE is 90%.

Thus, although paramount interest lay with total mortality as the original endpoint in SAVE, recruitment considerations required its combination with deterioration in LV ejection fraction.

Additional endpoints of SAVE were to evaluate (a) the effects of captopril on cardiovascular mortality and cause-specific mortality; (b) frequency of decline in LV function as measured by radionuclide angiography; (c) development of heart failure severe enough to clinically require open-label ACE inhibition or a hospitalization for the management of heart failure (Table 3). Other important cardiovascular events for post-MI patients, such as risk for recurrent MI and clinical use of coronary revascularization procedures were evaluated. The SAVE study would also evaluate the possible adverse effects of chronic captopril therapy.

4. *Statistical Analyses*

All analyses in SAVE were performed on an intention-to-treat basis (14). The intention-to-treat component of the analysis is critical as it does not allow reasons for changes in study drug compliance or drug discontinuation during the course of the study to influence the measurement of the effect size. All *P* values were two sided, allowing for the possibility of unanticipated deleterious effects of the study medication on the primary trial outcome. The comparability of baseline characteristics in the two treatment groups was ascertained by chi-square tests for categorical variables and standard normal (z) tests for continuous variables. Kaplan-Meier estimates for the distributions of time from randomization to the clinical events of interest were computed. For the comparisons of the captopril and placebo groups with respect to endpoints, reductions in risk, *P* values, and confidence intervals were directly determined from the proportional hazards analyses. A proportional hazards regression model with time-dependent covariates was used to assess the relative risk of death for patients who had heart failure requiring either open-label therapy with an ACE inhibitor or hospitalization. The combined endpoint of death or survival with a major decline in LV function was assessed though a modification of the Gehan procedure (15) for those patients who had a follow-up ejection fraction measurement. The small number of patients who survived the trial but did not have a follow-up ejection fraction were censored.

5. *Echocardiographic Component*

An important issue in SAVE was whether there would be an increase in LV size after infarction, and if this change could be attenuated by the use of captopril. To examine this issue, 773 patients randomized to SAVE agreed to participate in this substudy requiring baseline and follow-up echocardiograms. The data obtained in each of these analyses would be reviewed for quality in the SAVE echocardiogram core laboratory. This quality control consisted of the echocardiographic images being accepted only if there were at

Table 3 SAVE Endpoints

Primary endpoints
Total mortality
Total mortality and/or ≥9 unit reduction in left ventricular ejection fraction
Secondary endpoints
Cause-specific mortality
Recurrent myocardial infarction
Severe congestive heart failure requiring open label ACE inhibitor therapy
Severe congestive heart failure requiring hospitalization
Cardiovascular mortality or the occurrence of recurrent myocardial infarction or severe congestive heart failure

Abbreviation: *SAVE*, Survival and Ventricular Enlargement; *ACE*, angiotensin-converting enzyme.

least three technically quantitative acceptable views. On completion of this quality review, 512 of the 773 patients had baseline studies that were deemed technically acceptable (16). These patients would receive repeat echocardiograms at 3 months, 1 year, and 2 years after randomization. Thus, it would be possible to assess the relationship between echocardiographic measures of LV enlargement and the incidence of adverse cardiovascular events and to evaluate whether the effects of captopril therapy on clinical outcome would be related to changes in echocardiographic measures of LV dysfunction.

6. Operations

The participating units of the trial—45 clinical centers, a clinical coordinating center, a data coordinating center, an RVG quality control laboratory, an electrocardiograph coding laboratory, and the sponsor were administratively linked by the study's principal investigator to encourage effective communication and to maintain the smooth operation of the trial. Each of the units was involved in the planning and development phase of the trial and contributed to the writing of the SAVE protocol and manual of operations. A steering committee, composed of the SAVE principal investigators of each of the clinical centers, was the decision-making apparatus for the scientific and technical conduct of the study. The clinical centers were the units that randomized the participants and those that dispense study medication. They conducted follow-up visits with the patients and completed the study forms for transmission to the data coordinating center.

A data and safety monitoring committee was composed of scientists who were experts in clinical cardiology and biostatistics. This committee would periodically review and evaluate study progress, which included recruitment data, quality control, adverse effects of medication, and fatal and nonfatal events. The data and safety monitoring committee made recommendations, as appropriate, regarding the safe conduct and continuation of the study, guided by statistical monitoring rules based on stochastic curtailment principles.

The clinical coordinating center was responsible for protocol modifications, financial disbursements, and monitoring clinical care decisions regarding adverse events. Each of the clinical units notified the clinical coordinating center when, based on the patient's clinical history and lack of response to nonvasodilator therapy for heart failure, they believed their patient required open-label captopril therapy. However, the clinical coordinating center received no information with respect to therapy group assignments. The data coordinating center was responsible for performing the actual randomization of patients to SAVE. It received all study forms, monitored the compliance of each of the clinical units with the protocol, and maintained the integrity of the database. Unblinded information was presented by the data coordinating center only to the data and safety monitoring committee. In the rare event that a patient's clinical center requested that patient be unblinded, the data coordinating center, after investigating the circumstances, informed the patient's physician of the therapy group assignment. Neither the clinical coordinating center, study physician, nor the patient were given this information.

The sponsor (Bristol Myers-Squibb) was informed of all logistical operations of the trial and attended the regularly scheduled steering committee meetings. The sponsor had direct responsibility for the disbursement of study medication and study forms. The sponsor received information on the occurrence of serious adverse drug reactions to meet their mandated reporting responsibilities but did not receive information about the identity of the patient's study medication unless there was a specific requirement by the government regulatory agency (Food and Drug Administration). Because the sponsor did not attend the meetings of the data and safety monitoring committee, the sponsor had no knowledge of either therapy assignment or unblinded results.

During the course of the trial, the clinical and data coordinating centers together monitored the performance of the clinical centers, with issues of protocol adherence being jointly adjudicated by frequent telephone contacts. In addition, monthly conference calls were made between the chairman of the steering committee, the clinical coordinating center, the data coordinating center, and the sponsor during which operational and logistical issues of the trial were discussed. Reports were presented by the data coordinating center and clinical coordinating center to all center investigators and the sponsor during steering committee meetings held three times a year.

In addition, there was an electrocardiogram core laboratory (responsible for documenting MI occurrence both at baseline and during follow-up), and a RVG core laboratory (permitting an assessment of RVG quality and confirming the presence of a low ejection fraction). The ancillary trials and publications committee reviewed all applications for additional research involving SAVE study participants. A mortality committee using the endpoint review committee was established using SAVE investigators to standardize the classification of deaths in SAVE.

IV. THE SAVE EXPERIENCE

A. Screening

The SAVE participants were randomized in equal numbers and in a double-blind manner to either captopril or placebo. The randomization process was stratified by age (older than 70 years) and ejection fraction (less than 20%), guaranteeing that the small subset of patients at the highest risk for reduced survival were allocated evenly between therapy groups. In addition, randomization was also stratified for participating centers. Screening for SAVE commenced in January 1987 and was completed in January 1990. This process revolved around the continued surveillance of SAVE clinical center intensive care and coronary care units, an examination undertaken by 45 clinical centers and their 112 satellite facilities in the United States and Canada. Only patients in the early (3 to 16 days postinfarction) convalescent period of MI were considered.

A SAVE MI was considered to have occurred if the patient experienced either (a) acute changes in an electrocardiogram (Q or QS finding plus ST elevation and/or T-wave inversion plus absence of left bundle branch block or Wolf-Parkinson-White syndrome) obtained shortly after the infarction with the attendant clinical symptoms and elevation in myocardial enzymes, or (b) the patient had an elevation of myocardial enzymes that were twice as high as normal levels and typical symptoms of an MI were present. The patients were then evaluated for SAVE inclusion and exclusion criteria (Table 4).

The patients who were not excluded then had their RVG-EF measured. Objective evidence of LV dysfunction was defined as a resting RVG demonstrating an RVG-EF of less than 40%. The SAVE screening experience is summarized in Table 4. Between 1987 and 1990, 95,856 coronary care unit patients were screened, of which 36,630 (38.2%) sustained an MI based on the attending physician's judgment. Of these, 31,010 survived the initial 72 hours in the hospital and were age eligible. Of these 31,010 patients, 18,935 (61.1%) had ejection fractions greater than 40% (as determined by either clinical assessment, RVG, echocardiographic, or contrast ventriculography), and 575 patients (1.9%)

Table 4 SAVE Screening Experience, January 27, 1987 to January 31, 1990

95856	Coronary Care Unit Admissions Screened		
	Patients Excluded		Reason
	→	59226	no clinical MI
36630			
	→	5620	death or age exclusion
31010	Clinical MI Survived 72 hours		
	→	18935	LVEF > 40%
	→	575	no SAVE MI
	→	2562	>16 days after MI
8938	SAVE exclusions		
	→	25	women of childbearing age
	→	64	previous captopril hypersensitivity
	→	10	neutropenia
	→	35	systemic lupus erythematosus
	→	702	serum creatinine > 2.5 mg/dl
	→	625	congestive heart failure requiring vasodilation
	→	104	hypertension requiring vasodilation
	→	911	other illness precludes patients involvement
	→	294	unstable post myocardial infarction course
	→	1750	patient unwilling or unable to cooperate
	→	125	excluded for other reason
	→	218	death during screening
4065	No exclusions		
	→	1178	already on ACE inhibitor
	→	367	ischemia not evaluated in 16 days
	→	270	no informed consent
	→	19	adverse reaction to test dose
2231	Randomized to SAVE		

Abbreviations: *SAVE*, Survival and Ventricular Enlargement; *MI*, myocardial infarction; *LVEF*, left ventricular ejection fraction; *ACE*, angiotensin-converting enzyme.

did not meet the SAVE criteria for MI and were excluded. There were 2562 patients (8.3%) who could not be randomized during the 16-day window (13).

The exclusion reasons are provided in Table 4. There were 4065 patients who had a SAVE-eligible MI, did not have any specific exclusion criteria, and had a nuclear ejection fraction of less than 40%. Some of the prominent reasons for exclusion were 625 patients had already experienced clinical heart failure and 1178 were already taking an ACE inhibitor. In 367 patients, ischemia was either manifested clinically or by exercise testing, and an invasive evaluation was not pursued within the 16-day window for randomization. Two hundred seventy patients did not consent to participate in the trial. All 2250 consenting patients were required to receive a single test dose of open-label captopril (6.25 mg). Nineteen patients (0.8%) were excluded because of either orthostatic or ischemic symptoms attributed to administration of study medication. This left 2231 patients for randomization into the trial.

Patients were first scheduled for follow-up examinations 2 weeks after randomization. Subsequent follow-up visits were every 3 months during the first year and every 4 months thereafter. At each visit, a history and physical examination, including functional capacity, were obtained. Interim clinical events since the last visit were elicited and recorded on study forms. In addition, possible adverse reactions were recorded. The evaluation of compliance to medication would be ascertained by pill counts. If symptomatic heart failure developed after recruitment, physicians had the option of using open-label captopril for patients not responding to conventional therapy. When this option was chosen, the clinical coordinating center was notified, confirming that the treating physician believed the patient required ACE inhibition for heart failure that was refractory to the conventional therapy of diuretics, digitalis, or both. The recently proven effective therapy of the combination of hydralazine and nitrates was also recommended. The clinical decision to start open-label ACE inhibitor therapy for symptomatic heart failure did not result in unblinding the clinical investigator.

V. THE PRIMARY FINDINGS OF SAVE

A. SAVE Follow-Up

There were no significant differences before randomization in the characteristics of the patients in the two treatment groups (Table 5). Of the 2231 patients enrolled in the trial, the survivors were followed up for an average (± SD) of 42 ± 10 months (range, 24 to 60). Upon completion of this follow-up period, the vital status of six patients (four in the placebo group and two in the captopril group) was unknown. Blood pressure increased in both groups from baseline to 3 months, but to differing extents; systolic and diastolic pressures were both significantly higher in the placebo group than in the captopril group at 3 months after randomization. This difference was maintained during follow-up values at the 1-year visit, 125 ± 18/77 ± 10 mm Hg for placebo and 119 ± 18/74 ± 10 mm Hg for captopril ($P < 0.001$ for both systolic/diastolic pressures). The mean heart rate for both groups at 1 year was 72 beats per minute.

B. Compliance with Therapy in SAVE

The number of patients taking their assigned study medication at 1 year was similar in the placebo group (808 of 985, or 82%) and the captopril group (787 of 1001, or 79%). At the last study visit, 73% of the surviving patients in the placebo group (612 of 841) and 70% of those in the captopril group (619 of 887) were still taking the study drug. Of these patients, 90% of those in the placebo group (549 of 612) and 79% of those in the captopril group (486 of 619) reached the target dose of 150 mg per day after randomization.

C. Primary Endpoint—Mortality

There were 503 deaths during the study: 275 of the 1116 patients (25%) in the placebo group and 228 of 1115 (20%) in the captopril group; the reduction in the risk of death from all causes was 19% (95% confidence interval [CI], 3 to 32%; $P = 0.019$) (Fig. 1). Of the deaths, 84% (422 of 503) were from cardiovascular causes (234 in the placebo group vs 188 in the captopril group); the reduction in risk was 21% (95% CI, 5 to 33%; $P = 0.014$) (Table 6). Within this category, the significant reduction in mortality was

Table 5 Baseline Characteristics of SAVE Participants

Characteristic	Placebo (n = 1116)	Captopril (n = 1115)
Mean age (yrs)	59.5	59.3
Age > 70 yrs (%)	15	15
Sex ratio M/F %	82/18	83/17
Clinical history of presentation		
Previous MI	35	36
Diabetes mellitus	23	21
Hypertension	42	44
Current smoker	53	53
Means days to randomization	11	11
Events between MI and randomization		
Highest serum creatinine kinase	13.6	13.8
Killip class I	59	60
Thrombolytic therapy (%)	32	34
Cardiac catheterization (%)	54	57
PTCA (%)	17	17
Coronary artery bypass surgery (%)	8	10
Infarct type and location		
Anterolateral Q wave	54	56
Inferoposterior Q wave	17	18
Both	12	11
Non-Q wave	10	10
Other	7	5
Mean radionuclide ejection fraction	31	31
Medication use within 24 hours of randomization		
Antiarrhythmic drugs	11	14
Anticoagulant agents	28	28
Aspirin	59	59
Other antiplatelet agents	14	14
Beta-blockers	36	35
Calcium channel blockers	42	42
Digitalis	27	25
Diuretics	35	35
Nitrates	53	50
Mean blood pressure (mm Hg)		
Systolic	113	112
Diastolic	70	70
Mean heart rate (beats/min)	78	78

Abbreviations: *SAVE*, Survival and Ventricular Enlargement; *MI*, myocardial infarction; *PTCA*, percutaneous transluminal coronary angioplasty.

attributed to progressive heart failure in the captopril group as compared with the placebo group (38 vs 58 deaths, respectively). The reduction in the risk of progressive heart failure was 36% (95% CI, 4 to 58%; $P = 0.032$). These 96 deaths included the 12 patients who underwent cardiac transplantation (seven assigned to placebo and five to captopril). Deaths from noncardiovascular causes (16%) were distributed evenly between the two treatment groups. No differences were noted between the two groups with regard to deaths from

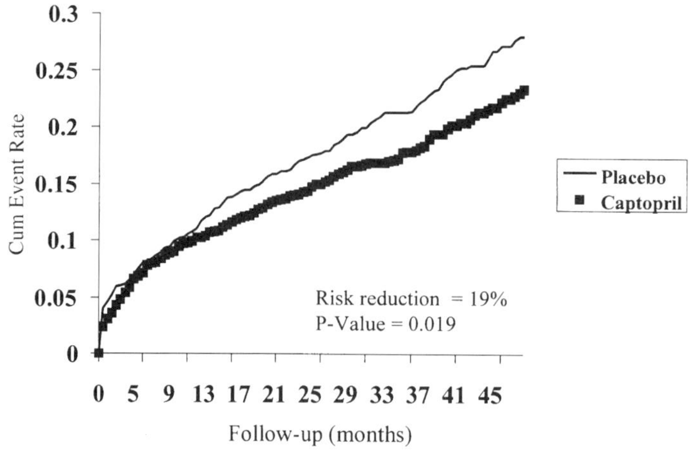

Fig. 1 Effect of captopril on total mortality in SAVE.

cancer, including gastrointestinal cancer. Repeat ejection fractions were obtained in 96% of the surviving patients randomly assigned to placebo (806 of 841) and in 95% of those assigned to captopril (838 of 887) toward the end of the observation period. A deterioration of 9 or more units was noted in 16% of the surviving patients in the placebo group (125 of 806) and 13% of those in the captopril group (110 of 838) ($P = 0.168$). When this measure of progressive LV dysfunction was combined with mortality from all causes, this prospectively defined endpoint was reached in 36% of the patients assigned to placebo (400 of 1116) and 30% of the patients assigned to captopril (338 of 1115); the reduction in risk was 15% (95% CI, 5% to 25%; $P = 0.006$).

Table 6 Cause of Death in Study Participants

Cause of death	Placebo	Captopril	Risk reduction	95% CI	P-value
Cardiovascular	234	188	21	5–35	0.014
Atherosclerotic heart disease	222	174	23	6–37	0.009
Progressive heart failure	58	38	36	4–58	0.032
Sudden with preceding symptoms	50	43			NS
Sudden, unexpected	75	62			NS
Acute myocardial infarction	25	24			NS
Cardiac procedures	9	5			NS
Other cardiac	5	2			NS
Vascular	12	14			NS
Noncardiovascular	41	40			NS
Cancer	20	14			NS
Infection or gastrointestinal bleeding	18	16			NS
Traumatic or unknown	3	10			NS
All	275	228	19	3–32	0.019

Abbreviation: *CI*, confidence interval.

D. Morbidity from Cardiovascular Causes

1. Heart Failure

The incidence in the development of symptomatic heart failure clinically requiring open-label therapy with an ACE inhibitor became more frequent over time, with 13% of the overall population (297 of 2231) developing this degree of heart failure. Regardless of therapy assignment, the need for open-label therapy with an ACE inhibitor was associated with an increased risk of death: 37% of patients with this degree of heart failure died during the trial (110 of 297), whereas only 20% of patients who did not require an ACE inhibitor died (393 of 1934) (relative risk, 4.5; 95% CI, 3.6 to 5.6; $P < 0.001$). However, the patients randomly assigned to receive captopril were significantly less likely to have this form of treatment failure than those assigned to placebo (118 of 1115 [11%] vs 179 of 1116 [16%], respectively; reduction in risk, 37%; 95% CI, 20 to 50 percent; $P < 0.001$). The group randomly assigned to captopril therapy also had a considerable reduction in the number of patients who died after starting open-label therapy with an ACE inhibitor (39/118 patients vs 71/179 in the placebo group; reduction in risk, 47%; 95% CI, 21% to 64%; $P = 0.002$).

Treatment failure that resulted in the need for hospitalization to treat heart failure was an even worse prognostic sign. Regardless of therapy assignment, such hospitalizations, which occurred in 15% of the study population (346 of 2231), were associated with a highly increased risk of death. Among the patients with this degree of heart failure, 47% (164 of 346) died during the trial, whereas among the patients not hospitalized for heart failure, 18% (339 of 1885) died (relative risk, 6.4; 95% CI, 5.3 to 7.8; $P < 0.001$). With captopril therapy, the proportion of patients who required hospitalization for heart failure was reduced (to 14%, or 154 of 1115 patients, vs 17 percent, or 192 of 1116 patients, with placebo; risk reduction, 22%; 95% CI, 4% to 37%, $P = 0.019$). The captopril group also had significantly fewer patients who were hospitalized for heart failure and who later died (64/154 patients vs 100/192 in the placebo group; reduction in risk, 38%; 95% CI, 15% to 54%; $P = 0.003$).

2. Recurrent MI

After randomization, 303 patients had at least one clinically reported (fatal or nonfatal) MI (170 patients in the placebo group and 133 in the captopril group; reduction in risk, 25%; 95% CI, 5% to 40%; $P = 0.015$) (Fig. 2). Of these patients, 129 assigned to placebo and 108 assigned to captopril had the specified levels of creatinine kinase or were designated as having a fatal MI by the mortality classification committee (reduction in risk, 19%; 95% CI, −4% to 37%; $P = 0.102$). In the captopril group, there was also a substantial reduction in the number of patients who had recurrent clinical MIs and subsequently died (56/108 vs 80/129 in the placebo group; reduction in risk, 32%; 95% CI, 4% to 51%; $P = 0.029$). Coronary revascularization procedures during the follow-up period were also less likely to occur in patients randomized to captopril therapy (195/1116 for the placebo group vs 154/1115 for the captopril group; reduction in risk 24%; 95% CI 6 to 39%; $P = 0.010$).

3. Combined Clinical Endpoint

The number of patients who either died of cardiovascular causes or had major nonfatal events (heart failure requiring ACE therapy, heart failure requiring hospitalization, or recurrent MI) was reduced with captopril therapy (from 448 of 1116 patients [40%] in the

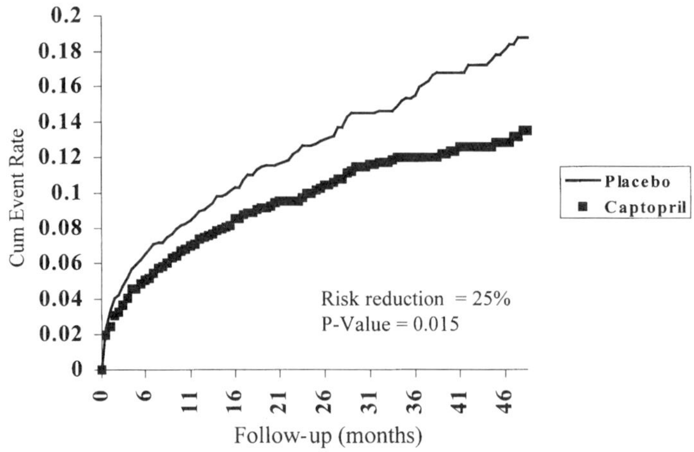

Fig. 2 Effect of captopril on recurrent myocardial infarction in SAVE.

placebo group to 359 of 1115 patients [32%] in the captopril group; risk reduction, 24%; 95% CI, 13% to 34%; $P < 0.001$). If 1000 patients were treated with captopril therapy for 3 years, 80 major cardiovascular events would be prevented. The effect on mortality from all causes and on cardiovascular mortality and morbidity of major, prospectively specified, prerandomization characteristics known to influence survival after MI was as anticipated, that is, regardless of treatment assignment, advanced age, history of MI, lower LV ejection fraction, and higher Killip classification were each associated with a higher incidence of adverse events. When these subgroups were analyzed, captopril therapy showed a consistent benefit, although to varying degrees, in reducing both mortality from all causes and mortality and morbidity from cardiovascular causes.

A proportional hazards model for mortality from all causes demonstrated a significant influence of captopril in reducing mortality independently of age, ejection fraction, history of MI, sex, base-line arterial blood pressure, and use of thrombolytic therapy, aspirin, or beta-blockers ($P = 0.013$). An important point is that the use of captopril produced additive benefits when used in conjunction with other previously proven therapies.

4. Echocardiography Results

The two-dimensional echocardiograms from 512 patients were accepted for quantitative analysis. These were obtained at a mean of 11.1 ± 3.2 days after the index MI. Thirteen patients died during the follow-up period from noncardiovascular causes, leaving a cohort of 499 patients. There were 55 deaths within the first year before the follow-up echocardiogram (24 in the placebo and 31 in the captopril group, $P = 0.275$). Four hundred twenty of these survivors (95%) had repeat two-dimensional echocardiograms that were judged acceptable for quantitative analysis at 1 year.

The clinical features of the patients in the echocardiographic substudy resembled those in the overall trial. Furthermore, patients randomly assigned to placebo or to captopril within the echocardiographic substudy were similar except for the peak creatinine phosphokinase levels, which were significantly higher in the captopril-treated group.

Baseline LV end-diastolic and end-systolic areas and percent change in area were all strong, independent predictors of cardiovascular mortality. Total mortality increased with increasing end-diastolic volume when end-diastolic volume was assessed in quartiles (Fig. 3). These baseline echocardiographic variables were added individually to the multivariate model for survival, which included factors well known to influence survival (age, sex, diabetes, hypertension, prior infarction, thrombolysis, and radionuclide ejection fraction). When added to this model, echocardiographic LV end-systolic area and percent change in LV area emerged as some of the strongest independent predictors of clinical outcome.

Left ventricular end-diastolic and end-systolic areas and percent change in LV area at baseline were similar in the captopril and the placebo treatment groups. At 1 year, LV end-diastolic and end-systolic areas had increased in both treatment groups, but the increases in areas were significantly greater in the placebo patients than in those treated with captopril ($P = 0.023$ for diastole, $P = 0.021$ for systole). This greater increment resulted in larger LV areas in the 1-year survivors in the placebo-treated group ($P = 0.038$ and $P = 0.015$, respectively). Percent change in LV area was significantly greater at 1 year in the captopril-treated group compared with placebo ($29 \pm 8\%$ vs $27 \pm 7\%$, $P = 0.005$). The change in diastolic area over time by therapy group is depicted (Fig. 4).

One hundred eleven of the 420 (26.4%) 1-year survivors with 1-year echo measurements sustained at least one major cardiovascular event (defined as cardiovascular death, heart failure requiring either hospitalization or open-label captopril therapy, or recurrent infarction) during late follow-up. The event rate was higher in the placebo treatment group (31.8%) compared with the captopril treatment group (20.7%), indicating a risk reduction of 35% ($P = 0.010$). Patients who sustained adverse cardiovascular events irrespective of treatment assignment had more than a threefold greater increase in end-systolic areas from baseline to 1 year compared with patients who experienced no adverse cardiovascular

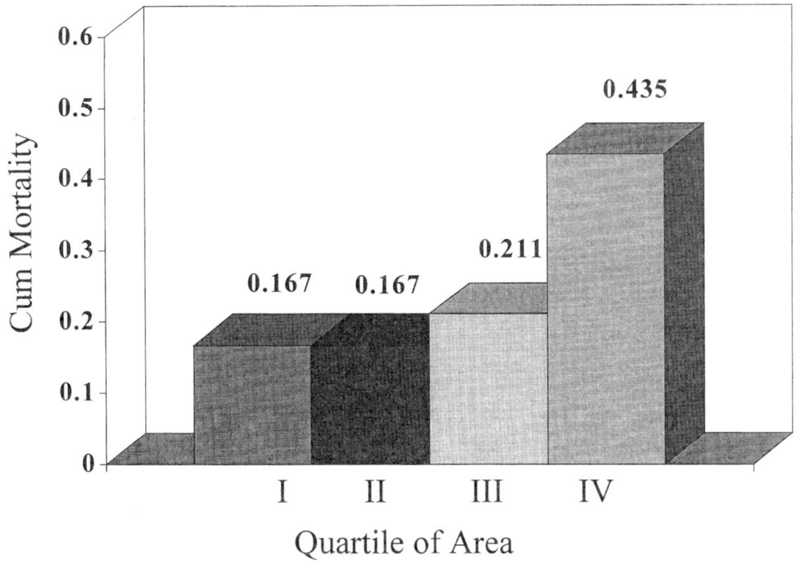

Fig. 3 Relationship of end diastolic volume at baseline to total mortality in SAVE.

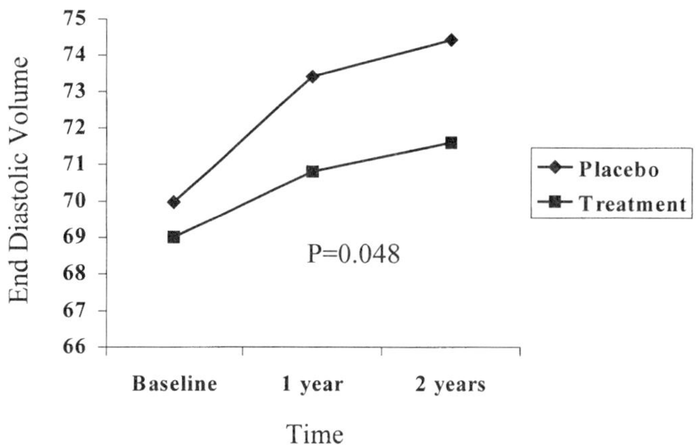

Fig. 4 Change in end diastolic volume over time by therapy group in SAVE.

events (5.35 ± 9.88 vs 1.48 ± 9.01 in diastole, $P < 0.001$, and 6.37 ± 10.29 vs 1.35 ± 9.62 systole, $P < 0.001$). Furthermore, the interval change in percent change in LV area at 1 year was significantly lower in patients who sustained adverse cardiovascular events compared with patients who did not (−3 ± 6% vs 0 ± 7%, $P < 0.001$) (17).

Captopril therapy resulted in a trend toward less deterioration in the percent change in area (−1.3 ± 7.0 vs −0.1 ± 7.0, $P = 0.105$; placebo vs captopril). Among patients who did not sustain adverse cardiovascular events, the increase in LV area was much less in the captopril-treated group both in diastole (0.38 ± 9.21 vs 2.67 ± 8.67 cm^2, $P = 0.02$) and in systole (0.26 ± 9.98 vs 2.53 ± 9.11 cm^2, $P = 0.038$). Although captopril reduced the number of patients with cardiovascular events, the changes in LV cavity areas in the captopril-treated patients with cardiovascular events were similar to patients treated with placebo who experienced adverse cardiovascular events. However, effective failure of the therapy to reduce ventricular enlargement was associated with no reduction in the risk for major cardiovascular events.

E. Subgroup Analyses

The position taken by Yusuf (18) is to use the overall trial results to indicate the likely effect of therapy in a particular subgroup. If this stance is taken for SAVE, we would conclude that captopril significantly reduces all-cause mortality and cardiovascular mortality/morbidity in each of the subgroups. However, providing the individual analyses for the subgroup strata can provide important information if the environment for its correct interpretation is provided. This includes the clear understanding that the subgroup analysis is exploratory and a useful exercise in hypothesis generation. The presence of an interaction effect, revealing the differential effect of captopril in a subgroup would be an important finding worthy of confirmation. However, the absence of a specific trial design methodology incorporation into the trial to capture the subgroup effect of interest must be and is acknowledged.

1. Demographics

In each of the subgroup strata—age 61 or older, male gender, USA origin, and white race—the data suggest that captopril may appear to confer a benefit for mortality. For

Table 7 Subgroup Analysis in SAVE—Demographics

				Total mortality			Cardiovascular mortality/morbidity		
Variable	Level	Pts Placebo	Pts Captopril	Risk Red	CI	Power	Risk Red	CI	Power
Age	< 61	528	558	−4	−40 to 23	0.314	16	−5 to 32	0.66
	≥ 61	588	557	28	10 to 42	0.682	29	15 to 41	0.895
Gender	male	912	929	22	6 to 36	0.744	28	16 to 38	0.949
	female	204	186	2	−53 to 37	0.174	4	−32 to 30	0.371
Country	USA	789	785	17	−3 to 32	0.652	20	6 to 32	0.919
	Canada	327	330	25	−4 to 46	0.332	35	15 to 50	0.55
Race	white	1002	991	18	1 to 32	0.747	24	12 to 34	0.956
	nonwhite	114	124	27	−21 to 56	0.168	28	−7 to 51	0.323

Abbreviations: *SAVE*, Survival and Ventricular Enlargement; *CI*, confidence interval.

these same strata and, in addition, for subjects younger than 61, and randomization in a Canadian center, a benefit tended to be conferred for the occurrence of the combined endpoint. The subgroup strata of women and nonwhite race provide insufficient power for interpretation of the relative risks, making the relative risks uninterpretable (Table 7).

2. *Clinical History*

The SAVE database provided important clinical history of the randomized patients before the index SAVE MI (19). Regarding total mortality, captopril tended to be effective in patients who had an index MI before the SAVE MI as well as in those patients for whom the SAVE MI was the first heart attack (8). The trend for a captopril effect was also apparent within four of the five subgroups for the location of the SAVE index MI and for those patients randomized more than 7 days after the SAVE MI. Each of the Goldman and New York Heart Association (NYHA) classes demonstrated a trend to captopril benefit for total mortality. The trend for a mortality benefit conferred by captopril is also apparent for patients without diabetes and patients without hypertension. Point estimates for captopril benefit support the notion of a uniform captopril effect in both the presence and absence of hypertension, diabetes, and a family history of heart disease. Patients without history of cardiac catheterization, cardiac surgery, thrombolysis, or percutaneous transluminal coronary angioplasty (PTCA) each had interpretable results for total mortality and demonstrated a trend to benefit from mortality by captopril.

The trend for captopril to protect from the occurrence of either cardiovascular mortality or cardiovascular morbidity was apparent for patients regardless of the presence of an MI before the SAVE MI and for patients with electrocardiographic changes indicative of both an anterior and inferior MI at baseline. This trend to captopril benefit was also apparent for patients who were randomized more than 7 days after the infarction, patients in Goldman classes I, II, and III, patients in NYHA classes 1 and 2, patients with and without diabetes by history, patients with and without hypertension, patients with and without a family history of heart disease, and patients without a history of cardiac catheterization, cardiac surgery, thrombolysis, or PTCA.

3. *Index Infarction Hospitalization History*

In each of the subgroups for Killip class where the power is above 50%, there is a trend to captopril benefit for each of total mortality and the combined cardiovascular mortality/morbidity endpoint (Table 8). There is a trend to benefit in patients who had heart failure between the SAVE MI and randomization and in those patients without thrombolysis and without either PTCA or coronary artery bypass surgery. Patients without hypotension requiring intervention also demonstrated a trend toward captopril benefit to prevent total mortality. A trend to protection from cardiovascular mortality/morbidity was observed for patients in each of Killip classes I and II, patients regardless of the occurrence of heart failure at baseline, and in patients without a history of thrombolysis or revascularization (either PTCA or coronary artery bypass surgery) between the SAVE MI and randomization. This trend was also observed in patients regardless of whether they suffered from hypotension requiring intervention in the immediate post-index infarction period.

Treating physicians in SAVE were encouraged to use all medications according to the accepted practice of medicine in the postinfarction-prerandomization period. The substrate strata were interpretable (i.e., had prior power of 50% or higher) and demonstrated a trend to captopril benefit for total mortality for patients who did not use beta-blockers, patients regardless of aspirin use, patients who did not use antiarrhythmic agents, and patients who did not use non-ACE inhibitor vasodilators, or sympathetic blockers, digoxin, or anticoagulants (Table 9). This same trend to captopril benefit was observed in patients in whom diuretics were used. A trend to benefit from cardiovascular mortality/morbidity was observed in patients either on or off beta-blockers, aspirin use, diuretic use, calcium channel blockers, digoxin, or anticoagulants. This trend was observed in patients on antiarrhythmic agents, non-ACE inhibitor vasodilators, and sympathetic blockers.

Our conclusions after multiple analyses of these subgroups is that within SAVE, there was no strong evidence of a differential effect of captopril within any subcohort. All subgroups appeared to uniformly benefit from captopril therapy.

4. Adverse Events

After randomization, the use of beta-blockers, aspirin, digitalis, and nitrates was similar in the two groups. There was, however, more use of diuretic therapy among the patients taking placebo (38% vs 32% for captopril, $P = 0.002$), a finding consistent with the higher incidence of symptomatic heart failure in this group. The following symptoms were reported: dizziness (5%), alteration in taste (2%), cough (6%), and diarrhea (2%). The following numbers of patients discontinued the study medication at the time of these adverse events: 25 in the placebo group and 32 in the captopril group who had dizziness (P not significant); 5 and 9, respectively, who had taste alteration (P not significant); 9 and 27 with cough ($P = 0.003$); and none with diarrhea. Cost effectiveness studies (20,21) demonstrated that the captopril therapy was both life and cost saving. An examination was carried out in two models. The persistent-benefit model assumed that the survival benefit associated with captopril therapy would persist beyond 4 years. The limited-benefit model assumed that captopril therapy incurred costs but no survival benefit beyond 4 years. In the limited benefits analyses, the incremental cost-effectiveness of captopril therapy ranged from $3600/quality adjusted life-year for 80-year-old patients to $60,800/quality-adjusted life-year for 50-year-old patients. In the persistent-benefit analyses, incremental cost-effectiveness ratios ranged from $3,700 to $10,000/quality-adjusted life-year, depending on the age. The SAVE investigators concluded that the cost-effectiveness of captopril therapy for 50- to 80-year-old survivors of MI with a lower ejection fraction compares favorably with other interventions for survivors of MI.

F. Secondary Results

Although the responsibility of clinical trial workers is to focus on the primary mission of the research effort, opportunities to use the dataset to examine other relevant public health and clinical issues often abound and have proven themselves impossible to ignore. These same opportunities were available in SAVE; thus, although the SAVE workers concentrated on testing the prospectively stated primary hypothesis of the trial, other issues of interest to the medical community were also examined. However, several words of caution must be offered before describing these ancillary SAVE findings.

1. Hazards of Secondary Analyses

Using clinical trial data to explore issues other than those for which the trial is designed raises important issues in result interpretation. Most every disciplined investigator has acknowledged the conflicting forces of data interrogation (the desire to measure many

Table 8 Subgroup Analysis in SAVE—Baseline Morbidity

Variable	Level	Pts Placebo	Pts Captopril	Total mortality Risk Red	Total mortality CI	Total mortality Power	Cardiovascular mortality/morbidity Risk Red	Cardiovascular mortality/morbidity CI	Cardiovascular mortality/morbidity Power
Prior MI	No	721	718	22	0 to 39	0.506	21	4 to 35	0.758
	Yes	395	397	16	−8 to 35	0.533	29	14 to 42	0.881
Infarct type	Anterior	605	624	9	−19 to 29	0.431	16	−3 to 31	0.711
	Posterior	193	201	16	−32 to 46	0.187	27	−2 to 48	0.372
	Both	135	126	38	2 to 61	0.232	34	6 to 54	0.434
	Non-Q-wave	110	106	36	−10 to 62	0.171	33	−2 to 56	0.281
	Other	73	58	−2	−64 to 38	0.193	16	−32 to 46	0.332
Days to randomization	3–7 Days	197	177	11	−35 to 42	0.208	16	−16 to 39	0.381
	>7 Days	919	938	20	3 to 34	0.724	26	13 to 36	0.948
Goldman scale	Class 1	627	659	17	−10 to 37	0.393	24	6 to 38	0.71
	Class 2	265	259	19	−11 to 41	0.367	19	−6 to 37	0.571
	Class 3	204	180	22	−8 to 44	0.371	35	14 to 51	0.636
NYHA	Class 1	731	740	12	−13 to 31	0.463	20	3 to 34	0.781
	Class 2	317	299	30	6 to 47	0.468	31	13 to 45	0.755
	Class 3	65	75	28	−29 to 53	0.205	34	−4 to 58	0.306
Diabetes	No	857	882	20	2 to 35	0.639	26	12 to 37	0.898
	Yes	259	233	12	−21 to 36	0.355	17	−6 to 36	0.651
Hypertension	No	708	686	19	−3 to 36	0.535	29	14 to 41	0.809
	Yes	408	429	20	−4 to 38	0.493	20	2 to 35	0.809
Family history heart disease	No	593	603	12	−13 to 31	0.476	15	−4 to 30	0.764
	Yes	516	510	26	5 to 42	0.544	33	18 to 45	0.828

Pre-MI Cath	No	838	831	21	2 to 36	0.619	23	9 to 35	0.89
	Yes	278	284	16	−13 to 38	0.394	30	10 to 45	0.676
Pre-MI PTCA	No	1073	1078	19	4 to 32	0.791	25	13 to 35	0.973
	Yes	43	37	13	−152 to 70	0.063	9	−92 to 57	0.102
Pre-MI thrombolysis	No	1081	1078	18	2 to 31	0.784	24	12 to 34	0.972
	Yes	35	37	54	−34 to 84	0.08	41	−28 to 72	0.12
Pre-MI cardiac surgery	No	980	994	20	3 to 34	0.72	25	13 to 36	0.946
	Yes	136	121	6	−44 to 38	0.22	18	−15 to 42	0.423
Pre-MI revascularization	No	954	970	2	4 to 35	0.716	25	13 to 36	0.943
	Yes	162	145	7	−41 to 38	0.223	17	−15 to 40	0.435
Killip class	Class 1	672	676	25	4 to 42	0.499	25	8 to 38	0.765
	Class 2	366	355	18	−10 to 38	0.42	26	7 to 41	0.733
	Class 3	62	62	−21	−101 to 30	0.151	11	−40 to 44	0.277
	Class 4	16	22	16	176 to 74	0.064	47	−27 to 78	0.13
CHF	No	648	647	31	11 to 48	0.474	27	10 to 40	0.748
	Yes	466	467	7	−18 to 26	0.555	23	6 to 36	0.863
Thrombolysis	No	761	739	17	−1 to 32	0.715	25	11 to 36	0.933
	Yes	355	376	22	−14 to 47	0.238	23	−1 to 41	0.497
Revascularization	No	854	815	22	6 to 36	0.756	28	16 to 38	0.956
	Yes	262	300	−13	−79 to 28	0.156	4	−32 to 30	0.336
Hypotension req intervention	No	886	859	19	1 to 33	0.688	24	11 to 35	0.93
	Yes	229	256	21	−14 to 45	0.279	27	3 to 45	0.504

Abbreviations: *SAVE*, Survival and Ventricular Enlargement; *CI*, confidence interval; *MI*, myocardial infarction; *NYHA*, New York Heart Association; *PTCA*, percutaneous transluminal coronary angioplasty.

Table 9 Subgroup Analysis in SAVE—Medication Within 24 Hours of Randomization

				Total mortality			Cardiovascular mortality/morbidity		
Variable	Level	Pts Placebo	Pts Captopril	Risk Red	CI	Power	Risk Red	CI	Power
Beta blockers	No	718	724	14	−5 to 30	0.682	24	10 to 35	0.928
	Yes	398	391	33	4 to 53	0.295	26	4 to 43	0.531
Aspirin	No	463	458	14	−10 to 33	0.521	29	13 to 43	0.797
	Yes	653	657	24	2 to 41	0.502	20	4 to 34	0.805
Antiarrhythmics	No	989	962	14	−4 to 30	0.698	23	11 to 34	0.942
	Yes	127	153	42	13 to 62	0.293	33	7 to 52	0.494
Non-ACE vasodilators	No	1106	1109	18	2 to 31	0.793	24	12 to 34	0.976
	Yes	10	6	74	−124 to 97	0.056	73	−129 to 97	0.067
Sympathetic	No	1112	1108	19	3 to 32	0.798	24	13 to 34	0.977
	Yes	4	7	23	−769 to 93	0.042	23	−769 to 93	0.042
Diuretics	No	725	724	22	−1 to 39	0.482	23	7 to 36	0.782
	Yes	391	391	17	−7 to 35	0.564	26	10 to 40	0.853
Calcium	No	648	643	19	−7 to 38	0.567	26	11 to 39	0.85
	Yes	468	472	19	−4 to 33	0.447	22	3 to 37	0.731
Digoxin	No	818	835	16	−4 to 33	0.575	26	12 to 38	0.87
	Yes	298	280	21	−5 to 41	0.453	19	−2 to 36	0.73
Nitrates	No	529	553	16	−10 to 36	0.423	18	−2 to 34	0.675
	Yes	587	562	20	−1 to 36	0.587	29	15 to 41	0.887
Anticoagulation agents	No	801	798	26	8 to 30	0.675	22	8 to 34	0.906
	Yes	315	317	0	−39 to 28	0.296	30	9 to 46	0.601

Abbreviations: *SAVE*, Survival and Ventricular Enlargement; *CI*, confidence interval; *ACE*, angiotensin-converting enzyme.

different clinical assessments at the end of the experiment) versus interpretive parsimony (the alpha level and, therefore, the success of the trial rest on the interpretation of the primary endpoint), each force pulling in the opposite direction, bedeviling investigators as they plan and execute their experiments. Although guidance for the selection of endpoints in clinical trials is available (12), this area remains controversial (22–27). Baseline analyses are perhaps best described as epidemiologic cross-sectional studies. Although they are illuminating, the identification of a cause that is antecedent to an effect can be problematic if the variables are measured simultaneously. Analysis examining the relationship between baseline measures and events that the patients experience during the post-randomization follow-up period can be illuminating as well, but the use of only a subcohort (subset analysis) and *P* value multiplicity vitiates the conclusive strengths of these evaluations. So, although clinical trials can generate much interesting data and shed light on relationships involving comorbidity and clinical sequelae, this light is dimmed by design and interpretation conundrums. The findings are best interpreted when viewed as exploratory or hypothesis generating.

With these caveats, SAVE provided interesting and timely information on several public health issues. The issue of sex bias in the treatment of women rose to the forefront in the 1980s. Even though coronary artery disease was the leading cause of death among women, previous studies demonstrated that physicians were perhaps less likely to aggressively pursue coronary artery disease in women. A cross-sectional study in SAVE involving baseline data examined the nature and severity of anginal symptoms and the use of antianginal/anti-ischemic medications before enrollment of men and women into SAVE. The data revealed that, although women were just as likely as men to have angina and to be treated with antianginal medications and that women complained of greater functional disability from angina, fewer women had had cardiac catheterization or coronary artery bypass surgery before randomization in SAVE. Furthermore, although men and women were equally likely to undergo bypass procedures after a cardiac catheterization, women were half as likely as men to undergo an invasive cardiac procedure. This result remained, even after adjusting for important baseline differences between men and women as measured by variables obtained at baseline (28).

A similar examination of selection issues in SAVE involved the use of thrombolytic therapy in acute MI. A cross-sectional analysis of baseline data revealed that although the SAVE population was selected from a population of patients with LV dysfunction, the majority of patients who were judged as clinically unsuitable for thrombolytic therapy were at higher risk for adverse cardiovascular events (29). This analysis in the early thrombolytic era raised the question of the use of this therapy in high-risk groups.

Continuing in the vein of public health, as the debate over managed health care as an alternative health care system grew in the United States in the 1980s, major differences in the organization of the health care systems in Canada and the United States were recognized. The SAVE trial exploited the fact that it randomized patients from the United States and Canada by examining differences in post-randomization clinical events rates by the patient's randomization country. The execution of this embedded, forward observational design on the SAVE dataset concluded that coronary arteriography was more commonly performed in the United States than in Canada (66% vs 35%) and the revascularizations procedures before randomization were also more frequent (31% vs 12%). When these patients were followed prospectively during the post-randomization follow-up period in SAVE, patients randomized from the United States and Canada had the same total mortality rate and the same rate of recurrent MI. However, patients randomized in Canada did have a higher frequency of activity-related angina (30). Finally, an important contribution made by the subsidiary analyses executed in SAVE involved neurohormones. Previous studies had indicated that patients with an acute MI have significant activation of all neurohumoral systems on admission to the hospital. However, this activation began to subside within the first 72 hours after MI so that, after several days, all plasma neurohormones returned to normal. The only exception to this observation was in patients with LV dysfunction and overt heart failure, in whom both plasma renin activity and atrial natriuretic peptide increased, and in patients with LV dysfunction but no obvious heart failure, in whom only atrial natriuretic peptide was increased. In SAVE, 522 patients had plasma neurohumeral levels measured 12 days mean time after index MI. The results demonstrated that a subgroup of patients without overt heart failure sustained persistent neurohumeral activation at the time of postinfarction hospital discharge. Because patients with persistent neurohumoral activation are in all likelihood at greater risk of developing complications and perhaps more likely to benefit from pharmacological therapy blunting the effects of neurohumoral activation, SAVE demonstrated that measurement of predischarge neurohumoral activation may be useful. Furthermore, N-terminal pro atrial natriuretic factor (ANF) was found to be a potent predictor of survival, even stronger than ANF itself, and remained important, after adjusting for age, gender, prior MI, hypertension, diabetes, use of thrombolysis, Killip class, the location of the MI, and LV ejection fraction (31–34).

VI. DISCUSSION

The SAVE trial demonstrated that the long-term administration of the ACE inhibitor, captopril, to recent survivors of MI with LV dysfunction resulted in reduced total mortality, cardiovascular mortality, and morbidity. An important strength of SAVE was the breadth and depth of its findings. The consistent findings of the effect of therapy among its endpoints bolster the contribution of ACE inhibitor therapy in the post-MI setting. The attenuation of LV enlargement associated with captopril identified in SAVE's echocardiographic component supported the mechanistic understanding of the pathophysiology of LV dysfunction, providing assurance of the stability of the SAVE findings through corroboration of the mechanism of captopril action.

Although the major focus of SAVE was the examination of ACE inhibitor therapy on mortality, interest remained high throughout the trial on captopril's ability to influence secondary endpoints. These endpoints included recurrent MI, heart failure, and radionuclide ventriculograms. For each of these endpoints, SAVE supported the conclusion of a produced benefit.

The breath of SAVE's assessment of clinical outcome extended through extensive subgroup analyses. A reasoned examination of the subgroup analyses from SAVE suggests that the benefits of captopril therapy were relatively uniform in the SAVE study, indicating that therapy benefit was not confined to one particular subgroup.

A. Strengths and Weaknesses of SAVE

An additional strength in SAVE was its investigator team. Throughout SAVE, continued pressure was brought to bear to use new therapies. These new therapies potentially affect SAVE by creating a bias to the null, deflating both captopril and placebo event rates to a point that would blur statistical distinctions between them. A strength of the protocol was to allow each of these procedures to be used during the course of the trial in a blinded fashion. The investigators were free to use all new therapies on an individual basis for their patients. By doing this, patients in the trial were assured of getting the best and newest approved therapies for their medical and health conditions. Second, this process assured that the positive findings of SAVE could be applied ''on top of'' current medical therapy. Angiotensin-converting enzyme inhibitor use after infarction could be applied with full expectation of benefit from the newest therapy available for the treatment of LV dysfunction.

A weakness of SAVE was recruitment. Its initial sample size was to be 4000 patients. Unfortunately, several months after SAVE randomizations began, it became clear that recruitment would fall short of its goal, and after 9 months of slower than expected recruitment, some trial adjustments were considered. Because of fears that an underrecruited SAVE would be underpowered to detect a total mortality effect with statistical significance, interest was generated in the computation of a combined endpoint (total mortality and a reduction in ejection fraction). At the conclusion of SAVE, each of these endpoints was statistically significant ($P = 0.019$ for total mortality, $P = 0.016$ for the combined endpoint). Although application of the most stringent multiple endpoint testing rules (34) would show that the consideration of both does not inflate the type I error above the 0.05 boundary, chronic recruitment difficulties plagued SAVE throughout is randomization period.

The SAVE study encompassed a lab bench-to-bedside approach, proving that this new use of captopril could save lives and reduce untoward cardiovascular events. As such, it has favorably changed the practice of medicine. As with any good research experience, it also provided useful observations for other studies. The reduction in coronary events in the ACE inhibitor-treated group was somewhat unexpected. This observation, coupled with similar findings in SOLVD, generated the rationale for the National Heart, Lung and Blood Institute (NHLBI) trial, Prevention of Events—Angiotensin Converting Enzyme inhibitor (PEACE) trial (35), which is a direct extension of SAVE, testing whether coronary events can be reduced by use of an ACE inhibitor in patients with coronary artery disease.

APPENDIX OF PERSONNEL

Principal Investigator: Marc A. Pfeffer, MD, PhD

Chairman, Steering Committee: Eugene Braunwald, MD

Policy board: Richard Gorlin, MD, Mount Sinai Medical Center, New York, NY; William W. Parmiey, MD, University of California San Francisco, San Francisco, CA; James Ware, PhD, Harvard School of Public Health, Boston, MA; Karl T. Weber, University of Missouri-Columbia, Columbia, MO.

Data coordinating center: University of Texas Health Science Center, Houston, TX: Denese Alsmeyer, Cynthia Ang, Christina Cole Berryhill, Wanda Bradshaw, Evelyn Butcher, Robert Byington, Celia L. Canales, Bobbie Carroll, Young-Ha Cho, Lisa Clemons, Charles Cooper, Larry Cormier, Barry R. Davis, MD, PhD, Lori Cole Diman, Rhonda Evans, Pamela Gilman, Patrick Grealy, Roberta Haglund, Peggy Hamm, PhD, C. Morton Hawkins, ScD, Susan Henley, Toweilla Henry, Corina Hernandez, Delores Hernandez, Leticia Johnson, Sherol Jordan, Homai Khajautia, Nita Lafayette, John Lara, Susan Le Blanc, Jone-Ing Lin, Brad Marshall, Alice Martinez, Lemuel A. Moyé, MD, PhD, Lynne

Mutchler, Mutuku Mwanthi, Melanie Palmer, Denise Patterson, Janet Pyle, Joyce M. Randolf, Barbara Raslan, Glenn Schreyer, Lara Simpson, Leona Thomas, Gordon Tsai, Sandy Uresti, Terri Vincent, Ava Ware, Barbara Wooten, Lori Zigich.

Clinical coordinating center: Brigham and Women's Hospital, Boston, MA: Marc A. Pfeffer, MD, PhD, Gervasio A. Lamas, MD, John D. Rutherford, MD, L. Howard Hartley, MD, Kathleen Connors, RN, Angela Perry.

Mortality/Endpoints Committee: Milton Packer, MD, Chairman, Mount Sinai Medical Center, New York, NY; Victoria Bernstein, MD, University of British Columbia, Vancouver, British Columbia, Canada; Thomas E. Cuddy, MD, University of Manitoba, Winnipeg, Manitoba, Canada; Barry R. Davis, MD, PhD, The University of Texas at Houston, Houston, TX; Kirk Jacobson, MD, Sacred Heart Hospital, Eugene, OR; Gervasio A. Lamas, MD, Brigham and Women's Hospital, Boston, MA; Sandra Lewis, MD, Oregon Heart Institute, Portland, OR; John McCans, MD, Jewish General Hospital, Montreal, Quebec, Canada; Otelio Randall, MD, Howard University Hospital, Washington, DC; Bruce Sussex, MD, University of Newfoundland, Newfoundland, Canada; St. John's, John H. Wertheimer, MD, Albert Einstein Medical Center, Philadelphia, PA.

Ancillary trials/publications committee: Edward M. Geltman, MD, Chairman, Washington University School of Medicine, St. Louis, MO; John C. Alexander, MD, Bristol-Myers Squibb Co., Princeton, NJ; Eugene Braunwald, MD, Brigham and Women's Hospital, Boston, MA; Bernard J. Gersh, MD, Mayo Clinic, Rochester, MN; C. Morton Hawkins, ScD, The University of Texas, Houston, TX; Milton Packer, MD, Mount Sinai Medical Center, New York, NY; Marc A. Pfeffer, MD, PhD, Brigham and Women's Hospital, Boston, MA.

Catheterization Core laboratory: Gervasio A. Lamas, MD, Gary Mitchell, MD, Gregory Flaker, MD, Richard Webel, MD, Sidney C. Smith Jr, MD.

Echocardiography Core laboratory: Martin St. John Sutton, MD, Theodore Plappert, Kathleen Connors, RN, Marc A. Pfeffer, MD, PhD.

Radionuclide Ventriculography Core laboratory: Frans J.T. Wackers, MD, Jennifer Mattera, Barry Zaret, MD, Mark Saari, Donna Natali, Diane Errico, Edward Levine.

Electrocardiography Core laboratory: John Rutherford, MD.

SAVE study centers: *Albany Medical Center*: Theodore L. Biddle, MD, Joseph Sacco, MD, Debra, L. Herault, Martha Power, Maureen Curran. *Albert Einstein Medical Center*, N.D.: John H. Wertheimer, MD, FACP, FACC, Clifford Stauss, DO, Ellen Liedel, Joanne Ackler, RN, Jill Stunkard, RN, Scott Deron, DO, Marguerite Ambrose, Deborah McClary, RN. *Bowman Gray School of Medicine*: Henry S. Miller Jr, MD, Deborah Wesley, RN. *Brigham and Women's Hospital*: Gervasio A. Lamas, MD, L. Howard Hartley, MD, Marc A. Pfeffer, MD, PhD, John Rutherford, MD, Barton Heller, MD, Ralph Bevivino, MD, Raymond Zick, MD, Robert Rimmer, MD, Michael Hession, MD, Charles Gaughan, MD, Gary Mitchell, MD, Martin St. John Sutton, MD, Solomon Gabbay, MD, Francis E. Hubbard, MD, Gerard Gaughan, MD, Paul E. Boinay, MD, Carole Chapin, RN, Kathleen Connors, RN, Mary Wade, RN, Pam Gillispie, RN, Marilou Dorman, RN, Margo Mandano-O'Malley, RN, Robert English, Harvey Stone, Lowell Martin, Mary Beth Bi. *Iowa Heart Center*: David Gordon, MD, Sir Will. Wickerneyer, MD, Mark Polich, Kate Elphic. *Ginger Medical Center*: Francis J. Menapace Jr, Richard J. Butcher, MD, Thomas

Modesto, MD, M. Kleman, RN, Marianne Gorcsan, RN. *Hospital Sacred-Coeur, Montreal*: Jean-Lucien Rouleau, N. Marc Klein, MD, Real LeBeau, MD, Ginette Gaude RN, Jocelyne Fouguette. *Hopital Notre Dame, Montreal*: Francois Sestier, MD, PhD, Daniel Savard, N. Pierre Laramee, MD, Jacques Lenis, MD, Lauj Belanjer, Celine Roy, Colette Lemay. *Hospital of Medical College of Pennsylvania*: Peter R. Koury, MD, Michael Crawford, MD, Seth J. Rials, MD, Roger Marinchak, MD, Michael Koslow, MD, Ted Frieh, MD, Arthur Belber, MD, Brenda Esopi, RN, Patricia Bernard, RN, Lucy Smith, RN, Lynn Cunningham, I Kathy O'Connors. *Howard University Hospital*: Otelio S. Randall, MD, James Diggs, MD, Charles Cu, MD, Prafulla P. Mehrotra, MD, Yuyue Wong, Rcsea Associate; Zhenqui Huang, MD, Betty Deen, Bart Alexander, PhD. *The Jackson Clinic Foundation*: John Firnham, John H. Morledge, MD, Paul H. Hinderaker, A.D.), Gene Musser, MD, Donald Logan, Daniel Danahy, MD, Beth Sommerfield, RN, C; Shanle, Janice Burks; Dorothy Admas, Diane How, Norcric Streicher, Karen Woods, CNMT. *Jewish General Hospital*: John McCans, MD; David Langleben, MD; Claude Maranda, MD; Eileen Shalit; Elizabeth Graham; Gyongyi Belfer. K. *Kingston General Hospital*: John O. Parker, MD; Lynda Reid, Karen Lahey, RN; Kathy Webb; Micheline LaPlante; *LAVAL Hospital Quebec Heart Institute*: Gilles R. Dagenais, MD, Jacques Rouleau, MD; Claude Nadeau, MD; Francois DeLage, MD; Diane LaForge, Paule Bariville; Michael Sampson. *Lutheran General Hospital*: Richard Sorkin, MO); David H. Cooke, MD. Michael J. Rosen, MD; Tri Young, RN, Andi Schaechter, RN. *Massachusetts Medical Center*: Costas T. Lambrew, MD; Paul Sweeney, MD; Peter Shaw, MD; Pam Birmingham, RN; Suzanne Vermilya, *Massachusetts General Hospital*: Randall Zusman, MD; Joyce Higgins, RN; Denise Mullaney, RN, Donna Christensen, RN. *Mayo Clinic*: David Haves, Bernard J. Gersh, MD; Ian Clements, MD; Ann McLaughlin, RN; BSN; Judy A. Fletcher, RN. *Memorial University of Newfoundland*: Bruce A. Sus., MD; Mark Furey, MD: Bruce Josephson, MD; AI Williams; Bonnie S. Cochrane, RN; Bernadette Ingersoll. *Mount Sinai Medical Center*: Dale Adler, Donna Cramer; Barbara Leidner, PA-C. *Mount Sinai Medical Center, New York*: Milton Packer, MD; Joanna Maravel, BA; Richard Steingart, MD, Kantrowitz, MD; Stanley Katz, MD; Marrick L. Kukin, MD; Zeev Neuwirth, MD; Ramesh Dharawat, MD, Gerald Neuberg, MD, David Pinsky, MD; Meyer H. Abittan, MD; Peter Wilson, MD; William Sclwa MD; Josephine A. Sollano, RN; Mary Ellen Coglianese, RN; Suzanne Bilocleau, RN; Deborah Ahern, Nancy S. Hulhoff, RN; Mary Taylor, RN; George Titus Josef Michac. MD; Joseph Skarzynski, MD. *Oregon Heart Institute*: Sandra Lewis, MD; Carol Cook; Jane Huber, RN; Beth Moore, RN. *Sacred Heart Hospital*: Kirk Jacobson, MD; Loren C. Barlow, MD; Mark S. Heerema, MD; Frank H. Littell, MD; Mary P. Pugsley; Steven N. Butt; Cathy Hendrickson; Mary Jean Jacobson; Mareie Moore, RN; Susan Edwards. *Sharp Hospital*: Sidney C. Smith, Jr, MD; Peter Hoagland, MD, Irene Lama; Roberta Rogowski; Celene Peters; Hillary Kimes; Leann Chow; Tammy Finger; Debbie Nelson. *State University of New York*: Edward J. Brown, Jr, MD; Richard Joseph, MD; Fulvio Maxxucchi, MD; John Mannisi, Michael Zema, MD; Laura Teplitz. *Tulsa Heart Center*: Lofty L. Basta, MD; Arthur D. Hagan, MD; Gary Gershony; Judy King, RN, CCRN; Jolene Durham, RN. *University of Arizona/V.A. Medical Center, Tucson*: Steven Goldman, MD; Herschel Richter, MD; Julie Brandt, MSRN; Edwin Holcombe, LPN; Debbi Carrol, RN; Susan Bigda, RN; Cynthia Krome, RN; Mark Wenzell, RN. *University of Arkansas Medical School*: Ha Dinh, MD; Joseph Bissett, MD, Bonnie J. Baker, MD; Marvin L. Murphy, MD; Masood Khan, MD; Norma Tellez; Barbara Cotter, LPN; Ginny Hullihan. RN; Betty Allen; Stephanie Van Arsdale, RN; Sherry Killingsworth. *University of British Columbia*: Victoria Bernstein, MD; Susan Mooney. *University of California,*

Davis Medical Center: Ezra Amsterdam, MD; Robert Martschinske, MD; Linda Palmer; Doreen Arons; Larry Baker; Sherryl Kubel. *University of Connecticut Health Center*: W. David Hager, MD; Sharon Larkin, RN; Laura Kearney, RN; Arthur L. Riba, MD; Karen L. Waters, RN; Jeanne Mitchell, Milton J. Sands, Jr.; Martha Radford, MD; Joanne Folger, RN; Patricia Malone, Bernard Clark, MD. *University of Louisville*: Joel Kupersmith, MD; Jean Corwin, RN, MS. *University of Manitoba*: Thomas E. Cuddy, MD; Robert Hoeschen, MD; Michael Frais, MD; Pat Courcelles; Dale Bedard, RN, Angela Wiebe. *University of Maryland School of Nursing*: Stephen S. Gottlieb, MD; Mark Effron, MD; Michelle Weinberg, RN; Ken Tyler. *University of Massachusetts Medical School*: Joseph S. Alpert, MD; Joel Gore, MD: Joshua M. Creenberg, MD; Mary Ryan. RN; Cathy Mahan, RN. *University of Missouri*: Gregory C. Flaker, MD; RicharJ Webel, MD; William Wright; Barbara Russell, RN; Sondra Flaker, MD. *University of New Mexico*: Jonathan Abrams, MD; Bruce Shively, MD; Dolores Garcia, RN. *University of South Florida*: Stephen P. Glasser, MD; Douglas Schocken, MD;U.R. Shettigar, MD; Cameron L. Priesmeyer, RN. *University of Tennessee, Memphis*: Bela Hackman, MD; Edgar Shick, Jr, Ph.D; Jay M. Sullivan, MD; David Mirvis, MD; Jerald Insel; Beate Griffin, RN; Gene Frulla; Mary Mills; Susic Burnette, RN; Marsha Fulton-Crizer. *University of Texas at Galveston*: John M. Wallace, MD; Rajinder K. Bhalla, MD. *University of Toronto*: Patricia McEwan, MD; Zion Sasson, MD; Charles Lefkowitz; Paul Daly, MD; Kim Lunn; Beverly Carlyle; Mary Ann Christensen; Patricia Robertson, RN. *University of Wisconsin at Madison*: Neville Bittar, MD, Margaret Spatola; Yi-Jun Wu. *Victoria Hospital*: Malcolm Arnold, MD; Gail Burton; Lebarado Melenday, MD; Gilbert Hurwitz, MD; Keith Finnie, MD; John Imrit, MD; Michael Weingert, MD; Jane White. *Wadsworth Veterans Administration Hospital*: Bramah N. Singh, MD, PhD; Koonlawee Nademanee, MD; Maru N. Josephson, MD; Alison Fast, Mary Laska-Schoenbaum, RN. *Washington University School of Medicine*: Edward M. Geltman, MD; Allan S. Jaffe, MD; Julio E. Perez, MD; Daniel Bauwens, MD; Scott A. Brodarick, MD; Tom Martin, MD; Nancy Ricciotti, Colleen Schaab, RN; Jolene Buscetto.

REFERENCES

1. Hammermeister KE, DeRouen TA, Dodge HT. Variables predictive of survival in patients with coronary artery disease. Circulation 1979; 59:421–430.
2. Norris RM, Barnaby PF, Brandt PWT, Geary GG, Whitlock RMI, Wild CJ, Barratt-Boyes BJ. Prognosis after recovery from first acute myocardial infarction. Determinants of reinfarction and sudden death. Am J Cardiol 1984; 53:408–413.
3. The Multicenter Post-Infarction Research Group. Risk stratification and survival alter myocardial infarction. N Engl J Med 1983; 309:331–336.
4. Hutchine GM, Bulkley BH. Infarct expansion versus extension: two different complications of acute myocardial infarction. Am J Cardiology 1978; 41:1127–1132.
5. Easton LW, Weiss JL, Bulkley BH, Garrison JB, Weisfedlt ML. Regional cardiac dilitation after acute myocardial infarction. N Engl J Med 1979; 300:57–62.
6. Erlebackher JA, Weiss JL, Eaton LW, Kullman C, Weisfeldt ML, Bulkley BH. Late effects of acute infarct dilitation on heart size: a two dimensional echocardiographic study. Am J Cardiol 1982; 49:1120–1126.
7. McKay RG, Pfeffer MA, Pasternak RC, Markai JE, Come PC, Nakao S, Alderman JD, Ferguson JJ, Safian RD. Left ventricular remodeling after myocardial infarction: a corollary to infarct expansion. Circulation 1986; 74:693–702.
8. Fletcher PJ, Pfeffer JM, Pfeffer MA, Braunwald E. Left ventricular diastolic pressure-volume

relations in rats with healed myocardial infarction effects on systolic function. Circ Res 1981; 49:616–626.
9. Pfeffer JM, Pfeffer MA, Braunwald E. Progressive ventricular remodeling in rat with myocardial infarction. Am J Physiol 1991; 260:H1406–H1414.
10. Pfeffer JM, Pfeffer MA, Braunwald E. Influence of chronic captopril therapy on the infarcted left ventricle of the rat. Circ Res 1985; 57:84–95.
11. Pfeffer MA, Pfeffer JM, Steinberg CR, Finn P. Survival after an experimental myocardial infarction: beneficial effects of long-term therapy with captopril. Circulation 1985; 72:406–412.
12. Pfeffer MA, Lamas GA, Vaughan DE, Parisi AF, Braunwald E. Effect of captopril on progressive ventricular dilatation after anterior myocardial infarction. N Engl J Med 1988; 319:80–86.
13. Moyé LA, for the SAVE Cooperative Group. Rationale and design of a trial to assess patient survival and ventricular enlargement after myocardial infarction. J Am Cardiol 1991; 68:700–790.
14. Pfeffer MA, Braunwald E, Moyé LA, Basta L, Brown EJ Jr, Cuddy T, Davis BR, Geltman EM, Goldman S, Flaker GC. Effect of captopril on mortality and morbidity patients with left ventricular dysfunction after myocardial infarction—results of the Survival and Ventricular Enlargement Trial. N Engl J Med 1992; 327(10):669–677.
15. Moyé LA, Davis BR, Hawkins CM. Analysis of a clinical trial involving a combined mortality and adherence dependent interval censored endpoint. Stat Med 1992; 11:1705–1717.
16. Sutton MSJ, Pfeffer MA, Plappert T, Rouleau JL, Moyé LA, Dagenais GR, Lamas GA, Klein M, Sussex B, Goldman S, Menapace FJ, Parker JO, Lewis S, Sestier F, Gordon DF, McEwan P, Bersnsetin V, Braunwald E, for the SAVE Investigators. Quantitative two dimensional echocardiographic measurements are major predictors of adverse cardiovascular events following acute myocardial infarction. Circulation 1994; 89:68–75.
17. Sutton MSJ, Pfeffer MA, Moyé LA, Plappert T, Rouleau JL, Lamas G, Rouleau J, Parker JO, Arnold MO, Sussex B, Braunwald E, for the SAVE Investigators. Cardiovascular death and left ventricular remodeling two years after myocardial infarction: baseline predictors and impact of long term use of captopril: information from the survival and ventricular enlargement (SAVE). Circulation 1997; 96:3294–3299.
18. Yusuf S, Wittes J, Probstfield, Tyroler HA. Analysis and Interpretation of Treatment Effects in Subgroups of Patients in Randomized Clinical Trials. JAMA 1991; 2266:93–98.
19. Moyé LA, Pfeffer MA, Wun CC, Davis BR, Geltman E, Hayes D, Farntam DJ, Randall OS, Dinh H, Arnold JM. Uniformity of captopril benefit in the post infarction population: subgroup analysis in SAVE. Eur Heart J 1994; 15:(suppl B) 2–8.
20. Tsevat J, Duke D, Goldman L, Pfeffer M, Lamas G, Soukup J, Kuntz K, Lee T. Cost-effectiveness of captopril therapy after myocardial infarction. J Am Coll Cardiol 1995; 26:914–919.
21. Michel BC, Ai MJ, Remme WL, Kingma JH, Kragten JA, van Nieuwenhuizen R, van Hout BA. Economic aspects of treatment with captopril for patients with asymptomatic left ventricular dysfunction in The Netherlands. Eur Heart J 1996; 17:731–740.
22. Dubey SD. Adjustment of p-values for multiplicities of interconnecting symptoms. In: Buncher RC, Tsay JY, eds. Statistics in the Pharmaceutical Industry. 2d ed. New York: Marcel Dekker, 1994:513–527.
23. Gnosh BK, Sen PK. Handbook of Sequential Analysis. New York: Marcel Dekker Inc.,
24. Miller RG. Simultaneous Statistical Inference. 2d ed. New York: Springer-Verlag, 1981.
25. Rothaman RJ. No adjustments are needed for multiple comparisons. Epidemiology 1990; 1: 43–46.
26. Friedman L, Furberg C, DeMets D. Fundamentals of Clinical Trials. 3d ed. Mosby 1996:308.
27. Moyé, LA. P-value interpretation and alpha allocation in clinical trials. Ann Epidemiol 1998; 8:351–357.
28. Steingart RM, Packer M, Hamm P, Coglianese ME, Gersh B, Geltman E, Sallano J, Katz S,

Moyé L, et al. Sex differences in the management of coronary artery disease. N Engl J Med 1991; 325:226–230.
29. Pfeffer MA, Moyé LA, Braunwald E, Basta L, Brown EJ Jr, Cuddy TE, Dagenais GR, Flaker GO, Geltman EM, Gersh BJ. Selection bias in the use of thrombolytic therapy in acute myocardial infarction. JAMA 1991; 266(4):528–532.
30. Rouleau JL, Moyé LA, Pfeffer MA. A comparison of management patterns after acute myocardial infarction in Canada and the United States. US vs. Canada. N Engl J Med 328:779–784.
31. Rouleau JL, Champlain JD, Klein M, Bichet D, Moyé LA, et al. Activation of Neurohumoral Systems in Postinfarction Left Ventricular Dysfunction. Accepted. J Am Coll Cardiol 1993; 22:390–398.
32. Hall CH, Rouleau JL, Moyé LA, de Champlain I, Bichet D, Klein M, Sussex B, Packer M, Rouleau J, Arnold MO. N-Terminal proatrial natriuretic factor—an independent predictor of long term prognosis after myocardial infarction. Circulation 1994; 89:1934–1942.
33. Rouleau JL, Packer M, Moyé LA, de Champlain J, Bichet D, Klein M, Rouleau JR, Sussex B, Arnold JM, Sestier F. ‘‘Prognostic value of neurohumoral activation in patients with an acute myocardial infarction: effect of captopril.’’ J Am Coll Cardiol 1994; 24:583–591.
34. Vantrimpont P, Rouleau J, Ciampi A, Harel F, de Champlain J, Bicher D, Moyé L, Pfeffer M for the SAVE Investigators. Two-year time course and significance of neurohumoral activation in the Survival and Ventricular Enlargement (SAVE) study. Eur Heart J 1998; 10:1552–1563.
35. Pfeffer MA, Bomanski M, Rosenberg Y, Verter J, Geller N, Albert P, Hsia J, Braunwald E. Prevention of events with angiotensin-converting enzyme inhibition (the PEACE study design). Am J Cardiol 1998; 82:25H–30H.

20

STOP-Hypertension-2: The Swedish Trial in Old Patients with Hypertension-2

LENNART HANSSON

University of Uppsala, Uppsala, Sweden

LARS H. LINDHOLM

Umeå University Hospital, Umeå, Sweden

I. INTRODUCTION

The benefits of treating hypertension in the elderly, in terms of achieving reductions in cardiovascular morbidity and mortality, have been well documented in several prospective intervention studies (1–7). One of these trials, the Swedish Trial in Old Patients with Hypertension (STOP-Hypertension) (4), can be regarded as an immediate predecessor and a source of inspiration for the present trial, STOP-Hypertension-2 (8).

In 1991, a question had been raised regarding the usefulness of newer antihypertensive agents, specifically angiotensin-converting enzyme (ACE) inhibitors and calcium antagonists, in the prevention of cardiovascular morbidity in elderly hypertensives. To investigate this issue the present trial, STOP-Hypertension-2, was designed and initiated in 1991. It was decided to use virtually the same inclusion criteria as in STOP-Hypertension, that is, hypertensive men and women ages 70 to 84 with blood pressure 180 mm Hg systolic or higher, 105 mm Hg diastolic or higher, or both (Table 1). The only difference between the two trials was that patients with isolated systolic hypertension could be included in STOP-Hypertension-2. This was based on the positive findings in patients with isolated systolic hypertension treated with diuretics that were presented in 1991 in the Systolic Hypertension in the Elderly Program (SHEP) study (3), results that have later been

Table 1 Inclusion and Exclusion Criteria in the STOP-Hypertension-2 Study

Inclusion criteria
Men and women
Ages 70–84 years
Essential hypertension
Blood pressure $\geq$ 180 mm Hg systolic or $\geq$ 105 mm Hg diastolic, or both
Exclusion criteria
Secondary hypertension
Stroke or myocardial infarction less than 6 months before inclusion
Insulin-treated diabetes mellitus
Malignancy
Alcoholism
Dementia or other serious mental disorder

Abbreviation: *STOP*, Swedish Trial in Old Patients.

supported by two trials based on calcium antagonist therapy: the Systolic Hypertension in Europe (Syst-Eur) trial (6) and the Systolic Hypertension in China (Syst-China) trial (7).

The primary aim of the STOP-Hypertension-2 study was to compare cardiovascular mortality during conventional antihypertensive therapy, that is, diuretics, beta-blockers, or both, using exactly the same compounds as in STOP-Hypertension, to the effect of newer therapies, such as ACE inhibitors or calcium antagonists, in this regard (Table 2). For obvious ethical reasons, a long-term placebo control group was not contemplated. A secondary aim was to compare the three therapeutic alternatives—conventional therapy versus ACE inhibitors versus calcium antagonists in terms of their effect on cardiovascular mortality.

The scientific background and rationale of STOP-Hypertension-2 have already been described in some detail, as has a progress report focusing on the similar antihypertensive efficacy of the three therapeutic modalities (9,10).

II. METHODS

Baseline values in the study population at randomization are given in Table 3. The PROBE design (11) (Prospective Randomized Open Blinded Endpoint) was used, which is similar to routine clinical practice. Patients were randomized to one of three groups. In the first group they received conventional antihypertensive therapy, using diuretics or beta-blockers. Exactly the same drugs as in STOP-Hypertension (4) were used, that is, atenolol

Table 2 Endpoints in the STOP-Hypertension-2 Study

Primary endpoint
Fatal cardiovascular disease
Secondary endpoints
Fatal + nonfatal strokes and myocardial infarcts + other cardiovascular mortality
Diabetes mellitus
Atrial fibrillation
Congestive heart failure

Abbreviation: *STOP*, Swedish Trial in Old Patients.

Table 3 STOP-Hypertension-2: Baseline Characteristics at Randomization (Mean Values and %)

	All	Conventional therapy	ACE inhibitors	Calcium antagonists
Patients (n)	6614	2213	2196	2205
Age (years)	76.5	76.5	76.6	76.4
Males (%)	33.2	32.0	33.7	34.0
Recruited from				
STOP-Hypertension (%)	6.2	5.8	6.2	6.7
Supine BP (mm Hg)	194/98	194/98	194/98	194/98
Standing BP (mm Hg)	187/101	187/101	187/101	187/101
BMI (kg/m^2)	26.7	26.7	26.7	26.7
S-cholesterol (mmol/L)	6.4	6.4	6.4	6.5
S-triglycerides (mmol/L)	1.7	1.7	1.7	1.7
B-glucose (mmol/L)	5.6	5.6	5.6	5.5
Smokers (%)	9.0	8.8	9.4	8.8
History of				
Myocardial infarction (%)	3.1	3.3	2.7	3.4
IHD (%)	8.0	8.4	9.4	8.8
Stroke (%)	3.9	4.0	3.9	3.8
CHF (%)	1.9	1.5	2.3	2.0
Atrial fibrillation (%)	4.7	4.7	5.3	4.1
Other CVD (%)	5.1	5.2	5.2	4.8
Diabetes mellitus (%)	10.9	11.4	10.7	10.5

Abbreviations: *STOP*, *Swedish Trial in Old Patients*; *BMI*, body mass index; *BP*, blood pressure; *IHD*, ischemic heart disease; *CHF*, congestive heart failure; *CVD*, cardiovascular disease. (From Ref. 8.)

or metoprolol CR or pindolol or the fixed-ratio combination of hydrochlorothiazide plus amiloride (Moduretic®). In the second group, two ACE inhibitors were used, enalapril or lisinopril, and in the third group two calcium antagonists, felodipine or isradipine were used. The choice between the two ACE inhibitors or the two calcium antagonists was not randomized, nor was the allocation to any of the beta-blockers or the diuretic in the conventional treatment group.

The aim was to reach a supine blood pressure of 160/95 mm Hg or below. If this goal was not achieved with the first step of medication supplementary treatment was given (8). All endpoints were assessed by an independent endpoint committee, using strict and prespecified criteria for the approval of endpoints (9). The members of this committee were blinded to the treatment and the blood pressure levels of the patients with reported endpoints. Randomly selected centers were audited by an independent auditor.

The study was designed to have a statistical power of 90% to detect a 25% difference in cardiovascular mortality in a two-sided test at 5% significance between patients treated with conventional therapy or newer agents. This would provide an 80% power to detect a similar difference between any of the three therapeutic alternatives. As it turned out, there were more primary endpoints than expected and there was actually sufficient statistical power at the 80% level to show a 20% superior effect with any of the therapies, had there been one.

Analysis was by intention to treat. Cox regression analysis used time since randomization as a nonparametrically modeled time variable. The model adjusted for gender, for

Table 4 Supine Blood Pressure (mm Hg)

	Conventional	ACE inhibitors	Calcium antagonists
Randomization	194/98	194/98	194/98
1 month	173/88	174/89	172/88
6 months	165/85	167/86	167/85
12 months	165/85	167/86	167/85
24 months	163/84	164/84	165/84
36 months	161/83	163/83	163/82
48 months	161/82	162/82	162/82
54 months	158/81	159/81	159/80

Abbreviation: *ACE*, angiotensin-converting enzyme.
(From Ref. 8.)

baseline values of age and diastolic blood pressure, and for baseline status of diabetes and smoking. All calculations used Stata software (version 5).

III. RESULTS

A. Effect on Blood Pressure

The three therapeutic regimens were virtually identical in their blood pressure-lowering effect (Table 4).

B. Adverse Events

The reported adverse events, based on a 40-item questionnaire used at every visit, are summarized in Table 5. Adverse events are reported as the percentage of patients in each

Table 5 Percentage of Patients Reporting Adverse Events

	Conventional therapy	ACE inhibitors	Calcium antagonists
Dyspnea	11.8	7.3	8.5
Palpitations	2.9	5.3	7.9
Flushing	1.6	2.2	9.7
Headaches	5.7	7.7	10.0
Cold hands and feet	9.1	3.3	2.5
Bradycardia	3.7	0.8	1.4
Nightmares	5.8	1.4	2.0
Dry mouth	4.4	2.0	2.7
Ankle edema	8.5	8.7	25.5
Insomnia	4.3	1.8	2.3
Dry cough	3.7	30.1	5.7
Vertigo	27.8	27.7	24.5

Twelve of the most commonly reported side effects symptoms during the study. Symptoms that were present at randomization have not been included unless they reappeared at visit number six or later.
Abbreviation: *ACE*, angiotensin-converting enzyme.
(From Ref. 8.)

	Relative risk (95% CI)*		p
Cardiovascular mortality	0·99	(0·84–1·16)	0·89
All myocardial infarction	1·04	(0·86–1·26)	0·69
All stroke	0·89	(0·76–1·04)	0·13
All major cardiovascular events	0·96	(0·86–1·08)	0·49
Total mortality	1·01	(0·89–1·14)	0·92
Frequency of diabetes mellitus	0·96	(0·75–1·23)	0·77
Frequency of atrial fibrillation	1·09	(0·92–1·31)	0·32
Frequency of congestive heart failure	0·95	(0·79–1·14)	0·55

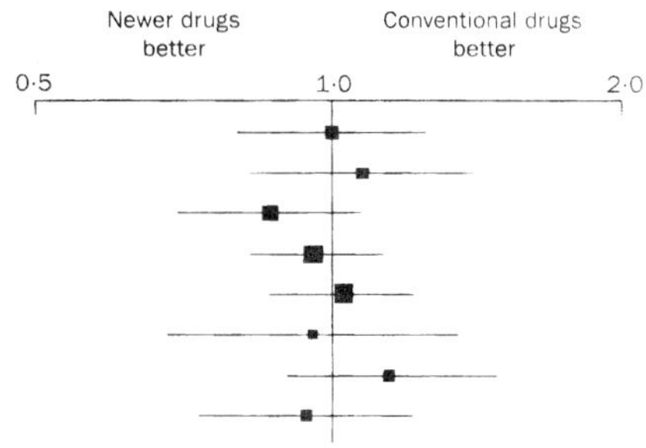

Fig. 1 Relative risk of cardiovascular mortality and morbidity for the newer drugs versus the conventional drugs. (From Ref. 8.)

of the three treatment groups who, at any time during the trial, reported the respective adverse event. To facilitate the presentation of these data, only the 12 most frequently reported adverse events or symptoms have been listed. Symptoms present at the time of randomization have not been included, unless they reappeared at visit number six or later. Extensive analysis of adverse effects will be presented in a separate publication.

C. Effect on Endpoints

Fatal cardiovascular events, the primary endpoint, occurred in 221 patients in the group treated with conventional therapy (19.8 per 1000 patient-years) and in 438 patients in the group treated with newer agents (19.8 per 1000 patient-years); relative risk 0.99 (95% confidence interval [CI] 0.84–1.16, $P = 0.89$).

Among the above-mentioned 438 fatal cardiovascular events, 226 occurred in patients taking ACE inhibitors (20.5 per 1000 patient-years) and in 212 patients taking calcium antagonists (19.2 per 1000 patient-years); the relative risks in comparison with conventional therapy were 1.01 (95% CI 0.84–1.22, $P = 0.89$) and 0.97 (95% CI 0.80–1.17, $P = 0.72$), respectively. The relative risk in the ACE inhibitor group, when compared with the calcium antagonist group, was 1.04 (95% CI 0.86–1.26, $P = 0.67$).

Fatal cardiovascular events in the three therapy groups, compared two at a time, are shown in Figures 1 to 4.

The combined endpoint of fatal and nonfatal stroke and fatal and nonfatal myocardial infarction plus other cardiovascular mortality occurred in 460 patients treated with

	Relative risk (95% CI)*		p
Cardiovascular mortality	1·01	(0·84–1·22)	0·89
All myocardial infarction	0·90	(0·72–1·13)	0·38
All stroke	0·90	(0·74–1·08)	0·24
All major cardiovascular events	0·94	(0·82–1·07)	0·32
Total mortality	1·02	(0·89–1·18)	0·76
Frequency of diabetes mellitus	0·96	(0·72–1·27)	0·77
Frequency of atrial fibrillation	1·15	(0·94–1·41)	0·18
Frequency of congestive heart failure	0·83	(0·67–1·03)	0·095

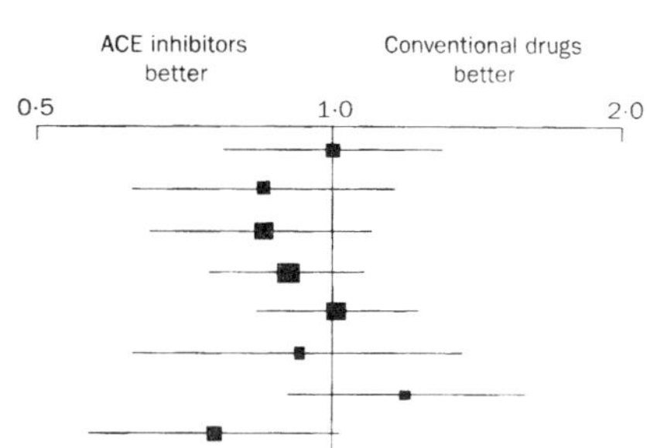

Fig. 2 Relative risk of cardiovascular mortality and morbidity for the ACE inhibitors versus the conventional drugs. (From Ref. 8.)

	Relative risk (95% CI)*		p
Cardiovascular mortality	0·97	(0·80–1·17)	0·72
All myocardial infarction	1·18	(0·95–1·47)	0·13
All stroke	0·88	(0·73–1·06)	0·16
All major cardiovascular events	0·99	(0·87–1·12)	0·85
Total mortality	0·99	(0·86–1·15)	0·90
Frequency of diabetes mellitus	0·97	(0·73–1·29)	0·83
Frequency of atrial fibrillation	1·04	(0·85–1·29)	0·68
Frequency of congestive heart failure	1·06	(0·87–1·31)	0·56

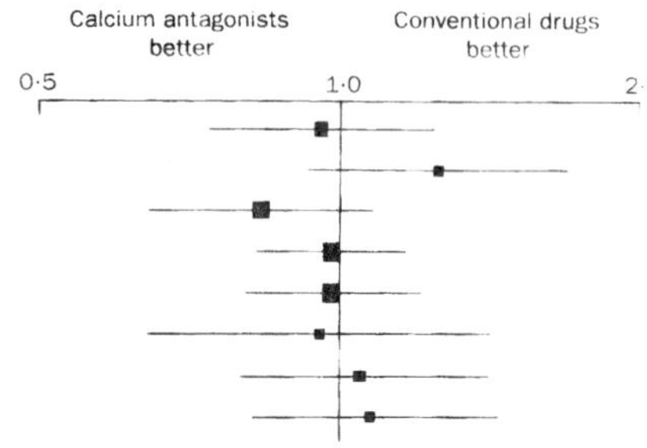

Fig. 3 Relative risk of cardiovascular mortality and morbidity for the calcium antagonists versus the conventional drugs. (From Ref. 8.)

conventional therapy (44.1 per 1000 patient-years) and in 887 patients treated with newer agents (42.8 per 1000 patient-years); relative risk 0.96 (95% CI 0.86–1.08, $P = 0.49$).

Of the 887 patients with the combined endpoint while taking newer therapy, 437 occurred in the ACE inhibitor group and 450 in the calcium antagonist group. The relative risks in comparison with conventional therapy were 0.94 (95% CI 0.82–1.07, $P = 0.32$) and 0.99 (95% CI 0.87–1.12, $P = 0.85$), respectively. The relative risk for patients treated with ACE inhibitors, as compared with those given calcium antagonists, was 0.95 (95% CI 0.83–1.08, $P = 0.42$).

This combined endpoint in the three therapy groups, compared two at the time, is shown in Figures 1 through 4.

No difference was seen in the incidence of fatal and nonfatal stroke between the three therapeutic regimens, nor was there any difference in the incidence of myocardial infarction when comparing conventional therapy against the other two regimens. However, there were significantly fewer fatal and nonfatal myocardial infarctions during ACE inhibitor treatment as compared with calcium antagonist treatment (12.8 per 1000 patient-years vs 16.7 per 1000 patient-years); relative risk 0.77 (95% CI 0.61–0.96, $P = 0.018$). Linked to this, and statistically not independent, there was also a lower incidence of congestive heart failure in the ACE inhibitor arm as compared with the calcium antagonist arm.

Total mortality and other secondary endpoints, such as the incidence of diabetes mellitus, atrial fibrillation, and congestive heart failure are shown in Figures 1 through 4.

	Relative risk (95% CI)*		p
Cardiovascular mortality	1·04	(0·86–1·26)	0·67
All myocardial infarction	0·77	(0·61–0·96)	0·018
All stroke	1·02	(0·84–1·24)	0·84
All major cardiovascular events	0·95	(0·83–1·08)	0·42
Total mortality	1·03	(0·89–1·19)	0·71
Frequency of diabetes mellitus	0·98	(0·74–1·31)	0·91
Frequency of atrial fibrillation	1·10	(0·90–1·34)	0·37
Frequency of congestive heart failure	0·78	(0·63–0·97)	0·025

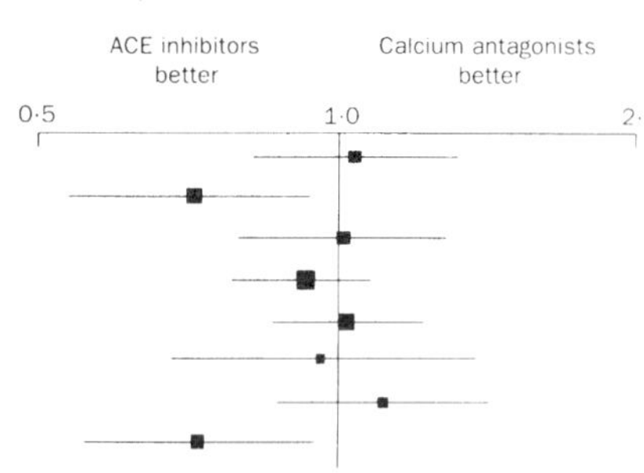

Fig. 4 Relative risk of cardiovascular mortality and morbidity for the ACE inhibitors versus the calcium antagonists. (From Ref. 8.)

The incidence of fatal and nonfatal cancer will be analyzed in detail and compared with the data of the National Cancer Register in Sweden. This will take the form of a special report.

IV. DISCUSSION

In this prospective intervention trial in 6614 elderly hypertensive patients, none was lost to follow-up. This was also the case in STOP-Hypertension (4), but the present trial was considerable longer and recruited more than four times as many patients.

More primary endpoints than expected were obtained, resulting in a statistical power of 94.6%, rather than the intended 90% for the principal analysis. Treatment with conventional antihypertensive agents, such as diuretics and beta-blockers, reduced blood pressure equally well as the newer classes of compounds, ACE inhibitors, and calcium antagonists. The prevention of cardiovascular mortality, the primary endpoint of the study, was also virtually identical when comparing the different therapies, the relative risks when comparing the various therapeutic alternatives being between 0.97 and 1.04 with narrow confidence intervals.

The fact that all the three therapies showed virtually no difference in their ability to prevent cardiovascular mortality and major cardiovascular morbidity is in agreement with the previously published Captopril Prevention Project (CAPPP), which showed no difference in major cardiovascular events in 11,018 hypertensive patients randomized to treatment with either conventional antihypertensive agents or an ACE inhibitor-based regimen (12). In CAPPP, there was some suggestion that an ACE inhibitor-based therapy might be less protective against stroke than conventional treatment with diuretics or beta-blockers (12). Although a plausible explanation that this was not the case was provided, it is reassuring that the present trial found no difference between the three therapeutic regimens in their protective effect against stroke.

The finding that calcium antagonists were not less effective than diuretics/beta-blockers in preventing cardiovascular events is a new observation. Previous intervention trials in hypertension in which calcium antagonists have been shown to reduce cardiovascular morbidity have all been comparisons with placebo (6,7,13).

The observation that fatal and nonfatal myocardial infarctions and congestive heart failure occurred at a significantly lower rate in patients treated with ACE inhibitors than in those receiving calcium antagonists can be seen as supporting the published results from the substudy of the Adequate Blood Pressure Control in Diabetes (ABCD) study (14). However, this observation should be interpreted with some caution, as 48 statistical comparisons were performed. Thus, the possibility of a chance finding cannot be excluded. In no other regard did the calcium antagonists prevent cardiovascular events less effectively than conventional antihypertensive agents or ACE inhibitors. This finding should put an end to any remaining concerns about safety of calcium antagonist when used appropriately, an opinion that has already been put forward (15,16).

It can be concluded that the STOP-Hypertension-2 results add information to the already accepted view that elderly hypertensive patients benefit from antihypertensive treatment in terms of showing reduced cardiovascular morbidity and mortality. Both older antihypertensive agents, such as diuretics and beta-blockers as well as newer agents, such as ACE inhibitors and calcium antagonists are useful in this regard. The choice between the various alternatives will obviously have to be related to other factors such as cost, side effects, and comorbid conditions. All these factors will be addressed in future papers based on the STOP-Hypertension-2 database. Thus, the preparation of reports on health economy aspects, cancer morbidity and mortality, and a detailed adverse events analysis have already been initiated. The report on adverse events will obviously also list these in relation to the ''on-treatment'' incidence, which may be more relevant than the ''intention-to-treat'' incidence provided here.

REFERENCES

1. Amery A, Birkenhäger W, Brixko P, Bulpitt C, Clement D, De Schaepdryver A, Dollery C, Fagard R, Forette F, Forte J, Hamdy R, Henry JF, Joossens JV, Leonetti G, Lund-Johansen P, O'Malley K, Petrie J, Strasser T, Tuomilehto J, Williams B. Mortality and morbidity results from the European Working Party on High Blood Pressure in the elderly trial. Lancet 1985; 1:1351–1354.
2. Coope J, Warrender TS. Randomised trial of treatment of hypertension in elderly patients in primary care. BMJ 1986; 293:1145–1151.
3. SHEP Cooperative Research Group. Prevention of stroke by hypertensive drug therapy in older persons with isolated systolic hypertension: Final results of the systolic hypertension in the elderly program. JAMA 1991; 265:3255–3264.
4. Dahlöf B, Lindholm LH, Hansson L, Scherstén B, Ekbom T, Wester P-O. Morbidity and mortality in the Swedish Trial in Old Patients with Hypertension (STOP-Hypertension). Lancet 1991; 338:1281–1285.
5. MRC Working Party. Medical Research Council trial of treatment of hypertension in older adults: principal results. BMJ 1992; 304:405–412.
6. Staessen JA, Fagard R, Thijs L, Celis H, Arabidze GG, Birkenhäger WH, Bulpitt CJ, de Leeuw PW, Dollery CT, Fletcher AE, Forette F, Leonetti G, Nachev C, O'Brien ET, Rosenfeld J, Rodicio JL, Tuomilehto J, Zanchetti A, for the Systolic Hypertension in Europe (Syst-Eur) Trial Investigators. Randomized double-blind comparison of placebo and active treatment for older patients with isolated systolic hypertension. Lancet 1997; 350:757–764.
7. Liu L, Wang JG, Gong L, Liu G, Staessen JA, for the Systolic Hypertension in China (Syst-China) Collaborative Group. Comparison of active treatment and placebo for older Chinese patients with isolated systolic hypertension. J Hypertens 1998; 16:1823–1829.
8. Hansson L, Lindholm LH, Ekbom T, Dahlöf B, Lanke J, Scherstén B, Wester P-O, Hedner T, de Faire U, for the STOP-Hypertension-2 study group. Randomized trial of old and new antihypertensive drugs in elderly patients: cardiovascular mortality and morbidity in the Swedish Trial in Old Patients with Hypertension-2 study. Lancet 1999; 354:1751–1756.
9. Dahlöf B, Hansson L, Lindholm LH, Scherstén B, Wester P-O. Ekbom T, Hedner T, De Faire U. STOP-Hypertension-2: a prospective intervention trial of ''newer'' versus ''older'' treatment alternatives in old patients with hypertension. Blood Press 1993; 2:136–141.
10. Lindholm LH, Hansson L, Dahlöf B, Ekbom T, Hedner T, De Faire U, Scherstén B, Wester P-O. The Swedish Trial in Old Patients with Hypertension (STOP-Hypertension-2): a progress report. Blood Press 1996; 5:300–304.
11. Hansson L, Hedner T, Dahlöf B. Prospective Randomized Open Blinded End-point (PROBE) Study: A novel design for intervention trials. Blood Press 1992; 1:113–119.
12. Hansson L, Lindholm LH, Niskanen L, Lanke J, Hedner T, Niklason A, Luomanmäki K, Dahlöf B, de Faire U, Mörlin C, Karlberg BE, Wester PO, Björck J-E, for the Captopril Prevention Project (CAPPP) Study Group. Effect of angiotensin-converting-enzyme inhibition compared with conventional therapy on cardiovascular morbidity and mortality in hypertension: the Captopril Prevention Project (CAPPP) randomised trial. Lancet 1999; 353:611–616.
13. Gong L, Zhang W, Zhu Y, Zhu J, 11 collaborating centres in the Shanghai area, Kong D, Pagé V, Ghadirian P, DeLorier J, Hamet P. Shanghai Trial of Nifedipine in the Elderly (STONE). J Hypertens 1996; 14:1237–1245.

14. Ad Hoc Subcommittee of the Liaison Committee of the World Health Organization and the International Society of Hypertension. Effects of calcium antagonists on the risks of coronary heart disease, cancer and bleeding. J Hypertens 1997; 15:105–115.
15. van Zwieten PA, Hansson L. Calcium antagonists and safety: the turning of the tide. Blood Press 1999; 8:5–8.
16. Staessen JA, Birkenhäger WH, Fagard RH. Dihydropyridine calcium-channel blockers for the treatment of hypertensive diabetic patients. Eur Heart J 2000; 21:2–7.

STEERING COMMITTEE

For the Swedish Hypertension Society:

Lennart Hansson MD, Uppsala (principal investigator), Björn Dahlöf MD, Göteborg (coordinator), Tord Ekbom MD, Lund (coordinator), Thomas Hedner MD, Göteborg, Ulf de Faire MD, Stockholm, Lars H Lindholm MD, Lund (secretary), Bengt Scherstén MD, Lund, and P-O Wester MD, Umeå.

For the sponsors:

Gunilla Eneroth, MSD, Christina de Flon, Hässle Läkemedel, Per-Erik Hörnkvist, Zeneca, Håkan Köhlmark, Sandoz, Christer Larsson, Hässle Läkemedel, Erland Linjer, Zeneca, Nils-Bertil Nilsson, MSD, Anders Tjerngren, Sandoz, and John Wengren, PharMed.

Study Secretary
Anita Holmner, Göteborg

Safety committee
Mats Ribacke MD, Stockholm, Hans Wedel PhD, Göteborg, and Lars Wilhemsen MD, Göteborg.

Endpoint committee
Kjell Asplund MD, Umeå, Leif Erhardt MD, Malmö, and Bengt Göran Hansson MD, Halmstad.

Statistician
Jan Lanke PhD, Lund.

Data auditor
Ola Samuelsson MD, Göteborg.

Coordinating center
Department of Medicine, Östra Hospital, Göteborg

Data handling center
Department of Community Health Sciences, Lund University

21

The Controlled ONset Verapamil INvestigation of Cardiovascular Endpoints (CONVINCE) Trial

WILLIAM J. ELLIOTT and HENRY R. BLACK

Rush-Presbyterian-St. Luke's Medical Center, Chicago, Illinois

JAMES D. NEATON and GREGORY GRANDITS

University of Minnesota, Minneapolis, Minnesota

T. DANIEL FAKOUHI

G. D. Searle & Co., Skokie, Illinois

I. INTRODUCTION

The Controlled ONset Verapamil INvestigation of Cardiovascular Endpoints (CONVINCE) trial is a randomized, double-blind, parallel-group, two-arm, actively controlled, multicenter, international, 5-year clinical trial involving 16,602 hypertensive patients with at least one additional cardiovascular risk factor. The CONVINCE trial was designed to compare the rate of fatal or nonfatal myocardial infarction (MI), fatal or nonfatal stroke, or cardiovascular disease-related death in two antihypertensive treatment regimens. One treatment arm begins with Controlled Onset Extended Release (COER™)-verapamil, which has its major antihypertensive effect 6 to 12 hours after administration. The other (''standard of care,'' SOC) arm begins with either hydrochlorothiazide (HCTZ) or atenolol, one of which is preselected by the investigator for an individual patient before randomization.

The enrolled patient population included hypertensive (blood pressure [BP] ≥ 140/90 on two occasions, or taking antihypertensive drug therapy) men or women, at least 55 years of age, with an established second risk factor for cardiovascular disease. Initial medications were: COER-verapamil (180 mg/day), HCTZ (12.5 mg/day), or atenolol (50 mg/day). Initial doses were doubled if BP did not reach goal (systolic BP $<$ 140 mm and diastolic BP $<$ 90 mm Hg). If BP was not controlled by the higher dose of the initial medication, HCTZ was added to COER-verapamil, or the SOC choice not initially selected was added in the SOC arm. An angiotensin-converting enzyme (ACE) inhibitor was recommended (although nearly any open-label medication was allowed) as the third step for patients whose BP was not adequately controlled, or if there was a contraindication to one of the two SOC medications. Patients take two sets of tablets daily, one in the morning and one in the evening. Although most patients switched from an established antihypertensive medication to randomized treatment, untreated patients with stages I to III hypertension (systolic blood pressure [SBP] between 140 and 190, or diastolic blood pressure [DBP] between 90 and 110 mm Hg) were also eligible. Outcomes were monitored by an independent data and safety monitoring board. Enrollment began in 1996, finished in 1998, and follow-up is expected to be completed in 2002.

II. OBJECTIVES OF CONVINCE

The primary and secondary objectives of CONVINCE are shown in Table 1. The CONVINCE trial is unusual in that its power calculation is based on the principle of demonstrating "equivalence" of the two therapeutic regimens in preventing the primary endpoint: nonfatal MI, nonfatal stroke, or cardiovascular disease-related death, whichever occurs first for a given patient. The secondary objectives of CONVINCE include both efficacy (#1 to 5 of Table 1) and safety issues (#5 to 13 of Table 1).

III. STUDY PROTOCOL

The design of CONVINCE is illustrated in Figure 1 (1). Eligible patients were randomized in a 1 : 1 ratio to either the COER-verapamil or SOC arm. Before randomization, the investigator decided which of two SOC drugs (HCTZ or atenolol) he or she thought was the better choice for that individual patient, should the patient be assigned to the SOC arm.

Randomization was stratified by clinical site and SOC choice within site. To maintain the double-blind nature of the study, a double dummy strategy was used: patients initially received two bottles of blinded tablets, one containing placebo and the other active medication. The SOC tablet (or matching placebo) was taken in the morning; the COER-verapamil tablet (or matching placebo) was taken at bedtime.

After randomization, patients were monitored monthly until goal BP ($<$ 140 mm Hg systolic AND $<$ 90 mm Hg diastolic) was achieved. If not, the dose of initial medication was doubled (step I, level 2; see Fig. 1). If goal BP was not achieved after a further month of blinded therapy, another blinded medication was added (step II, level 1): HCTZ + COER-verapamil or both SOC agents. The dose of the added medication may be doubled (step II, level 2) after a further month if BP remained uncontrolled.

Open-label medication may be added if blinded study medication was not tolerated, or if goal BP was not achieved, with step II medication. An ACE inhibitor was recommended as the initial open-label or step III drug. For patients with a history of cough or other problem with an ACE inhibitor, any antihypertensive medication was acceptable other than a nondihydropyridine calcium antagonist, beta-blocker, or thiazide diuretic. If step III treatment did not control the patient's BP, the investigator could switch to another

Table 1 Primary and Secondary Objectives of CONVINCE

Primary objective: To compare regimens starting with either COER-verapamil or a JNC-V-defined SOC drug (HCTZ or atenolol) for the prevention of the combined endpoint of nonfatal MI, nonfatal stroke, or cardiovascular disease-related death over a 5-year average period of follow-up.

Secondary objectives: To compare the two regimens for:

1. fatal or nonfatal stroke
2. fatal or nonfatal MI
3. death from cardiovascular disease
4. primary endpoints occurring between 6:00 AM and 12:00 noon.
5. nonfatal MI, nonfatal stroke, cardiovascular disease-related death, or hospitalization caused by one of the following: coronary artery revascularization or heart transplant, transient ischemic attack or carotid endarterectomy, angina pectoris, congestive heart failure, accelerated or malignant hypertension, renal failure (acute or chronic), or renal artery revascularization
6. all-cause mortality
7. incidence of cancer (excluding nonmelanoma skin cancers)
8. hospitalization because of bleeding (except intracerebral bleeding)
9. serious adverse events (as defined by the U.S. FDA)

In addition, because of concerns about safety and tolerability of the agents being studied, comparisons across regimens are planned for:

10. multiple event profiles over the course of the study*
11. proportion of patients using each step of treatment
12. average BPs and the proportion of patients at or below goal BP at each follow-up visit
13. the occurrence of withdrawal from blinded medication at each step of treatment.

* This secondary objective provides for statistical evaluation of patients who suffer sequential events (e.g., a nonfatal stroke followed by a nonfatal MI the next day, and an extension of the infarction 2 weeks later). The Kaplan-Meier method of comparing time-to-event curves censors all data after the first qualifying event, which necessitates a different method of comparing overall event rates.

Abbreviations: *CONVINCE*, Controlled ONset Verapamil INvestigation of Cardiovascular Endpoints; *COER*, controlled onset extended release; *JNC*, Joint National Committee; *SOC*, standard of care; *HCTZ*, hydrochlorothiazide; *MI*, myocardial infarction; *FDA*, Food and Drug Administration.

step III agent, increase the dose of the previously chosen agent, or add another open-label agent. If an agent that could be added at step II was contraindicated, step II could be omitted and open-label medication added to the step I regimen.

IV. ANALYSIS OF SAMPLE SIZE CALCULATIONS AND POWER ESTIMATES

The CONVINCE trial is a direct comparison of a proven versus a newer pharmacological agent with a chronobiologically based delivery system (2, 3). It followed the new paradigm for large, simple trials (4), that is, data collection is minimal and focused on the clinical endpoints of interest, and sample size was chosen to ensure that moderate differences between COER-verapamil and SOC in the primary endpoint would be ruled out if no significant difference was found between treatment groups. The analysis and monitoring plans are based on confidence intervals of the treatment hazard ratio (COER-verapamil vs SOC).

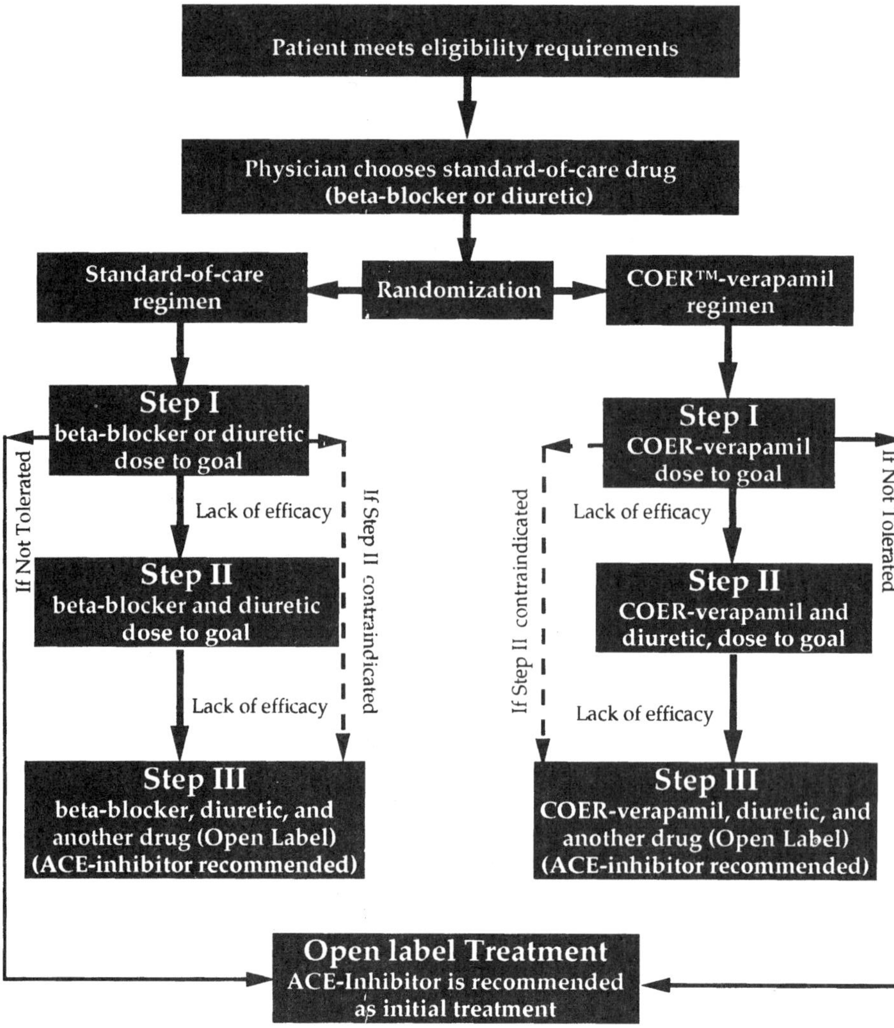

Fig. 1 Outline of treatment regimens for the Controlled ONset Verapamil INvestigation of Cardiovascular Endpoints (CONVINCE) trial. Note that if either hydrochlorothiazide (HCTZ) or atenolol is contraindicated, step II can be skipped (and the contraindicated medication would be omitted in step III treatment). There are two dose levels in each step of treatment.

A. Sample Size

Two key parts of the sample size calculation are the efficacy of the SOC regimen and the treatment difference between regimens to be detected. Several sources were used to estimate the former:

1. The meta-analysis of Collins et al. (5) indicated that BP treatment was associated with a 42% reduction in the odds of fatal/nonfatal stroke and a 14% reduction in the odds of fatal/nonfatal coronary heart disease (CHD), based on 773 strokes and 1442 coronary events. Combining these two endpoints by weighting the separate odds ratios by the number of events results in a 25% reduction in the odds of fatal/nonfatal stroke or CHD.

2. Since the overview by Collins et al. and the design of CONVINCE, three large placebo-controlled trials in the elderly were published (6–8) that have a pooled reduction in the odds of fatal/nonfatal cardiovascular disease (CVD) of 27.5%. If these three trials are combined with the overview of Collins et al., the pooled reduction is 26%.

3. These results do not specify the type of antihypertensive treatment. All but one (9) of these trials have used either a diuretic or beta-blocker initially. Our estimates for the odds of fatal/nonfatal CVD reduction for individual therapies agree with those of Psaty et al: (10) diuretic 28%; beta-blocker 12%; but far fewer trials using beta-blockers as initial therapy have been performed (11). If the choice of SOC in CONVINCE is estimated at 75% HCTZ and 25% atenolol, the weighted percentage reductions in the odds of fatal/nonfatal CVD is 24%.

This review of the clinical efficacy of SOC treatment led us to estimate that SOC would reduce the primary endpoint of CONVINCE by 24% to 28%, compared with no treatment.

The alternative hypothesis for the study was specified to ensure that a 50% loss of this efficacy of SOC with COER-verapamil (12% to 14%) could be detected with a high probability. This corresponds to a hazard ratio of COER-verapamil versus SOC between 1.16 (0.88/0.76) and 1.19 (0.86/0.72). For purposes of sample size, because the stated hypothesis is two-sided, for the alternative hypothesis, we considered alternatives ranging from 0.84 (1/1.19) to 0.86 (1/1.16) for the hazard ratio.

B. Other Sample Size Assumptions

1. The 5-year estimated CVD event rate in the SOC group is between 12.5 and 17.5%. In the Systolic Hypertension in the Elderly Program (SHEP), the 5-year SOC event rate was 8.9%. In an overview of nine trials in the elderly with few baseline CVD risk factors, there were 572 coronary or stroke events in approximately 32,000 years of follow-up (1.8 per 100 person-years). This gives an estimated 5-year rate of 8.5%. Because CONVINCE required at least one other CVD risk factor, we assumed the SOC event rate would be at least one third and possibly up to twofold higher, than this estimate. We also assumed that the event rate in the SOC group would increase by 6% each year.

2. The minimum follow-up was 4 years for each participant.

3. Enrollment was completed in 2 years; thus, the average period of follow-up was 5 years and some participants will be followed up for as long as 6 years.

4. Noncompliance to COER-verapamil was estimated at 7.5% in the first year and 3% each subsequent year. This rate of noncompliance was observed in the Treatment of Mild Hypertension Study (TOMHS) for the calcium antagonist, amlodipine (12).

5. Losses to follow-up for reasons other than death resulting from non-CVD were estimated at 1% per year.

6. Losses to follow-up because of non-CVD mortality were estimated at 1% per year, which was the rate in STOP-Hypertension, SHEP, and MRC studies (6–8).

7. No adjustments were made for noncompliance, as these rates were based on intent-to-treat analyses from the trials used. We assumed the level of compliance to SOC in CONVINCE should be similar to that observed in other hypertension trials in the elderly.

Table 2 gives sample size estimates for three hypothesized relative risk estimates (0.84, 0.85, and 0.86) and for three estimates of the 5-year fatal/nonfatal CVD event rate in the SOC group (12.5%, 15%, and 17.5%), based on a computer program developed by

Table 2 Sample Size for Two Groups (and Power for a Combined Sample Size of 15,000) for Three Levels of the 5-Year Event Rate in the SOC Group and for Three Hypothesized Relative Risks

	Sample size* (power for 2N = 15,000)		
Hypothesized relative risk† (COER-verapamil/SOC)	5-year event rate in SOC (%) 12.5	15.0	17.5
0.84	12,143 (0.88)	10,098 (0.93)	8,637 (0.96)
0.85	13,887 (0.83)	11,550 (0.89)	9,879 (0.93)
0.86	16,024 (0.77)	13,328 (0.84)	11,402 (0.90)

* Type I error = .05 (two-sided); power = 0.80; 10% lost to follow-up; 19.5% noncompliance to verapamil.
† Before consideration of noncompliance to COER-verapamil.
Abbreviations: *SOC*, standard of care; *COER*, controlled onset extended release.

Shih and Lakatos (13, 14). Power estimates are given in parentheses, assuming a combined sample size of 15,000.

In summary, if the 5-year event rate is 15% in the SOC group, CONVINCE is powered at 0.84 to detect a relative risk of 0.86 with 15,000 patients. The target number of events for this set of parameters is 2024. After taking into account noncompliance to COER-verapamil, losses, and the pattern of events in the SOC group, the realized relative risk corresponding to this set of parameters is 0.89. Thus, CONVINCE is very well powered to detect small, but clinically meaningful, treatment differences.

C. Planned Analysis and Monitoring

The approach to establishing equivalence is based on confidence intervals of the hazard ratio (COER-verapamil vs SOC) as described by Fleming (15). For interim analyses, the Lan-DeMets implementation (16) of the O'Brien-Fleming guideline (17) is used to formulate repeated confidence intervals. This approach allows for flexibility in frequency of interim analyses. It requires specification of the number of events in advance, which was originally estimated at 2024 for CONVINCE.

Monitoring guidelines are based on these confidence intervals. If the lower limit of the adjusted interval lies above 1.0, COER-verapamil would be inferior to SOC, as it is associated with greater risk of a primary endpoint. If the upper limit lies below 1.00, COER-verapamil is superior. If the interval includes 1.00 and is narrow, with its upper limit below 1.16 and its lower limit above 0.86, the treatment would be equivalent. If the interval contains 1.00 but is broader than that above, then the comparison is inconclusive.

D. Modifications to Original Sample Size

In the course of its regularly scheduled meetings, the CONVINCE data and safety monitoring board (DSMB) has assessed the progress of CONVINCE in meeting its various goals, including recruitment and statistical power. Because of a higher than originally anticipated rate of withdrawal from blinded study medications, the CONVINCE executive committee (on the recommendation of the DSMB) increased the number of enrolled patients to 16,600, and the target number of events to 2246. This upward adjustment of the numbers of patients and events needed was expected to maintain the statistical power of the study as originally planned. Although this modification of the original sample size obviously increased the cost and possibly the length of the study, it was implemented to assure appropriate statistical power in this equivalence study, which obviously would be threatened by an unanticipated increase in the numbers of patients not taking blinded study medication, which tends to bias toward the null hypothesis. Should the necessary numbers of events not occur by the planned end of the trial, the additional approach of increasing the average time of follow-up for patients could be implemented.

V. ELIGIBILITY CRITERIA FOR CONVINCE

The CONVINCE trial was designed according to the paradigm of the large simple trial (4) to maximize enrollment and generalizability of the conclusions to usual clinical practice, and to minimize exclusions, inconvenience, and cost of the study. Essentially any hypertensive person who has achieved his/her 55th birthday and has one additional traditional cardiovascular risk factor is eligible (see Table 3 for a list of inclusion and exclusion criteria). The exclusion criteria are simple, straightforward, and expected for a study that randomizes patients to blinded therapy with either verapamil, atenolol, or hydrochlorothiazide.

VI. MAIN RESULTS

The results of CONVINCE are expected in 2002. Preliminary data from the 16,602 patients enrolled in CONVINCE by 661 centers in 15 countries over 809 days have been presented (18). The participating population has an average age of 65.6 ($\pm$ 7.4 SD) years; 55.8% were women; 83.5% were taking antihypertensive drug therapy at randomization. Eighty-five percent were white, 7.3% black, 5.6% Hispanic, 1.7% Asian, and 0.5% ''other ethnicity.'' Average BP at enrollment was 150.0/86.6 mm Hg but was significantly higher among those not taking antihypertensive drug treatment (160.7/93.7 mm Hg). Atenolol or HCTZ was chosen as the standard-of-care choice for 52.3% or 47.7% of the patients, respectively. The percentages of patients with each concomitant traditional risk factor for cardiovascular disease were: overweight ($\geq$ 25% over ideal body weight or body mass index [BMI] $>$ 28.5 kg/m^2, 49.7%), dyslipidemia (31.7%), cigarette use (22.6%), diabetes (19.8%), known vascular disease (17.1%), left ventricular hypertrophy (11.7%), previous MI (7.8%), vascular bruit (4.9%), previous stroke (4.7%), or previous transient ischemic attack (2.1%). Fully 48.9% of the patients had more than one traditional cardiovascular risk factor (excluding hypertension and gender) at randomization.

VII. WHY CONVINCE WAS DONE

There are four major reasons why CONVINCE was done: (1) to provide evidence for a specific, novel formulation of a widely used calcium antagonist as an effective preventive agent against MI, stroke, or cardiovascular death in high-risk hypertensive patients; (2) to provide evidence from randomized, multicenter clinical trials that addresses suggestions from epidemiological and case-control studies that calcium antagonists are associated with an increased risk of MI, death, bleeding, or cancer; (3) to provide evidence that chronotherapeutically oriented blood pressure lowering may reduce the increase in cardiovascular events seen during the early morning hours; and (4) modern technology had matured to the point where it became feasible and economically possible to plan and launch this large, simple effectiveness trial for a chronic disease such as hypertension.

Table 3 Inclusion and Exclusion Criteria for CONVINCE

Inclusion Criteria for CONVINCE

1. Age ≥ 55 years
2. Current treatment for hypertension or diagnosed with hypertension: either
   Currently taking antihypertensive medication(s) for at least the last 2 months AND have SBP < 175 mm Hg and DBP < 100 mm Hg at the qualifying visit

OR

   Not taking antihypertensive medications OR medications for less than 2 months AND have 140 ≤ SBP ≤ 190 mm Hg or 90 ≤ DBP ≤ 110 mm Hg at the qualifying visit

3. Presence of at least one of the following conditions:
   History of MI > 12 months before randomization
   History of stroke > 6 months before randomization
   History of cigarette use (current or within the last 3 years)
   Type II diabetes mellitus (fasting plasma glucose > 140 mg/dL, [>7.8 mmol/L] on two occasions, or nonfasting plasma glucose > 200 mg/dL [> 11.1 mmol/L])
   Left ventricular hypertrophy by echocardiogram or electrocardiogram (either of which is already on file)
   Low HDL (< 35 mg/dL [< 0.9 mmol/L]), high LDL (> 159 mg/dL [> 4.11 mmol/L]), or high total cholesterol (> 250 mg/dL [> 6.46 mmol/L]) on two occasions in the 5 years prior to randomization
   History of transient ischemic attack with hospitalization
   Body weight ≥ 25% above ideal
   Presence of any known atherosclerotic vascular disease
   Presence of a vascular bruit
4. Written informed consent must be obtained before admission to CONVINCE

Exclusion Criteria for CONVINCE

1. History of congestive heart failure, NYHA classification II–IV
2. Cardiac dysrhythmias requiring medical treatment (such as beta-blocker, a calcium channel blocker, or other antiarrhythmic)
3. Secondary hypertension from any cause (such as pheochromocytoma, coarctation of the aorta, or renal insufficiency)
4. Sick sinus syndrome, heart block greater than first degree, bradycardia (heart rate < 55 BPM), or presence of Wolff-Parkinson-White or Lown-Ganong-Levine syndrome
5. Other contraindications to either COER-verapamil or **BOTH** HCTZ **AND** atenolol. A person with contraindication to either HCTZ or atenolol is eligible
6. Working an evening, night, or alternating shift
7. Known MI within 12 months or stroke within 6 months of randomization date
8. Known renal impairment (serum creatinine ≥ 2.0 mg/dL [≥ 177 μmol/L] or creatinine clearance < 30 ml/min)
9. Factors suggesting noncompliance with the protocol, such as current alcohol or drug abuse, clinical dementia, or history of missing appointments or doses
10. A disease likely to cause death within 5 years, such as untreated malignancy
11. The investigator's clinical judgment that the patient will not achieve adequate BP control using a three-drug regimen (diuretic, verapamil, or beta-blocker, and one other agent)
12. Any patient currently not receiving antihypertensive medication with SBP > 190 mm Hg or DBP > 110 mm Hg
13. Any patient with a medical condition at screening requiring treatment with any of the specific study medications (HCTZ, verapamil, or atenolol)
14. Previous admission to the study
15. Participation in another clinical trial of antihypertensive medications within 30 days of randomization

Abbreviations: *CONVINCE*, Controlled ONset Verapamil INvestigation of Cardiovascular Endpoints; *SBP*, systolic blood pressure; *DBP*, diastolic blood pressure; *MI*, myocardial infarction; *HDL*, high-density lipoprotein; *LDL*, low-density lipoprotein; *NYHA*, New York Heart Association; *BPM*, beats per minute; *HCTZ*, hydrochlorothiazide.

A. Do Calcium Antagonists Reduce Cardiovascular Morbidity/Mortality?

At the time that CONVINCE was planned, there was genuine equipoise in the scientific and medical community about whether any of the antihypertensive agents besides diuretics or beta-blocking agents were effective in primary prevention of cardiovascular events, including acute MI, stroke, or cardiovascular disease-related death. The Fifth Report of the Joint National Committee on Detection, Evaluation, and Treatment of High Blood Pressure preferred diuretics or beta-blockers and considered other (generally newer) agents to be alternative therapies (19). This distinction (although not the nomenclature) was reaffirmed in Joint National Committee (JNC) VI with reference to ''uncomplicated hypertension'' (20). At the time that CONVINCE was designed, very little evidence existed that calcium antagonists could reduce morbidity or mortality from cardiovascular events, despite their widespread clinical use for angina pectoris or hypertension (21). Many authorities decried the situation seen for many antihypertensive drugs: there appears to be an inverse relationship between revenue from sales and benefits demonstrated in clinical trials. Although this may be changing (22), concern still flourished that the newer agents typically have more heavily advertised putative advantages but fewer long-term studies demonstrating benefits in the important outcomes of cardiovascular morbidity or mortality.

Since 1995 (when CONVINCE was planned), several long-term, randomized studies have shown both primary and secondary prevention of cardiovascular events with calcium antagonists. For ethical reasons, only two of these studies have been placebo-controlled (23, 24), nearly all the others have active control arms, typically using one traditional treatment strategy. In the largest trial of active antihypertensive drug therapy to date, nearly 19,000 patients were treated to one of three diastolic BP goals: 90 mm Hg or lower, 85 mm Hg or lower, or 80 mm Hg or lower. Contrary to the hypothesis that BP must have a point below which further lowering is harmful, the Hypertension Optimal Treatment (HOT) study showed no significant worsening of prognosis in those with the lowest treatment goal; indeed, in diabetics, the best results were obtained with the diastolic BP of 80 mm Hg or lower (see Chapter 15). Although this study was not designed to test the efficacy of a calcium antagonist-based treatment regimen in reducing cardiovascular morbidity or mortality, follow-up had to be lengthened substantially because the rate of cardiovascular events in the treated patients was much lower than anticipated. This study supports the initial choice of calcium antagonists in reducing cardiovascular morbidity and mortality [especially in diabetic hypertensives (25)], although two smaller studies pitting an initial calcium antagonist against an ACE inhibitor noted worse outcomes in the diabetics randomized to the former (26, 27). The potential role of calcium antagonists in secondary prevention has been even less well explored in clinical trials in patients with angina pectoris, previous MI, or known cardiovascular disease. Although amlodipine has shown promise in subgroup analyses in recent trials in heart failure (28) or recurrent coronary ischemic events (29), the nondihydropyridine calcium antagonists, verapamil (30–33) or diltiazem (34, 35) have improved prognosis after an initial MI (36, 37).

B. Are Calcium Antagonists Safe in Long-Term Use?

For at least 3 years beginning on March 11, 1995, public and media attention was repeatedly drawn to multiple reports from epidemiological and case-control studies suggesting that, apart from not having shown the expected reduction in cardiovascular morbidity and mortality in hypertensive patients, calcium antagonists were actually associated with an *increased* risk of acute MI (38), death (39), bleeding (40), or cancer (41–43). This issue has been intensely debated (44–52), with accusations of conflicts of interest (53) and media manipulation by special interest groups (54), and has resulted in a moratorium being placed on further publications on this topic in some journals until and unless prospective data are gathered (55). Because approximately 28% of hypertensive Americans are currently taking calcium antagonists, the interests of the public health would be well served if this question could be easily answered, soon. As is perhaps typical of alarming medical news, later contradictory reports, which tend to be reassuring to the population, garner less media attention.

The Antihypertensive and Lipid Lowering [Prevention of] Heart Attack Trial (ALLHAT), the largest trial of antihypertensive agents so far undertaken, will provide some of the prospective, randomized clinical trial data needed to address these important questions about the safety of calcium antagonists (see Chapter 22) (56). However, only 20% or less of the enrolled patients are likely to receive amlodipine for 5 years; the expected incidence of bleeding, cancer, or death from other causes is expected to be small and, therefore, of limited statistical power (57). The planned analyses of the WHO/ISH Collaborative Clinical Trialists will certainly be helpful (22), but there may be differences in homogeneity among these trials because of the different pharmacology of the dihydropyridine and nondihydropyridine calcium antagonists [verapamil is often given before chemotherapy for its putative benefits in reducing the emergence of drug-resistant clones of cancer cells (58)]. Thus, data derived from a blinded, randomized clinical trial to assess the long-term safety of verapamil, a very widely used agent for many cardiovascular and other conditions, will be welcome.

C. Is Chronotherapeutics a Useful Concept for Preventing Cardiovascular Events?

A third reason CONVINCE was done using a novel formulation of verapamil was the growing body of evidence in support of chronobiology and its importance in many clinical conditions. The work of Halberg (59), Smolensky (2), Muller (60–62), and others has made clear that many biological phenomena have a clear circadian variation. Recent meta-analyses of the world's literature on acute MI, sudden cardiac death, and stroke have shown a 40%, 29%, and 49%, respectively, increased risk of these events during the early morning (6:00 AM–12:00 PM) hours (63, 64). Many believe these phenomena, as well as angina pectoris, silent myocardial ischemia, and cardiac arrest, have their origins in a similar circadian variation in BP, heart rate, plasma catecholamines, platelet aggregability, and clotting factors, all of which also peak in the early morning hours (3).

Apart from making this compelling pathophysiological link, the concept of chronobiology has recently been extended into ''chronotherapeutics,'' which can be defined as an attempt at matching the delivery of a medication to the timing of the illness (2). Thus, several therapies for asthma reduce the typical nighttime increase in episodes of reactive airways (65), H_2-blockers have improved efficacy and fewer adverse effects when given at night (when gastric acid secretion is unopposed by buffering food (66), and the first positive results in the primary prevention of cardiovascular events were obtained when an HMG-CoA reductase inhibitor was given after dinner, when both the intake and synthesis of cholesterol are maximal (67).

A new preparation of verapamil, the first long-acting calcium antagonist approved for the treatment of hypertension in the U.S., is based on this principle of chronotherapeutics. COER-verapamil evolved from the Gastro-Intestinal Therapeutic System (GITS) and incorporates a ''delay-coat'' into the tablet that prevents gastrointestinal fluid absorption by the pill until 4 to 8 hours after oral administration (68–70). Taking the tablets at bedtime effectively prevents delivery of verapamil during the night, when BP is at its nadir, and leads to maximal plasma levels of verapamil in the early morning hours, when BP and pulse are the highest of the day. When verapamil is administered by the COER-24 delivery system to appropriate patients, there is a dose-related lowering of BP (71) and prevention of angina pectoris (72, 73). One of the important secondary outcomes of great interest in CONVINCE is the comparison of regimens and their ability to prevent the stroke, MI, or cardiovascular disease-related death that appears to be greatest in the early morning hours. It might be predicted that the regimen beginning with COER-verapamil (designed to have its greatest effect at this time of day) might be more effective in reducing both BP and heart rate than another medication (e.g., HCTZ or atenolol), which is ingested after arising, when both BP and heart rate have already nearly peaked (74). To address this question, all CONVINCE investigators are being asked to provide the time of day of occurrence for all primary endpoints; this is also the reason for excluding shift workers, whose increase in BP occurs before their awakening, not at the typical 6:00 AM to 12:00 PM period seen in those who arise between 6:00 AM and 8:00 AM.

D. Can Large, Simple Trials Be Done Cost Effectively over the Long-Term in Hypertension?

The concept of performing large, simple trials has been pioneered by the Oxford Group, typically observing for a short time many thousands of simple to enroll, high-risk patients into randomized treatment at many clinical sites (4). Obviously, the logistics and cost-effectiveness of this style of trial are more favorable in secondary prevention (e.g., survivors of acute MI) than in primary prevention, and with only a single intervention (e.g., thrombolysis) as compared with sustained treatment. Until recently, when considering a hypertension study, the many thousand pages of case report forms, the millions of pills needed, and the thousands of person-hours of monitoring the study were essentially insurmountable barriers to all but the most courageous, intrepid, and well-funded agencies.

In this era of evidence-based medicine, it is extremely important to provide proof of treatment strategies derived not only from the traditional efficacy studies performed by specialists in research clinics, but also effectiveness studies done by generalist physicians treating patients in the standard fashion in traditional medical settings. The idea of large simple trials was pioneered to provide such data (4) but has not been possible to implement over the long term in primary prevention studies because of the increased cost and complexity. The CONVINCE trial may be one of the first large simple trials of treatment of a chronic disease that attempts to make the research study: (a) as much like clinical practice as feasible for a double-blind, randomized trial; (b) maximize recruitment and generalizability of the conclusions; and (c) minimize exclusion criteria, data to be collected (especially regarding endpoints), and the ultimate cost of the trial (4).

The CONVINCE trial was designed when a large number of technological steps made possible a much more cost-effective study design than would have previously been conceivable. The use of a central computer, accessed by the common telephone keypad and an interactive voice response system (IVRS), for enrollment, drug dispensing, monitoring, and quality assurance has greatly simplified the management of this trial (1). The IVRS is estimated to have saved approximately 50% of the storage space and 60% of the dispensed pills, compared with the traditional single complete package per patient. The IVRS has taken over much of the day-to-day inventory, dispensing, and quality control work, which involves six different languages, 15 countries, 12 time zones, and 15 possible combinations of randomized pills. The initial provision of the physician-directed choice of HCTZ or atenolol as the SOC choice would have been much more difficult and costly without the IVRS.

Technological progress has also allowed a great deal of the paperwork associated with clinical trials to be minimized. The case report forms for CONVINCE have been streamlined into a maximum of 6 pages, which are transmitted by facsimile to a centralized data registry where they are entered into a database. Clinical site training has also been modernized, with two instructional videotapes, an Internet site for posting and distribution of study-related information (e.g., the protocol, manual of operations and procedures, sample informed consent document, and newsletter), and frequent teleconferences to maintain morale and dedication of clinical site personnel.

VIII. STRENGTHS AND WEAKNESSES OF CONVINCE

The major strength of CONVINCE is the large number of patients enrolled by a dedicated corps of investigators to address questions about the efficacy and safety of a novel formulation of a calcium antagonist in the long-term treatment of high-risk hypertensive patients. The CONVINCE trial may allow us to get around some of the limitations of most efficacy trials while yet retaining the gold standard characteristics of double-blind, multicenter clinical trials (75).

Black and Crocitto (75) recently called attention to the disparity between smaller complex trials and general clinical practice, and the fact that the conclusions derived from the older-style small complex trials were rarely generalizable to most patients. They proposed a solution for this dichotomy, namely the large simple trial, which can be compared favorably to the traditional small complex trial across several important parameters (Table 4). The major advantages of this type of large simple trial are: such trials accurately reflect the real world of clinical practice; they are much less expensive than the small complex trial; they address issues of the value of treatment for conditions in which the best treatment is uncertain; and they enroll all of the subgroups of patients who are likely to receive the therapy in broad medical practice. The disadvantages are that because only a small amount of information is collected in a large simple trial, there is little possibility of adequately examining questions after data collection has begun; such trials may miss the value of treatment in specific subgroups not adequately identified in the planning stage; there is

Table 4 Comparisons of Small, Complex Trials and Large, Simple Trials

Parameter	Small, complex trials	Large, simple trials
Sample size	Small to moderate	Very large
Setting	Specialized clinics	General practice offices
Training	Trained researchers	General physicians
Exclusions to enrollment	Many	Few
Cost per patient	Expensive	Inexpensive
Proof derived	Efficacy ("it can work")	Effectiveness ("it does work")
Conclusions	Focused	Generalizable

little academic or financial incentive for investigators and relatively few benefits to subjects; and the possibility exists that study conduct may be abbreviated, attention may suffer, and the trial may be characterized as sloppy.

The weaknesses of CONVINCE have yet to be fully revealed, primarily because enrollment has just been completed. The two disappointments to date are the relatively large proportion of patients who have discontinued blinded study medication (which had to be overcome by increasing the number of enrolled patients over the originally projected 15,000 to maintain study power), and the relatively slow accrual of primary and secondary study events. It is likely that the latter problem will also be overcome, particularly since the spotlight of study monitoring can soon be turned away from recruitment and onto the very important issue of timely reporting of outcome events.

One important attribute of CONVINCE, which is both a strength and weakness, is the preselection process performed by the investigator to use either the diuretic or beta-blocker as standard of care choice for the individual patient. During the design of CONVINCE, much discussion involved which medication should be mandated for the SOC arm (1). Many experts favor initiating treatment in the elderly with low-dose thiazide diuretics (20, 76, 77), but many practicing physicians instead prefer beta-blockers (21, 78, 79), despite little favorable evidence from clinical trials for primary prevention in this at-risk population (11). This dilemma was solved for CONVINCE in a truly Solomonic fashion by allowing investigators to choose either agent for each individual (as they would normally do in routine clinical practice). Although this policy is totally in keeping with the principles of a large simple trial, it opens the trial to post hoc criticism if too large a proportion of the patients have the (presumably less effective, based on current evidence) beta-blocker as their SOC choice. This may be yet another example that few practicing physicians follow guidelines promulgated by national or international authorities (21, 77–82). Preliminary data indicate that atenolol was the more common choice (52.3%) over HCTZ. This may be slightly at odds with the baseline assumptions used in the sample size calculation but is unlikely to threaten the validity of the entire study. The strength of CONVINCE in this area is that it has documented exactly what choices practicing physicians make. The weakness is that there may not be sufficient statistical power in CONVINCE for comparisons of outcomes of patients who received either the beta-blocker or the diuretic as the SOC choice. This potential deficiency will likely be overcome in analyses planned across classes of antihypertensive agents for the individual patient-based registry of international hypertension trials (22). The fact that the majority of physicians chose atenolol for the CONVINCE SOC arm may turn out to have been unfortunate if recently summarized data about the reduced efficacy of beta-blockers in preventing cardiovascular events in elderly hypertensives is verified (11). If, however, beta-blockers are actually more effective than the efficacy trials indicate (a view consistent with the 661 experienced physicians choosing therapy for patients in this study), CONVINCE may break new scientific ground. There may even be the possibility of a post hoc analysis comparing each of the two SOC regimens with the COER-verapamil arm, as roughly half the patients were treated initially with HCTZ and half with atenolol.

The anticipated difficulties with different cultural, national, and language barriers have largely been overcome because of the recognition of hypertension as a major risk factor for poor clinical outcomes in all CONVINCE countries. The technological advances of the last few decades in telephone, computer, and communications technology have all assisted in overcoming many of the common and expensive barriers to implementation of large clinical studies. Finally, the dedication and perseverance of many investigators, clinical site personnel, patients, and decision-making officials of the sponsor (who delegated responsibility for actually running the study to the fully independent executive committee) are likely to be rewarded in a few years when the final results of CONVINCE are known.

APPENDIX

CONVINCE Research Group Investigators

The committees and investigators at the clinical sites of CONVINCE are listed below.

Executive committee: Henry R. Black, M.D., Chair (primary principal investigator); Robert J. Anders, Pharm.D. (ex-officio); Tracy Lucente, CONVINCE senior project director (ex-officio); Richard H. Grimm Jr., M.D., Ph.D.; Lennart Hansson, M.D., Ph.D., Yves Lacoucière, M.D., James Muller, M.D., James D. Neaton, Ph.D. (ex-officio); Peter Sleight, M.D., Michael A. Weber, M.D., William B. White, M.D., Gordon Williams, M.D., Janet Wittes, Ph.D., Alberto Zanchetti, M.D., and a PAREXEL representative (ex-officio).

Endpoints committee: William B. White, M.D., Chair; William C. Cushman, M.D., William A. Frishman, M.D., Norman K. Hollenberg, M.D., Ph.D., Thomas G. Pickering, M.D., D. Phil., Thomas R. Price, M.D., and Dominic A. Sica, M.D.

Publications and ancillary studies committee: Richard H. Grimm Jr., M.D., Ph.D., Chair; Stephen P. Glasser, M.D., Gregory M. Grandits, M.S., Suzanne Oparil, M.D., Ronald M. Prineas, M.B.B.S., Ph.D., and Carolyn Kong (ex-officio).

Data safety and monitoring board: Lawrence S. Cohen, M.D., Chair; Lawrence M. Brass, M.D., David DeMets, Ph.D., Charles K. Francis, M.D., Daniel M. Kolansky, M.D., and Richard C. Pasternak, M.D.

CONVINCE principal investigators (by country, with country leader listed first):

Brazil: Décio Mion Jr., Fernando Antonio de Almeida, Iran Castro, Kátia Coelho Ortega.

Bulgaria: Tihomir Dascalov, Atanas Djurdjev, Anna Elenkova, Mladen Grigorov, Vallentina Grigorova, Roumiana Kermova-Grigorova, Christo Kojukharov, Georgi Kussitassev, Svoboda Lovdjieva, Stefan Mantov, Choudomir Nachev, Nikolay Penkov, Svetla Torbova, Christo Tsekov.

Canada: Yves Lacourcière, Carl Abbott, Michael Alexander, Don Allan, Ronnie Aronson, John Atherstone, Marie-Claude Audet, Murray Awde, Gordon Bailey, Robert Beattie, Michael Bentley-Taylor, Bruno Bernucci, Peter Bolli, Remi Bouchard, Ted Brankston, Ellen Burgess, Mathew Burnstein, Denis Callaghan, J. Harry Callaghan, Douglas Carmody, Richard Casey, Josette Castel, Martyn Chilvers, Paolo Costi, Benoit Coulu, David Crowley, I. Dan Dattani, John Davies, Jacquest de Champlain, Eric Deemsted, Sanjay Dhingra, Frank Doane, Peter Dzongowski, Connie Ellis, Neil Filipchuk, Daniel Garceau, Roger Hamilton, Paul Handa, Roy Harding, Kenneth Heaton, Breet Hennefant, James Hii, Kkandker Hoque, Marc Houde, William Hughes, Jamie Hynd, Saul Isserow, Christopher Janz, Martin Juneau, David Kendler, Carter Kennedy, Mahesh Khurana, Jan Kornder, Simon Kouz, Christopher Lai, Daniel Landry, High Langley, Pierre Larochelle, Claude Lauzon, Jacobson Le Roux, Roland Leader, Monique LeBlanc, Larry Leiter, Jacquest Lenis, Richard Lewanczuk, John Li, Robert Luton, Patrick Ma, Jonathan MacKenzie, Jamuna Makhija, Dan Malone, Jean-Marie Martel, Murray Matangi, Grant Matheson, Guiseppe Mazza, Tom McAvinue, Sheila McGrath, William McKeough, Jeanne McNeill, Pravine Mehta, Adrien Melanson, Karim Merali, Phil Morris, Robert Morrison, Shah Nawaz, Robert Nitkin, Brian O'Kelly, William O'Mahony, Robert Orchard, Yves Pesant, Robert Petrella, Denis-Carl Phaneuf, Eric Poulin, Brendan Quinn, J. Lloyd Reddington, Maurice Roy, Terrance Ruddy, Luis Salgado, Michel Sauve, Daniel Savard, Gulshan Sawhney, Larry Schmidt, Vyta Senikas, Daniel Shu, Duncan Sinclair, Randell Smith, David Spence, Richard St-Hilaire, James A. Stone, Bruno St-Pierre, Jim Swan, Paul Talbot, Kim-Weng Tan, Sheldon Tobe, Luc Trudeau, Alain Vanasse, Pradeep K. Vohora, Lorne Weiner, Richard Whatley, Paul Whitsitt, Mark Wilkinson, Noel Wright, Henry Wu.

Czech Republic: Renata Cifkova, Ivan Gregar, Petr Jansky, Milena Kubickova, Helena Nemcova, Petr Petr, Ivana Popdrapska, Borivoj Semrad, Jarmila Siegelova, Miroslav Soucek, Zdenek Vomacka, Eva Zidkova.

Germany: Karl Heinz Rahn, Stefan Gesenhues, Ranier Häge, Holger Kinkernagel, Roland Schmieder, Jürgen Steinhauer, Henning Wiswedel, Wolfram Zingler.

Hungary: Csaba Farsang, Miklos Csanady, Istvan Edes, Katalin Fugedi, Tamas Gexatesi, Czuriga Istvan, Tarjan Jeno, Ilona Pap, Andras Papp, Julit Rapi, Gyorgy Sallai, Matyas Sereg, Ferenc Szaboki, Sandor Timar, Peter Valyi, Gabor Veress.

Israel: Reuven Viskoper, Lora Bregman, Henya Brenner, Hedi Feibel, A. Feldman, Jos' Fidel, Horla Flandra, Cilia Furman, Uzi Gafter, Jihad Ghanem, Adiv Goldhaber, Israel Hochman, Adrian Iaina, Gennady Katz, Eldad Kisch, Israel Lupinski, Alon Margalit, Oscar Minuchin, Joseph Mishael, Olga Moskovich, Shmuel Oren, Ester Paran, Eduardo Podjarni, R. Prilug, Joseph Rosenfeld, Eli Rottenstreich, Roza Schneider, Pessah Shvartsman, Eugene Shveydel, Natali Shveydel, Naftali Stern, Alexander Strolovich, Joshua Weissgarten, Yoram Yagil, Chaim Yosefy, Hoze Zabludowski.

Italy: Alberto Zanchetti, Paolo Alboni, Ettore Ambrosioni, Santo Branca, Alberto Caiazza, Agostino Colli, Giuseppe Crippa, Antonio D'Avanzo, Umberto De Martino, Giuseppe De Venuto, Ezio Degli Esposti, Valter Donadon, Giovanbattista Ippoliti, Giuseppe Licata, Francesco Locatelli, Carlo Martines, Andrea Mezzetti, Lucio Mos, Ernesto Mossuti, Angelo Musco, Carlo Pasotti, Carlo Passaglia, Francesco Pellegrini, Alessandro Rappelli, Piera Recalcati, Esio Ronchi, Ermanno Rossi, Paolo Saba, Antonio Salvetti, Mauro Sasdelli, Giuseppe Seghieri, Andrea Semplicini, Umberto Senin, Ernesto Sgarbi, Evandro Tascione, Alvaro Vaccarella, Enrico Vincenzo Valvo, Luigi Vigna.

Mexico: Roberto Z. Bravo, Pedro C. Fajardo, Francisco J.M. Guerrero, Jorge A. Herrera, Demetrio G. Kosturakis, José Luis P. Leyva, Humberto R. Rodriguez, Eugenio Z. Ruesga, Gerardo R. Velasco.

Poland: Barbara Krupa-Wojciechowska, Marianna Janion, Krystyna Jaworska, Marek Jedras, Alicja M. Kostecka-Pokrysko, Barbara Kusnierz, Michal Ogorek, Wojciech Sodolski, Henryk Swierzy, Eugeniusz Szmatloch, Bozena Raszeja Wanic.

Slovakia: Jan Murin, Andrej Dukát, Jozef Gonsorcík, Gabriela Kaliská, Soña Kiñová, Mária Radomská, Alexander Ruttkay, Rafael Rybár.

Spain: Luis Miguel Ruilope, Jose-Javier Antón, Joaquin Aracil, Pedro Aranda-Lara, Julián Arenas, Andrés Ariza, Juan-Francisco Ayala, Manuel Barcariza, José Barber, M. Jesús Barreda, Manuel-Carlos Barreiro, Joan Bayó, Pedro Cabrera, Carlos Calvo-Gómez, Isable Camé, Jesús Chamorro, Josep Closas, Antonio Coca-Payeras, Natividad Cordero, Rodrigo Córdoba, Juan-Ramón Cuervo, Antoni Dalfó, José-Javier De-Castro, Alberto-J. del-Alamo, V. del-Yerro, Rafael Durá, Severo Fernandez, Angel-Pedro Fernández, Ramón Ferrer, Juan-Eugenio Forcada, Vidal Francisco-Javier, José-Javier Garcia, Blas Gil-Extremera, Manuel Gómez, Apolo Gonzáles, Gonzol Iriarte, Juan-Jose Jimenez, Jose-Ignacio Jimenez, Pedro Jimenez, Jose Luis Llisterri, Jesús López, Carlos López, Juan-Carlos López, Francisco-Javier Lora, Alberto-J. Ma-Jesus, Agustin Martinez, Jesús

Martin-Garcia, Fernando Mato, Agustin Minguez, José-Ramón Moliner, Francisco Morales, Manuel Nieto, Javier Nieto-Iglesias, Esther Nuñez, Diego Nuñez, Josefina Oliván-Martinez, Francisca Paniagua, Juan-Carlos Pedrosa, José-Francisco Pensado, Julio Perete, Alvaro Pérez, Pablo Pérez-Luengo, Ascunción Peset, Jaume Plana, M. Angeles Pontes, Miguel-Angel Prieto, Luis-Antonio Ramilla, Salvador Rey, Mercedes Rodriguez, Carlos Rodriguez, Rafael Roldan, Victor Romero, Montserrat Roures, Manuel Royo, Antonio Ruiz, Jaime Ruiz, Aldjandro Salanova, M. Amor Sanchez, Javier Sobrino, Josep Soler, José-Luis Tena, Fernando Torguet, José Torres, Irama Valero, Fernando Veiga, Jose-Félix Zuazagoitia.

Sweden: Lennart Hansson, Valeria Ahgren, Hakan Ahlander, Thomas Angerbjörn, Lars-Erik Bergdahl, Hillevi Blom-Pfeiffer, Mats Boström, Thomas Brydolf, Bo Erik Kristensson, Georg Dahlen, Kent Ekenbratt, Ulla Britt Ericsson, Birger Fagher, Lars Fröberg, Magnus Geirsson, Juha Harju, Thomas Hedner, Christer Höglund, Thomas Hoheisel, Stefan Hofvendahl, Gunilla Johnasson, Saima Jönsson, Ingemar Luttu, Hans Nerell, Jan Ostergren, Jan Östergren, Lars Ostling, Anna Maria Ottosson, Martin Rosengren, Aru Sandanam, Sigge Strid, Bengt Svensson, Lars Svensson, Bengt-Olov Tengmark, Thomas Thulin, Claes de Verdier, Per Westerholm.

United Kingdom: Peter Sleight, David Birrell, Mark Blagden, Ian Clark, David Dutchman, Iain Gordon, Nigel Guest, Michael Haughney, David Huggan, Mokshad Kansagra, James Kay, Brian Lennox, Graham Martin, Grant McHattie, Douglas McKeith, Peter Mooney, Michael Mutch, Derek Neilson, Mark Reid, Christopher F. Rose, John Ross, Daya Sugar, Pauline Shearer, Barry Silvert, Roger Snook, Rory C. F. Symons, John Vernon, J. Zachariah.

United States: Henry R. Black, Ali Abdul, Marwan Adjan, Allen B. Adolphe, Jorge Luis Aguilera-Montalvo, Alexander Alverez, Larry Amacker, Jay Anders, Coleen Andruss, Jose S. Aponte, Jeffrey T. Apter, Peter Arcuri, H. Morgan Ashurst, Gerard P. Aurigemma, Herman Ayvazyan, James Bates, Mark A. Becker, John Bennett, Paul Benson, Lynn Bentson, Joan Benz, James Bergthold, Manick Bhardwaj, Dennis Bloomfield, Zachary T. Bloomgarden, Merle Bolton, Jeffrey L. Boone, Kenneth Boren, Ira R. Braverman, Carlos L. Brown, III, Nate Brown, Robert Burns, Bruce Burtenshaw, David A. Calhoun, James R. Campbell, Barry Caparoso, Mark Capkin, Raymond Carlson, Barry L. Carter, Inge R. Carter, Richard S. Castaldo, Robert Cesarec, C. Kohler Champion, Tien C. Cheng, Andrew Chubick, Robert Ciemiega, Mehmood A. Ckan, Irving M. Cohen, Selwyn A. Cohen, Harry T. Colfer, Salvatore Conte, Clinton N. Corder, Marcelo Corpuz, Bruce Corser, Robert E. Cronin, Thomas Crouch, Jairo B. Cruz, Rebecca Dailey, Michael Daniels, Richard H. Davis, Donald M. Denmark, Dolph Martel Denny, Bart G. Denys, Marcus A. DeWood, Edward J. Diamond, Richard Dickstein, Phillip M. Diller, Steven Dorfman, Steven L. Duckor, Gary Dunkerley, Donald C. Durbeck, M. El Shahawy, Samer Helm Ellahham, William J. Elliott, Georg Emlein, Gary P. Erdy, Michael Famularo, James Farrell, Hebert Fendley, Paul Fenster, James I. Fidelholtz, Justus J. Fiechtner, Larry Fields, Eugene C. Fletcher, Rex W. Force, Carl Franzetti, Francisco Fuentes, Lonnie E. Fuller Sr., John T. Funai, Marvin Galler, Walter Gaman, Garo S. Garibian, Gumaro Garza, M.R. Gedeon, Michael J. Germain, Steven Glasser, Richard L. Glenn, Sudheer T. Gogte, Ivan L. Goldsmith, Robert J. Goldstein, G.M. Gollapudi, Stephen L. Goss, Atul Goswami, Richard D. Goulah, Ray Graf, Alan Graff, Daniel Gremillion, Clarence Grimm, Colby H. Grossman, Ambrish Gupta, Narendra K. Gupta, Alexander Halkos, Robert J. Harriman, Clyde Harris, Jennifer Hedgepeth, Lynn Helmer, Mario Henriquez, Bradley T. Heppner, Donald K. Hickey, James R. Hill, Matthew Hilmi, Jon Hobson, Judith S. Hochman, Susan Hole, Joanne J. Holland, Lynne Hopkins, Mark Houston, Donald Hunninghake, Carmen

D. Irizarry, Sima Issen, Syed Jafri, Avanindra Jain, Michael J. Jamieson, Oswaldo Jimenez, Joseph P. Johns, Kjel Johnson, Wayne H. Kaesemeyer, Richard O. Kamrath, Roy Kaplan, Ronald Karlsberg, H.B. Karunaratne, Gerald Keightley, James Kern, Chet Kessler, Rashid A. Khairi, Vithal Kinhal, Timothy Klein, Gary E. Kolb, Michael J. Koren, Gregory Koshkarian, Marc Kozinn, Jeffrey Kramer, Seth Krauss, Barry Kricsfeld, Steven Kulback, Peter Kurzweil, Niranjan Lal, Victor Lamin, John A. Larry, Gary M. Lattin, Robert Lee, Theodore E. Lefton, Peter M. Lemis, James Lewis, Loren Lipson, Thomas Little, Peter A. Lodewick, Charles Lucas, Sofia X. Scholar Luisa, Jane Lyssy, Gregory MacDonald, Adrian Magee, Frank Maggiacomo, Craig Maltman, Richard A. Margolin, Charles Margolis, Allan Markus, Barry L. Marmorstein, David G. Marsh, Thomas Martin, Michael Marzec, Daniel Masacarenhas, Brian McCarroll, Mary P. McGowan, Kenneth G. McGrath, Robert D. McInroy, Michael E. McIvor, Timothy Menelly, Franz Messerli, Delbert H. Meyer, Donald W. Middleton, Jr., Felise Milan, Michael Miller, Kelly Mills, Mahendra Mirani, Michael J. Mirro, C. Brendan Montana, Marc Morse, Herbert Moskow, Harvey A. Mossman, William Mroczek, Andrew Muckle, Cynthia Mulrow, Marc A. Munger, Uttam O. L. Munver, David Nash, Jeffrey Newman, Albert Olash Jr., Roger On, John Ondrejicka, Stephen Ong, Ramin Oskoui, Meenakshi Patel, Tushar C. Patel, Andres Patron, Davita Persaud, Subhash Popli, R. Walter Powell, Rajendra Prasad, William Prechel, Dustan F. Pulle, John Pullman, Gary P. Reams, Jerry A. Reed, Harvey Resnick, Arthus Riba, Ralph W. Richter, Kenneth Rictor, Dennis Riff, Peter Ripley, Terry A. Riske, Daniel Risser, Ernesto Rivera, Jose R. Rivera del Rio, Mohammad Rizwan, Douglas Roberts, Jerry W. Robinson, Thomas Rocco, Daeyoung Roh, Robert S. Rood, Steven J. Rosansky, Herman Rose, Eli M. Roth, Robert Rouchon, Michael R. Rubin, Michael C. Ruddy, Kenneth Russ, Philip Sager, Bradley R. Sakran, Gilbert Salazar, Tariq Saleem, Albert M. Salomon, Raul Sanchez-Ramos, Milton Sands, Francisco A. Santini-Oliveri, Deepak Sant-Ram, Frederick W. Schaerf, Frederick Schaller, Ricky Schneider, John F. Seaworth, Eric Seyferth, Rajnikant Shah, Louis Shane, Jeffrey G. Shanes, Charles J. Sigmund, Anthony Silvagni, Stuart J. Simon, Satesh C. Singh, Sudeep Singh, Stan F. Slabic, John Sobolski, William Sokol Jr., John C. Somberg, Devendra Soni, John Sorensen, Neal B. Sorensen, Vincent Sorrell, Miguel Sosa-Padilla, Daniel Sporn, Allan Stahl, Gregg W. Stone, Henry Stratman, Danny Sugimoto, John E. Sutherland, Louise A. Taber, Addison Taylor, Carmen Texidor, Gerald Timmis, Steven R. Towner, Steven R. Turner, Gregory S. Uhl, Jeffrey R. Unger, Raymond Urbanski, Russell N. Vanhouzen, Jose B. Vazquez-Tanus, Jose Vero-Miro, Michael J. Voyack, Wyatt Voyles, Robert C. Watkins Jr., Mervyn Weerasinghe, Robert Weinstock, Marion R. Wofford, Nathan D. Wong, Laurence G. Yellen, Ralph Yung, Miguel Zabalgoita, Franklin J. Zieve.

REFERENCES

1. Black HR, Elliott WJ, Neaton JD, Grandits G, Grambsch P, Grimm RH Jr, Hansson L, Lacourcière Y, Muller J, Sleight P, Weber MA, White WB, Williams G, Wittes J, Zanchetti A, Fakouhi TD, for the CONVINCE Research Group. Rationale and design for the Controlled ONset Verapamil INvestigation of Cardiovascular Endpoints (CONVINCE) Trial. Control Clin Trials 1998; 19:370–390.
2. Smolensky MH, D'Alonzo GD. Medical chronobiology: concepts and applications. Am Rev Resp Dis 1993; 147:S2–S19.
3. Straka RJ, Benson SR. Chronopharmacologic considerations when treating the patient with hypertension: a review. J Clin Pharmacol 1996; 36:771–782.
4. Peto R, Collins R, Gray R. Large-scale randomized evidence: large, simple trials and overviews of trials. J Clin Epidemiol 1995; 48:23–40.

5. Collins R, Peto R, MacMahon S, Hebert P, Fiebach NH, Eberlein KA, Godwin J, Qizilbash N, Taylor JO, Hennekens CH. Blood pressure, stroke, and coronary heart disease, Part 2. Short-term reductions in blood pressure: overview of randomized drug trials in their epidemiological context. Lancet 1990; 335:827–838.
6. Dahlöf B, Lindholm LH, Hansson L, Scherstén B, Eckbom T, Wester P-O. Morbidity and mortality in the Swedish Trial in Old Patients with Hypertension (STOP-Hypertension). Lancet 1991; 338:1281–1285.
7. SHEP Cooperative Research Group. Prevention of stroke by antihypertensive drug treatment in older persons with isolated systolic hypertension: final results of the Systolic Hypertension in the Elderly Program. JAMA 1991; 265:3255–3264.
8. MRC Working Party. Medical Research Council trial of treatment of hypertension in older adults: principal results. BMJ 1992; 304:405–412.
9. Wolff FW, Lindeman RD. Effects of treatment of hypertension in the elderly in primary care. BMJ 1986; 293:1145–1151.
10. Psaty BM, Smith NL, Siscovick DS, Koepsell TD, Weiss NS, Heckbert SR, Lemaitre RN, Wagner EH, Furberg CD. Health outcomes associated with antihypertensive therapies used as first-line agents: a systematic review and meta-analysis. JAMA 1997; 277:739–745.
11. Messerli FH, Grossman E, Goldboourt U. Are beta-blockers efficacious as first-line therapy for hypertension in the elderly: a systematic review. JAMA 1998; 279:1903–1907.
12. Neaton JD, Grimm RH Jr, Prineas RJ, Stamler J, Grandits GA, Elmer PJ, Cutler JA, Flack JM, Schoenberger JA, MacDonald R. Treatment of Mild Hypertension Study: final results. JAMA 1993; 270:713–724.
13. Shih JH. Sample size calculation for complex clinical trials with survival endpoints. Control Clin Trials 1997; 16:395–407.
14. Lakatos E. Sample sizes based on the log-rank statistic in complex clinical trials. Biometrics 1988; 44:229–241.
15. Fleming T. Evaluation of active control trials in AIDS. J Acquir Immune Defic Syndr 1990; 3 (suppl 2):S82–87.
16. Lan KKG, DeMets DL. Discrete sequential boundaries for clinical trials. Biometrika 1983; 70:659–663.
17. O'Brien PC, Fleming TR. A multiple testing procedure for clinical trials. Biometrics 1979; 35:549–556.
18. Black HR, Elliott WJ, Grandits G, Fakouhi TD. Baseline characteristics of the 16,605 patients enrolled in the CONVINCE Study [abstract]. Am J Hypertens 1999; 14:141A.
19. The fifth report of the Joint National Committee on Detection, Evaluation, and Treatment of High Blood Pressure (JNC V). Arch Intern Med 1993; 153:154–183.
20. Sheps SG, Chair. The sixth report of the Joint National Committee on prevention, detection, evaluation, and treatment of high blood pressure. Arch Intern Med 1997; 157:2413–2446.
21. Siegel D, Lopez J. Trends in antihypertensive drug use in the United States: do the JNC V recommendations affect prescribing? JAMA 1997; 278:1745–1748.
22. Protocol for prospective collaborative overviews of major randomized trials of blood-pressure-lowering treatments. World Health Organization International Society of Hypertension Blood Pressure Lowering Treatment Trialists' Collaboration. J Hypertens 1998; 16:127–137.
23. Staessen JA, Fagard R, Thijs L, Celis H, Arabidze GG, Birkenhäger WH, Bulpitt CJ, de Leeuw PW, Dollery CT, Fletcher AE, Forette F, Leonetti G, Nachev C, O'Brien ET, Rosenfeld J, Rodicio JL, Tuomilehto J, Zanchetti A. Randomised double-blind comparison of placebo and active treatment for older patients with isolated systolic hypertension. The Systolic Hypertension in Europe (Syst-Eur) Trial Investigators. Lancet 1997; 350:757–764.
24. Liu L, Wang J, Gong I, Liu G, Staessen JA, for the Systolic Hypertension in China (Syst-China) Collaborative Group. Comparison of active treatment and placebo in older Chinese patients with isolated systolic hypertension. J Hypertens 1998; 16:1823–1829.
25. Toumilehto J, Rastenyte D, Birkenhäger WH, Thijs L, Antikainen R, Bulpitt CJ, Fletcher AE,

Forette F, Goldhaber A, Palatini P, Sarti C, Fagard R, for the Systolic Hypertension—Europe (Syst-Eur) Trial Investigators. Effects of calcium channel blockade in older patients with diabetes and systolic hypertension. N Engl J Med 1999; 340:677–684.
26. Estacio RO, Jeffers BW, Hiatt WR, Biggerstaff SL, Gifford N, Schrier RW. The effect of nisoldipine as compared with enalapril on cardiovascular outcomes in patients with non-insulin dependent diabetes and hypertension. N Engl J Med 1998; 338:645–652.
27. Tatti P, Pahor M, Byington RB, Di Mauro P, Guarisco R, Strollo G, Strollo F. Outcome results of the Fosinopril versus Amlodipine Cardiovascular Events randomized Trial (FACET) in patients with hypertension and NIDDM. Diabetes Care 1998; 21:597–603.
28. Packer MA, for the PRAISE Study Group. Final results of the Prospective Randomized Amlodipine Ischemia and Survival Evaluation Study. N Engl J Med 1996; 335:1107–1111.
29. Raizner AE, Oesterle S, Waksman R, et al. The PREVENT trial. A feasibility study of intracoronary brachytherapy in the prevention of restenosis: an interim report [abstract]. Circulation 1998; 98:I–651.
30. Danish Study Group on Verapamil in Myocardial Infarction (DAVIT-I). Verapamil in acute myocardial infarction. Eur Heart J 1984; 5:516–528.
31. Danish Study Group on Verapamil in Myocardial Infarction. Effect of verapamil on mortality and major events after acute myocardial infarction. The Danish Verapamil Infarction Trial II (DAVIT-II). Am J Cardiol 1990; 66:779–785.
32. Rengo F, Carbonin P, Pahor M, De Caprio L, Bernabei R, Ferrara N, Carosella L, Acanfora D, Parlati S, Vitale D. A controlled trial of verapamil in patients after acute myocardial infarction: results of the calcium antagonist reinfarction Italian study (CRIS). Am J Cardiol 1996; 77:365–369.
33. Hansen JF, Hagerup L, Sigurd B, Pedersen F, Mellemgaard K, Pedersen Bjergaard O, Mortengen LS. Cardiac event rates after acute myocardial infarction in patients treated with verapamil and trandolapril versus trandolapril alone. Danish Verapamil Infarction Trial (DAVIT) Study Group. Am J Cardiol 1997; 79:738–741.
34. Gibson RS, Boden WE, Theroux P, Strauss HD, Pratt CM, Gheorghiade M, Capone RJ, Crawford MH, Schlant RC, Kleiger RE. Diltiazem and reinfarction in patients with non-Q-wave myocardial infarction. Results of a double-blind, randomized, multicenter trial. N Engl J Med 1986; 315:423–429.
35. The effect of diltiazen on mortality and reinfarction after myocardial infarction. The Multicenter Diltiazem Postinfarction Trial Research Group. N Engl J Med 1988; 319:385–392.
36. Sleight P. Calcium antagonists during and after myocardial infarction. Drugs 1996; 51:216–225.
37. Messerli FH, Boden WE, Fischer HJ, Schechtman KB. Heart-rate lowering calcium antagonists in hypertensive post-MI patients [abstract]. J Hypertens 1996; 14(suppl 1):S220.
38. Psaty BM, Heckbert SR, Koepsell TD, Siscovick DS, Raghunathan TE, Weiss NS, Rosendaal FR, Lemaitre RN, Smith NL, Wahl PW. The risk of myocardial infarction associated with antihypertensive drug therapies. JAMA 1995; 274:620–625.
39. Furberg CD, Psaty BM, Meyer JV. Nifedipine: dose-related increase in mortality in patients with coronary heart disease. Circulation 1995; 92:1326–1331.
40. Pahor M, Guralnik JM, Furberg CD, Carbonin P, Havlik R. Risk of gastrointestinal haemorrhage with calcium antagonists in hypertensive persons over 67 years old. Lancet 1996; 347: 1061–1065.
41. Pahor M, Guralnik JM, Salive ME, Corti M-C, Carbonin P, Havlik RJ. Do calcium channel blockers increase the risk of cancer? Am J Hypertens 1996; 9:695–699.
42. Pahor M, Guralnik JM, Ferrucci L, Corti MC, Salive ME, Cerhan JR, Wallace RB, Havlik RJ. Calcium channel blockade and incidence of cancer in aged populations. Lancet 1996; 348: 493–498.
43. Fitzpatrick AL, Daling JR, Furberg CD, Kronmal RA, Weissfeld JL. Use of calcium channel blockers and breast cancer risk in postmenopausal women. Cancer 1997; 80:1438–1447.

44. Furberg CD, Psaty BM. Should calcium antagonists be used as first-line drugs in the treatment of hypertension? The con side. Arch Intern Med 1995; 155:2157–2161.
45. Furberg CD, Psaty BM. Calcium antagonists: not appropriate as first line antihypertensive agents. Am J Hypertens 1996; 9:122–124.
46. Epstein M. Calcium antagonists should continue to be used for first-line treatment of hypertension. Arch Intern Med 1995; 155:2150–2156.
47. Messerli FH. Case-control study, meta-analysis, and bouillabaisse: putting the calcium antagonist scare into context [editorial]. Ann Intern Med 1995; 123:888–889.
48. Epstein M. Calcium antagonists: still appropriate as first-line antihypertensive agents. Am J Hypertens 1996; 9:110–121.
49. Fagan TC. Calcium antagonists and mortality: another case of the need for clinical judgment [editorial]. Arch Intern Med 1995; 155:2145.
50. Mancia G, van Zwieten PA. How safe are calcium antagonists in hypertension and coronary heart disease? J Hypertens 1996; 14:13–17.
51. Parmley WW. A delayed answer to the calcium blocker question [editorial]. J Am Coll Cardiol 1996; 27:510–511.
52. Hansen JF. Is the safety and efficacy of calcium antagonists now established? Cardiovascular Drugs Ther 1998; 12:145–147.
53. Stelfox HT, Chua G, O'Rourke K, Detsky AS. Conflict of interest in the debate over calcium-channel antagonists. N Engl J Med 1998; 338:101–106.
54. Deyo RA, Psaty BM, Simon G, Wagner EH, Omenn GS. The messenger under attack—intimidation of researchers by special-interest groups. N Engl J Med 1997; 336:1176–1180.
55. Frohlich ED, Zanchetti A. Antihypertensive therapy: safety and efficacy of drugs and publications. J Hypertens 1996; 14:273–275, and Hypertension 1996; 26:317–318.
56. Davis BR, Cutler JA, Gordon DJ, Furberg CD, Wright JT Jr, Cushman WC, Grimm RH, LaRosa J, Whelton PK, Perry HM, Alderman MH, Ford CE, Oparil S, Francis C, Proschan M, Pressel S, Black HR, Hawkins. Rationale and design for the Antihypertensive and Lipid Lowering Treatment to Prevent Heart Attack Trial (ALLHAT). Am J Hypertens 1996; 9:342–360.
57. Elliott WJ. ALLHAT: the largest and most important clinical trial in hypertension ever done in the U.S.A. [editorial]. Am J Hypertens 1996; 9:409–411.
58. Bennis S, Ichas F, Robert J. Differential effects of verapamil and quinine on the reversal of doxorubicin resistance in human leukemia cell line. Int J Cancer 1995; 62:283–290.
59. Johansson BB, Norrving B, Widner K, Wu J, Halberg F. Stroke incidence: circadian and circaseptan (about weekly) variations in onset. Prog Clin Biol Res 1990; 341A:427–436.
60. Muller JE, Ludmer PL, Willich SN, Tofler GH, Aylmer G, Klangos I, Stone PH. Circadian variation in the frequency of sudden cardiac death. Circulation 1987; 75:131–138.
61. Muller JE. Morning increase in cardiovascular disease. Drug Ther 1988; 18:58–67.
62. Muller JE, Mangel B. Circadian variation and triggers of cardiovascular disease. Cardiology 1994; 85 (suppl 2):3–10.
63. Cohen MC, Rohtla KM, Lavery CE, Muller JE, Mittleman MA. Meta-analysis of the morning excess of acute myocardial infarction and sudden cardiac death. Circulation 1997; 79:1512–1515.
64. Elliott WJ. Circadian variation in the timing of stroke onset: a meta-analysis. Stroke 1998; 29:992–996.
65. D'Alonzo GE, Smolensky MH, Feldman S, Gnosspelius Y, Karlsson K. Bambuterol in the treatment of asthma. A placebo-controlled comparison of once-daily morning vs evening administration. Chest 1995; 107:406–412.
66. Primrose JN, Rogers MJ, Holmfield JH. The effects of 300 mg ranitidine at night, twice daily, and four times daily on intragastric acidity in normal subjects. Aliment Pharmacol Therap 1993; 7:287–291.
67. Shepherd J, Cobbe SM, Ford I, Isles CG, Lorimer AR, McFarlane PW, McKillop IH, Packard

CJ. Prevention of coronary heart disease with pravastatin in men with hypercholesterolemia. West of Scotland Coronary Prevention Study Group. N Engl J Med 1995; 333:1301–1307.
68. Gupta SK, Atkinson L, Tu T, Longstreth JA. Age and gender related changes in stereoselective pharmacokinetics and pharmacodynamics of verapamil and norverapamil. Br J Clin Pharmacol 1995; 40:325–331.
69. Gupta SK, Yih MY, Atkinson L, Longstreth J. The effect of food, time of dosing, and body position on the pharmacokinetics and pharmacodynamics of verapamil and norverapamil. J Clin Pharmacol 1995; 35:1083–1093.
70. Elliott WJ, Prisant LM. Drug delivery systems for antihypertensive agents. Blood Press Monitoring 1997; 2:53–60.
71. White WB, Anders RJ, MacIntyre JM, Black HR, Sica DA. Nocturnal dosing of a novel delivery system of verapamil for systemic hypertension. Am J Cardiol 1995; 76:375–380.
72. Cutler NR, Anders RJ, Jhee SS, Sramek JJ, Awan NA, Buitas J, Lahiri A, Woroszylska M. Placebo-controlled evaluation of three doses of a controlled-onset, extended release formulation of verapamil in the treatment of stable angina pectoris. Am J Cardiol 1995; 75:1102–1106.
73. White WB, Black HR, Weber MA, Elliott WJ, Bryzinski B, Fakouhi TD. Comparison of effects of COER-verapamil at bedtime and nifedipine GITS on arising on early morning blood pressure, heart rate, and the heart rate-pressure product. Am J Cardiol 1998; 81:424–431.
74. Frishman WH, Glasser S, Stone P, Deedwania PC, Johnson M, Fakouhi TD. Comparison of controlled-onset, extended release verapamil with amlodipine and amlodipine plus atenolol on exercise performance and ambulatory ischemia in patients with chronic stable angina pectoris. Am J Cardiol 1999; 83:507–514.
75. Black HR, Crocitto MT. Number needed to treat: solid science or a path to pernicious rationing? Am J Hypertens 1998; 11:128S–134S.
76. Moser M. Why are physicians not prescribing diuretics more frequently in the management of hypertension? JAMA 1998; 279:1813–1816.
77. The World Health Organisation/International Society of Hypertension Guidelines for the Management of Hypertension. J Hypertens 1999; 17:151–185.
78. Psaty BM, Koepsell TD, Yanez ND, Smith NL, Manolio TA, Heckbert SR, Borhani NO, Gardin JM, Gottdiener JS, Rutan GH. Temporal patterns of antihypertensive medication use among older adults, 1989 through 1992. An effect of the major clinical trials on clinical practice? JAMA 1995; 273:1436–1438.
79. Manolio TA, Cutler JA, Furberg CD, Psaty BA, Whelton PK, Applegate WB. Trends in pharmacologic management of hypertension in the United States. Arch Intern Med 1995; 155: 829–837.
80. Gottlieb SS, McCarter RJ, Vogel RA. Effect of beta-blockade on mortality among high-risk and low-risk patients after myocardial infarction. N Engl J Med 1998; 339:489–497.
81. Kromholz HM, Radford MJ, Wang Y, Chen J, Helat A, Marciniak TA. National use and effectiveness of beta-blockers for the treatment of elderly patients after acute myocardial infarction. National Cooperative Cardiovascular Project. JAMA 1998; 280:623–629.
82. Avorn J, Monette J, Lacour A, Bohn RL, Monane M, Mogun H, LeLorier J. Persistence of use of lipid-lowering medications. A cross-national study. JAMA 1998; 279:1458–1462.

22

Rationale and Design for the Antihypertensive and Lipid-Lowering Treatment to Prevent Heart Attack Trial (ALLHAT)

JEFFREY A. CUTLER and DAVID J. GORDON

National Heart, Lung, and Blood Institute, National Institutes of Health, Bethesda, Maryland

BARRY R. DAVIS

University of Texas School of Public Health, Houston, Texas

JACKSON T. WRIGHT, Jr.

Case Western University School of Medicine, Cleveland, Ohio

CURT D. FURBERG

Wake Forest University School of Medicine, Winston-Salem, North Carolina

I. INTRODUCTION

A. Antihypertensive Treatment

An estimated 50 million people in the United States have elevated blood pressure (systolic blood pressure [SBP] of 140 mm Hg or higher or diastolic blood pressure [DBP] of 90 mm Hg or higher) or are taking antihypertensive medication (1). Hypertension is considerably more common among blacks than among whites, and its sequelae are more frequent and severe in the former. The sequelae can be substantially reduced by drug treatment but with a large aggregate cost to society. Variation in the cost of treating hypertension is, in large part, determined by the cost of the antihypertensive agents used. Given the number of patients treated (23 million in 1987), drug choice has substantial economic

This research is supported by DHHS Contract number (NO1-HC-35130) from the National Heart, Lung, and Blood Institute, National Institutes of Health, U.S. Department of Health and Human Services.

implications (2). For example, according to one analysis, if 1982 prescribing practices had been in effect in 1992, it was estimated that drug expenditures for that year would have been \$3.1 billion less (3).

Despite the known etiologic relationship of hypertension to coronary heart disease (CHD), individual large-scale randomized clinical trials in largely middle-aged subjects have usually not shown statistically significant reductions in rates of CHD death or nonfatal myocardial infarction with antihypertensive drug treatment (4). However, these trials have not been designed with adequate sample sizes to find effects of moderate size, and overviews of such hypertension trials have shown that antihypertensive treatment does lead to a reduction in CHD event rates (5). Still, the estimated reduction (14%) was less than expected based on epidemiological data (6). The cited overviews did not take into account the strongly positive results of the Systolic Hypertension in the Elderly Program (SHEP), in which diuretic-based treatment reduced major CHD events by 27% (95% confidence interval [CI] 4% to 43%) (7). Other trials in older persons with diastolic/systolic hypertension (8, 9) have reported at least a trend toward similar results. One possible explanation given for the failure of previous trials to demonstrate the expected degree of CHD reduction is that adverse effects of study drugs, particularly high-dose diuretics, may have offset the potential benefit of blood pressure reduction. These potential adverse effects include diuretic-induced hypokalemia, hypomagnesemia, hyperuricemia, hyperlipidemia, hyperglycemia, impaired insulin sensitivity, and increased ventricular ectopic activity (1, 10, 11). However, such side effects are minimal at currently recommended doses.

In the late 1970s and the 1980s, new and costlier antihypertensive agents—calcium antagonists, angiotensin-converting enzyme (ACE) inhibitors, and alpha-adrenergic blockers—were developed and approved for use in chronic antihypertensive therapy. However, evidence that might justify their use in preference to the older classes of drugs is limited. Only two moderately large, long-term randomized trials have compared representatives of all of these drug classes: the 1-year trial conducted by the Department of Veterans' Affairs Cooperative Study Group on Antihypertensive Agents (12), and the 4.4-year Treatment of Mild Hypertension Study (TOMHS) (13). Although these trials have reported some differences in blood pressure (BP) control, adverse effects, quality of life, biochemical effects, and target-organ changes, these differences did not present a pattern that consistently favored one class of drugs over others. Also, these trials did not have clinical endpoints as the primary outcome for comparisons of drug classes.

Other relevant data come both from animal experiments and clinical trials in patients with heart disease. Calcium channel blockers inhibit the development of atherosclerotic lesions in rabbit models, but clinical trial data on morbidity and mortality are conflicting. An overview of all post myocardial infarction (MI) trials with calcium channel blockers reported a 6% (95% CI, −4% to +18%) increase in mortality (14). An update of this overview that included three additional trials in patients with angina pectoris or MI also suggested unfavorable results, particularly with dihydropyridine calcium channel blockers (15). The increased mortality with the short-acting formulations of nifedipine and nicardipine occurred primarily in patients with a recent MI. This outcome might be different with a long-acting dihydropyridine such as amlodipine, and indeed, the recent positive results of the Syst-Eur trial in isolated systolic hypertension (using nitrendipine, a moderately long-acting dihydropyridine) (16) and suggestive results of Prospective Randomized Amlodipine Survival Evaluation Study (PRAISE) and The Vasodilator-Heart Failure Trial (VHeFT) III in heart failure patients (using amlodipine and felodipine) (17, 18) provide some support for the importance of pharmacokinetic factors. Nevertheless, findings for a variety of outcomes from both observational studies and clinical trials have kept the so-called calcium channel blocker controversy alive (19, 20). Furthermore, placebo-controlled trials do not directly address comparative benefits and risks versus other (including less expensive) agents.

The ACE inhibitors reduce mortality in both severe and less severe heart failure (21–23), and reduce morbidity, including CHD, in asymptomatic left ventricular (LV) dysfunction (24). Prevention of coronary lesions in the Watanabe rabbit model with captopril treatment has been demonstrated (25), perhaps because of effects on cellular proliferation in the vessel wall. The hypothesis that antiatherosclerotic effects of ACE inhibitors occur in humans in part of the rationale for more recent trials in CHD patients with preserved LV function (26, 27). Recently concluded and ongoing trials in hypertensive patients are, as in the Antihypertensive and Lipid-Lowering Treatment to Prevent Heart Attack Trial (ALLHAT), comparing ACE inhibitors with traditional drugs (see ''Discussion''), below.

The alpha-adrenergic blockers have had moderately favorable effects on lipid profile, particularly on high-density lipoprotein (HDL) cholesterol, low-density lipoprotein (LDL) cholesterol, and the LDL/HDL ratio (13, 28). Improvements in insulin resistance have also been reported with alpha-blockers, an observation that may be especially relevant to patients with type II diabetes mellitus (29). Finally, there is some evidence that these agents reduce platelet aggregability and stimulate tissue plasminogen activator (30–32).

These data from existing studies in humans and animal models do not provide definitive evidence as to whether newer drugs are superior, equivalent, or inferior to the older drugs in the treatment of hypertension and the prevention of its cardiovascular complications. Given the clinical, public health, and economic importance of this issue, large-scale comparative trials have long been needed to assess the role of newer versus older antihypertensive agents in cardiovascular disease prevention; the ALLHAT has been one response to this need.

B. Cholesterol-Lowering Treatment

Lowering high cholesterol levels has been clearly and repeatedly shown to reduce the incidence of CHD events in randomized trials (33). However, in trials completed before 1993, any reduction in CHD deaths was offset by an increase in non-CHD deaths, and there was no net reduction in mortality (34). More recent trials using the HMG CoA reductase inhibitors or ''statins'' have not shown any adverse trends in non-CHD mortality (35–40). Two large trials in patients with established CHD, the Scandinavian Simvastatin Survival Study (4S) (35) and the Long-Term Intervention with Pravastatin in Ischaemic Heart Disease (LIPID) study (39), have shown significant reductions in all-cause mortality, and a meta-analysis of 34 single-factor cholesterol-lowering trials of 3 or more years' duration shows a significant 10% reduction in mortality (40).

However, even after the establishment of the general safety and efficacy of the statins in the prevention and treatment of CHD without an offsetting increase in non-CHD mortality, some important practical questions about cholesterol lowering still remain unanswered. The ALLHAT study is also designed to address many of these remaining questions.

The pre-statin trials were done almost exclusively in middle-aged white men. Although the majority of statin trials do include women and extend the upper age limit beyond 60, randomized trial data in women, men older than age 70, and racial and ethnic minorities are still sparse. Subgroup analyses of the four large statin trials that included women all suggest that they benefit at least as much as men from cholesterol lowering, but women comprise only 10% to 20% of the patients in these studies (35, 37–39). Subgroup analyses of these trials and West of Scotland Coronary Prevention Study (WOSCOPS) (36) by age suggest that the older participants derive significant benefit from treatment, although the relative risk reduction tends to be smaller than in younger patients. This is in agreement with epidemiological data suggesting the diminution with increasing age of the regression coefficient relating cholesterol levels and CHD event rates (41). However, the upper age limits in these trials ranged from 64 to 75 years at entry, and they lacked power to address whether the benefits of cholesterol lowering extend beyond age 70. By contrast, the ALLHAT cholesterol trial has no upper age limit and has met its objectives of enrolling most study patients with age older than 65, approximately half female participants, and more than half who are racial or ethnic minorities.

More data are also needed on the efficacy of cholesterol lowering in specific conditions conferring high risk of CHD (diabetes, hypertension, renal failure), which have often been grounds for exclusion from randomized trials of cholesterol lowering. If cholesterol lowering confers similar relative risk reduction in the presence of these conditions as it does in their absence, then it may be a particularly valuable and cost-effective adjunct to the primary treatment of these conditions. By design, all ALLHAT participants are hypertensive, and patients with other risk factors such as diabetes were specifically enrolled.

There is also some ambiguity about the net benefit of cholesterol lowering in patients whose pretreatment level of cardiovascular risk is less than that of patients with established CHD, as even low-level drug toxicity may negate a beneficial effect on CHD mortality when the initial risk (that is, in the absence of treatment) of CHD death is relatively modest. In the meta-analysis of 34 cholesterol-lowering trials, reduction in all-cause mortality was confined to the 25 trials of secondary prevention (40). Mortality was not reduced in the nine primary prevention trials, despite a nonsignificant trend toward reduced all-cause mortality in primary prevention trials using statin drugs. In the Air Force-Texas Coronary Atherosclerosis Prevention Study (AFCAPS/TexCAPS) trial, persons with ''average'' cholesterol levels and no prior CHD derived significant benefit from 5 years of lovastatin treatment in terms of nonfatal CHD events but not in terms of mortality (38). This probably reflects the fact that the mortality rate in this trial was only 0.5% per year, and only 17% of those deaths were the result of CHD. A large majority of the participants in the ALLHAT cholesterol trial were free of established CHD at entry. Thus, it is mainly a primary prevention trial, although the high prevalence of non-lipid CHD risk factors confers a relatively high risk in relation to other primary prevention trials of cholesterol lowering.

Finally, subgroup analysis of the Cholesterol and Recurrent Events (CARE) trial (42) suggested that there may be a level of LDL cholesterol (approximately 125 mg/dl) below which cholesterol lowering confers no additional benefit. This apparent disassociation between cholesterol lowering and reduction of CHD event rates at low LDL cholesterol levels, also reported in WOSCOPS (43) but not 4S (44), is somewhat at odds with epidemiological observations that cholesterol is a continuous risk factor at least down to *total* cholesterol levels below 150 mg/dl (45, 46). A substantial portion of ALLHAT participants and all of those with CHD at entry can be expected to attain LDL-cholesterol levels below 125 mg/dl during pravastatin treatment.

Table 1 Anticipated Sample Size of ALLHAT Treatment Groups

Cholesterol-lowering trial (2 arms)	Antihypertensive trial (4 Arms)				
	Chlorthalidone	Amlodipine	Lisinopril	Doxazosin	Total
Pravastatin	3,655	2,115	2,115	2,115	10,000
Usual care	3,655	2,115	2,115	2,115	10,000
Not eligible	7,310	4,230	4,230	4,230	20,000
Total	14,620	8,460	8,640	8,460	40,000

Abbreviation: *ALLHAT*, Antihypertensive and Lipid-Lowering Treatment to Prevent Heart Attack Trial.

II. OBJECTIVES AND DESIGN

The ALLHAT, sponsored by the National Heart, Lung, and Blood Institute (NHLBI) in conjunction with the Department of Veterans' Affairs (DVA), is a practice-based, randomized clinical trial in high-risk hypertensive patients age 55 years and older, of whom approximately half are women and half are ethnic minorities, especially African-Americans. The trial was initially funded for protocol development and other preparatory work in August 1993 and conducted patient recruitment between February 1994 and May 1998. Follow-up is scheduled to end in March 2002.

The ALLHAT has two components. The antihypertensive component is a double-blind trial designed to determine whether the combined incidence of fatal CHD and nonfatal MI differs between traditional treatment, based on a thiazide-like diuretic, and regimens initiated with each of three alternative antihypertensive drug classes—a calcium antagonist, an ACE inhibitor, or an alpha-adrenergic blocker. The lipid-lowering component is an open-label trial designed to determine whether lowering serum cholesterol using an HMG CoA reductase inhibitor in older (at least age 55) men and women who are moderately hypercholesterolemic (a subset of those randomized into the antihypertensive trial) will reduce all-cause mortality as compared with a control group receiving "usual care."

Drugs to satisfy these design objectives were selected by the NHLBI from among the agents in the specified classes that had been approved by the Food and Drug Administration for once-daily administration. Outside advisors who eventually became members of ALLHAT's governing committees assisted NHLBI staff in compiling prioritized lists of acceptable drugs, and the final selections were among those in which a manufacturer expressed willingness to participate by supplying the agent. (It was, however, necessary to purchase a diuretic to be able to conduct the trial.)

A. Hypotheses and Statistical Design

The primary hypotheses of the antihypertensive trial component are that the combined incidence of fatal CHD and nonfatal MI (first or recurrent) will differ in hypertensive patients randomized to (a) a calcium antagonist (amlodipine), (b) an ACE inhibitor (lisinopril), or (c) an alpha-adrenergic blocker (doxazosin) as first-line therapy from the incidence in those randomized to a thiazide-like diuretic (chlorthalidone) as first-line therapy. Thus the statistical design accounted for three primary comparisons.

To maximize statistical power for the antihypertensive trial, 1.7 times as many patients have been assigned to its diuretic arm, as compared with each of the other three arms (Table 1). The rationale for the sample size, estimated at 40,000, was based on

Table 2 Secondary Hypotheses for the ALLHAT Trial Components

Antihypertensive trial—The following endpoints (or their incidence) will be different in patients randomized to receive amlodipine, lisinopril, or doxazosin relative to those receiving chlorthalidone:

1. All-cause mortality
2. Combined coronary heart disease (CHD or revascularization procedures or hospitalized angina)
3. Stroke
4. Combined cardiovascular disease (CHD or stroke or coronary revascularization procedures or angina [hospitalized or medically treated] or CHF [hospitalized or medically treated] or peripheral arterial disease [hospitalized or outpatient revascularization procedure]),
5. Left ventricular hypertrophy by ECG
6. Renal disease (slope of reciprocal of serum creatinine)
7. Health-related quality of life
8. Major costs of medical care

Lipid-lowering trial—The following endpoints (or their incidence) will be different in patients randomized to receive pravastatin relative to those receiving usual care:

1. The combined incidence of CHD death and nonfatal myocardial infarction, especially in certain subgroups, e.g., African Americans, patients older than age 65, type II diabetics, and women
2. Changes in the biennial study ECG indicative of myocardial infarction
3. Cause-specific mortality
4. Total and site-specific cancer incidence
5. Health-related quality of life
6. Major costs of medical care

Abbreviations: *ALLHAT*, Antihypertensive and Lipid-Lowering Treatment to Prevent Heart Attack Trial; *CHD*, coronary heart disease; *CHF*, congestive heart failure; *ECG*, electrocardiogram.

detecting a 20% theoretical benefit (16% after considering plausible rates of crossover) between the diuretic and alternate treatment arms with 80% to 85% power. More details are presented in the Appendix. Secondary hypotheses, including both additional endpoints (such as stroke, total mortality, renal function, and quality of life) and major subgroups to be evaluated, are listed in Table 2.

The primary hypothesis of the cholesterol-lowering trial component is that mortality from all causes will differ in hypertensive patients with LDL cholesterol levels between 100 and 189 mg/dl (within this range, higher for those without and lower for those with known CHD) who are randomized to receive pravastatin, plus advice to follow a cholesterol-lowering [National Cholesterol Education Program Step I (47)] diet, compared with mortality in those randomized to receive dietary advice only, with pharmacological treatment added only if subsequently judged by a personal physician to have become indicated. The sample size was originally estimated as 20,000 participants. It was subsequently reduced to 10,000, based on external trial data and initial recruitment experience, and is expected to provide 84% power to detect an observed (after drop-in and drop-out) 16% reduction in the primary endpoint and 80% power for a 20.6% reduction in fatal CHD or nonfatal MI. More details are presented in the Appendix. Secondary hypotheses for this component, mostly similar to those for the antihypertensive component, are also listed in Table 2.

III. ENROLLMENT AND FOLLOW-UP PROCEDURES

A. Recruitment and Baseline Visits

A total of 632 clinics in the United States, Puerto Rico, the U.S. Virgin Islands, and Canada, recruited through mass mailings and presentations at major professional meetings enrolled at least one patient in ALLHAT. This has resulted in randomization of 42,448 patients for the antihypertensive trial and 10,357 participants for the cholesterol trial. Patient recruitment for ALLHAT, which was completed for the antihypertensive and cholesterol components in January and May 1998, respectively, relied on a variety of methods, particularly chart review within the participating clinical sites, to identify patients who were potentially eligible for the trial components. Mass mailings and media were used to a limited degree to recruit potential patients from outside the participating clinics. The rate of overall recruitment was largely driven by continued accrual of new sites, which was expanded from an originally anticipated 250 to 300 sites and continued into early 1997. The rate of recruitment into the cholesterol component was a function of overall recruitment plus the lag required for application of the additional eligibility criteria. More details on both site and patient recruitment are presented in reports in progress (48, 49).

Eligibility for the antihypertensive trial component was determined at two prerandomization visits 1 day to 2 months apart (Table 3). The objective of visit 1 was to assess eligibility for and interest in ALLHAT and to begin withdrawing patients from beta-blockers and central alpha-agonists. Additional interim prerandomization visits were conducted as needed to step-down these medications. Because only patients who had been randomized to the antihypertensive trial component were considered for randomization to the cholesterol-lowering trial component, randomization to the latter could only take place at the first post-randomization visit for the antihypertensive trial—usually 4 weeks later—or at a subsequent visit.

Blood pressure eligibility criteria for the antihypertensive trial, listed in Table 4, were based on the patient's current treatment status and on the average of two seated BP measurements, using a standard mercury sphygmomanometer, at each of two visits. For untreated patients, the criteria used were the Joint National Committee (JNC) V/VI definitions of diastolic or systolic hypertension, stages I to II (1). For treated patients, the criteria were based on reasonable BP control on no more than two drugs, that is, 160 mm Hg or lower systolic and 100 mm Hg or lower diastolic at visit 1, and remaining 180 mm Hg or lower systolic and 110 mm Hg or lower diastolic at visit 2 (when medication may have been partially withdrawn).

Additional inclusion criteria and exclusion criteria for the antihypertensive and lipid-lowering trials are presented in Table 5. Because the eligibility for the hypertension trial was established first, these criteria applied to both trials. Beyond those related to diagnosis and previous treatment of hypertension, the primary intent was to enroll a cohort with a sufficiently high expected event rate to test the study hypotheses. This was the reason for the requirement for at least one other risk factor for CHD. Age is the most important such criterion; the initial lower age cutpoint was 60 years, but because of concerns about recruitment, this was reduced to 55 years when the trial leadership was satisfied that the effect on study power would be small. Although cigarette smoking was not an initial criterion because of knowledge that smoking cessation leads to a rather rapid improvement in CHD risk, it was later added with the understanding that success of cessation efforts is modest at best, even in older people.

Table 3 ALLHAT Patient Visit Schedule

Visit #	Months from visit 2	Purpose: Antihypertensive trial	Purpose: Cholesterol-lowering trial
—	−6.0 to 1 day	Identify potential participant	
1	−2.0 to 1 day	Assess eligibility and interest	
1a,b,c	As needed	Step down from prestudy antihypertensive drugs if on beta-blockers or central alpha-agonists	
2	0	Randomization, lab, diet/lifestyle counseling	Fasting LP profile*, ALT†
3	1	Routine data collection Dosage titration if needed	Randomization, fasting LP Profile, NCEP‡ Step 1 diet
4	3	Routine data collection Dosage titration if needed	Dosage titration if needed ALT, TC††
5, 6, 7	6, 9, 12 (more often if needed)	Routine data collection Dosage titration if needed	Routine data collection Dosage titration if needed
8, 9, 10	Every 4 months	Routine data collection	Routine data collection

Postrandomization visits are shaded.
* Total cholesterol, triglyceride, HDL, and LDL cholesterol levels. LDL calculated by the Friedewald formula (50).
† Alanine aminotransferase.
‡ NCEP, National Cholesterol Education Program (47).
†† Total cholesterol
Abbreviations: *ALLHAT*, Antihypertensive and Lipid-Lowering Treatment to Prevent Heart Attack Trial.

Table 4 ALLHAT Blood Pressure Eligibility Criteria

	Lower limit[1] (mm Hg)		Upper limit[2] (mm Hg)	
Status at visit 1 and visit 2	SBP	DBP	SBP	DBP
On 1–2 drugs for hypertension for at least 2 months	—	—	160[3] 180[4]	100[3] 110[4]
On drugs for <2 months or currently untreated	140	90	180	110

[1] SBP or DBP lower limit must be met at visit 1 and visit 2
[2] SBP and DBP upper limit must be met at visit 1 and visit 2
[3] Visit 1 only
[4] Visit 2 only

Abbreviations: *ALLHAT*, Antihypertensive and Lipid-Lowering Treatment to Prevent Heart Attack Trial; *SBP*, systolic blood pressure; *DBP*, diastolic blood pressure.

Table 5 Major ALLHAT Inclusion and Exclusion Criteria

Antihypertensive trial

1. *Inclusion*
   a. One or more manifestations of atherosclerotic cardiovascular disease- (i) old (> 6 months) or age-indeterminate myocardial infarction or stroke; (ii) history of revascularization procedure; (iii) documented atherosclerotic cardiovascular disease
   b. Type II diabetes mellitus (plasma glucose > 140 mg/dl [fasting] or 200 mg/dl [nonfasting] and/or on insulin or oral hypoglycemics)
   c. HDL-cholesterol < 35 mg/dl (on ≥ two determinations within past 5 years)
   d. Left ventricular hypertrophy on ECG or echocardiogram
   e. ST-T wave ECG changes indicative of ischemia
2. *Exclusion*
   a. Symptomatic MI or stroke within the past 6 months
   b. Symptomatic congestive heart failure and/or ejection fraction < 35%, if known
   c. Angina pectoris within the past 6 months
   d. Serum creatinine ≥ 2 mg/dl
   e. Requirement for thiazide-like diuretics, calcium antagonists, ACE inhibitors, or alpha-blockers for reasons other than hypertension
   f. Requirement for more than two antihypertensive drugs to achieve satisfactory blood pressure control
   g. Sensitivity or contraindications to any of the first-line study medications
   h. Factors suggesting a low likelihood of compliance with the protocol, e.g., plans to move or travel extensively
   i. Diseases likely to lead to noncardiovascular death over the course of the study
   j. Blood pressure > 180 mm Hg systolic or > 110 mm Hg diastolic on two separate readings during screening or step-down

Lipid-lowering trial

1. *Inclusion*
   a. Enrollment in the antihypertensive trial
   b. An LDL cholesterol of 120–189 mg/dl (100–129 mg/dl for patients with known CHD) with a triglyceride level ≤ 350 mg/dl
2. *Exclusion*
   a. Current use of prescribed lipid-lowering agents or large doses (≥ 500 mg/day) of nonprescription niacin
   b. Contraindications to HMG CoA reductase inhibitors (e.g., significant liver disease, ongoing immunosuppressive therapy, known allergy or intolerance to the study drug)
   c. Known untreated secondary cause of hyperlipidemia (e.g., hypothyroidism, nephrotic syndrome)
   d. Alanine aminotransferase (ALT) > 2.0 × upper limit of normal

Abbreviations: *ALLHAT* Antihypertensive and Lipid-Lowering Treatment to Prevent Heart Attack Trial; *HDL*, high-density lipoprotein; *ECG*, electrocardiogram; *MI*, myocardial infarction; *ACE*, angiotensin-converting enzyme; *LDL*, low-density lipoprotein.

B. Randomization

Patients meeting the ALLHAT eligibility criteria discontinued prior antihypertensive drugs the day of visit 2 and were randomized to one of the four ALLHAT treatment arms after giving informed consent. This visit was intended to take place between 1 day and 8 weeks after visit 1, depending on the length of time required to step down from prestudy medications or determine hypertension status. Patients initially taking no drugs, or those well-controlled on one drug, could be randomized as soon as 1 day after visit 1. Prolonged step-downs were discouraged (though not prohibited), because many patients who could not be withdrawn quickly from their prestudy regimens were expected to be more difficult to maintain on a simple regimen during the trial. All randomized patients were also to be given appropriate hygienic advice (on limiting dietary sodium and alcohol if excessive, increasing physical activity as appropriate, and restricting caloric intake if overweight), with reinforcement as needed during the trial.

Patients who indicated their interest in the cholesterol-lowering component at visit 1 and had not been treated with lipid-lowering drugs during the prior 2 months were considered as potential candidates. A fasting lipid battery (total cholesterol, triglycerides [TG], HDL cholesterol [HDL-C] calculated LDL cholesterol [LDL-C]) and serum ALT was obtained at visit 2. Patients with an LDL-C between 120 and 189 mg/dl (between 100 and 129 mg/dl for patients with known CHD) and fasting TG of 350 mg/dl or less at this visit were informed by telephone of their eligibility for the cholesterol-lowering trial component and told to fast overnight for visit 3. If the patient was eligible to participate in this ALLHAT component at visit 3, the investigator phoned the clinical trials center and received a random assignment to either pravastatin or usual care. Patients assigned to usual care, as well as those assigned to pravastatin, were advised to follow the National Cholesterol Education Program (NCEP) Step I diet ($< 30\%$ of calories from fat, $< 10\%$ of calories from saturated fat, < 300 mg cholesterol per day). A fasting lipoprotein profile was obtained at this visit as a baseline for each randomized participant in this trial component. The clinical trials center used the average total cholesterol (TC_0) and LDL (LDL_0) cholesterol levels from visits 2 and 3 to calculate a target TC level corresponding to a 25% fall in LDL cholesterol, according to the following formula: target $TC = TC_0 - (0.25 \times LDL_0)$. In addition, 10% of the pravastatin group and 5% of the usual care group are monitored at selected annual visits using fasting LDL cholesterol.

The main baseline characteristics of patients enrolled in the antihypertensive trial are as follows: mean age of 67 years and BP (visit 1) of 145/83 mm Hg (for the 9.8% previously untreated, 159/91 mm Hg); 46.8% are women; 35.6% African/American (3.3% were also Hispanic), 12.5% white Hispanic, and 47.1% white non-Hispanic. Baseline characteristics of those randomized into the cholesterol component are generally similar, and in this component, mean total, LDL, and HDL cholesterol levels were 224, 146, and 48 mg/dl, respectively (for the 11.5% with CHD at entry, 196, 120, and 45 mg/dl). Approximately 35% of participants in both components have diabetes mellitus.

IV. TREATMENT PROGRAM

A. Antihypertensive Intervention

The BP goal in all four arms is less than 90 mm Hg diastolic and less than 140 mm Hg systolic. The therapeutic goal is to achieve BP control on the lowest possible dosage of the first-line drug, but to use the maximum dose of the blinded drug before adding other drugs. The number and dose of study drugs prescribed in pursuit of these goals are guided by patient tolerance and clinical judgment, particularly in use of regimens of more than two drug. The dosage levels available for each drug are listed in Table 6.

The identity of the first-line drug is masked at each dosage level. To minimize the

Table 6 ALLHAT First- (Blinded), Second- (Open Label), and Third-Line (Open Label) Antihypertensive Drugs*

Step 1 agent	Initial dose	Dose 1	Dose 2	Dose 3
Chlorthalidone	12.5	12.5	12.5	25
Amlodipine	2.5	2.5	5	10
Lisinopril	10	10	20	40
Doxazosin	1	2	4	8
Step 2 and step 3 agents				
Reserpine		0.05 qd or 0.1 qod	0.1 qd	0.2 qd
Clonidine (oral)		0.1 bid	0.2 bid	0.3 bid
Atenolol		25 qd	50 qd	100 qd
Hydralazine (third-line)		25 bid	50 bid	100 bid

* Sources of the four step 1 agents are: chlorthalidone: Ogden Bioservices, Inc., Rockville, Maryland; amlodipine: Pfizer, Inc., New York, New York; lisinopril: AstraZeneca Pharmaceuticals Group, Wilmington, Delaware; and doxazosin: Pfizer, Inc., New York, New York.
Abbreviation: *ALLHAT*, Antihypertensive and Lipid-Lowering Treatment to Prevent Heart Attack Trial.

potential first-dose hypotension with doxazosin, the initial dosage level was used during the first week after randomization. For the other three drugs, the initial dose and step 1 dosages are identical. Also, to allow three dose levels for the other agents with maintenance of the blind, doses 1 and 2 of chlorthalidone are both 12.5 mg. Patients were expected to return at 1-month intervals for any necessary increase in dosage until both the systolic and diastolic goal pressures are reached. If the initial dose of the blinded drug is not tolerated, it is discontinued. A subsequent rechallenge with the medication is encouraged, if appropriate.

For patients in any of the four treatment arms who are unable to attain satisfactory BP control on the maximum tolerable dosage of their first-line drug, a choice of second- and third-line drugs are provided in open-label form for use in *addition to* (not substitution for) the first-line drug (Table 6). The choice of second-line drug(s) is at the discretion of the treating study investigator. Because the study investigators are blinded to the identity of the first-line drug to which each patient is assigned, it is likely that the frequency of use of each of the second-line drugs will be similar among the four treatment arms. Although in special cases, investigators may choose to prescribe second-line antihypertensive drugs other than those provided by the study, thiazide diuretics, calcium antagonists, ACE inhibitors, and alpha-adrenergic blockers are avoided unless maximum tolerated doses of a 3-drug regimen have been tried and are unsuccessful in controlling BP.

B. Cholesterol-Lowering Intervention

As noted above, the cholesterol-lowering component of ALLHAT was a randomized comparison of an HMG CoA reductase inhibitor (pravastatin) plus diet versus usual care plus diet in a subset of patients participating in the antihypertensive component of the study. The starting dosage of pravastatin was originally 20 mg, taken in the evening. For patients who did not attain a decrease in serum TC corresponding to at least a 25% decrease in LDL cholesterol after 2 months, the daily dosage was to be increased to 40 mg. After about 1000 participants were enrolled, the starting dose was changed to 40 mg to enhance the contrast with usual care. All participants in this ALLHAT component receive instruction in the Step I diet recommended by the NCEP (47) upon randomization into the study. Randomization into this trial component was supposed to occur 4 to 26 weeks after randomization into the antihypertensive component of ALLHAT but could occur after up to 52 weeks.

V. DETERMINATION OF OUTCOMES

A. Data Collection and Endpoint Classification

The outcomes that will be obtained and tabulated over the course of the study are listed in Table 7. Occurrences of clinical endpoints are documented by a checklist completed at each follow-up visit and supplemented by interim reporting as needed. Other than blood pressure and total serum cholesterol, outcomes based on continuous measurements (LV hypertrophy, renal function, quality of life) are based on data collected at selected annual visits. The study investigators are required to complete and submit to the clinical trials center a short questionnaire for each occurrence of a clinical endpoint identified at or between regular visits. For each endpoint involving a death or hospitalization, the investigator also submits a copy of the death certificate or hospital discharge summary upon which the diagnosis is based. For fatal events, the underlying cause of death is classified by the physician-investigator at the clinical site.

Table 7 ALLHAT Outcomes

1. Death
    a. definite myocardial infarction
    b. definite coronary heart disease
    c. possible coronary heart disease
    d. stroke
    e. congestive heart failure
    f. other cardiovascular disease
    g. cancer
    h. accident, suicide, or homicide
    i. other noncardiovascular cause
    j. unknown cause
2. Myocardial infarction
3. Stroke
4. Angina (hospitalized or treated)
5. Congestive heart failure (hospitalized or treated)
6. Peripheral arterial disease (hospitalized or treated)
7. New cancer diagnosis (hospitalized or treated)
8. Accident or attempted suicide (hospitalized or treated)
9. Left ventricular hypertrophy (biennial study ECG)
10. Renal function (slope of the reciprocal of serum creatinine level versus time)
11. Quality of life
12. Medical care utilization

Abbreviations: *ALLHAT*, Antihypertensive and Lipid-Lowering Treatment to Prevent Heart Attack Trial; *ECG*, electrocardiogram.

For a random (10%) subset of hospitalized (fatal and nonfatal) MIs and strokes, the clinical trials center requests more detailed information. For this subset, in-hospital electrocardiograms (ECGs) and enzyme levels (for MIs), neurologists reports, and computed tomographic (CT) or magnetic resonance imaging (MRI) reports (for strokes) are evaluated by the study endpoints committee, and the accuracy of the discharge diagnoses are assessed.

A National Death Index (NDI) search is being performed periodically to identify and document deaths that may have occurred among patients who are lost to follow-up. To identify nonfatal events in patients lost to follow-up and because of the time lag inherent in the NDI, other tracking methods, including Medicare hospitalization files (and, for selected participants, a private tracing service) are also being used or planned.

B. Data Analysis

The primary endpoint of the antihypertensive component of ALLHAT is combined fatal and nonfatal CHD. The primary response variable is time from randomization to development of this event. The log-rank test (51) will be used to compare each of the nondiuretic treatment groups to the diuretic one. For the secondary endpoints of all-cause mortality, stroke, and combined coronary and cardiovascular outcomes, the log-rank test will also be used. For the outcomes of left ventricular hypertrophy (LVH) by ECG and health-related quality of life, comparison of proportions will be used to see if there are differences in the treatment groups. For the outcome of renal disease, the reciprocal of a participant's creatinine values at baseline, 3 months, and year 2, 4, and 6 will be obtained. Using treatment group as a fixed effect and time as a random effect, a treatment-by-time interaction effect will be estimated using the longitudinal models of Laird and Ware (52).

The primary endpoint of the ALLHAT lipid-lowering component is all-cause mortality. The primary response variable is time from randomization to death. The log-rank test will be used to compare the group assigned to pravastatin plus diet to the group assigned to usual care plus diet. For the secondary endpoints of combined fatal and nonfatal CHD, fatal and nonfatal cancer, and cause-specific mortality, the log-rank test will also be used. In addition, the log-rank test will be used to compare treatments within each of the following subgroups for the outcome of combined fatal and nonfatal CHD: men, women, 65 years and older, younger than age 65, African Americans, non-African Americans, diabetics, and nondiabetics. For the outcome of health-related quality of life, comparison of proportions will be used to see if there are differences in the treatment groups.

Interim monitoring has focused on patient intake overall and within each clinical center; center adherence to protocol; baseline comparability of treatment groups; sample size assumptions with regard to event rates, crossover rates, competing risk and loss to follow-up; adverse effects data; and effects of treatment on the primary and secondary study outcomes. Interim analyses coincide with the meetings of the Data and Safety Monitoring Board (DSMB). Stochastic curtailment is being used for monitoring treatment differences in both the antihypertensive and the lipid-lowering studies (53, 54).

VI. ORGANIZATIONAL STRUCTURE

The ALLHAT study has an organizational structure that differs greatly from the usual NHLBI-supported clinical trial. This so-called large, simple trial model, implemented previously in the ISIS trials coordinated by Oxford University investigators (55) and first used by NHLBI in the Digitalis Investigative Group trial (56), is appropriate when the following conditions apply: (a) a very large sample size is needed, (b) a streamlined protocol is possible, (c) the targeted conditions are commonly encountered in clinical practice, and (d) there is widespread interest in the study question among clinicians.

The trial is being performed by a large number of practicing physician-investigators at 632 practice sites who are compensated on a per-capita basis for each patient enrolled and for follow-up visits according to a fixed payment schedule. These fees are expected to cover the costs of the data collection (step-down and titration visits, questionnaires, blood drawing, ECG recording) specified above. The fee does not include the cost of required laboratory work and ECG coding, which is performed by central facilities and paid for directly by the clinical trials center, or the costs of documenting study endpoints, for which there is separate reimbursement.

The clinical trials center, in addition to its conventional data handling and monitoring responsibilities, is responsible for identifying and paying these physician-investigators and for contracting with other academic institutions to provide regional coordinators (physicians, nurses, and other professionals with multicenter clinical trial experience) to assist clinics with recruitment and protocol compliance. Approximately 16% of study patients were recruited by DVA hospitals, which operate under separate agreement and funding from the NHLBI and constitute one of the nine ALLHAT regions. The clinical trials center was also responsible for awarding and supervising subcontracts for a drug distribution center, a central laboratory, and an ECG coding center. A steering committee of experts in the relevant subject areas has also been appointed by NHLBI; most members are also regional physician coordinators. The clinical trials center has overall responsibility for training and quality control. Staff from all clinical sites were required to attend a training session. The training session included orientation to the study protocol, blood pressure measurement training and certification, orientation to the ECG and laboratory procedures, and training in recruitment and retention of participants as well as completion and transfer of study forms. Periodic refresher training is held in conjunction with regularly scheduled study investigators' meetings. These refresher sessions include a review of correct blood pressure measurement procedures or any problem that may be identified through review of routine monitoring activities.

Responsibilities of the clinical trials center with regard to quality control include: (a) reviewing all forms for completeness and accuracy prior to data entry; (b) resolving problems by telephone or facsimile transmission with clinical sites (c) double data entry of forms; (d) cross-forms edits to identify missing forms and procedures; (e) monitoring the performance of study components and providing timely summary reports to the program office and to the steering committee; and (f) providing detailed and up-to-date statistical reports of study progress to the DSMB at their meetings.

The DSMB is responsible for monitoring all aspects of the study, including those that require access to blinded data. The DSMB and its chair were appointed by the director of NHLBI; they are experts who are not otherwise affiliated with the study. During the active recruitment phase, the DSMB monitored the progress of recruitment and the random allocation of participants to the various treatment arms. The DSMB may recommend modifications in (or termination of) one or both study components if the study design goals are not being met. The approval of the DSMB is required for any other significant changes in the protocol recommended by the steering committee during the course of the study.

At any time during the study, the DSMB may recommend discontinuation of any of the treatment arms of either study component on any of the following grounds:

1. Compelling evidence from this or another trial of a significant adverse effect of the study treatment(s) that is sufficient to override any potential benefit on CHD and preclude its further use in the target population.
2. Compelling evidence from this or another trial of a significant beneficial effect of a study treatment, such that its continued denial to the other study groups is ethically untenable.
3. A very low probability of successfully addressing the study hypotheses within a feasible time frame, because of inadequate recruitment, compliance, drug response, event rate, etc.

The director of the NHLBI will make the final decision on whether to accept the DSMB's recommendation to discontinue any component of the study.

VII. DISCUSSION

The initial era of large-scale hypertension treatment trials began with the Veterans Administration studies of the 1960s and largely concluded with the trials in elderly patients that reported results in the early 1990s. Such trials were designed to address the question of whether blood pressure reduction per se conferred morbidity and mortality benefits for a number of vascular outcomes in a variety of population groups (57). They used those treatment regimens—now termed ''traditional''—that were known to be efficacious and generally well-tolerated for reducing blood pressure. The trials on the whole have demonstrated broad and important benefits. An offshoot of the original issues addressed by such trials has been the question of how far to reduce blood pressure levels; trials of this question were conducted in the 1980s and continue currently.

With the wide acceptance and application of results of the first generation of trials, as well as other advances in prevention of cardiovascular diseases, CVD rates are much lower than formerly in North America, western Europe, and Australasia. This is part of the reason that the second generation of trials requires much larger sample sizes. Furthermore, the main question has evolved beyond that of *whether* to treat and is now *how* to treat, that is, trials comparing active treatments. Because the differences being tested are hypothesized to arise from what have been called *ancillary properties* of antihypertensive drugs, they are expected to be smaller than those produced by BP reduction. The sample size requirements have necessitated new approaches to organizing trials, as exemplified by ALLHAT. The challenges engendered, including recruitment of sites and patients, training of investigators and staff in clinical trial methods, monitoring and quality control, and the sheer size of such efforts, are daunting. Nevertheless, the initial tasks of clinic and patient recruitment have been successfully accomplished in ALLHAT.

A considerable number of other trials comparing active treatments have also been initiated, both before and subsequent to starting ALLHAT (58). Several of these comparing an ACE-inhibitor-based regimen with one based on diuretics, beta-blockers, or dihydropyridine calcium-channel blockers, have reported results, including findings of both differences and no differences for a variety of endpoints (59–62). Although there has been some suggestion of an advantage for ACE-inhibitors over other classes in the particular case of diabetic patients, results have been neither consistent nor conclusive. Hence, the questions that ALLHAT was designed to address remain unanswered (63, 64).

VIII. CONCLUSIONS

Hypertension is a frequent health problem in Americans, especially among older individuals and blacks. It is associated with a significantly increased risk of morbidity and mortality. At the time ALLHAT was initiated, only diuretics and beta-blockers had been shown to reduce this risk in long-term clinical trials. Whether newer and usually more costly antihypertensive agents confer increased benefit in terms of reduced incidence of cardiovascular disease is still unknown. Also unknown is the potential benefit of treating moderately hypercholesterolemic older men and women with an HMG CoA-reductase inhibitor, not only in terms of reduced coronary heart disease but also total mortality. The results of ALLHAT are expected to be available by the year 2002 and should help resolve these issues of major importance to medical practice and public health.

NOTE ADDED IN PROOF

The doxazosin arm of ALLHAT was terminated by decision of the Director, NHLBI, on January 24, 2000. The results leading to the termination are reported in JAMA 2000; 283: 1967–1975.

ACKNOWLEDGMENTS

The ALLHAT investigators acknowledge contributions of study medications supplied by Pfizer, Inc. (amlodipine and doxasozin), AstraZeneca (atenolol and lisinopril), and Bristol-Myers Squibb (pravastatin), and the financial support provided by Pfizer to NHLBI.

APPENDIX I

Considerations for Sample Size

The statistical power to test the primary hypothesis of the antihypertensive trial is approximately 82.5%, based on the following assumptions: (a) sample size of 40,000 (approximately 22,000 men and 18,000 women; (b) 6-year incidence of CHD events of 7.8% in the diuretic group (derived from the Framingham Study, the Hypertension Detection and Follow-Up Program [HDFP], and SHEP [personal communication]); (c) a 16.3% reduction in the CHD event rate after adjustment for noncompliance and losses to follow-up in each of the three nondiuretic treatment arms compared with the diuretic arm; (d) rates of crossover between each of the other study drugs and chlorthalidone or non-study medication of 2.75% in each of the first 3 years and 6% over the last 3 years of follow-up (rates derived from the TOMHS [personal communication]), yielding a cumulative 24% rate of patients crossing over to another medication at least once in 6 years; (e) CHD status undeterminable at the end of the study for 16.8% of patients because of competing risks (non-CHD death) or loss to follow-up; (f) a 25% reduction in CHD event rates (before adjustment for noncompliance and losses to follow-up) among the 10,000 patients randomized to the active treatment arm of the cholesterol-lowering trial component, and (g) a type I error of 0.05 (two-sided), corresponding to a critical Z-score of 2.37 after adjustment for multiple comparisons using the Dunnett procedure (65).

The original ALLHAT protocol used an age criterion of 60 or older and did not include current cigarette smoking as a risk factor. Lowering the entry age decreased the CHD event rate, but the addition of the smoking risk factor resulted in the CHD event rate estimate remaining at 1.35% per year. More pessimistic or optimistic assumptions were also considered. These include (a) event rates of 1.05%/year to 1.65% per year; (b) crossover rates of 22% to 26% and loss rates of 11.8% to 21.8%. Power estimates ranged from 77% to 86% under these assumptions.

Based on National Health and Nutrition Examination Survey (NHANES) II (66) data for ages 65 to 74 years, in which the LDL-C cutpoints for ALLHAT patients without CHD corresponded to the 25th and 86th percentile (men) and to the 14th and 76th percentile (women), just over 60% of patients in the ALLHAT study will be LDL-eligible for the cholesterol-lowering trial. It was assumed that about 80% of LDL-eligible patients (or 50% of all ALLHAT patients) would participate in the cholesterol-lowering trial. Slightly lower estimates (slightly under 60%) were later obtained in the more recent (1988–1991) NHANES III data (National Center for Health Statistics, personal communication), reflecting a general downward temporal trend in LDL cholesterol levels as well as the incorporation of more data from blacks and from persons aged 75 to 84 years.

The statistical power to test the primary hypothesis of the cholesterol-lowering trial is approximately 80%, based on the following assumption: (a) sample size of 10,000 allocated equally between pravastatin and usual care groups; (b) 6-year total mortality of 12.2% (2.15% per year) in the usual care group (derived from Framingham, HDFP and SHEP [personal communication]); (c) a 20% reduction in mortality in the pravastatin treatment arm before adjustment for dropouts and drop-ins; (d) a "dropout" rate (from pravastatin treatment to no treatment) of 6% in year 1, and 3% in all subsequent years, and a "drop-in" rate (from no treatment to pravastatin or a similar drug) of 2.5% per year—cumulative rate of 19.3% of pravastatin patients off treatment and 14.1% of usual care patients on treatment at the end of 6 years; (e) no losses to mortality follow-up; (f) a 10% reduction in mortality rate in each of the three nondiuretic treatment arms of the antihypertensive trial component; and (g) a type I error $\alpha = 0.05$ (two-sided), corresponding to a critical Z-score of 1.96.

The drop-in and drop-out rates were derived from several assumptions: (a) based on previous experience with HMG CoA reductase inhibitors, compliance was expected to be good, with the bulk of noncompliance occurring early in the trial; (b) in most cases, the study physician is the patient's primary care physician and thus, there is less concern about outside physicians changing patient's medicines than in a more conventional, university-based trial; (c) the patients being considered for the cholesterol-lowering trial have lower LDL-C levels than are typically treated in ordinary practice. Many patients in the United States who clearly need cholesterol-lowering drugs are not being treated despite higher LDL levels. Given the cost of lipid-lowering agents and the relatively modest lipid levels of the patients, not many patients assigned to no medication are expected to be taking active lipid-lowering medication; (d) ALLHAT physicians are advised not to randomize patients who are already receiving cholesterol-lowering drugs or who, in their opinion, should receive these drugs as part of their "usual care." Thus, potential crossovers to active treatment are, for the most part, not being randomized in the first place; (e) after the publication of the 4S results, the protocol was amended to exclude patients with established CHD, LDL-C above 130 mg/dl from the cholesterol-lowering trial. Also, the 4S study had a drop-in rate of 13% and a drop-out rate of 10% over the course of 5.4 years.

In the original ALLHAT protocol with an age criterion of 60 years or older and not including current cigarette smoking as a risk factor, we estimated a 2.35% per year mortality rate and an unadjusted treatment difference of 12.5%. With the protocol modifications and the results of the 4S study (adjusted 30% treatment difference), the new assumptions were felt to be reasonable.

APPENDIX 2

ALLHAT Research Group Investigators

Investigators at the clinical centers of the ALLHAT Research Group

Steering Committee
Michael H. Alderman, MD
Henry R. Black, MD
William C. Cushman, MD
Jeffrey A. Cutler, MD, MPH
Barry R. Davis, MD, PhD
Charles K. Francis, MD
Curt D. Furberg, MD (Chair)
Richard H. Grimm, Jr. MD, PhD
L. Julian Haywood, MD
John LaRosa, MD
Frans H. H. Leenen, MD
Suzanne Oparil, MD
H. Mitchell Perry, Jr. MD
Jeffrey L. Probstfield, MD
Paul K. Whelton, MD, MSc
Jackson T. Wright, Jr. MD, PhD (Vice Chair)

ALLHAT Project Office, Bethesda, Maryland
Jeffrey A. Cutler, MD, MPH
Debra Egan, MS, MPH
David Gordon, MD, PhD
Craig Miron
Chuke Nwachuku, MA, MPH
Gerald H. Payne, MD
Michael Proschan, PhD

ALLHAT Clinical Trials Center, Houston, Texas
Judy Bettencourt, BA
Barry R. Davis, MD, PhD
Charles E. Ford, PhD
Robert J. Hardy, PhD
C. Morton Hawkins, ScD
Barbara (Basia) Kimmel, MS, MS
Darwin R. Labarthe, MD, PhD
Christine Morvillo Lusk, MPH

Linda B. Piller, MD, MPH
Sara Pressel, MS

ALLHAT Drug Distribution Center, Rockville, Maryland
John Pelosi, RPh, MS

ALLHAT Central Laboratory, Minneapolis, Minnesota
Jean Bucksa, MT
John Eckfeldt, MD, PhD
Maren Nowicki, MT

ALLHAT ECG Coding Center, Minneapolis, Minnesota
Carmen O. Christianson
Richard S. Crow, MD

Pfizer, Inc.
Ann Barry, PhD
Patricia Walmsley, MD

Zeneca, Inc.
Melynda Esack, MD

Bristol-Myers Squibb, Inc.
Rene Belder, MD
Mark E. McGovern, MD
Margot Mellies, MD

ALLHAT Regional Physician and Study Coordinators
William C. Cushman, MD
Therese S. Geraci, MSN, RN, CS
H. Mitchell Perry, Jr. MD
Sandra M. Walsh, MA
Anne Juratovac, RN
Robert A. Pospisil, RN
Mahboob Rahman, MD
Jackson T. Wright, Jr., MD, PhD
Michael H. Alderman, MD
Kim Brennan, BS
Lillian Carroll, RN, MS
Sheila Sullivan, BA
Gail Barone, RN, BA
Henry R. Black, MD
Rudell (Rudy) Christian, MPH
Sharon Feldman, MPH
Julie Hynes, MS, RD
Tracy L. Lucente, MPH
Charrise (Sherry) O'Neill, RN, BS, CCRC
Kimberley L. Jenkins, MPH

Cora E. (Beth) Lewis, MD, MSPH
Peggy McDowell, RN
Suzanne Oparil, MD
Nivea I. Vazquez, BBA
Janice Johnson, BS
Connie Kingry, RN, BSN
Rebecca A. Letterer, RN, BSN
Jeffrey L. Probstfield, MD
Tanya Aldentaler
Richard H. Grimm, Jr., MD, PhD
Leslie Ann Holland, BA
Brenda Jaeger-Fox
Karen Margolis, MD
Laurie Quint Adler
Gail T. Louis, RN, BA
Pamela Ragusa, RN, BSN
Paul K. Whelton, MD, MSc
Jeff D. Williamson, MD, MHS
Angela Williard, RN, BSN
R.L. Sue Ferguson, RN
Frans H. H. Leenen, MD
Joanna Tanner

ALLHAT Data and Safety Monitoring Board
William B. Applegate, MD
Julie S. Buring, ScD
Richard Carleton, MD (Chair)
Edward Cooper, MD
Keith C. Ferdinand, MD, FACC
Marian Fisher, PhD
Raymond W. Gifford, Jr., MD
Sheldon Sheps, MD

VAMC Detroit, Detroit, Michigan
James R. Sowers, MD (PI)
Saib Gappy, MD
Lisa Bey-Knight, RN

Wade Park VAMC, Cleveland, Ohio
Eleni I. Pelecanos, MD, MPH (PI)
David Davidson, RN

Memphis VAMC, Memphis, Tennessee
Roger G. Smith, MD (PI)
Anita W. McKnight, BSN, RN

Miami VAMC, Miami, Florida
Richard Preston, MD (PI)
Gustavo Godoy, MD
MaryAlice S. Yoham, MSN, ARNP-C

New York VAMC, New York, New York
Lois Anne Katz, MD (PI)
Diane Zimmerman, PA-C

The Wellness Plan, Detroit, Michigan
Marc Keshishian, MD (PI)
Richard Miller, MD
Marlene Vaughn, RN

RUSH Prudential HMO, Van Buren Office, Chicago, Illinois
Vance Lauderdale, MD (PI)
Terese Bertucci, RN, MS

RUSH Prudential HMO, Anchor Evergreen, Evergreen Park, Illinois
Sandy Gibson, DO (PI)
Gail Floyd, MD

University of South Carolina, Columbia, South Carolina
Nowa A. Omoigui, MD, MPH (PI)
Ossoma Abdulrahman, MD
Peggy L. Jumper

People's Health Centers, St. Louis, Missouri
Gina Chan, MD (PI)
Carmel R. Boykin-Wright, MD
Tonia Willekes, MD
Clara Scott, BSW

UT-HHSC/MS Houston, Texas
Carlos Herrera, MD (PI)
Madeline Jewell, MSN

West Alabama Health Services, Inc, Eutaw, Alabama
Sandral Hullett, MD (PI)
Glenn Hughes, PhD
Queen Batch, LPN

West Alabama Health Services—Greensboro Center, Greensboro, Alabama
Sandral Hullett, MD (PI)
Glenn Hughes, PhD
Queen Batch, LPN

WAHS—Livingston Health Center, Livingston, Alabama
Sandral Hullett, MD (PI)
Glenn Hughes, PhD

WorkSite Treatment, New York, New York
Joaquin Negrette, MD (PI)
Virginia Littauer, RN

Storeworkers' Local #3, New York, New York
Joaquin Negrette, MD (PI)
Virginia Littauer, RN

University of Nevada School of Medicine, Las Vegas
Ambika Rao, MD (PI)
Roslyn M. Collins, RN

West Gastroenterology Group, Inglewood, California
Timothy C. Simmons, MD (PI)
Fred Gletten, MD
Donald Henderson, MD
Adebambo Ojuri, MD
Bisrat Yirgou

Newark Community Health Centers, Inc., Newark, New Jersey
Anita Vaughn, MD (PI)
Ernestine Blaine

Bedford-Stuyvesant Family Health Center, Brooklyn, New York
M. Monica Sweeney, MD (PI)
Anthony Greenidge, MD

Peekskill Area Health Center, Peekskill, New York
Peter Foster, MD (PI)
Jose Baez, MD
Helen Sandefur, LPN

Clinical Directors Network Inc., New York, New York
Jonathan N. Tobin, PhD (PI)
Flavio Rausei, MBA

Osteopathic Health Care Center, Philadelphia, Pennsylvania
Ronald Reinhard, DO (PI)
Shirley Combs

PCOM Cambria Street Healthcare Center, Philadelphia, Pennsylvania
Ronald Reinhard, DO (PI)
Oliver Bullock, DO
Suzanne Walker

Jackson-Hinds Comprehensive Health Center, Jackson, Mississippi
W.T. Crowell, MD (PI)
N. Shekoni, MD
Adonna James, RN

King/Drew Medical Center, Los Angeles, California
Harry J. Ward, MD (PI)
Barbara, Brackeen, RN

OCHC—Stone Mountain Medical Office, Stone Mountain, Georgia
Adel Mikhail, MD (PI)
Robert J. Anderson, PharmD

The Medical Center for Lane County, Springfield, Oregon
Randall G. Lorenz, MD (PI)
Laurie Lorenz, RN

Kaiser Permanente of Georgia, Tucker, Georgia
Joshua Barzilay, MD (PI)
Jeanne L. Jordan, RN, BSN

Candler Medical Group—Central Park, Savannah, Georgia
Paul S. Bradley, MD (PI)
Ray R. Maddox, PharmD
Wanda Kay North, RN, CCRC

Candler Medical Group, Savannah, Georgia
Paul S. Bradley, MD (PI)
Robert B. Remler, MD
Wanda Kay North, RN, CCRC

Candler Medical Group—Rincon, Rincon, Georgia
Paul S. Bradley, MD (PI)
Jack D. Heneisen, MD
David E. Sauers, DO
Wanda Kay North, RN, CCRC

Forest Hill Family Practice, Richmond, Virginia
Benjamin F. Zambrana, PhD, MD (PI)
Nancy Williams

AHEC Family Practice Center, Pine Bluff, Arizona
Herbert F. Fendley, MD (PI)
Ann Fendley, MD
J.E. ''Eddie'' Maples, Jr. RN, RRT

Cardiovascular Physicians, LTD, Milwaukee, Wisconsin
Burton J. Friedman, MD (PI)
Anne Friedman, RN

Albert Einstein Hospital, Bronx, New York
David Brown, MD (PI)
Madhavi Pamidi, MD
Mirian Zavala, RN

University Health Associates, Charleston, West Virginia
Stephen R. Grubb, MD, FACP (PI)
Whitney B. Robinson, RN, BSN

Ochsner Clinic—Baton Rouge, Baton Rouge, Louisiana
Jay Hollman, MD (PI)
Rajat Bhushan, MD
Deborah Mayeux, LPN

Mid Delta Family Practice Clinic, Cleveland, Mississippi
Nate Brown, MD (PI)
Alicia Williams Evans
Sarah Cooks

Westview Clinic, West St. Paul, Minnesota
James W. Haight, MD (PI)
Sue Hassing

Cook County Hospital, Chicago, Illinois
Arthur Hoffman, MD, MPH (PI)
Emma Edwards, RN, BSN

Ridgeview Research Center, Chanhassen, Minnesota
Roberta Midwinter, MD (PI)
Cecil Provence, MD
John Torseth, MD
Cheryl Blaser, CMA, CCRC

UCLA School of Medicine, Los Angeles, California
Ka Kit P. Hui, MD, FACP (PI)
Vladimir Bokarius, MD

University of Mississippi Medical Center, Jackson, Mississippi
C. Andrew Brown, MD, MPH (PI)
Catherine Adair, RN

Augusta Hypertension, PC, Augusta, Georgia
Wayne H. Kaesemeyer, MD (PI)
Sonya C. Holtkamp, RN, BSN

Hamilton Health Center, Harrisburg, Pennsylvania
Thomas M. Bryan, MD (PI)
Portia Bolen-Geter

Hamilton Health Center—Walnut Street, Harrisburg, Pennsylvania
Leilani Gyening, MD (PI)
Portia Bolen-Geter

Lehigh Valley Hospital, Allentown, Pennsylvania
Nelson Kopyt, DO (PI)
Mary Gallagher Sabo, BSN

Palomar Medical Group, Escondido, California
Emmet W. Lee, MD (PI)
Cary Hoover, CRC

Medical Clinic, San Juan, Texas
Rodolfo Nieto Trevino, MD (PI)
Maria Teresa Trevino, MD
Isela A. Martinez

Leo L. Altenberg, MD, PA, Euless, Texas
Leo L. Altenberg, MD (PI)
Alma Lozano

Wayne State University Health Center, Detroit, Michigan
Anita Moncrease, MD (PI)

Robert Mendelson, MD Private Practice, Jamaica, New York
Robert I. Mendelson, MD (PI)

Bowdoin Street Health Center, Dorchester, Massachusetts
Joseph A. Ingelfinger, MD (PI)

Codman Square Community Health Center, Boston, Massachusetts
Jonathan Pincus, MD (PI)
Joseph A. Ingelfinger, MD
Vivian Jimenez

The Ohio State University, Columbus, Ohio
Robert A. Murden, MD, FACP (PI)

Fleet/Burgdorf Health Center, Hartford, Connecticut
Ellen Olarsh Nestler, MD (PI)
Nellie Medina, RN

Wake Forest University School of Medicine, Winston-Salem, North Carolina
Frank S. Celestino, MD (PI)
John Summerson, MS

John Peter Smith Hospital, Fort Worth, Texas
Richard Young, MD (PI)

Harlem Hospital Center, New York, New York
Velvie Anne Pogue, MD (PI)
Michael Omoh, MD
Donna Dowie, MD

Trinity Hypertension Research Center, Carrollton, Texas
Henry A. Punzi, MD, FACIP (PI)
Dawn DeRoo, RN, WHCNP

John D. Stokes, MD, PA, Clearwater, Florida
John D. Stokes, MD (PI)
Jamie L. Rousseau

Medical Parameters, Martinez, Georgia
Robert B. Rhoades, MD (PI)
Shirley K. Wiley, MA, CCRC

Sutter Gould Medical Foundation, Modesto, California
George Chao, MD (PI)
Stephen Turitzin, MD
Gale F. Golden, RN, CRC

Providence Medical Center Heart Research Department, Portland, Oregon
Frank D. McBarron, MD (PI)
Stephanie MacKenzie

Richard Fowler, MD, PC, Mesa, Arizona
Richard F. Fowler, MD (PI)
Dianne Woods Fowler, RN

University of Illinois College of Medicine, Peoria, Illinois
James F. Graumlich, MD (PI)
Steven Belknap, MD
Susan Cole, MD
Nancy L. Novotny, RN, MS

Carver Family Health Center, Peoria, Illinois
James F. Graumlich, MD (PI)
James W. Barnett, MD
Nancy S. Novotny, RN, MS

The Cleveland Clinic Foundation, Cleveland, Ohio
Donald G. Vidt, MD (PI)
Joseph P. Frolkis, MD, FACP
Pamela S. Suhan, RN, CCRC

Clinic for Digestive and Nutritional Disorders, Tallahassee, Florida
Joseph Lee Webster, Sr, MD (PI)
Robin Byrd Webster

Cora Christian, MD—Private Practice, Frederiksted, St. Croix, Virgin Islands
Cora L. E. Christian, MD, MPH, FAAFP (PI)
Kathleen Bryan, MA

AHEC of South Arkansas Family Practice Clinic, El Dorado, Arizona
J. Douglas Owens, MD (PI)
Renee McCafferty, MS

Internal Medicine Clinic, National Naval Medical Center, Bethesda, Maryland
Gerald D. Denton, MD (PI)
Dianne Tesch, RNP

ALLHAT Clinical Center, Danville, Illinois
R. Sadiq, MD (PI)
Beth Mason, PharmD
Penny L. Sands, RN

Community Healthcare Clinic, Houston, Texas
Admerle Hall-Hoskins, DO (PI)
Netha Gardner

University Family Medicine Foundation, Cleveland, Ohio
George E. Kikano, MD (PI)
Darrell T. Hulisz, PharmD
Larraine Jacob, RN

Mercy Diagnostic and Treatment Center, Chicago, Illinois
Dan Vicencio, MD (PI)
Charlene Bermele, RN

R. Glenn Carter, MD—Private Practice, Hinesville, Georgia
R. Glenn Carter, MD (PI)
Yvonne B. Jones, MA

University of Oklahoma College of Medicine-Tulsa, Tulsa, Oklahoma
Martina J. Jelley, MD, MSPH (PI)
Tracy Lawson, RN

Heart and Lung Associates of the Finger Lakes, Newark, New York
Frederick T. Zugibe, Jr. MD (PI)
Anna R. Zugibe

Bronx Nephrology Hypertension PC, Bronx, New York
Mario A. Henriquez, MD, FACP (PI)
Ana Silvia Henriquez, MPH

Doctor's Office, Haverstraw, New York
Mario A. Henriquez, MD, FACP (PI)
Olga Garcia

East Albany Medical Center, Albany, Georgia
Phillip R. Poulos, MD (PI)
Ron Malcolm, PA
Jani Dennis, RN

Baker County Primary Health Center, Newton, Georgia
Phillip R. Poulos, MD (PI)
James Womack, PA
Madeleine (Madge) Holm, BSN

Lee Medical Arts Center, Leesburg, Georgia
Phillip R. Poulos, MD (PI)
Michael Hardy, PA-C
Madeleine (Madge) Holm, BSN

Edison Medical Center, Edison, Georgia
Phillip R. Poulos, MD (PI)
Cynthia Earl, PA-C
Madeleine (Madge) Holm, BSN

Redwood Family Practice, Eureka, California
Lawrence J. Wieland, MD (PI)
Douglas Jornlin, RN

Clearwater Cardiovascular Consultants, Clearwater, Florida
Jorge P. Navas, MD (PI)
Ann Gove, RN, BA

Baylor College of Medicine, Houston, Texas
Carlos Vallbona, MD (PI)
David Hyman, MD, MPH
Valory Pavlik, PhD
Glori Chauca, MD

Bay Hill Family Care, Orlando, Florida
Nasirdin H. Madhany, MD (PI)
Marion Brewster, LPN

Loma Linda Faculty Medical Offices, Loma Linda, California
Denise Jackson Townsend, MD (PI)
Leslie Albert, RN

Altru Hospital, Grand Forks, North Dakota
Noah N. Chelliah, MD (PI)
Kelly Hagen, RN

Martha Flowers, MD—Private Practice, Pine Bluff, Arizona
Martha Ann Flowers, MD (PI)
Johnnie Miller, BS, FNP

UT Southwestern Medical Center, Hypertension Division, Dallas, Texas
Nina Radford, MD (PI)
Ronald Victor, MD
Shannon Daly, RN

ALLHAT Clinical Center, Gahanna, Ohio
Albert M. Salomon, DO (PI)
Andree Welsh

Pulsifer Medical Associates PC, Rochester, New York
David Dobrzynski, MD (PI)
Joyce Hackemer, RPA-C

Primary Care Internal Medicine Clinic, El Paso, Texas
Jo Anne Neubauer, MD (PI)
Price Stanley, PharmD
Debra Manghane, RN

Valley Medical Group, Bakersfield, California
Carlos A. Alvarez, MD (PI)
Kent Simmons, RN, FNP

South Carolina Heart Center, Columbia, South Carolina
William Lawrence Schoolmeester, MD (PI)
Jacqueline Sheriod, BSN

The Mt. Sinai Medical Center, Cleveland, Ohio
Laurie Sadler, MD, FACP (PI)
Robert L. Haynie, MD, PhD
Julian Isakow, MD
Ellen S. Cooper, RN

Fanno Creek Clinic, Portland, Oregon
Scott W. Falley, MD (PI)

Mayo Clinic, Division of Hypertension, Rochester, Minnesota
Vincent J. Canzanello, MD (PI)
John W. Graves, MD
Lois Klein

Cardiology Foundation of Lankenau, Wynnewood, Pennsylvania
James F. Burke, MD (PI)

Michael Duzy, DO
Susan Heaney, RN, MSN

Fairbury Medical Associates BPMC, Fairbury, Illinois
Nikhi Kothari, MD (PI)
Shirley Ifft

Voice of Calvary Family Health Center, Jackson, Mississippi
Andrea Phillips, MD (PI)
Dilshad Fakhruddin, MD
Teresa Polk, CFNP

Voice of Calvary Family Health Center, West, Jackson, Mississippi
Andrea Phillips, MD (PI)
Dilshad Fakhruddin, MD
Teresa Polk, CFNP

Voice of Calvary—Nazareth Church, Jackson, Mississippi
Andrea L. Phillips, MD (PI)

VAMC Augusta, Augusta, Georgia
Thomas J. Hartney, MD (PI)
Nanci McPhail, MD
Nancy London, RN

VAMC Baltimore, Baltimore, Maryland
Bruce P. Hamilton, MD (PI)
Jennifer H. Hamilton, MD
Acquanetta Lancaster, NP
Yvonne B. Ferguson

VAMC Kansas City, Kansas City, Missouri
Thomas B. Wiegmann, MD (PI)
Dana Smith, RN, BSN

VAMC Bronx, Bronx, New York
Clive Rosendorff, MD, PhD (PI)
Steven A. Atlas, MD
Jean Baruth, RN

VAMC Buffalo, Buffalo, New York
James Lohr, MD (PI)
Kenneth A. Kellick, PharmD
Peggy Gugliuzza, RN, NP

VAMC East Orange, East Orange, New Jersey
Sithiporn Sastrasinh, MD (PI)

VAMC Houston, Houston, Texas
Gabriel B. Habib, MD (PI)
Patricia Tibbits

VAMC Louisville, Louisville, Kentucky
Vasti L. Broadstone, MD (PI)
Eloise U. Campbell, RN, BSN, CDE

VAMC Milwaukee, Milwaukee, Wisconsin
Mahendr S. Kochar, MD (PI)
Gloria Kotecki, LPN

VAMC New Orleans, New Orleans, Louisiana
Vecihi Batuman, MD (PI)
Patricia Willhoit, RN, NP

VAMC Kansas City, MO, Kansas City, Missouri
Santosh Sharma, MD (PI)
Phyllis Hannah, MD
Terri Finnigan, RN, BSN

VAMC St. Louis, St. Louis, Missouri
Stephen J. Giddings, PhD, MD (PI)
Sharon Carmody

VAMC St. Louis, St. Louis, Missouri
Stephen J. Giddings, PhD, MD (PI)
Shantiel Fleming

VAMC Washington, DC, Washington, DC:
Vasilios Papademetriou, MD (PI)
Puneet Narayan, MD
Aldo Notargiacomo, BS

VAMC Alexandria, Alexandria, Louisiana
Jerome M. Sampson, MD (PI)
Clement FX Carroll, MD
Kamalendia Mondal, MD
Janet Schmitt, PharmD

VAMC Battle Creek, Battle Creek, Michigan
Ireneo Diaz, MD (PI)

VAMC Bay Pines, Bay Pines, Florida
Ramon Lopez, MD (PI)
Jacques Durr, MD
Tatiana Webster, MD
Debra Williams, RN

VAMC Brooklyn, Brooklyn, New York
William L. Green, MD (PI)
Amal Farag, MD
Helena A. Guber, MD
Estelita Anteola, RN

VAMC Charleston, Charleston, South Carolina
Jan N. Basile, MD (PI)

Irene Coley
Allston A. Kitchens
Jennifer McFaddin
Deborah Ham, BS

VAMC Dayton, Dayton, Ohio
Mohammed Saklayen, MD (PI)
Anil Kumar Mandal, MD
Helen J. Neff, RN

Carl Vinson VAMC, Dublin, Georgia
K. J. Upadhya, MD (PI)
Meenakshi M. Ram, MD
Lauri Wilkes, BS

VAMC Lake City, Lake City, Florida
Girish Bhaskar, MD (PI)
Ut Van Tran, MD
Gloria C. Duren, LPN

VAMC Jackson, Jackson, Mississippi
Kent Kirchner, MD (PI)
Rajesh Patel, MD
Ardell Hinton, MS, CCRC

VAMC North Little Rock, North Little Rock, Arkansas
William J. Carter, MD (PI)
Miriam Rose Oakum, MD
Mary E. Lynch, MT

VAMC Loma Linda, Loma Linda, California
Paul G. St. John Hammond, MD (PI)
Dana A. Shriver, RN, BSN

VAMC Long Beach, Long Beach, California
Joel Neutel, MD (PI)
Deanna G. Cheung, MD
Stanley Franklin, MD
Gaurang Shah, MD
Eric Bowes

VAMC Minneapolis, Minneapolis, Minnesota
Jordan Holtzman, MD (PI)
Kara Rebeck, RN, MA, MA

VAMC Murfreesboro, Murfreesboro, Tennessee
Dharapuram Venugopal, MD (PI)
Regina Cassidy, PharmD
Rimda Gupta, MD

VA Medical Center, Nashville, Tennessee
Ghodrat A. Siami, MD, PhD (PI)
Hayden Ross-Clunis, MD
Flora Sandra Siami, BS

VAMC Northport Medical Services, Northport, New York
Joanne Holland, MD (PI)
Christine Spiller, RN

Carl T. Hayden VA Medical Center, Phoenix, Arizona
James V. Felicetta, MD (PI)
Nicollette Estrada, FNP
Halina Roznowski, RN-CRC

VAMC Richmond, Richmond, Virginia
Pramod Mohanty, MD (PI)
James Schmitt, MD
Edie Earley, RN

VAMC Salisbury, Salisbury, North Carolina
Samuel M. Fox, PharmD (PI)
Lateena Loggans, RN

VAMC-1 San Francisco, San Francisco, California
Barry Massie, MD (PI)
Denise Van Ostaeyen, RNP

VAMC-2 San Francisco, San Francisco, California
Barry Massie, MD (PI)
Denise Van Ostaeyen, RNP

VAMC San Juan, San Juan, Puerto Rico
Jose Luis Cianchini, MD (PI)
Jean DaMore, RN

VAMC Columbia, Columbia, South Carolina
Alberto Saenz, MD (PI)
Ken Jones

VAMC Tucson, Tucson, Arizona
Steven Goldman, MD (PI)
Janice Christensen, MD
Hoang Thai, MD
Janet Ohm, RN, BSN, CCRN, CCRC

VAMC North Chicago, North Chicago, Illinois
Jen-Chieh Cheng, MD (PI)
Janice L. Gilden, MD
Sant P. Singh, MD
Maria Lesko, RN

VAMC Oklahoma City, Oklahoma City, Oklahoma
Udho Thadani, MBBS, MRCP, FRCP(C), FACC (PI)
Barbara A. Parker, RN, BSN

VAMC Leavenworth, Leavenworth, Kansas
Donald L. Courtney, MD (PI)
Dorinda Wilson

VAMC Shreveport, Shreveport, Louisiana
W. Ronald Skowsky, MD (PI)
Ann Leitz, RN, MSN

VAMC Pittsburgh, Pittsburgh, Pennsylvania
Melissa McNeil, MD (PI)
Laurie Trilli Carradine, PharmD
Lisa Hirosky

VAMC Tampa, Tampa, Florida
Alfredo Peguero-Rivera, MD (PI)
Nancy Rolbiecki, LPN

Camden Internal Medicine Associates, PA, Camden, South Carolina
James C. McAlpine, Jr. MD (PI)
Darlene Weathers, LPN

Raleigh Internal Medicine Associates, PA, Raleigh, North Carolina
Christopher M. Perkins, MD (PI)
James O'Rourke, MD
Lynda E. Seal, RN

Morehouse School of Medicine, Atlanta, Georgia
David W. Anderson, MD (PI)
Tim Briscoe, PharmD

Morehouse Medical Associates, Atlanta, Georgia
Elizabeth Ofili, MD (PI)
Claudette Mitchell-Ali LPN/CVT

E.O. Family Health Center, Inc., Miami, Florida
Fatima Zafar, MD (PI)
Patricia A. Seabrooks, ARNP, C, DNSc

Family Practice Group, Pocatello, Idaho
Michael S. Baker, MD (PI)
Todd Gillespie, PA-C

New Britain General Hospital, New Britain, Connecticut
James L. Bernene, MD (PI)
Anthony Lachman, MD
John Lawson, MD
Linda Ciarcia, RN

ALLHAT Clinical Center, Unionville, Connecticut
James L. Bernene, MD (PI)

John Lawson, MD
Linda Ciarcia, RN

Jeffrey M. Kagan, MD—Private Practice, Newington, Connecticut
James L. Bernene, MD (PI)
Jeffrey M. Kagan, MD
Kathryn Horman, PA-C, BS

ALLHAT Clinical Center, Shreveport, Louisiana
Byron Andra M. Jackson, MD (PI)

Marshfield Clinic, Marshfield, Wisconsin
Richard Dart, MD (PI)
Douglas Duffy, MD
Dawn David

Lakeland Center—Marshfield Clinic, Minocqua, Wisconsin
Richard Dart, MD (PI)
Mark Rassier, MD
Peg Bodmer, RN

MediQuest Research Group Inc., Ocala, Florida
Robert L. Feldman, MD (PI)
Shari Strickland, LPN

Blackstone Cardiology Associates, Pawtucket, Rhode Island
Kenneth A. LaBresh, MD (PI)
Catherine Alteri

Chinatown Service Center Family Health Clinic, Los Angeles, California
Jin Sim Khoo, MD (PI)
Y. C. Huang

Bassett Healthcare, Cooperstown, New York
Anne N. Nafziger, MD, MHS (PI)
Anne Menhinick, RN, BSN

1199 Worksite Wellness Programs, New York, New York
Celia Shmukler, MD (PI)
Susan Gedan, RN

Interfaith Medical Center, Brooklyn, New York
Devendra K. Shrivastava, MD (PI)
Debbie DeJesus, EMT

University of South Dakota, Sioux Falls, South Dakota
Angelina Trujillo, MD (PI)
Cheryl Ageton, RN

University Physicians—Rapid City, Rapid City, South Dakota
Angelina Trujillo, MD (PI)
Steve Haas, MD
Judy Haas, RN, BSN

Ogden Research Foundation, Ogden, Utah
C. Basil Williams, MD (PI)
Cynthia L. Slot, CRC

Northwestern Medical Faculty Foundation, Chicago, Illinois
Martin J. Arron, MD (PI)

Victor E. Battles, MD, Fort Worth, Texas
Victor E. Battles, MD (PI)
Judy Hill, RN

Erickson Medical Clinic, Park Rapids, Minnesota
Vern E. Erickson, MD (PI)
Janice Heegard

Centro Cardiovascular de Caguas, Caguas, Puerto Rico
Pedro J. Colon, Sr, MD, FACC (PI)
Nivea I. Vazquez, BBA

Comerio Medical Center, Comerio, Puerto Rico
Luis Gonzalez-Bermudez, MD (PI)
Maria A. Collazo, MD
Ricardo Martinez, MD
Emilio Rivera, MD
Carmen Sanchez, RN
Grisel I. Martinez

Woodland Avenue Health Center, Philadelphia, Pennsylvania
Brenda D. Rogers, MD (PI)
Shradhdha Patel, RN

Columbia Medical Plan, Columbia, Maryland
Michael Kelemen, MD (PI)
Eileen E. Brightwell, BS

Southwest Medical Associates, Las Vegas, Nevada
James W. Synder, MD (PI)
Ruth E. Parr, RN, BSN

Lake Charles Memorial Heart and Vascular Center, Lake Charles, Louisiana
James S. Dunnick, MD (PI)
Tammy Hughes, LPN

CCOM Medical Group, Inc, Muskogee, Oklahoma
Yee Se C. Ong, MD (PI)
Viola Christy, RN

East Side Internists, Inc, Providence, Rhode Island
Richard J. Ruggieri, MD (PI)

Sigurds Janners, MD, PC, Hancock, Michigan
Sigurds Janners, MD (PI)
Candace E. Koski Janners, RN, BSN

University of Kansas Medical Center, Kansas City, Kansas
David B. Wilson, MD (PI)
Di DeVore, RN

Cardiology Associates, Port Charlotte, Florida
Louis D. Rosenfield, MD (PI)
Paul Eubanks, CMA

The Lindner Research Center, Cincinnati, Ohio
Robert Toltzis, MD (PI)
Chris Blanck, RN

Truman Medical Center UMKC School of Medicine, Kansas City, Missouri
Nathaniel Winer, MD (PI)
Annette M. Quick, MD
Carol J. Tudor

Atlantic Cardiology Associates, Exter, New Hampshire
Mark I. Jacobs, MD (PI)
Joyce Aliseo, RN

Myers Foundation Family Health Center of Tchula, Tchula, Mississippi
Ronald V. Myers, Sr, MD (PI)
Elvis James, MA

Myers Foundation—Family Health Center of Yazoo City, Yazoo City, Mississippi
Ronald V. Myers, Sr, MD (PI)
Sylvia H. Myers

Myers Foundation Family Health Center of Belzoni, Belzoni, Mississippi
Ronald V. Myers, Sr, MD (PI)
Barbara Bell, CNA

Howard S. Ellison, MD, PC, Conyers, Georgia
Howard S. Ellison, MD (PI)
Gail Lowe, MT

Maimonides Primary Care, Brooklyn, New York
Justine Ngheim, MD (PI)
Mila Yevdayeva

St. Agnes Adult Ambulatory Care Center, Baltimore, Maryland
Hanna Rachocka, MD (PI)
Max Kawalec, MD
Sharon Silverman, MD
Debbie Som, MD
Karen Thompson

Tatum Family Health Clinic, Gary, Indiana
David E. Ross, MD (PI)
Henedina W. Macabalitaw, MD
Lorraine Leavy

Medical Diagnostics Center, Indianapolis, Indiana
John Howard Pratt, MD (PI)
Kathy Byrd

Johns Hopkins Geriatrics Center, Baltimore, Maryland
Peter Vietas Vaitkevicius, MD (PI)

Health Trends Research LLC, Baltimore, Maryland
Boris Kerzner, MD (PI)
Susan E. Childs, BS, BSN, MS
Dan Yetter

Winona Memorial Hospital, Indianapolis, Indiana
Jack H. Hall, MD (PI)
Dottie Fausset, MBA, RN

Medical Research Consortium—Lebanon, Lebanon, Indiana
Jack H. Hall, MD (PI)
Elaine Habig, MD
Susan S. Taylor, RN

Faculty-Resident Group Practice, Michael Reese Hospital, Chicago, Illinois
Kevin E. Hunt, MD (PI)
Hallie Howard, RN

All Saints Health Care, Racine, Wisconsin
Gregory A. Shove, MD (PI)
Jeralyn Scales, Medical Assistant

Maricopa Medical Center, Phoenix, Arizona
William Dachman, MD (PI)
Jeff Parker, MD
Cindy Foley, EMT, CRC

Creighton Cardiac Center, Omaha, Nebraska
Syed M. Mohiuddin, MD (PI)
Lois A. Rasmussen, RN, BSN

Montefiore Medical Center, Bronx, New York
Janet U. Gorkin, MD (PI)
Amy Erlich, MD

Cardiovascular Medical Specialists, PA, Hollywood, Florida
Jonathan R. Jaffe, MD (PI)
Lisa Nitzberg, MD

Intermedic Health Center, Port Charlotte, Florida
Terence P. Connelly, MD (PI)
Charlotte Bould, RN

Family Health Center of West Town, Chicago, Illinois
Michael Friedman, MD (PI)

Naresh K. Parikh, MD, PC, Chamblee, Georgia
Naresh K. Parikh, MD (PI)
Rekha Singh, MD

Department of Family Practice & Family Practice Residency Program, Yonkers, New York
Lauren DeAlleaume, MD (PI)
Joseph L. Halbach, MD, MPH
Catherine L. Hopkins, MS, RN, FNP

Lutheran Senior Health Services, Fort Wayne, Indiana
Kavita S. Persaud, MD (PI)
Deborah Mielke, RN

Abi Rayner, MD PSC, Madisonville, Kentucky
Abi V. Rayner, MD (PI)
Connie R. Tyler, RN

Wyman Park Medical Associates, Baltimore, Maryland
Sandra W. Hairston, MD (PI)
Marilyn Partlow, LPN

Westfield Family Physicians, PC, Sherman, New York
Donald Brautigam, MD (PI)
Chris Flanders, RN, BSN

Allina Health System—United Family Health Center, St. Paul, Minnesota
Katherine F. Guthrie, MD (PI)
Carol Ann M. Kubajak, PharmD, MS

Kenneth H. Williams and Associates, Baltimore, Maryland
Kenneth H. Williams, MD (PI)
J. William Cook, MD
Stephanie Linder, MD
Barbara Socha, MD
Mary Carol Gary, RN

Deaconess Hospital—Center Campus, St. Louis, Missouri
Madan Chilappa, MD (PI)
M. Renee Kelley, RMA

Cardiology Division, New Bellevue, New York, New York
Richard I. Levin, MD, FACP, FACC (PI)

Northern Counties Health Care Inc., Hardwick, Vermont
Brendan N. Buckley, MD (PI)
Tonya H. Howard, RN, FNP
Fay Gallant

Danville Health Center, Danville, Vermont
Brendan N. Buckley, MD (PI)
Timothy Tanner, MD
Penelope Courchesne, RN

Northern Counties Health Care Inc.—Concord, Vermont
Brendan N. Buckley, MD (PI)
Bradford Armstrong, MD
Pat Cushman, RN

Northern Counties Health Care Inc.—Island Pond, Vermont
Brendan N. Buckley, MD (PI)
Robert Primeau, MD
Janet Osborne, RN

Valley Medical Center, Kettering, Ohio
Meenakshi Patel, MD (PI)
Jackie Tucker, CMA

Ringrose Clinic, Inc, Guthrie, Oklahoma
Robert E. Ringrose, MD (PI)
Karen Walters, RNC

Altus Medical Clinic, Altus, Oklahoma
Joe Leverett, MD (PI)
Lonnie Scholl, PA-C

Cardiology Associates of Johnstown, Johnstown, Pennsylvania
Charles J. Oschwald, MD, FACC (PI)
Noelle Potts, RT

Lancaster Heart Foundation, Lancaster, Pennsylvania
Seth J. Worley, MD, FACC (PI)
Joann Tuzi, RN

Family Medicine, Brent Clark, MD, Pittsburgh, Pennsylvania
Brent Clark, MD (PI)

Sant Ram Medical Associates, West Grove, Pennsylvania
Deepak Sant Ram, MD (PI)
Bernice Springer

Family Medical Center, Johnstown, Pennsylvania
Jeanne Spencer, MD (PI)
Loretta Nagy, LPN

Associates in Diagnostic Internal Medicine, Pittsburgh, Pennsylvania
Peter P. Tanzer, MD (PI)

Cardiology Outpatient Clinic—University of Pittsburgh, Pittsburgh, Pennsylvania
Galal M. Ziady, MD (PI)
David Nace, MD
Marsha L. MacIntyre, RN

Idaho State University Department of Family Medicine, Pocatello, Idaho
Rex W. Force, PharmD, BCPS (PI)
Mimi Macdonald, LPN

Excelsior Medical Clinic, Sumter, South Carolina
Joseph C. Williams, MD (PI)
Beverly Hill, Medical Assistant

Mid-South Clinical Research Institute (CRI), Memphis, Tennessee
Howard W. Marker, MD (PI)
Michael Herr, RN

Clinical Cardiology Research Center, Dallas, Texas
Cara East, MD (PI)
Elizabeth Soltero, CCRC

University of Texas Health Center at Tyler, Tyler, Texas
David R. Shafer, MD (PI)
Barbara Hiltscher, RN, BSN

Madrona Medical Group, Bellingham, Washington
Grant E. Deger, MD (PI)
Jeanette Anderson, RN

University of Arkansas for Medical Sciences—Endocrinology, Little Rock, Arkansas
Debra L. Simmons, MD (PI)
Phil Kern, MD
Kathy Riordan, RN, CDE

Tower Medical Associates, Los Angeles, California
William T. Young, MD (PI)
Valerie Thibideaux

Howard University Hypertension and Lipid Clinic, Washington, DC
Tamrat M. Retta, MD, PhD (PI)
Shichen Xu, MD

Internal Medicine Associates, Washington, DC
Jerry M. Earll, MD (PI)
Laraine Doyle, RN
Nancy Knowlan, RN

Christiana Care Health System, Newark, Delaware
G. Stephen DeCherney, MD (PI)
James Lenhard, MD
Deborah Crane, RN, CCRC

Palm Beach Center for Clinical Investigation, West Palm Beach, Florida
Lee A. Fischer, MD (PI)
Holly Hadley, MD

Uchenna A. Okoronkwo, II, MD, PC, Oakland, California
Uchenna A. Okoronkwo, II, MD (PI)
Gloria J. Joseph

LSU Clinics, New Orleans, Louisiana
Henry Rothschild, MD, PhD (PI)
Ann D. McKendrick, MSW

LSU Hypertension Research Clinic, New Orleans, Louisiana
Efrain Reisin, MD (PI)
Gertie Smith, LPN

Vernon A. Valentino, MD, APMC, Lafayette, Louisiana
Vernon A. Valentino, MD (PI)
Lisa Bass, LPN

Androscoggin Cardiology Associates, Auburn, Maine
Robert J. Weiss, MD, FACC, FACP (PI)
Tami Gosselin, MA

MCP-Hahnemann University, Philadelphia, Pennsylvania
Steven P. Kutalek, MD, FACC (PI)
Christina Ann Baessler, RN

Medical College of Pennsylvania Hospital, Philadelphia, Pennsylvania
Steven P. Kutalek, MD, FACC (PI)
John M. Fontaine, MD

Chapel Hill Internal Medicine, Chapel Hill, North Carolina
Paula F. Miller, MD (PI)
Whitman L. Reardon, MD

Family Practice Center, Columbus, Georgia
Michael F. Walsh, MD (PI)
Lauren C. Duty, PharmD
Lynn Stevenson, PharmD

Ambulatory Care Pharmacy, Columbus, Georgia
Michael F. Walsh, MD (PI)
Lauren C. Duty, PharmD
Lynn Stevenson, PharmD

MSU-KCMS Internal Medicine, Kalamazoo, Michigan
Anne Cavanagh, MD (PI)
Kathy S. Church, BSN, CEN

Danny M. Anderson, MD, Inc, Sonora, California
Danny M. Anderson, MD (PI)
Judith Joy Boggess, MD
Barbara Christianson, CMA

St. Thomas Medical Group, Nashville, Tennessee
Mark C. Houston, MD (PI)
Laurie Hays, RN

Heart Center of Salt Lake, Salt Lake City, Utah
J. Joseph Perry, MD (PI)
Wendy Schvaneveldt, RN

Cardiovascular Associates, PC—Montclair, Birmingham, Alabama
Russell C. Reeves, MD, FACC (PI)
Judy L. Swindell

Central North Alabama Health Services, Inc., Huntsville, Alabama
Arthur Williams, MD (PI)
Kristy Moorehead, LPN

East Tennessee Medical Group, Maryville, Tennessee
Alan Lee Smuckler, MD (PI)
Vickie Rhule, RN

Horizon Physicians Group, Knoxville, Tennessee
Alan Lee Smuckler, MD (PI)
Lee R. Dilworth, MD
Vickie Rhule, RN

Baptist Health Center, Talladega, Alabama
Clay Davis, MD (PI)
Joan Aultman, NP

Clinical Hypertension Center, Los Angeles, California
Vincent DeQuattro, MD (PI)
Debora DePing Li, MD

Brevard Cardiology Group, Merritt Island, Florida
Khalid H. Sheikh, MD, FACC (PI)
Eugene Killeavy, MD, FACC
Ursula Anderson, ARNP

Midatlantic Cardiovascular Associates—Plumtree Road, Bel Air, Maryland
Sidney O. Gottlieb, MD, FACC (PI)
Lois Nelson, PA
David Lowry, MPH, DrPH

Midatlantic Cardiovascular Associates, Baltimore, Maryland
Sidney O. Gottlieb, MD, FACC (PI)
Loriane Black

Washington County Internal Medicine, PC, Sandersville, Georgia
William Rawlings, MD (PI)
Jessica Heldreth, LPN

Indiana University—Methodist Family Practice Center, Indianapolis, Indiana
David L. Fryman, MD (PI)
Julie Koehler, PharmD

Cardiovascular Clinics, PC, Merrillville, Indiana
Harish A. Shah, MD (PI)
T. Nguyen, MD
Shah Vijay, MD
Dave Vijay, MD
Erica Johnston, RCVT

The Heart Clinic PA, Kansas City, Kansas
Nalini G. Premsingh, MD (PI)
Kathy Schroepfer

Kaiser Permanente Largo Medical Center, Largo, Maryland
John S. Golden, MD (PI)
Donna J. Mateski, MS, RD

ALLHAT Clinical Center, Bridgewater, New Jersey
Alexander B. Kudryk, MD (PI)
Susan Yuchnovitz, LPN

ALLHAT Clinical Center, Mount Holly, New Jersey
R. Bruce Denniston, MD, FACP (PI)
Marylyn Reppert

Primary Care Center, Sandersville, Georgia
Earle M. Taylor, MD (PI)
Mike Loraditch, MD
Talesha W. Phillips, LPN

Family Medical Center, Seattle, Washington
Allan J. Ellsworth, PharmD (PI)
Bill Neighbor, MD

Carolina Family Care (Denmark), Denmark, South Carolina
Robert M. Jones, MD (PI)
Angela L. Hampton, PA-C
Randi K. Popp, MD
Barbara S. Boineau, MA

Family Medicine Center, Charleston, South Carolina
Angela G. Wilson, PharmD (PI)

WNC Hypertension Prevention and Treatment Center, Asheville, North Carolina
Ronald R. Caldwell, MD (PI)
Kymberly M. Caldwell

The Union Memorial Hospital, Baltimore, Maryland
F. Michael Gloth, III, MD, FACP (PI)
C. E. Smith, C-CRC

Illinois Center for Clinical Trials, Chicago, Illinois
Glen A. Sussman, PhD (PI)
Robert June, MD, PhD
Leslie Zun, MD, MBA, FACEP
Tamara Hemphill, RN

San Diego Cardiovascular Associates, Encinitas, California
George W. Dennish, III, MD, FACC (PI)
Nancy Horton, LVN, CRC

North General Hospital, New York New York
Myo Maw, MD (PI)
Kevin Martin, MD

Charles F. Scott, MDPC, East Point, Georgia
Charles F. Scott, MD (PI)
Corine Munroe

Memorial Health University Medical Center, Savannah, Georgia
Lloyd S. Goodman, MD (PI)
Raymond Earl Stanford, RN, CCRC

W. Murray Yarbrough, MD—Private Practice, Birmingham, Alabama
W. Murray Yarbrough, MD (PI)
Elizabeth N. Yarbrough

Indianapolis Cardiovascular Research Office, Indianapolis, Indiana
Bradley A. Weinberg, MD (PI)
Beth Viellieu-Fischer, RN

East Carolina University School of Medicine, Greenville, North Carolina
Mark D. Darrow, MD (PI)
Lisa Rodebaugh, RN

Selma Medical Associates, Winchester, Virginia
Randolph H. Renzi, MD (PI)
Linda Stollings Thompson, RN

Naval Medical Center San Diego, San Diego, California
CDR Peter E. Linz, MC USN (PI)
Ker Boyce, MD
Janet Kozlowski, RN

Thomas A McKnight, MD, PC, Fremont, Nebraska
Thomas A. McKnight, MD (PI)
Jean K. Schafersman, CMA

ALLHAT Clinical Center, Philadelphia, Pennsylvania
Pasquale F. Nestico, MD (PI)
Olivia Ranalli

Mobile Diagnostic Center, Mobile, Alabama
Thomas A. Kessler, MD (PI)
Nancy P. Wettermark

Truman Medical Center-East, Kansas City, Missouri
Beth E. Rosemergey, MD (PI)
Kelly Gorman

Ong Medical Center, Oxon Hill, Maryland
Stephen T. Ong, MD, MPH (PI)
Daryl Fraley

St. John Family Practice, St. Petersburg, Florida
Hugo A. St. John, MD (PI)
Teresa St. John, BSN

Internal Medicine Center of Akron, Akron, Ohio
Joseph A. Finocchio, MD (PI)
Irene Chenowith, MD
Amy Law, RN

UMDNJ-New Jersey Medical School, Newark, New Jersey
Maya P. Raghuwanshi, MD (PI)
Aloysius B. Cuyjet, MD, FACC
Friedrick Nash, MD
Sarah Suarez, BA

Doctors Office Center (DOC), Newark, New Jersey
Maya P. Raghuwanshi, MD (PI)
Friedrick Nash, MD
Sarah Suarez, BA

Beaumont Internal Medicine Associates, PA, Beaumont, Texas
Carlos Arroyo, MD (PI)
Donna Richard

VAMC East Orange, East Orange, New Jersey
Suat Akgun, MD (PI)
Eileen Moser, MD
Linda Condit, RN

VAMC Las Vegas, Las Vegas, Nevada
Joseph Chinn, MD (PI)
Carol A. King, DrPH

Stratton VA Medical Center, Albany, New York
James T. Higgins, MD (PI)
Robert Garris, PharmD
Kerry Johnston, RPh
Benoit A. Tonneau, MD
James A. Begley, MS

VAMC Providence, Providence, Rhode Island
Satish Sharma, MD (PI)
Mary L. Beliard, RN

VAMC Batavia, Rochester, New York
Krishna Sharma, MD (PI)
Phyllis Gehring, RN

VAMC Marion, Marion, Illinois
Mohammed Mansuri, MD (PI)
Gayle Deeter, RN

VAMC Des Moines, Des Moines, Iowa
Russell Glynn, MD (PI)
Beth Hargens, RN

VAMC Salt Lake City, Salt Lake City, Utah
Christof Westenfelder, MD (PI)
Jeanie O'Donnell, MSN

VAMC Fargo, Fargo, North Dakota
Babu Eladasari, MD (PI)
Emily Garten, RN

VAMC Decatur, Decatur, Georgia
Mary Ellen Sweeney, MD (PI)
W. Virgil Brown, MD
Mary Ellen Sweeney, MD

VAMC Montgomery, Montgomery, Alabama
Avinash C. Pradhan, MD (PI)
Gail Palmgren, PharmD
Dolores E. Reed, RN, BSN

Cleveland Clinic Florida, Ft. Lauderdale, Florida
Jerry O. Ciocon, MD, FACP, FACA, AGSF (PI)
Erlinda Capili-Rosenkranz, MD
Gregory Cohn, MD
Fernando Stancampiano, MD
Renee (Maureen) Miller, RA

Botsford General Hospital, Farmington Hills, Michigan
Nicholas Z. Kerin, MD (PI)
Bernadette Letzring, RN

Diabetes and Metabolism Associates, APMC, New Orleans, Louisiana
Jonathan K. Wise, MD, FACP (PI)
Skye N. Noble, LPN

L.B. Price, MD, PA, Quincy, Florida
Ira B. Price, MD (PI)
Patricia Walden

Family Practice Center, Ottumwa, Iowa
Robert H. Schneider, MD (PI)
Pam Van Antwerp, RN

Family Practice Residency Florida Hospital, Orlando, Florida
David G. Pocock, MD (PI)
Stephanie Gold

Marc S. Posner, MD, PA, Baltimore, Maryland
Marc S. Posner, MD (PI)
Cyndy Compton

ALLHAT Clinical Center, Portsmouth, Virginia
Doris M. Rice, MD (PI)
Alice Williams, RN

Deaconess Billings Clinic Research Division, Billings, Montana
Susan English, MD (PI)
Lana Sokoloski, RN

Richard Castaldo, MD, PC, Buffalo, New York
Richard S. Castaldo, MD (PI)
Deborah J. Castaldo

Medicine II Clinic E.A. Conway Hospital, Monroe, Louisiana
Barbara Beard, DO (PI)

Springfield Medical Center, Panama City, Florida
Misal Khan, MD (PI)
Gulafshan Khan

Cardiology Consultants, Pensacola, Florida
Brent D. Videau, MD (PI)
Sheila Bennett, RN

The Bowling Green Study Center, Bowling Green, Ohio
William E. Feeman, Jr, MD (PI)
Gwenda Sue Schroeder

Comprehensive Adult Risk Evaluation (CARE), Oakland, California
General K. Hilliard, MD (PI)
Barbara Holmes, MA

Health Care Plan, West Seneca, New York
Brian D. Snyder, MD (PI)
Kelly Thomas, RN

Eastwick Medical Associates, Philadelphia, Pennsylvania
Donald Fox, MD (PI)
Robert A. Centrone, DO
Steven A. Feinstein, MD
Harvey A. Soifer, DO
Kathleen T. Devine, PA-C

Andre K. Artis, MD, PC, Gary, Indiana
Andre K. Artis, MD (PI)
Mary Hutchinson

Warrior Family Practice, Tuscaloosa, Alabama
H. Joseph Fritz, MD (PI)

Kathleen Broderick, MD, FACP—Internal Medicine, Naples, Florida
Kathleen Broderick, MD, FACP (PI)

Michael Stein, MD, PA, West Palm Beach, Florida
Michael J. Stein, MD (PI)
Karen Odom Dudley, LPN

ALLHAT Clinical Center, New York, New York
Mahshid Arfania Assadi, MD, FACP (PI)
Cyrus Assadi, MD
Mahshid Arfania Assadi, MD, FACP

Alexian Brothers Senior Health Center, St. Louis, Missouri
Francois R. Charles, MD (PI)
Mary L. Gregory, DA

University of Arizona Health Sciences Center, Tucson, Arizona
Charles Y. Lui, MSc, MD, FACC, FACA (PI)
Lupita Aguirre

Family Medicine Clinic, PC, Onawa, Iowa
Curtis A. Mock, MD (PI)
Rhonda R. Gibson, RN, BS

Gunnar Medical Group, Berwyn, Illinois
Charles J. Bareis, MD (PI)
Terri Flegel, RN, BSN

Gunnar Medical Group, Chicago, Illinois
Charles J. Bareis, MD (PI)
Peter P. Mayock, MD
Pamela Porcelli, RN, BSN

MacNeal Center for Clinical Research Site C, Newark, Illinois
Charles J. Bareis, MD (PI)
Lloyd Flatt, MD
Terri Flegel, RN, BSN

Herman Rose, MD, PA, Fort Worth, Texas
Herman Rose, MD, FACP (PI)
Maxine Pickard

Drs. Samuels and Huddleston APMC, Chalmette, Louisiana
Bruce S. Samuels, MD (PI)
André G. Smith, LPN

Drs. Samuels and Huddleston APMC Lakeland, Chalmette, Louisiana
Bruce S. Samuels, MD (PI)
André G. Smith, LPN

Athens Internal Medicine, Athens, Alabama
Nauman Qureshi, MD (PI)
Theresa Tucker, RN

Aspen Medical Group, East Lake Street, Minneapolis, Minnesota
David A. Berman, MD (PI)
Pamela Snyder, RN

ALLHAT Clinical Center, Williamsville, New York
Joseph L. Maddi, MD (PI)
Mary Anne Neary, RN

The Heart Group Inc, Cuyahoga Falls, Ohio
Alfred I. Narraway, DO, FACC (PI)
Cynthia Griffin, RN

Huntington Memorial Hospital, Pasadena, California
Neil E. Doherty, III, MD (PI)
Donna Ujiiye, RN, MN

Falmouth Cardiology Associates, PC, Falmouth, Massachusetts
Thomas Sbarra, MD (PI)
Mary Cassidy, NP

UCI Heart Disease Prevention Program, Irvine, California
Nathan D. Wong, PhD (PI)
Stanley Franklin, MD
Julius M. Gardin, MD, FACC

Frank E. Sessoms, MD, Inc., Pittsburgh, Pennsylvania
Frank E. Sessoms, MD (PI)
Sailaja Keduri
Dawn Whyte, RT

Oakridge Medical Clinic, Lake Oswego, Oregon
H. Freeman Harris, MD (PI)
Susan E. Murray, CCRC

Daryl R. Dizmang, MD, Napa, California
Daryl R. Dizmang, MD (PI)
Dan Lyle, RN

OSF Medical Group—Fairway Drive, Bloomington, Illinois
Paul Pedersen, MD (PI)
Kurt Stevens, RN

VA Medical Center, Houston, Texas
Horacio J. Adrogue, MD (PI)
Debby S. Verrett

Maria L. Rios, MD (Private Practice), Humacao, Puerto Rico
Maria L. Rios, MD (PI)
Marisol Rios

Primary Health Care Practices PC, Macon, Georgia
David Crowder, MD (PI)

Michigan Medical PC, Kentwood, Michigan
Marian E. Oleszkowicz, MD (PI)
Kyle A. Rasikas, MD
Barb Dobbs, RN

Lionel B. Katchem, DO, PC, Ontario, California
Lionel B. Katchem, DO (PI)
Arlene J. (Penny) Katchem

Mountainside Hospital Clinic, Montclair, New Jersey
Ruth Wong-Liang, MD (PI)
Raymond Y. Liang, MD
Paula Baran, RN, BSN

Center for Family Medicine, Greenville, South Carolina
Palmira S. Snape, MD (PI)
Stephanie Brundage, MD
Steven Eggleston, PharmD

Richmond Area High Blood Pressure Center, Richmond, Virginia
Dean C. Williams, MD (PI)
Linda Macklin, RN

Howard S. Yager, MDPC, Atlanta, Georgia
Howard S. Yager, MD (PI)
Jan Dantzler

Stevens Health Clinic, Edmonds, Washington
Stephen R. Yarnall, MD, FACP, FACC (PI)
Angelika Micketti, CMA

Goshen Medical Center—Plainview Site, Rose Hill, North Carolina
Betsy Jones, DO (PI)

Long Island College Hospital Family Care Center, Brooklyn, New York
Charles Berk, MD (PI)
Joan Fleischman, MD
Virginia Robertson, MD
Elizabeth Schwartzburt, MD
Mary Zachary, MD
Mary McCormack, MSN, MPH, FNP

New York Methodist Hospital, Brooklyn, New York
C.V. Ramana Reddy, MB, BS (PI)
Thayyullathil Bharathan, MD
Mithilesy Kumar Das, MD
Muthuswamy Krishnamurthy, MD, FACP
G.M. Tadros, MD

UHSCOM—Excelsior Springs, Excelsior Springs, Missouri
James R. LaSalle, DO (PI)
Debbie Douglas-Wood, CMA

UHSCOM, Kansas City, Missouri
James R. LaSalle, DO (PI)
J. Lewis Alderman, PhD
Robbi Arenson, RT (R)

Pitman Internal Medicine Associates, Pitman, New Jersey
Michael A. Farber, MD (PI)
Lewis John DeEugenio, MD, FACP
Bruce J. McGann, MD
Susan Ferguson, LPN

Pitman Internal Medicine Associates, Mullica Hill, New Jersey
Michael A. Farber, MD (PI)
Lewis John DeEugenio, MD, FACP
Bruce J. McGann, MD
Susan L. Ferguson, LPN

University of Iowa Hospitals, Iowa City, Iowa
William Lawton, MD (PI)
Mary Jo Roberts, RN

Department of Internal Medicine/Medical Education, Macon, Georgia
Paul H. D'Amato, MD (PI)
David E. Mathis, MD
David C. Parish, MD, MPH, FACP
Allison Scheetz, MD
Bobbye M. Wieman, RN

Department of Internal Medicine/Medical Education, Macon, Georgia
Paul H. D'Amato, MD (PI)
David E. Mathis, MD
David C. Parish, MD, MPH, FACP
Allison Scheetz, MD
Bobbye M. Wieman, RN

Pavilion Medical Associates, Baltimore, Maryland
James H. Mersey, MD (PI)
Eugene Obah, MD
Mary Rykiel, RN

GBMC Weinberg Community Health Center, Baltimore, Maryland
James H. Mersey, MD (PI)
Juan Carlos Palacios, MD
Rosemary C. Weatherley, RN, CNOR

Elliott N. Schwartz, MD, PC, Oakland, California
Elliott N. Schwartz, MD (PI)
Patricia Ellen Schwartz, RN

CoMedPro, North Andover, Massachusetts
Albert Sobrado, MD (PI)
Janet Pellegrino, FNP

VAMC Hampton, Hampton, Virginia
Regina Lemly, MD (PI)
Laura Gendron, RPh

VAMC Black Hills, Hot Springs, South Dakota
Sheila Eckrich, MD (PI)
James Woehl, CNP

VAMC Black Hills, Fort Meade, South Dakota
Sheila Eckrich, MD (PI)
Janet H. Wegenke, BSN

VAMC Biloxi, Biloxi, Mississippi
Ashok Kanade, MD (PI)
Gwendolyn Owens-Harrison, PharmD

Donald W. Doucet MD—Internal Medicine, New Roads, Louisiana
Donald W. Doucet, MD (PI)
Madeline L. Doucet

Russell W. Simpson, MD, PC and Associates, Denver, Colorado
Russell W. Simpson, MD (PI)
Peter Nicholson, MD
Pamela Lowe, MA

Hamilton B. Mizer Primary Care Center, Niagara Falls, New York
Jerome Andres, MD (PI)
Gordon Wang, MD
Christine R. Lynott, LPN

Medical Arts Clinic, Corsicana, Texas
Kent E. Rogers, MD (PI)
Brooke Glicksman, PA-C

Cardiac Center, Kenmore, New York
Donald P. Copley, MD (PI)
Marie A. Price, RN

San Joaquin General Hospital, French Camp, California
Ramesh Dharawat, MD, FACC (PI)
Ali Usman, MD

The Brooklyn Hospital Center, Brooklyn, New York
Kenneth Ong, MD (PI)
Samuel Chan, MD
Walter J. Pierce, MD
Jose Rivero, MD
Jo Ann Varvatsas

REFERENCES

1. The fifth report of the Joint National Committee on detection, evaluation, and treatment of high blood pressure (JNC V). Arch Intern Med 1993; 153:154–183.
2. Stason WB. Cost and quality trade-offs in the treatment of hypertension. Hypertension 1989; 13 (suppl I):I-145–I-148.
3. Manolio TA, Cutler JA, Furberg, CD, Psaty BM, Whelton PK, Applegate WB. Trends in

pharmacologic management of hypertension in the United States. Arch Intern Med 1995; 155: 829–837.
4. MacMahon SW, Culter JA, Furberg CD, Payne GH. The effects of drug treatment for hypertension on morbidity and mortality from cardiovascular disease: a review of randomized controlled trials. Prog Cardiovasc Dis 1986; XXIX (3, suppl 1):99–119.
5. Collins R, Peto R, MacMahon S, Hebert P, Fiebach NH, Eberlein KA, Godwin J, Quizilbash N, Taylor JO, Hennekens CH. Blood pressure, stroke, and coronary heart disease. Part 2. Short-term reductions in blood pressure: overview of randomized drug trials in their epidemiological context. Lancet 1990; 335:827–838.
6. MacMahon S, Peto R, Cutler J, Collins R, Sorlie P, Neaton J, Abbott R, Godwin J, Dyer A, Stamler J. Blood pressure, stroke, and coronary heart disease. Part 1. Prolonged differences in blood pressure: prospective, observational studies corrected for the regression dilution bias. Lancet 1990; 335:765–774.
7. SHEP Cooperative Research Group. Prevention of stroke by antihypertensive drug treatment in older persons with isolated systolic hypertension: final results of the Systolic Hypertension in the Elderly Program (SHEP). JAMA 1991; 265:3255–3264.
8. Dalhlof B, Lindholm LH, Hansson L, Schersten B, Ekbom T, Wester PO. Morbidity and mortality in the Swedish Trial in Old Patients with Hypertension (STOP-Hypertension). Lancet 1991; 338:1281–1285.
9. MRC Working Party. Medical Research Council of treatment of hypertension in older adults: principal results. BMJ 1992; 304:405–412.
10. Cohen JD, Neaton JD, Prineas RJ, Daniels KA, for the MRFIT Research Group. Diuretics, serum potassium, and ventricular arrhythmias in the Multiple Risk Factor Intervention Trial. Am J Cardiol 1987; 60:548–554.
11. Ferrari P, Rosman J, Weidman P. Antihypertensive agents, serum lipoproteins, and glucose metabolism. Am J Cardiol 1991; 67:26B–35B.
12. Materson BJ, Reda DJ, Cushman WC, Massie BM, Freis ED, Kochar MS, Hamburger RJ, Fye C, Lakshman R, Gottdiener J, Ramirez EA, Henderson WG, for the Department of Veterans Affairs Cooperative Study Group on Antihypertensive Agents. Single-drug therapy for hypertension in men: a comparison of six antihypertensive agents with placebo. N Engl J Med 1993; 328:914–921.
13. Neaton JD, Grimm RH Jr, Prineas RJ, Stamler J, Grandits GA, Elmer PJ, Cutler JA, Flack JM, Schoenberger JA, McDonald R, for the Treatment of Mild Hypertension Study Research Group. Treatment of Mild Hypertension Study: final results. JAMA 1993; 270:713–724.
14. Held PH, Yusuf S, Furberg CD. Calcium channel blockers in acute myocardial infarction and unstable angina: an overview. BMJ 1989; 299:1187–1192.
15. Yusuf S, Held P, Furberg C. Update of effects of calcium antagonists in myocardial infarction or angina in light of the second Danish Verapamil Infarction Trial (DAVIT-II) and other recent studies. Am J Cardiol 1991; 67:1295–1297.
16. Staessen JA, Fagard R, Thijs L, et al., for the Systolic Hypertension in Europe (Syst-Eur) Trial Investigators. Morbidity and mortality in the placebo-controlled European Trial on Isolated Systolic Hypertension in the Elderly. Lancet 1997; 360:757–764.
17. Packer M, O'Connor CM, Ghali JK, Pressler ML, Carson PE, Belkin RN, Miller AB, Neuberg GW, Frid D, Wertheimer JH, Cropp AB, DeMets DL. Effect of amlodipine on morbidity and mortality in severe chronic heart failure. N Engl J Med 1996; 335:1107–1114.
18. Cohn JN, Ziesche S, Smith R, Anand I, Dunkman WB, Loeb H, Cintron G, Boden W, Baruch L, Rochin P, Loss L, for the Vasodilator-Heart Failure Trial. Effect of the calcium antagonist felodipine as supplement vasodilator therapy in patients with chronic heart failure treated with enalapril: V-HeFT III. Circulation 1997; 96:856–863.
19. Ad Hoc Subcommittee of the Liaison Committee of the World Health Organisation and the International Society of Hypertension. Effects of calcium antagonists on the risk of coronary heart disease, cancer and bleeding. J Hypertens 1997; 15:105–115.

20. Psaty BM, Furberg CD. Clinical implications of the WHO/ISH statement on calcium antagonists. J Hypertens 1997; 15:1197–1200.
21. The SOLVD Investigators. Effect of enalapril on survival in patients with reduced left ventricular ejection fractions and congestive heart failure. N Engl J Med 1991; 325:293–302.
22. Pfeffer MA, Braunwald E, Moye LA, Basta L, Brown EJ Jr, Cuddy TE, Davis BR, Geltman EM, Goldman S, Flaker GC. The effect of captopril on morbidity and mortality in patients with left ventricular dysfunction following myocardial infarction. N Engl J Med 1992; 327: 699–677.
23. The Acute Infarction Ramipril Efficacy (AIRE) Study Investigators. Effects of ramipril on mortality and morbidity of survivors of acute myocardial infarction with clinical evidence of heart failure. Lancet 1993; 342:821–828.
24. The SOLVD Investigators. Effect of enalapril on mortality and the development of heart failure in asymptomatic patients with reduced left ventricular ejection fractions. N Engl J Med 1992; 327:685–691.
25. Chobanian AV, Haudenschild CC, Nickerson C, Drago R. Anti-atherogenic effect of captopril in the Watanabe heritable hyperlipidemic rabbit. Hypertension 1990; 15:327–331.
26. The HOPE Study Investigators. The HOPE (Heart Outcome Prevention Evaluation) Study. The design of a large simple randomized trial of an angiotensin converting enzyme inhibitor (ramipril) and vitamin E in patients at high risk of cardiovascular events. Can J Cardiol 1996; 12:127–137.
27. Pfeffer MA, Domanski M, Rosenberg Y, Veter J, Geller N, Albert P, Hsia J, Braunwald E. Prevention of events with angiotensin-converting enzyme inhibition (The PEACE Study Design). Am J Cardiol 1998; 82:25H–30H.
28. Pool JL. Effects of doxazosin on serum lipids: a review of the clinical data and molecular basis for altered lipid metabolism. Am Heart J 1991; 121:251–259.
29. Lithell H. Effects of antihypertensive drugs on insulin, glucose and lipid metabolism. Diabetes Care 1991; 14:203–209.
30. Hernandez RH, Carvajal AR, Pajuelo JG, Armas de Hernandez MJ, Armas Padilla MC, Barragan O, Boada Boada JJ. The effect of normotensive subjects and patients with hypertension: an in-vitro study. Am Heart J 1991; 121:389–394.
31. Hernandez RH, Pajuelo JRG, Carvajal AR, Armas Padilla MC, Armas de Hernandez MJ, Barragan O, Boada Boada JJ. Evidence of an antiplatelet aggregation action of doxazosin in patients with hypertension: an ex-vivo study. Am Heart J 1991; 121:395–401.
32. Jansson JH. Effects of doxazosin and atenolol on the fibrinolytic system in patients with hypertension and elevated serum cholesterol. Eur J Clin Pharmacol 1991; 40:321–326.
33. Law MR, Wald NJ, Thompson SG. By how much and how quickly does reduction in serum cholesterol concentration lower risk of ischaemic heart disease? BMJ 1994; 308:367–373.
34. Gordon DJ. Cholesterol lowering and total mortality. In: Rifkind BM, ed. Contemporary Issues in Cholesterol Lowering: Clinical and Population Aspects, New York; Marcel Dekker, 1995: 33–48.
35. Scandinavian Simvastatin Survival Study Group. Randomised trial of cholesterol lowering in 4444 patients with coronary heart disease: the Scandinavian Simvastatin Survival Study (4S). Lancet 1994; 344:1383–1389.
36. Shepherd J, Cobbe S, Ford I, Isles C, Lorimer AR, Macfarlane PW, McKillop JH, Packard CJ, for the West of Scotland Coronary Prevention Study Group. Prevention of coronary heart disease with pravastatin in men with hypercholesterolemia. N Engl J Med 1995; 333:1301–1307.
37. Sacks FM, Pfeffer MA, Moye LA, Rouleau JL, Rutherford JD, Cole TG, Brown L, Warnica JW, Arnold JMO, Wun CC, Davis BR, Braunwald E, for the Cholesterol and Recurrent Events Investigators. The effect of pravastatin on coronary events in patients with average cholesterol levels. N Engl J Med 1996; 335:1001–1009.
38. Downs JR, Clearfield M, Weis S, Whitney E, Shapiro DR, Beere PA, Langendorfer A, Stein

EA, Kruyer W, Gotto AM, for the AFCAPS/TexCAPS Research Group. Primary prevention of acute coronary events with lovastatin in men and women with average cholesterol levels. Results of the AFCAPS/TexCAPS Trial. JAMA 1998; 279:1615–1622.
39. The Long-Term Intervention with Pravastatin in Ischaemic Disease (LIPID) Study Group. Prevention of cardiovascular events and death with pravastatin in patients with coronary heart disease and a broad range of initial cholesterol levels. N Engl J Med 1998; 339:1349–1357.
40. Gordon DJ. Cholesterol lowering reduces mortality. In: Grundy SM, ed. Cholesterol Lowering Therapies 1999. New York: Marcel Dekker, Inc. 1999: 299–311.
41. Gordon DJ, Rifkind BM. Cholesterol-lowering and the older patient. Am J Cardiol 1989; 63: 48H–52H.
42. Sacks FM, Moyé LA, Davis BR, Cole TG, Rouleau JL, Nash DT, Pfeffer MA, Braunwald E. Relationship between plasma LDL concentrations during treatment with pravastatin and recurrent coronary events in the Cholesterol and Recurrent Events Trial. Circulation 1998; 97:1446–1452.
43. West of Scotland Coronary Prevention Study Group. Influence of pravastatin and plasma lipids on clinical events in the West of Scotland Coronary Prevention Study (WOSCOPS). Circulation 1998; 97:1440–1445.
44. Pedersen TR, Olsson AG, Færgeman O, Kjekshus J, Wedel H, Berg K, Wilhelmsen L, Haghfelt T, Thorgeirsson G, Pyörälä K, Miettinen T, Christophersen B, Tobert JA, Musliner TA, and Cook TJ. Lipoprotein changes and reduction in the incidence of major coronary heart disease events in the Scandinavian Simvastatin Survival Study (4S). Circulation 1998; 97:1453–1460.
45. Stamler J, Wentworth D, Neaton JD. Is the relationship between serum cholesterol and risk of premature death from coronary heart disease continuous and graded? Findings in 356,222 primary screenees of the Multiple Risk Factor Intervention Trial (MRFIT). JAMA 1986; 256: 2823–2828.
46. Chen Z, Peto R, Collins R, MacMahon S, Lu J, Li W. Serum cholesterol and coronary heart disease in a low-cholesterol population: positive relationship with no evidence of a threshold. BMJ 1991; 303:276–282.
47. Expert Panel on Detection, Evaluation, and Treatment of High Blood Cholesterol in Adults. Summary of the second report of the Nation Cholesterol Education Program (NCEP) Expert Panel on Detection, Evaluation, and Treatment of High Blood Cholesterol in Adults (Adult Treatment Panel II). JAMA 1993; 269:3015–3023.
48. Wright JT, Cushman WC, Davis B, for the ALLHAT Group. The Antihypertensive and Lipid Lowering Treatment to Prevent Heart Attack Trial (ALLHAT): Clinical Center Recruitment. Submitted.
49. Pressel S, Davis BR, Louis G, et al. Participant Recruitment in the Antihypertensive and Lipid-Lowering Treatment to Prevent Heart Attack Trial (ALLHAT). Submitted.
50. Friedewald WT, Levy RI, Fredrickson DS. Estimation of the concentration of low-density lipoprotein cholesterol in plasma without use of the preparative ultracentrifuge. Clin Chem 1972; 18:499–502.
51. Mantel N. Evaluation of survival data and two new rank order statistics arising in its consideration. Cancer Chemother Rep 1966; 50:163–170.
52. Laird NM, Ware JH. Random effects models for longitudinal data. Biometrics 1982; 38:963–974.
53. Lan KKG, Wittes J. The B-value: a tool for monitoring data. Biometrics 1988; 44:579–585.
54. Davis BR, Hardy RJ. Upper bounds for type I and type II error rates in conditional power calculations. Comm Stat 1990; A19(10):3571–3584.
55. Sleight P. Trials and tribulations: the ISIS experience. Aust N Z J Med 1992; 22(5 suppl): 583–586.
56. Williford WO, Collins JF, Garg R, Gorlin R, Yusuf S. Design and implementation of the NHLBI and the VA Cooperative Studies Program Collaborative Study ''Trial to evaluate the effect of digitalis on mortality in heart failure.'' Control Clin Trials 1992; 13:386.

57. Cutler JA, Psaty BM, MacMahon S, Furberg CD. Public health issues in hypertension control: what has been learned from clinical trials? In: Laragh JH, Brenner BM, eds. Hypertension Pathophysiology, Diagnosis and Management. 2d ed. New York: Raven Press Ltd., 1995.
58. World Health Organization-International Society of Hypertension Blood Pressure Lowering Treatment Trialists' Collaboration. Protocol for prospective collaborative overviews of major randomized trials of blood-pressure-lowering treatments. J Hypertens 1998; 16:2:127–137.
59. Estacio RO, Jeffers BW, Hiatt WR, Biggerstaff SL, Gifford N, Schrier RW. The effect of nisoldipine as compared with enalapril on cardiovascular outcomes in patients with non-insulin-dependent diabetes and hypertension. N Engl J Med 1998; 338; 10:645–652.
60. Tatti P, Pamor M, Byington RP, Malro PD, Guarlsco R, Strollo G, Strollo F. Outcome results of the fosinopril versus amlodipine cardiovascular events randomized trial (FACET) in patients with hypertension and NIDDM. Diabetes Care 21; 4:597.
61. UK Prospective Diabetes Study Group. Efficacy of atenolol and captopril in reducing risk of macrovascular and microvascular complications in type 2 diabetes: UKPDS 39. BMJ 1998; 317:713–720.
62. Hansson L, Lindholm LH, Niskanen L, Kabje Hm Gedber T, Niklason A, Luomanmaki K, Dahlof B, de Faire U, Morlin C, Karlberg BE, Wester PO, Bjorck JE. Effect of angiotensin-converting-enzyme inhibition compared with conventional therapy on cardiovascular morbidity and mortality in hypertension: the Captopril Prevention Project (CAPPP) randomized trial. Lancet 1999; 353:611–616.
63. Cutler JA. Calcium-channel blockers for hypertension-uncertainty continues. N Engl J Med 1998; 338:679–681.
64. Cutler J. Which drug for treatment of hypertension? Lancet 1999; 353:604–605.
65. Dunnett CW. A multiple comparisons procedure for comparing several treatments with a control. J Am Stat Assoc 1995; 60:573–583.
66. Vital and Health Statistics. Serum Lipids of Adults 20–74 Years: United States, 1976–80. Series II: Data from the National Health Survey, No. 242, DHHS Publication No. (PHS) 93-1692, Hyattsville, MD, 1993.

23

The 2nd Australian National Blood Pressure Study (ANBP2)

C. M. REID

Baker Medical Research Institute, Melbourne, Australia

P. RYAN

University of Adelaide, Adelaide, Australia

L. M. H. WING*

Flinders University, Adelaide, Australia

I. INTRODUCTION AND BACKGROUND TO ANBP2

The Australian Therapeutic Trial in Mild Hypertension was one of the first trials to demonstrate the benefit of lowering blood pressure with antihypertensive therapy in reducing morbidity and mortality from cardiovascular disease in a population of mild-to-moderate hypertensive subjects (1). Since the conduct of this first Australian National Blood Pressure Study (detailed in Chapter 4), the management of hypertension in Australia has shifted from the domain of specialist clinics to that of the family practitioner (2). In addition, family practitioners have been given a wider selection of therapeutic options with which to manage hypertension.

The appropriate selection of treatment strategies based on evidence from clinical trials remains a difficulty in the management of hypertension, both because of the limited range of agents subjected to outcome-based clinical trials and the lack of outcome data related to nonpharmacological treatments. For example, until 1997, no published outcome trial in hypertension had demonstrated the benefit of angiotensin-converting enzyme (ACE) inhibitor or calcium channel blocker therapy. Despite the lack of evidence, the use of these agents for the management of hypertension has been steadily increasing for the past 10 to 15 years to the point where they are now the most common agents prescribed for hypertension in most population groups, including the elderly (3).

---

* ANBP2 Management Committee: L. M. H. Wing, C. M. Reid, L. J. Beilin, M. A. Brown, G. L. R. Jennings, C. I. Johnston, J. J. McNeil, J. E. Marley, T. O. Morgan, P. Ryan, M. J. West.

The rationale for the widespread use of these newer agents hinges in part on the results of the earlier outcome trials using mainly diuretic- and beta-blocker-based therapy. Although the expected benefits of blood pressure reduction have been achieved in terms of stroke reduction (40%), the reduction of risk from coronary heart disease has been less than that predicted from epidemiological studies (4–8). It has been proposed that this reduced efficacy with respect to coronary heart disease risk may be related to the agents used, as diuretics and beta-blockers have some adverse effects on cardiovascular risk factors, such as lipids. On a theoretical basis, some properties of the newer agents, in particular the ACE inhibitors, suggest they may be more beneficial for reducing coronary heart disease risk. These include the lack of any effect on circulating lipids (9), a reduction in left ventricular hypertrophy (10), improved survival in the presence of cardiac failure (11), or reduced left ventricular function (12) and enhanced insulin sensitivity (13). Whether any of these putative additional properties will have any influence on outcome in the treatment of hypertension is still unknown.

Obtaining such information is considered vital, as the cost of antihypertensive therapy has a major impact on community and personal resources worldwide. In the Australian context, current government subsidy for antihypertensive drugs under the Australian Pharmaceutical Benefits Scheme is approximately AUS$375M per annum (14). This figure contains a disproportionate contribution from the newer agents (40% to 50% total antihypertensive prescriptions) for which the costs are 3 to 15 times greater than with a diuretic or a beta-blocker.

II. PRIMARY AIMS AND OBJECTIVES

The ANBP2 was conceived as a cardiovascular outcome trial based on the initial selection of therapeutic agent in older hypertensives. The primary aim is to determine, in hypertensive subjects aged 65 to 84, whether there is any difference in total cardiovascular events (fatal and nonfatal) over a 5-year treatment period between antihypertensive treatment with an ACE inhibitor-based regimen and treatment with a diuretic-based regimen.

The secondary objectives are to compare the difference between the two treatment regimens for total mortality, cardiovascular and noncardiovascular mortality, fatal and nonfatal cardiovascular events, total fatal and nonfatal strokes, total fatal and nonfatal coronary events, total fatal and nonfatal cardiovascular events other than strokes and coronary events, final drug regimens, and postrandomization blood pressure. The aims and objectives are summarized in Table 1.

III. STUDY DESIGN AND SAMPLE SIZE

The study is being conducted in Australian general (family) practices using a PROBE design, that is, prospective randomized open-label with blinding of end-point assessment (15). The PROBE design was chosen because of its suitability for the general practice environment.

Six thousand subjects (3000 in each group) were required, over a 5-year follow-up period (on average), at the 5% level of significance and with a power of 90%, to detect a 25% difference in total cardiovascular events (including cardiovascular deaths) between treatment regimens. The sample size includes an allowance of an extra 700 subjects to account for dropouts and crossover to the alternative regimen. The difference of 25% in

Table 1 ANBP2 Main Aim and Objectives

Main aim:	To determine in hypertensive subjects aged 65–84 years whether there is any difference in total cardiovascular events (fatal and nonfatal) over a 5-year treatment period between subjects treated with a diuretic-based regimen or ACE inhibitor-based regimen.
Secondary objectives:	To compare the difference between the two treatment regimens for:
	Mortality (total, CVD and non-CVD)
	Cardiovascular events (fatal and nonfatal)
	Stroke (total, fatal, nonfatal)
	Coronary events (total, fatal, nonfatal)
	"Other" CVD events (total, fatal, nonfatal)
	Postrandomization blood pressure
	Final drug regimens

Abbreviations: *ANBP2*, 2nd Australian National Blood Pressure Study; *ACE*, angiotensin-converting enzyme; *CVD*, cardiovascular disease.

total cardiovascular events between the two treatment groups will, if present, be of real clinical significance.

The sample size calculation was based on the number of cardiovascular events (approximately 20 per 1000 patients per year) observed in the groups receiving active drug treatment reported in the Systolic Hypertension in the Elderly (SHEP) (6) and Medical Research Council (MRC) elderly (8) studies. Initial sample size estimations were based on Fisher's exact test using cumulative event rates of 0.105 and 0.0788 over 5 years for the diuretic and ACE groups, respectively. We also calculated sample sizes based on the log-rank test for comparison of survival experience and subsequently refined this using Palta and McHugh's methods of adjusting for withdrawal and noncompliance because of crossovers (16). There was close agreement between the methods. The final analysis of data is planned after 30,000 patient-years of observation, that is, 6000 subjects followed up for at least 5 years.

A. Involving General (Family) Practitioners

General (family) practitioner (GP) participation was considered to be a crucial factor in the likely success of ANBP2. A network of participating GPs throughout Australia needed to be established to allow the study to proceed. An initial feasibility study was conducted to ensure that practitioner and patient recruitment strategies were satisfactory (17). An academic GP (regional medical coordinator) was appointed in each of five centers (based in Australian mainland states) to conduct peer-to-peer recruitment of GPs who might be interested in participating in the study. General practitioners were initially approached by letter and then received a telephone call from the regional medical coordinator, who explained the study and the implications for the GP. Those GPs indicating a willingness to receive more information were sent an information package about the study, and an appointment was made to discuss the study with the regional medical coordinator and one of the study nurses.

The conduct of ANBP2 in Australian general (family) practice has yielded more than 1900 participating GPs from approximately 1000 practices. This has now formed the basis of a GP research network for the conduct of other large-scale trials in Australian general practices.

B. Study Population

To identify potential subjects for the study, each general practitioner was asked to allow one of the study nurses to have access to the list of patients attending the practice. The nurse then identified all patients on the list who were ages 65 to 84. After review of the list by the GP, all individuals who were considered physically able to attend were sent a letter inviting them to attend a blood pressure screening program at the practice office. At this initial screening, blood pressure was measured by the study nurse, willingness of the patient to participate was ascertained, and information relating to exclusion criteria was sought. Untreated patients satisfying the initial visit criteria proceeded to the study entry phase. For those patients on antihypertensive therapy and interested in continuing, a consultation with the GP was arranged to commence withdrawal of current therapy according to predetermined guidelines. When the subject was free of drug therapy for at least 1 week, and if no new major symptoms had developed, the subject proceeded to the study entry phase. The study entry phase involved two further visits with the study nurse, together with satisfaction of the inclusion/exclusion criteria for the trial (Table 2).

Table 2 Enrollment Protocol and Inclusion/Exclusion Criteria for ANBP2

- Enrollment protocol
  - Identify all practice patients aged 65–84 years.
  - Letter of invitation to BP screening program at the practice.
  - BP screening conducted by study nurse.
  - All treated and any untreated subjects (with entry level blood pressure) reviewed by GP to satisfy inclusion/exclusion criteria and willingness for study.
  - Treated patients withdraw from medication and are drug free for at least 1 week.
  - Treated and untreated subjects have two additional weekly visits to satisfy BP eligibility criteria.
  - Average of last two visits BP readings taken as study entry value.
- Inclusion criteria
  - Men or women aged 65–84 years of age.
  - Have no history of recent cardiovascular morbidity.
  - Are capable of and willing to give informed consent.
  - Are ambulant and able to attend their GPs practice throughout the study.
  - Average untreated sitting blood pressure on the second and third screening visits of the study $\geq$ 60 mm Hg systolic or $\geq$ 90 mm Hg diastolic (if systolic $>$ 140 mm Hg).
- Exclusion criteria
  - Any life threatening illness considered to be likely to cause death within the study's observation period (5 years).
  - An absolute contraindication to an ACE inhibitor or diuretic.
  - Plasma creatinine concentration $>$ 0.2 mmol/L. The measurement should have been within the past 12 months or, if this is not available, will be undertaken at the initial screening visit.
  - Presence of any previous nonfatal cardiovascular event which defines an endpoint for the study in the past 6 months (see #5).
  - Accelerated or malignant hypertension.
  - Dementia.
  - Consideration by the subject's GP that the subject is unsuitable for the study.

Abbreviations: *ANBP2*, 2nd Australian National Blood Pressure Study; *BP*, blood pressure; *GP*, general practitioner; *ACE*, angiotensin-converting enzyme.

Each nurse participated in a training and validation program related to blood pressure measurement techniques before commencing work on the screening program. Blood pressure was taken after at least 5 minutes rest in the sitting position using a standard mercury sphygmomanometer. The subject's arm was free of any constricting clothing and comfortably supported at the level of the heart. The arm in which the recording was made was noted. Appropriate cuff choice was made on the basis of arm circumference measurements. Systolic blood pressure was taken as the pressure at which the Korotkoff sounds are first heard (phase 1), and diastolic pressure was taken at the disappearance of the Korotkoff sounds (phase 5).

On each occasion, three blood pressure measurements were taken. The average of the second and third blood pressure measurements was recorded as the blood pressure for that occasion. If these two blood pressure measurements differed by more than 10 mm Hg systolic or more than 6 mm Hg diastolic, further measurements were taken until two consecutive measurements were within these limits. At subsequent screening visits, blood pressure was taken by the same observer (where possible) as on the first occasion using the same arm and the same technique.

C. Randomization

Central randomization was achieved by telephoning the data management center at the conclusion of each randomization visit. Data were verified, and subjects satisfying all inclusion criteria were allocated to either ACE inhibitor or diuretic groups. Randomization was stratified for age (older or younger than age 75) and state of origin.

D. Drug Treatments

Once randomized, subjects commenced either ACE inhibitor- or diuretic-based treatment. Subsequent treatment adjustments to achieve goal blood pressures (Table 3) were made according to each supervising GPs usual practice, but broad guidelines on treatment were provided (Table 4). The target goal blood pressures focus on obtaining a systolic blood pressure of less than 140 mm Hg or a diastolic blood pressure of less than 90 mm Hg corresponding to current guidelines (22).

Table 3 Goal Blood Pressure for ANBP2

Goal blood pressure	
For entry systolic blood pressure $\geq$ 160 mm Hg	Reduction of systolic blood pressure by at least 20 mm Hg to a value $<$ 160 mm Hg. For subjects whose systolic blood pressure $>$ 160 mm Hg was the entry criterion, further reduction of systolic blood pressure to $<$ 40 mm Hg should be attempted wherever possible if tolerated by the subject.
For entry diastolic blood pressure $\geq$ 90 mm Hg	Reduction of diastolic blood pressure by at least 10 mm Hg to a value $<$ 90 mm Hg For subjects whose diastolic blood pressure $>$ 90 mm Hg was the entry criterion, further reduction of diastolic blood pressure to $<$ 80 mm Hg should be attempted wherever possible if tolerated by the subject.

Abbreviation: *ANBP2*, 2nd Australian National Blood Pressure Study.

Table 4 Drug Regimens and Goal Blood Pressures for ANBP2

Ace inhibitor group	Diuretic group
Step 1: ACE inhibitor (enalapril)	Step 1: Diuretic
Step 2: Beta-blocker or calcium channel antagonist or alpha blocker	Step 2: Beta-blocker, or calcium channel antagonist, or alpha blocker
Step 3: Drug from a class not used in step 2 or a diuretic	Step 3: Drug from a class not used in step 2
Step 4: Drug from a class not used in steps 2 or 3	Step 4: Drug from a class not used in steps 2 or 3

Abbreviations: *ANBP2*, 2nd Australian National Blood Pressure Study; *ACE*, angiotensin-converting enzyme.

The group initially receiving a diuretic had been advised not to receive an ACE inhibitor at any stage but may have the addition or substitution of drugs from any other class of antihypertensive agent if required. The group initially receiving an ACE inhibitor may also have the addition or substitution of drugs from other commonly used classes of antihypertensive agents if required, including, if necessary, a diuretic.

For subjects randomized to the ACE inhibitor arm of the study, GPs were advised to prescribe enalapril (Renitec™) as the ACE inhibitor, although GPs wishing to prescribe a different ACE inhibitor were at liberty to do so. For each antihypertensive drug, the starting dose was at the lower end of the recommended dose range for older subjects as stated in the drug's official product information. In the case of thiazide and thiazide-like diuretics, the starting dose was recommended at half of the usual daily dose, for example hydrochlorothiazide 25 mg, bendrofluazide 2.5 mg, and chlorthalidone 12.5 mg. For all drugs, dose increments and maximum daily doses also were as recommended in the appropriate product information. The cost of all drugs was subsidized through the Australian Government Pharmaceutical Benefits Scheme.

If a patient has been intolerant of a particular agent, it has been recommended that a substitute agent from the next step in the particular randomization arm for that subject should be prescribed. Additional therapy to achieve goal blood pressures has been suggested by following the steps in the specific randomization group to which the subject has been allocated.

E. Subject Follow-Up and Study Endpoints

The frequency of patient follow-up visits has been determined by the practitioner's usual practice for stabilization and follow-up of hypertensive patients, with the proviso that each patient be seen at least every 6 months throughout the study. The practitioner was asked to document on each occasion in the medical record the patient's blood pressure and drug treatment, particularly noting doses and treatment alternations. Every 6 months, a study nurse reviewed outcome information for each subject in terms of study endpoints (Appendix 1), drug dosing, and blood pressure.

If an endpoint occurred, copies of any available clinical information relating to that endpoint were collected, such as hospital discharge summaries, results of investigations undertaken by the GP, consultants' letters, death certificates, and autopsy reports. These data relating to study endpoints were forwarded to the data management center, where all subject identifiers apart from the subject's coded study number were removed before presentation to the endpoint committee.

F. Data Analysis

Comparability of baseline characteristics between the two treatment groups will be assessed by chi-square tests for categorical variables and t-tests (or the nonparametric equivalent) for continuous variables. The primary endpoint of interest is total cardiovascular events (including cardiovascular deaths). Secondary endpoints include death and coronary heart disease events. Both the final and interim analyses will include safety as well as efficacy analyses. All comparisons between treatments will be on an intention-to-treat basis. For the primary analysis, we will use the methods of Cook and Lawless to calculate a robust test statistic for recurrent events based on the cumulative expected number of events (18). The test statistic is adjusted for one interim analysis, as requested by the independent data monitoring committee, using an O'Brien-Fleming error spending function. The test will have a power of 58% and 81% at the interim and final analyses, respectively.

G. Study Organization

The organization established for ANBP2 is shown in Figure 1. The study has been coordinated by a management committee appointed by the High Blood Pressure Research Council of Australia. This committee provides overall policy for and direction of the project. The ethics review committee of the Royal Australian College of General Practitioners has approved the study.

H. Planned Substudies

In addition to the main trial, four substudies are being conducted. The substudies focus on specific aspects of hypertension, including left ventricular hypertrophy, health econom-

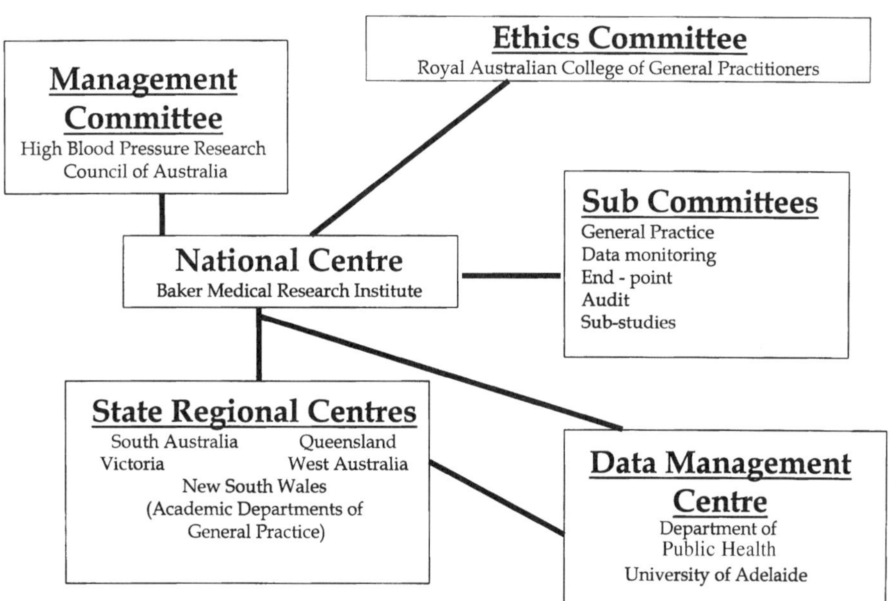

Fig. 1 Study organization.

ics and quality of life, ambulatory blood pressure monitoring, and genetic determinants. Each substudy has a coordinating committee and separate study protocol detailing sample size requirements. Each study is being conducted in a different location to reduce the demand on participating subjects and GPs within ANBP2.

1. Left Ventricular Hypertrophy

The primary aim of this study is to determine whether any difference in total mortality and morbidity from cardiovascular events between the two treatment groups can be related to entry echocardiographic parameters (e.g., left ventricular mass); secondly, to compare the effects on cardiac structure and function of treatment with an ACE inhibitor- or a diuretic-based treatment over a 3-year period; and finally, to determine whether any change in cardiac structure or function after treatment with an ACE inhibitor or a diuretic over a 3-year period is associated with the occurrence of cardiovascular events.

2. Health Economics and Quality of Life

The specific objectives in this study are to compare the alternative regimens in terms of opportunity costs to Australian society, including the costs of the management of side effects and adverse events and cost-effectiveness. The impact on patients' health-related quality of life while taking medication is also being assessed. The quality of life instruments being used are the SF36 (19), Rosser's classification of illness scale and the Symptom Distress Index (20). These instruments were chosen primarily for their suitability for use in a general practice situation.

3. Ambulatory Blood Pressure Monitoring

The main aim of this study is to determine whether blood pressure, assessed by ambulatory monitoring at study entry, is more closely related to cardiovascular outcome at 5 years than office blood pressure at study entry in a population of older hypertensives managed by their general practitioners. In addition, the study aims to determine whether elderly subjects with "white coat hypertension" at study entry, who then receive antihypertensive medications, have different cardiovascular outcomes than those without white-coat hypertension.

4. Genetic Study

The genetic study is intended to determine whether there is a relationship between specific genotypes related to blood pressure control and cardiovascular outcomes in elderly hypertensive patients. In addition, the association between these genotypes and response to antihypertensive drug therapy will also be examined. Initially, genotype frequencies for the ACE, angiotensinogen, and alpha-adducin genes will be compared between patients who are enrolled as part of the ANBP2 and age- and sex-matched normotensive controls who will be selected from the Victorian Family Heart Study (21). To ensure sufficient genetic contrast, controls will have blood pressure values below the median for their age and sex. As it has been suggested that some genetic markers are associated with varying degrees of hypertension, the cases will be stratified in secondary analyses according to entry blood pressure levels. As more predictive genetic markers become established, their relationship to outcome will also be examined in the study population.

Table 5 General Practitioner Participation in ANBP2

State	Practices	GPs
New South Wales	193	299
Queensland	193	378
South Australia	153	353
Victoria	373	665
West Australia	96	243
Total	962	1938

Abbreviations: *ANBP2*, 2nd Australian National Blood Pressure Study; *GP*, general practitioner.

I. Study Progress

1. Recruitment and Baseline Characteristics

The ANBP2 pilot study commenced in two states (Victoria and South Australia) in April 1995. General practitioner involvement was acceptable in these two states and the study was expanded in October 1995. Final GP involvement in the study is shown in Table 5. This figure represents 10.7% of all registered GPs in Australia.

Patient recruitment to the trial closed on June 30, 1998 with 6083 patients being randomised. A total of 54,399 subjects were screened for entry into the trial providing a randomization rate of 11%. Figure 2 illustrates the total number screened and randomized in each participating state.

The flow of subjects through to randomization is shown Figure 3 of randomized

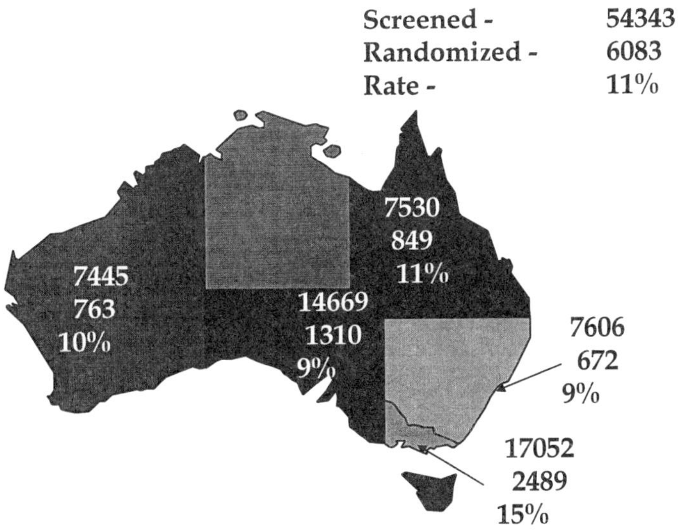

Fig. 2 Screening and randomization figures in the five participating centers of the 2nd Australian National Blood Pressure Study (ANBP2).

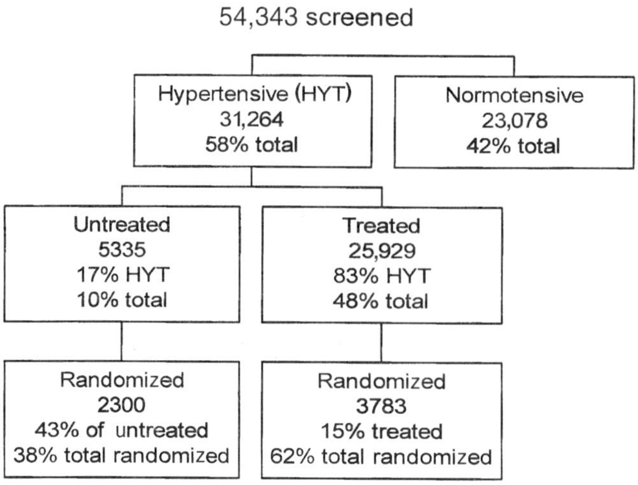

Fig. 3 Flow of subjects from identification to randomization into the 2nd Australian National Blood Pressure Study (ANBP2).

subjects who had been on previous antihypertensive medication. The baseline characteristics of the 6083 patients randomized are shown Table 6.

2. *Blood Pressure Control and Endpoint Accumulation*

At August 1999, more than 99% of subjects had had at least one 6-month review of follow-up case notes. Target systolic blood pressure of less than 160 mm Hg has been achieved by 63% of subjects, with 26% achieving less than 140 mm Hg. Diastolic blood pressure lower than 90 mm Hg has been achieved by 67% of subjects, with 19% achieving less than 80 mm Hg. However, only 24% of subjects are achieving the current International Society of Hypertension target of both systolic and diastolic blood pressure less than 140/90 mm Hg (22). The mean systolic and diastolic blood pressure and the percentage achieving target levels (systolic < 160 mm Hg and diastolic < 90 mm Hg) over the course of the follow-up period is also shown in Figure 4.

Table 7 shows the number and current rate of endpoints after approximately 10,380 of the planned 30,000 patient-years of observation.

IV. DISCUSSION

Previous trials have clearly demonstrated that in an older hypertensive population, cardiovascular outcomes are significantly reduced with antihypertensive therapy (6–8, 23). The question being addressed by ANBP2 is not whether treatment is beneficial, but whether the choice of newer agents (ACE inhibitors) as first line therapy confers additional benefit to that derived from older drugs (diuretics).

Since their release onto the Australian market in 1986, there has been a steady and rapid increase in the use of ACE inhibitors, primarily for the control of blood pressure and a steady decrease in the use of diuretics and beta-blockers (3). As ACE inhibitors are more expensive, the increase and rate of increase in the use of these agents accounts for a large proportion of the current and increasing costs attributed to antihypertensive agents

Table 6 Baseline Characteristics of ANBP2 Study Cohort (n = 6083)

Male:Female (%)	51:49
Age: mean	71.9 years
65–74 years	70%
75–84 years	30%
Blood pressure (mm Hg)	167 ± 13/91 ± 8
Previously treated	62%
Body mass index	27 ± 4 kg/m^2
Smoking current	7%
ex-smoker	44%
Alcohol current	69%
ex-drinker	6%
Physically active	75%
Coronary heart disease	10%
MI, angina, CABG, PTCA	
Cerebrovascular disease	5%
Stroke, TIA	
Other vascular disease	2%
Diabetes mellitus	7%
Hypercholesterolemia	36%
treated	13%

Abbreviations: *ANBP2*, 2nd Australian National Blood Pressure Study; *MI*, myocardial infarction; *CAB6*, coronary artery bypass graft; *PTCA*, percutaneous transluminal coronary angioplasty; *TIA*, transient ischemic attack.

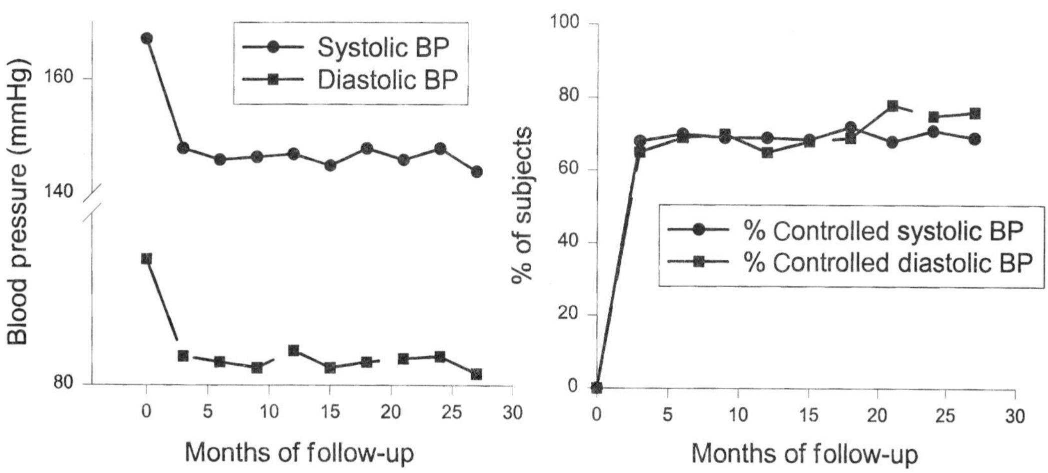

Fig. 4 Proportion of subjects achieving goal systolic and diastolic blood pressure during the follow-up phase of the 2nd Australian National Blood Pressure Study (ANBP2).

Table 7 Endpoint Accumulation After 10379 Patient-Years of Observation in ANBP2

Endpoint*	Number	Rate (x 1000 per year)
Sudden cardiac death	21	2.0
Rapid cardiac death	2	0.2
Heart failure or other coronary death	5	0.5
Fatal myocardial infarction	7	0.7
Fatal stroke	12	1.2
Nonfatal myocardial infarction	47	4.5
LV or heart failure	48	4.6
PTCA or CABG	75	7.2
Other coronary syndromes	39	3.8
Other cardiovascular events	3	0.3
Nonfatal stroke	64	6.2
TIA	32	3.1
TOTAL	355	34.2

* Numbers represent the total number of events (first and subsequent).
Abbreviations: *ANBP2*, 2nd Australian National Blood Pressure Study; *LV*, left ventricular; *PTCA*, percutaneous transluminal coronary angioplasty; *CABG*, coronary artery bypass graft; *TIA*, transient ischemic attack.

(3). From a community perspective, assessment of the value of ACE inhibitor use in comparison to other less expensive drug treatments is needed to justify the cost-effectiveness of current prescribing patterns.

Since the commencement of ANBP2 in 1994, only one trial has been published that compares the effects of newer and older therapies on cardiovascular outcomes in hypertension (24). The Captopril Prevention Project (CAPPP) study overall found that ACE inhibition was as effective as conventional diuretic β-blocker therapy in the prevention of cardiovascular morbidity and mortality in a population aged 25 to 66; however, stroke reduction was greater in the conventional therapy group. In an elderly population in which the risk of stroke is greater, clarification of the role of ACE inhibition as the initial choice of agent to reduce coronary heart disease and stroke risk is needed, and the results of ANBP2 will thus contribute important data.

In developing the protocol for ANBP2, it was important that the study design should reflect the setting in which hypertension is most commonly managed in Australia, namely general (family) practice. Although double-blind, randomized, controlled trials may be the most rigorous design for determining whether interventions are effective, they may not be the most appropriate to determine efficacy in the ''real world of general practice.'' An alternative to the double-blind, randomized controlled design that is being increasingly utilized in outcome studies, and which is being used in ANBP2, is the PROBE design (15). The advantage of this design is that it enables major questions related to the long-term impact of interventions to be assessed in the manner in which they are used.

One of the unique aspects of ANBP2 is that it is first cardiovascular outcome trial to be conducted entirely in a general practice setting in Australia. More than 2000 general practitioners have been involved in the project, which incorporates approximately 1 in 10 general practitioners in the nation. A potential advantage of general practice-based research is that GPs are the major prescribers of medication for the management of hypertension and, as such, it is likely that the results of the trial will be readily accepted by this group. It has been well recognized that major difficulties have occurred in the transition of clinical trial results to influencing patient management in practice, and involving such a large number of primary health care providers may assist in disseminating results.

However, conducting research in general practice according to the standards outlined by the Australian Therapeutic Goods Administration's *Guidelines for Good Clinical Research Practice* (25) has been a major challenge (17). Although the screening and randomization steps in ANBP2 were conducted by study nurses trained objectively to identify the hypertensive cohort, subsequent follow-up is blended with routine patient management in the actual setting of general practice by GPs and as such, protocol adherence is an important issue (26). Strategies adopted include peer-to-peer GP training and support, individual performance feedback to each site, and reviewing of case records by study nurses for endpoint data on a 6-monthly basis. To date, these strategies have provided endpoint data suitable for adjudication by the independent endpoint committee ($n = 355$), minimal loss to follow-up ($< 1\%$), and high levels of adherence to drug treatment protocol ($> 70\%$).

The instigation of this trial has also led to the establishment of a unique partnership between the Australian government and the pharmaceutical industry in terms of the funding arrangements for ANBP2. The funding arrangement involves the provision of study medications through the Australian government scheme for subsidy of pharmaceuticals, the Pharmaceutical Benefits Scheme (PBS), and the costs of general practice consultations for patients being claimed through the Australian universal health care scheme, Medicare. Merck, Sharp and Dohme (Australia) Pty. Ltd. provided support for infrastructure including nursing staff, data collection and analysis, and coordinating personnel for the project.

Since the commencement of ANBP2, additional partnerships have been added to the joint venture funding arrangements. The Australian National Heart Foundation and SpaceLabs Pty. Ltd. are providing support for the conduct of the ambulatory blood pressure monitoring substudy; the National Health and Medical Research Council of Australia for the independent data monitoring committee and the genetic substudy; the Victorian Health Promotion Foundation for evaluation of the efficacy and long-term safety of drug withdrawal before the screening phase. This additional support (at relatively low cost for each individual sponsoring agency) has provided the opportunity to add further value to government and industry support for ANBP2.

Evidence-based medical practice hinges on the use of "current best evidence" to make decisions about the appropriate management of individual patients (27). With limited and highly competitive resources, the opportunity for outcome trials to be funded through the government support is limited. The design of ANBP2, its unique funding arrangements, and the strategies implemented for ongoing patient monitoring and protocol adherence are enabling health outcomes research for the management of hypertension in Australia to be conducted in the course of current practice. The true winners will be the Australian public who will have "added value" to the costs incurred with the use of current medication.

ACKNOWLEDGMENTS

The ANBP2 acknowledges the contributions of the following host institutions: Baker Medical Research Institute and Department of Community Medicine and General Practice,

Monash University (Victoria); Department of General Practice and Department of Public Health, University of Adelaide (South Australia); Department of General Practice, University of Western Australia (West Australia); Department of General Practice, University of Sydney (New South Wales); Department of Social and Preventive Medicine, University of Queensland (Queensland). The authors also acknowledge the contribution of all participating GP investigators and subjects on the project and those who contributed to the numerous study committees listed below.

Management committee: L. M. H. Wing, C. M. Reid, L. J. Beilin, M. A. Brown, G. L. R. Jennings, C. I. Johnston, J. J. McNeil, J. E. Marley, T. O. Morgan, P. Ryan, M. J. West.
Finance committee: G. L. R. Jennings, C. I. Johnston, L. M. H. Wing, C. M. Reid, G. Macdonald
Left ventricular hypertrophy committee: G. L. R. Jennings, P. Fletcher, M. Feneley, E. Dewar, C. M. Reid.
Genetic committee: M. West, S. Harrap, L. Beilin, C. I. Johnston, C. Reid, P. Ryan.
Health economic and quality of life committee: J. Marley, J. Moss, P. Glasziou, F. Boyle, J. Primrose, C. M. Reid.
Independent data monitoring and safety committee: J. Chalmers, S. MacMahon, C. Silagy, J. Whitworth.
Ambulatory blood pressure monitoring committee: M. Brown, L. Beilin, L. M. H. Wing, C. M. Reid.
Data audit committee: J. McNeil, G. L. R. Jennings, L. M. H. Wing, C. M. Reid, J. Marley.
Endpoint committee: T. Morgan, L. M. H. Wing, D. Hunt, G. Donnan.
GP advisory committee: I. Steven, L. Piterman, F. deLooze, J. Dickinson, J. Gambrill, P. Joseph, C. M. Reid.

APPENDIX 1 ANBP2 Endpoint Definitions and Required Evidence

1. Death-cardiovascular
Coronary artery disease death

Endpoint	Supporting information
Myocardial infarction Autopsy or death certificate diagnosis, with definite or suspected diagnosis of myocardial infarction within 4 weeks of death.	1. Death certificate 2. Autopsy report (if available) 3. Hospital records 4. GP records
Sudden cardiac death Death occurring within 1 hour of the onset of new cardiac symptoms (ischemic chest pain or sudden collapse); OR Unwitnessed death after last being seen without new cardiac symptoms, and in each case, *without* any noncoronary disease (clinically or at autopsy) that could have been rapidly fatal.	1. Death certificate 2. Autopsy report (if available) 3. Hospital records 4. GP records
Rapid cardiac death (death after possible myocardial infarction) 1. Death within 1–24 hours of the onset of severe cardiac symptoms unrelated to other known causes. 2. Death in hospital with possible myocardial infarction (i.e., patients who have had typical ischemic pain and whose electrocardiogram	1. Death certificate 2. Autopsy report (if available) 3. Hospital records 4. GP records

Coronary artery disease death—Continued

Endpoint	Supporting information
and enzyme results do not fulfill the criteria for definite myocardial infarction and in whom there is no good evidence for another diagnosis for the event), e.g. resuscitated sudden deaths who live for a few hours often fall into this category.	
Cardiac failure (with coronary cause) Death resulting from heart failure (prior grade 3–4 dyspnea New York Heart Association), without any defined noncoronary cause.	1. Death certificate 2. Autopsy report (if available) 3. Hospital records 4. GP records
Other coronary death Any death in which the underlying cause is certified as coronary (and in which there is no evidence for a noncoronary cause of death, clinically or at autopsy) e.g., perioperative death after coronary artery grafts may fall into this category.	1. Death certificate 2. Autopsy report (if available) 3. Hospital records 4. GP records

Other cardiovascular deaths

Endpoint	Supporting information
Cardiac failure Death resulting from heart failure (prior grade 3–4 dyspnea New York Heart Association), with any defined noncoronary cause.	1. Death certificate 2. Autopsy report (if available) 3. Hospital records 4. GP records
Other vascular deaths Any death certified as caused by vascular but not cardiac disease, e.g., ruptured aortic aneurysm, dissecting aortic aneurysm, malignant hypertension, renovascular disease, complications of peripheral vascular disease.	1. Death certificate 2. Autopsy report (if available) 3. Hospital records 4. GP records
Noncoronary cardiac Any death in which the underlying cause is certified as the result of noncoronary cardiac disease, e.g., rheumatic heart disease.	1. Death certificate 2. Autopsy report (if available) 3. Hospital records 4. GP records

Cerebrovascular death

Endpoint	Supporting information
Stroke Any death resulting from the rapid onset of a new neurological deficit attributed to obstruction or rupture in the arterial system.	1. Death certificate 2. Autopsy report (if available) 3. Hospital records 4. GP records

Noncardiovascular deaths

Endpoint	Supporting information
Noncardiovascular death Any other death Cancer	1. Death certificate 2. Autopsy report (if available)

Noncardiovascular deaths—Continued

Endpoint	Supporting information
Trauma Suicide Renal failure Any other cause	3. Hospital records 4. GP records

2. Nonfatal Cardiovascular Events
Coronary artery disease

Endpoint	Supporting information
Myocardial infarction Any two of the following three a. History of typical ischemic pain lasting for at least 15 minutes and unresponsive to sublingual nitrates (if given); b. Elevation of creatine kinase (CK) enzymes to more than twice the upper limit of normal (for the laboratory), *and* more than twice the level shown by the patient in the routine test either immediately before or after the attack; c. Electrocardiographic changes of: new Q waves ≥ .03 sec in ≥ 2 leads of same group, *or* evolution of ST-T changes with ST elevation of 2 mm or more in anterior leads or 1 mm or more in inferior or lateral leads, followed by T-wave inversion of 1 mm or more in the same group of leads. Evolution over time, therefore, requires a minimum of two traces taken at least 1 day apart.	1. Hospital notes 2. GP notes 3. Electrocardiogram of event at beginning (admission) and 24 hours. 4. Laboratory report confirming peak CK
Lead groups for the purposes of the above definitions are: lateral site (leads I, aVL, V6) inferior site (leads II, III, aVF) anterior site (leads V1, V2, V3, V4, V5)	
Angina The onset of retrosternal chest pain with or without typical radiation to the arms and jaw usually precipitated by exertion or emotion.	1. Hospital discharge summary (if available) 2. GP notes
Coronary artery therapeutic procedures Hospital discharge diagnosis of coronary artery bypass grafting or coronary angioplasty.	1. Hospital discharge summary
Cardiac failure (left ventricular or congestive) (i) Hospital discharge diagnosis of cardiac failure **OR** (ii) Characteristic chest x-ray appearance **OR** (iii) At least two of the following three definite physical signs crackles in lung fields raised jugular venous pressure ankle edema	1. Hospital notes 2. GP notes 3. Copy of X-ray
Other coronary syndromes (e.g., unstable angina) The onset of severe retrosternal chest pain at rest or with minimal exertion, which may be associated with electrocardiogram changes (ST depression, T-wave flattening or inversion) but no enzyme rise.	1. Hospital discharge summary (if available) 2. GP notes 3. Electrocardiograms of event

Other cardiovascular endpoints	
Endpoint	Supporting information
Ruptured aortic or dissecting aneurism Onset of accelerated or malignant hypertension Acute occlusion of a major feeding artery in any vascular bed other than cerebral or coronary.	1. Hospital discharge summary or notes 2. GP notes
Cerebrovascular events	
Endpoint	Supporting information
Stroke Rapid onset of a new neurological deficit attributed to obstruction or rupture in the arterial system. The defined deficit must persist for at least 24 hours unless death supervenes and must include specific localizing findings confirmed by neurological examination or CT head scan with no evidence of an underlying nonvascular cause.	1. Hospital discharge summary or notes 2. GP notes
Transient cerebral ischemic attack Rapid onset of a focal neurological deficit lasting less than 24 hours, presumed caused by cerebral ischemia with no evidence of an underlying nonvascular cause.	1. Hospital discharge summary or notes 2. GP notes

REFERENCES

1. Australian National Blood Pressure Study Management Committee. The Australian Therapeutic Trial in Mild Hypertension. Lancet 1980; i:1261–1267.
2. Australian Bureau of Statistics. 1989–90 National Health Survey. Consultation with health professionals, Australia. Canberra: Australian Bureau of Statistics, 1992.
3. Henry D. Patterns of antihypertensive drugs in Australia 1986–93. Aust Prescriber 1994; 17(supp 1):32–36.
4. MacMahon S, Peto R, Cutler J. Blood pressure, stroke, and coronary heart disease. Part 1. Prolonged differences in blood pressure: prospective observational studies corrected for the regression dilution bias. Lancet 1990; 335:765–774.
5. Collins R, Peto R, MacMahon S. Blood pressure, stroke and coronary heart disease. Part 2. Short-term reductions in blood pressure:overview of randomised drug trials in their epidemiological context. Lancet 1990; 335:827–838.
6. SHEP Co-operative Research Group. Prevention of stroke by antihypertensive drug treatment in older persons with isolated systolic hypertension. JAMA 1991; 265:3255–3264.
7. Dahlof B, Lindholm LH, Hansson L, Schersten B, Ekbom T, Wester PO. Morbidity and mortality in the Swedish Trial in Old Patients with Hypertension (STOP Hypertension). Lancet 1991; 338:1281–1285.
8. MRC Working Party. Medical Research Council trial of treatment of hypertension in older adults: principal results. BMJ 1992; 304:405–412.
9. Weidmann P, Uehunge D, Gerber A. Antihypertensive treatment and serum lipoproteins. J Hypertens 1985; 3:297–306.
10. Dahlof B, Pennert K, Hansson L. Reversal of left ventricular hypertrophy in hypertensive patients: a meta-analysis of 109 treatment studies. Am J Hypertens 1992; 5:95–110.
11. The CONSENSUS Trial Study Group. Effects of enalaparil on mortality in severe congestive heart failure: results of the Cooperative North Scandinavian Enalapril Survival Study (CONSENSUS). N Engl J Med 1987; 316:1429–1435.
12. The SOLVD Investigators. Effect of enalapril on survival in patients with reduced left ventricular ejection fractions and congestive heart failure. N Engl J Med 1991; 325:293–302.

13. Pollaire T, Lithell H, Berne C. A comparison of the effects of hydrocholorothiazide and captopril on glucose and lipid metabolism in patients with hypertension. N Engl J Med 1989; 321: 868–873.
14. PBS Analysis Section Report. Pharmaceutical Benefits Branch: expenditure and prescriptions–12 months to 30 June 1997. Canberra: Commonwealth Department of Health and Family Services, 1998.
15. Hansson L, Hedner T, Dahlof B. Prospective Randomized Open Blinded End-point (PROBE) Study. A novel design for intervention trials. Blood Press 1992; 1:113–119.
16. Palta M, McHugh R. Planning the size of a cohort study in the presence of both losses to follow-up and non-compliance. J Chronic Dis 1980; 33:501–512.
17. Reid C, Nelson M, Beckinsale P, Ryan P, Wing LM, Beilin LJ, Brown MA, Jennings GL, Johnston CI, Marley J, Holyilj J, Morgan TO, Shaw J, Steven ID, West MJ. Feasibility of conducting cardiovascular outcome research in Australian General Practice—results from the ANBP2 Pilot Study. Clin Exp Physio Pharmacol 1997; 24:370–373.
18. Cook R, Lawless J. Interim monitoring of longitudinal comparative studies with recurrent event responses. Biometrics 1996; 52:1311–1321.
19. Ware JE, Sherbourne CD. The MOS 36-item short form health survey (SF-36): conceptual framework and item selection. Med Care 1992; 30:473–483.
20. Croog S, Levine S, Testa M, Brown B, Bulpitt C. The effects of antihypertensive therapy on the quality of life. N Engl J Med 1986; 314:1657–1664.
21. Deague J, Wilson C, Wrigg L, Harrap S. Discrepancies between echocardiographic measurements of left ventricular mass in a healthy adult population. Clin Sci 1999; 97:377–383.
22. Guidelines Subcommittee. 1999 WHO-ISH Hypertension guidelines for the management of hypertension. J Hypertens 1999; 17:151–183.
23. Staessen JA, Fagard R, Thijs L, Celis H, for the Syst-Eur Trial Investigators. Randomised double-blind comparison of placebo and active treatment for older patients with isolated systolic hypertension. Lancet 1997; 350(9080):757–764.
24. Hansson L, Lindholm L, Niskanen L, Lanke J, for the CAPPP study group. The Captopril Prevention Project: a prospective intervention trial of angiotensin converting enzyme inhibition in the treatment of hypertension. J Hypertens 1999; 8:985–990.
25. Commonwealth of Australia. Guidelines for Good Clinical Research Practice (GCRP) in Australia. Canberra: Department of Health and Family Services, 1991.
26. Management Committee. Second Australian National Blood Pressure Study. Clin Exp Physiol Pharmacol 1997; 24:188–192.
27. Silagy C. Evidence based medicine—effectiveness versus efficiency. Aust Epidemiologist 1996; 3(3):14–17.

24

Losartan Intervention For Endpoint Reduction in Hypertension: The LIFE Study

BJÖRN DAHLÖF

Sahlgrenska University Hospital/Östra, Göteborg, Sweden

RICHARD DEVEREUX

New York Hospital-Cornell Medical Center, New York, New York

ULF de FAIRE

Karolinska Hospital, Stockholm, Sweden

FREJ FYHRQUIST and MARKKU S. NIEMINEN

Helsinki University Central Hospital, Helsinki, Finland

HANS IBSEN

Glostrup University Hospital, Glostrup, Denmark

STEVO JULIUS

University of Michigan Medical Center, Ann Arbor, Michigan

SVERRE KJELDSEN

Ullevål Hospital, Oslo, Norway

KRISTER KRISTIANSON

MRL Scandinavia, Stockholm, Sweden

OLE LEDERBALLE-PEDERSEN

Viborg Hospital, Viborg, Denmark

The investigation is sponsored by Merck & Co., Inc.

LARS H. LINDHOLM

Umeå University Hospital, Umeå, Sweden

PER OMVIK

Hankeland Hospital, Bergen, Norway

SUZANNE OPARIL

University of Alabama at Birmingham, Birmingham, Alabama

HANS WEDEL

The Nordic School of Public Health, Göteborg, Sweden

I. BACKGROUND

Electrocardiographic (ECG) evidence of left ventricular hypertrophy (LVH) is almost ten times more common in individuals with blood pressures above 160/95 mm Hg than in normotensive persons (1). In a report from the Glasgow Blood Pressure Clinic, ECG-LVH was found in 35% of men and 22% of women with nonmalignant hypertension and a mean age of 50 years (2). Using echocardiographic criteria, the average prevalence of LVH in a hypertensive population is approximately 40% and increases with age (3, 4).

The importance of the structural changes in the cardiovascular system that accompany hypertension—in particular LVH—in conferring risk for cardiac complications is widely recognized. Whether assessed by ECG or echocardiography, LVH is a powerful, independent risk factor for an adverse cardiovascular outcome, yielding prognostic information beyond that derived from traditional cardiovascular risk factors, including high blood pressure, smoking, and lipid levels (1, 2, 5). In both the Framingham Heart Study (5) and a study conducted at the New York Hospital-Cornell Medical Center (6), left ventricular mass and age were the strongest predictors of prognosis. Among hypertensive patients, the risk of myocardial infarction, stroke, angina pectoris, and heart failure was increased several-fold by the presence of LVH. The seriousness of LVH is underscored by the finding that, within 5 years of its appearance, one third of men and one fourth of women with LVH are dead, usually from coronary disease (7).

Reversal of LVH has long been considered an important objective in treating hypertension and is emerging as a potential key therapeutic goal for lowering coronary risk. Among the strongest evidence to date for improved prognosis after regression of LVH comes from data from the Cornell Medical Center, where 166 men and women with hypertension were followed up with serial echocardiography over 10 years. In these patients, regression of LVH was associated with a lowered rate of cardiovascular complications (e.g., myocardial infarction, sudden cardiac death, stroke) (8). Data from the Framingham Heart Study similarly showed a definite reduction in cardiovascular events in the cohort of patients with ECG-measured LVH regression (9). Additional studies using electrocardiography have also shown that patients in whom LV mass decreases during antihypertensive therapy have a more favorable prognosis than those in whom this does not occur (10–12).

It is well established that antihypertensive therapy can reverse LVH, although the mechanism(s) by which the various drugs effect this change is not entirely clear. Two recent meta-analyses suggest that monotherapy with inhibitors of the angiotensin-converting enzyme (ACE) is more effective in decreasing LV mass than treatment with other antihypertensive agents, such as β-blockers and diuretics and possibly calcium channel blockers, which also reduce LV mass (13, 14). This observation was supported by results of controlled trials in hypertension comparing enalapril with hydrochlorothiazide (HCTZ) (15), ramipril with atenolol or HCTZ (16, 17), and captopril with minoxidil (18), all of which showed a greater reduction in LV mass with the ACE inhibitor treatment.

Thus the renin-angiotensin system (RAS) seems to have a major role in the establishment and maintenance of LVH. The primary hormone of the RAS is angiotensin II. In addition to elevating blood pressure, angiotensin II has been reported to exert direct effects on cardiac structure and function, stimulating proliferation and growth of vascular smooth muscle cells and cardiac myocytes (19). Activation of intracardiac RAS promotes cardiac hypertrophy and interstitial fibrosis, the latter of which is of notable pathological importance (20, 21).

Therefore, it is not surprising that RAS blockade has been proposed as an additional explanation, apart from the fall in blood pressure, for the effectiveness of ACE inhibitors in reversing LVH. A multivariate analysis of results from a comparative enalapril-HCTZ study in previously untreated hypertensive patients suggested that reversal of cardiac hypertrophy was more related to changes in the RAS than to a reduction in blood pressure (15). Other supportive evidence linking RAS to LVH development comes from the observation that ACE inhibitors are effective in reducing cardiac hypertrophy, even when administered at doses that do not lower blood pressure (22).

In cardiac tissue, ACE inhibitors inhibit only a fraction of angiotensin II formed from angiotensin I (23), and alternate pathways (e.g., chymase) may generate angiotensin II, even in the presence of ACE inhibitors (24). In addition, when ACE inhibition is not 100% complete, stimulation of renin secretion may lead to very high angiotensin I levels, returning angiotensin II levels toward or even to pretreatment levels (25). This suggests that blocking the effect of angiotensin II at its specific receptor site would result in more complete inhibition of systemically and locally produced angiotensin II and thereby a more profound reversal of cardiac structural changes.

Losartan is the first of a new class of orally active, nonpeptide antagonists of the angiotensin II receptor. Losartan and its active metabolite E-3174 potently and selectively inhibit angiotensin II by specifically targeting the AT_1 subtype of the angiotensin II receptor (26). Thus losartan provides an attractive, novel approach to modifying the role of angiotensin II in hypertension, with the potential for more sustained and maintained inhibition of the RAS. Losartan's efficacy and tolerability in the treatment of human hypertension has been well established (27). In experimental models of hypertension, losartan prevented or decreased established cardiac hypertrophy (28, 29). The clinical experience with losartan in relation to reversal of LVH is limited but promising, with levels of reversal in at least the same range as ACE inhibition (30–32). Moreover, promising results have been seen with losartan on survival in heart failure (33).

Losartan provides a useful biologic probe to test whether direct, effective inhibition of the RAS can improve the outcome of hypertensive patients, especially with respect to prevention of adverse cardiovascular complications. Specifically, the Losartan Intervention for Endpoint (LIFE) reduction in Hypertension study was designed to test whether selective angiotensin II receptor blockade with losartan not only lowers blood pressure but reduces LVH more effectively than conventional therapy, and thus improves prognosis in patients with hypertension (34). It is the largest study ever undertaken in persons with LVH and one of the largest intervention studies to date in essential hypertension. The LIFE study is also unique in that it uses ECG criteria for LVH to recruit a large population of high-risk hypertensives. Enrollment into this large, prospective interventional study is complete, with 9194 subjects randomized and being treated long term with losartan or atenolol in adherence with the protocol (35).

II. STUDY DESIGN

The LIFE study is a prospective, multicenter, double-blind, double-dummy, randomized, active-controlled study with two parallel groups. The design, inclusion/exclusion criteria, methods, outcome measures, and planned analysis approach for the LIFE study have been detailed elsewhere (34) (Tables 1–6).

A. Study Objectives

The primary objective of the LIFE study is to compare the long-term effects of losartan with those of the β-blocker, atenolol, both at doses of 50 to 100 mg per day, on the combined incidence of cardiovascular mortality, nonfatal myocardial infarction, and nonfatal stroke in patients with essential hypertension and documented LVH (Table 1). Atenolol was selected as the comparative agent because β-blockers are known to be beneficial in both primary and secondary prevention and because atenolol is the most widely used β-blocker for the treatment of hypertension, and its efficacy and tolerability have already been compared with those of losartan (36). The treatment goal is less than 140 and SiDBP less than 90 mm Hg. For those patients whose blood pressure (BP) is not at goal, HCTZ might be increased or additional antihypertensive medication (excluding ACE inhibitors, angiotensin II [AII] antagonists, or β-blockers) should be added, unless contraindicated (Table 2).

The specific hypothesis to be tested in the LIFE study is that losartan will result in a lower incidence of cardiovascular mortality and morbidity in this specified patient population than atenolol. For this study, a clinically meaningful difference between the two antihypertensive treatments was defined a priori as a 15% (or more) reduction in the proportion of subjects experiencing a primary fatal or morbid cardiovascular event (as defined above) in the group receiving losartan compared with the group treated with atenolol.

Secondary and tertiary study objectives, as defined in the protocol and to be assessed only after testing of the primary hypothesis is complete, are listed in Table 1. Electrocardiographic findings are being validated within the study using echocardiograms obtained in a subpopulation of the LIFE study group, comprising approximately 10% of the enrolled subjects (37). Additional planned analyses will use echocardiography and ECG to evaluate in greater detail the effects of the two drugs on LVH and the relationship of LVH change to other variables, including the incidence of cardiovascular events and the impact of study medication on arterial functioning and insulin resistance.

Table 1 Protocol-Specified Objectives of LIFE Study

Primary objective	To compare the long-term effects (≥ 4 years) of losartan and atenolol in hypertensive patients with documented LVH on the combination of cardiovascular mortality and morbidity (nonfatal myocardial infarction, nonfatal stroke).
Secondary objectives	To compare the long-term effects of losartan and atenolol on: • Total mortality • Cardiovascular mortality • Fatal and nonfatal myocardial infarction • Fatal and nonfatal stroke • Hospitalization for angina pectoris • Hospitalization for heart failure • Regression of ECG-LVH • Relationship between regression of ECG-LVH and cardiovascular mortality and morbidity • Coronary and peripheral revascularization procedures • Silent myocardial infarction as evaluated by serial readings of annual ECGs • Safety and tolerability based on adverse experience profile and discontinuation rates because of adverse experiences
Tertiary objectives	Evaluate: • Relationship between blood pressure control and cardiovascular morbidity and mortality • Influence of various known risk factors on cardiovascular event rate • Long-term effects of losartan and atenolol on new-onset diabetes mellitus • Long-term effects of losartan and atenolol on health care resource utilization

Abbreviations: *LIFE*, Losartan Intervention for Endpoint Reduction in Hypertension; *LVH*, left ventricular hypertrophy; *ECG*, electrocardiogram.

Table 2 Suggested Titration Steps if SiSBP ≥ 140 and/or SiDBP ≥ 90 mm Hg

End of Month	Treatment
1	Losartan 50 mg or atenolol 50 mg
2	Losartan 50 mg or atenolol 50 mg plus HCTZ 12.5 mg
4	Losartan 100 mg or atenolol 100 mg and HCTZ 12.5 mg
6	Losartan 100 mg or atenolol 100 mg and HCTZ 12.5 mg plus other antihypertensive therapy (excluding ACEIs, AII-antagonists, or beta-blockers) The dosage of HCTZ might be increased.

Key: SiSBP, sitting systolic blood pressure; SiDBP = sitting diastolic blood pressure.
Abbreviations: HCTZ, hydrochlorothiazide; *ACEI*, angiotensin-converting enzyme I; *AII-antagonists*, angiotensin II-antagonists.

B. Patient Selection

Eligible subjects were men and women aged 55 to 80 years with previously untreated or treated hypertension and ECG-documented LVH (Table 3). To be enrolled into the study, subjects were required to have trough sitting DBP readings of 95 to 115 mm Hg or sitting SBP readings of 160 to 200 mm Hg after 1 and 2 weeks on single-blind placebo treatment. Inclusion and exclusion criteria are listed in Table 3; these included certain cardiovascular conditions and serious noncardiac diseases that could limit long-term survival or increase the likelihood of nonadherence to study medication.

Left ventricular hypertrophy was diagnosed by the core laboratory (Sahlgrenska

Table 3 Criteria for Inclusion and Exclusion of Entry into the LIFE Study

Inclusion criteria:

- Male or female
- 55–80 years of age
- SiDBP 95–115 and/or SiSBP 160–200 mm Hg
- Left ventricular hypertrophy must meet the Cornell Product or Sokolow-Lyon criteria specified below:

  Cornell Product:

  Men

  Cornell product = [QRS duration (in msec)] * [RaVL + SV3 (in mm)] > 2440 mm × msec

  Women

  Cornell product = [QRS duration (in msec)] * [RaVL + SV3 (in mm) + 6 mm] > 2440 mm × msec

  Sokolow-Lyon:

  The Sokolow-Lyon voltage requirement is SV1 + RV5 or V6 > 38 mm.

Exclusion criteria:

- Known secondary hypertension, malignant hypertension, or hypertensive encephalopathy
- Increase in diastolic blood pressure to >115 mm Hg or in systolic blood pressure to >200 mm Hg during the placebo period
- History of stroke or myocardial infarction within the previous 6 months
- Presence of heart failure or known left ventricular ejection fraction ≤ 40%
- Angina pectoris requiring treatment with a β-blocker or a calcium antagonist
- History of renal or hepatic disorders with severe impairment (serum creatinine >160 μmol/L or 1.8 mg/dL) or patients with a solitary kidney or renal transplant
- Significant known aortic stenosis (mean antegrade Doppler gradient ≥ 20 mm Hg)
- Known hypersensitivity or contraindication to losartan, atenolol, or hydrochlorothiazide
- A condition that, in the treating physician's opinion, requires treatment with losartan, atenolol or another β-blocker, hydrochlorothiazide, or an ACE inhibitor
- Serious disease expected to cause substantial deterioration of patient's health during the next 4 to 6 years
- Current or recent history of alcohol or other drug substance abuse
- Mental or legal incapacitation
- Participation in another investigational drug trial using a nonapproved drug either at present or during the 10 days before entry into the study
- Unwillingness to participate
- Low compliance at end of placebo period, as judged by the investigator

Abbreviations: *LIFE*, Losartan Intervention for Endpoint Reduction in Hypertension; *ACE*, angiotensin-converting enzyme. SiSBP = sitting systolic blood pressure; SiDBP = sitting diastolic blood pressure.

University Hospital/Östra in Göteborg, Sweden) from standard 12-lead ECGs obtained in all potential participants before randomization. Left ventricular hypertrophy was identified by the core laboratory using criteria based on the product of Cornell voltage × QRS duration product (38–40): (RaVL + SV_3) × QRS duration >2440 mm × msec. Based on early studies (41, 42), an adjustment of Cornell voltage by 8 mm was initially made in women. Data published after completion of LIFE's design (43, 44) indicated that the gender adjustment should be smaller; accordingly, the gender adjustment for Cornell voltage in women was revised to 6 mm in May 1996 after 2383 patients had been enrolled (35). At this time, a Sokolow-Lyon voltage combination (Sv_1 + RV_5 or V_6) >38 mm was accepted as an alternate criterion for LVH in both women and men.

C. Study Procedures

The study procedures are presented in Table 4. The LIFE study consists of a 2-week placebo run-in period followed by a minimum 4-year period of randomized, active, double-blind treatment. Active treatment will continue for 4 years after the last patient is enrolled, that is, until at least April 30, 2001, or until 1040 subjects experience a primary cardiovascular endpoint.

After 2 weeks of placebo treatment, subjects who met the criteria for entry into the LIFE study were randomized to once-daily treatment with losartan or atenolol, beginning at a dose of 50 mg. During the study, antihypertensive therapy is adjusted, as detailed in Table 2, to achieve a goal blood pressure of 140/90 mm Hg or lower. Clinic visits occur at frequent intervals during the initial 6 months of observation and at 6-month intervals thereafter. At each visit, BP and heart rate are measured at trough (i.e., 22 to 26 hours postdose) using a standardized technique after subjects have been seated for 5 minutes.

Laboratory tests are performed by the central laboratory and include determinations of hemoglobin, serum glucose, sodium, potassium, creatinine, alanine pyruvic transaminase (ALAT, SGPT), uric acid, total and HDL cholesterol, and in the urinalysis, microalbumin and creatinine (Table 5). These laboratory determinations are performed at the beginning of the double-blind treatment period and after each year of active therapy. After randomization, standard 12-lead ECGs are obtained before the first dose of double-blind treatment on day 1, after 6 months, and after each year of active therapy. Adverse events are monitored throughout the study; primary endpoints are not be reported as adverse experiences.

D. Administrative Structure of the Study

A roster of committees is presented in Table 6. An independent, blinded international steering committee has the ultimate responsibility for the scientific conduct of the LIFE study. In each participating country, a data collection and monitoring center is working under the supervision of the central office. As indicated above, a central ECG laboratory is responsible for classification of all ECGs and for the blinded interpretation of serial ECG changes.

An endpoint classification committee was established to review all events reported by the clinical centers to determine if they constitute an endpoint as defined in the protocol. Study endpoints include *morbidity*, defined as nonfatal, clinically evident acute myocardial infarction and nonfatal stroke, and *mortality*, defined as death resulting from a fatal myocardial infarction, fatal stroke, sudden death, progressive heart failure, or other cardiovascular causes.

Table 4 Study Summary Table

Procedure	Screening Prestudy <365 days	Placebo baseline period[l] Visit 1 Day 14	Visit 2 Day 7	Visit 3 Day 1	Triple-blind period Visit 4 Month 1	Visit 5 Month 2	Visit 6 Month 4	Visit 7 Month 6	Visit 8 Year 1	Visit 9 Year 1.5	Visit 10 Year 2	Visit 11 Year 2.5	Visit 12 Year 3	Visit 13 Year 3.5	Visit 14 Year 4*
Medical history		X													
Complete physical examination		X							X		X		X		X
Obtain informed consent	X[f]	X													
Sitting BP and HR	(X)	X	X	X[b]	X	X	X	X	X	X	X	X	X	X	X
Standing BP and HR				X		X[c]	X[c]	X[c]	X[c]	X[c]	X[c]	X[c]	X[c]	X[c]	
Laboratory safety tests[l]		X[k]		X	X[j]				X		X				X
ECG (12-lead)	X[e]	X[a]		X				X	X		X		X		X
AE evaluation			X	X	X	X	X	X	X	X	X	X	X	X	X
Discontinue all antihypertensive medication	X														
Dispense placebo baseline medication		X[i]													
Dispense double-blind medication				X[g]	X	X	X	X	X	X	X	X	X	X	
Add additional antihypertensives to treatment regimen if appropriate						X[d]	X[d]	X[d]	X[d]	X[d]	X[d]	X[d]	X[d]	X[d]	
Healthcare resource utilization assessment[h]				X				X	X	X	X	X	X	X	X

[a] To be sent to ECG Core Center for evaluation of LVH inclusion criteria. May be taken up to 30 days prior to visit 1.
[b] Mean SiDBP must be 95–115 and/or SiSBP 160–200 mm Hg at 2 consecutive visits separated by at least 1 week for patient to be eligible to continue in study.
[c] Standing BP and HR measurement only necessary if patient requires upward titration of study drug.
[d] Add additional antihypertensives to treatment regimen if mean SiDBP is ≥ 90 and/or SiSBP ≥ 140 mm Hg. Titration regimen is test agent 50 mg alone → test agent 50 mg plus HCTZ 12.5 mg → 2x dose of test agent plus HCTZ 12.5 mg → other antihypertensive agents (excluding ACEIs, AII antagonists, or beta-blockers) plus 2x dose of test agent plus HCTZ 12.5 mg or more.
[e] May be an old ECG (fewer than 12 months).
[f] If ECG or other study tests are performed or medication discontinued with the intent to participate in the study.
[g] The last placebo tablet should have been taken the previous morning, i.e., approximately 24 hours before this visit.
[h] As specified in Standard Operating Procedures and worksheets.
[i] Patients who do not qualify after 14 days on placebo may remain on placebo for up to 14 additional days. They must have two consecutive blood pressures separated by at least 1 week equal to SiDBP 95–115 and/or SiSBP 160–200 for randomization.
[j] Abbreviated. Serum sodium, potassium, and creatinine only.
[k] Abbreviated. Serum glucose and creatinine only.
[l] Glucose retesting may be necessary for the evaluation of new-onset diabetes mellitus.
* **Note**: Patients will continue in the study until year 4 or until the 1040 patients reach a primary cardiovascular event, whichever is last. For patients who continue beyond year 4, perform procedures outlined for year 1.5 and year 2 for biannual and annual visits, respectively. All procedures listed for year 4 will also be performed at the final visit.
Abbreviations: *BP*, blood pressure; *HR*, heart rate; *ECG*, electrocardiogram; *SiDBP*, sitting diastolic blood pressure; *SiSBP*, sitting systolic blood pressure; *HCTZ*, hydrochlorothiazide; *ACEI*, angiotensin-converting enzyme inhibitors; *AII*, angiotensin-II.

Table 5 Laboratory Tests

Hematology	Hemoglobin
Blood chemistry	Creatinine, SGPT (ALAT), glucose, uric acid, sodium, potassium, total cholesterol, HDL cholesterol
Urinalysis	Microalbumin, creatinine
New-onset diabetes mellitus	Patients who at visit 1 or at any other time point in the study thereafter have a fasting serum (plasma) glucose value ≥ 140 mg/dL will have a fasting plasma sample taken after 1 week. If the glucose value is between 120 and 140 mg/dL, the patient will undergo an oral glucose tolerance test. If the initial serum (plasma) sample is nonfasting and ≥ 144 mg/dL, the patient will have a fasting plasma sample taken after 1 week. If the repeat fasting sample also is ≥ 140 mg/dL, the patient's diagnosis of diabetes is confirmed. If the repeat fasting plasma glucose value is < 140 mg/dL, the patient must undergo an oral glucose tolerance test. If after a 75-g oral glucose load the 2-hour plasma glucose value is ≥ 200 mg/dL, this is diagnostic of diabetes.

Abbreviations: SGPT (ALAT), serum glutamate pyruvate transaminase (alanine aminotransesterase); *HDL*, high-density lipoprotein.

Table 6 Roster of Committees

Steering committee	Bjorn Dahlöf, Goteborg, Sweden (Chairman)
	Richard B. Devereux, New York, NY, USA (Vice-Chairman)
	Sverre E. Kjeldsen, Oslo, Norway (Scandinavia Coordinator)
	Stevo Julius, Ann Arbor, Michigan, USA (U.S. Coordinator)
	Gareth Beevers, Birmingham, UK
	Ulf de Faire, Stockholm, Sweden
	Frej Fyhrquist, Helsinki, Finland
	Hans Ibsen, Glostrup, Denmark
	Lars H. Lindholm, Umeå, Sweden
	Markku S. Nieminen, Helsinki, Finland
	Per Omvik, Bergen, Norway
	Suzanne Oparil, Birmingham, Alabama, USA
	Ole Lederballe-Pedersen, Viborg, Denmark
	Hans Wedel, Goteborg, Sweden
Endpoint classification committee	Kristian Thygesen, Arhus, Denmark
	Daniel Levy, Framingham, Massachusetts, USA
Data safety monitoring board	John Kjekshus, Oslo, Norway (Chairman)
	Lewis H. Kuller, Pittsburgh, Pennsylvania, USA
	Pierre Larochelle, Montreal, Quebec, Canada
	Giuseppe Mancia, Monza, Italy
	Joel Menard, Paris, France
	Stuart Pocock, London, England
	John L. Reid, Glasgow, Scotland
	Michael A. Weber, Brooklyn, New York, USA

E. Statistical Considerations

Based on event rates among subjects with LVH in recent prospective studies in hypertension, a 15% 5-year event rate for the primary endpoint of combined incidence of cardiovascular death or nonfatal myocardial infarction or stroke is projected in the atenolol group (Table 7). With a sample size of 8300 subjects, the LIFE study was calculated to have 80% power to detect at least a 15% further reduction to 12.5% in the primary endpoint. The calculation of sample size was based on the long-rank test, using an exponential survival model described by Lachin and Foulkes (45). Because the LIFE study will continue to a fixed number of events (n = 1040), the power of the trial will not be appreciably affected by either the larger-than-planned study enrollment or by a difference in the actual event rate. To account for the possibility that a lower than expected event rate could substantially prolong the duration of the trial, the steering committee will monitor the accumulating event rate and has the right to recommend an increase to the sample size (while maintaining the requirement of 1040 patients with a primary event). Any such recommendation will be based on blinded, pooled-group data only and must be made before any unblinded interim efficacy analyses.

An independent data and safety monitoring board (DSMB) receives unblinded data, advises the steering committee at regular intervals about ethical aspects of study continuation, and makes recommendations to the steering committee regarding the safety of continuing the study based on their reviews of unblinded data. A single statistician has access to the randomization code and will perform the scheduled interim analyses. This person is forbidden to have contact with other individuals involved in the study.

Two interim analyses are scheduled after one third (343) and two thirds (686) of the expected number of events has occurred to determine if early termination is warranted because of overwhelming efficacy. The a priori stopping rule for early discontinuation of the LIFE study requires *P* values of 0.004 or less and 0.013 or less respectively, at the two interim analyses, and a *P* value of less than 0.046 at the planned end of the study, to maintain an overall 5% significance level for testing the primary hypothesis. The DSMB recommended continuation of the LIFE trial in March, 1998 after the first of these interim analyses.

All efficacy and safety data will be analyzed using an intent-to-treat approach that includes all randomized subjects regardless of any protocol violation. The primary endpoint is the time from randomization to the patient's first confirmed nonfatal stroke, nonfatal myocardial infarction, or cardiovascular death. The planned analysis of the primary endpoint involves a Cox regression model. In addition to treatment, the protocol specifies that the model will include the other covariates: degree of LVH by ECG and Framingham Risk Score defined by the patient's baseline characteristics. Additional analyses will include analyses of the components of the primary endpoint, angina pectoris requiring hospitalization, heart failure requiring hospitalization, changes in blood pressure and degree of

Table 7 Endpoints

Primary endpoints	Secondary endpoints
Cardiovascular death, nonfatal myocardial infarction, nonfatal stroke	Probable myocardial infarction, angina pectoris requiring hospitalization, heart failure requiring hospitalization, coronary or peripheral arterial revascularization, resuscitated cardiac arrest, silent myocardial infarction

LVH, and an exploration of the impact of changes in BP and degree of LVH on the primary endpoint.

III. RESULTS

A total of 945 centers in Denmark, Finland, Norway, Iceland, Sweden, United Kingdom, and the United States enrolled patients in the LIFE study during the period from September 1995 to April 1997, when recruitment was stopped. At this time, 9223 patients met the BP and other inclusion and no-exclusion criteria and had provided informed consent. Irregularities were discovered at one center and the steering committee decided to exclude this site from further participation; a total of 9194 participants remain after removal of this center. The patients who were randomized comprise about 28% of all those screened for the study and 48.5% of all those who were approved based on their ECG readings.

The majority of the study centers are active in primary care, although in Denmark most LIFE participants were referred from primary care physicians to hospital-based centers. The average number of patients enrolled at each center was 9.7 (range: 1 to 148). Twenty-five centers enrolled 40 or more patients; 17.6% of the overall study population was enrolled by these larger centers.

The total number of patients enrolled in the LIFE Study is almost 900 more than the 8300 initially planned. Based on the actual number of participants and the observed frequency of endpoints thus far, the LIFE study is on target for completion in 2001.

A. Baseline Characteristics

The demographic and baseline disease characteristics of the randomized participants have been analyzed and reported previously (35) (Tables 8–11).

The LIFE study population of hypertensive patients (mean blood pressure of 174.4/97.8 mm Hg) with ECG-documented LVH is composed of predominately white (92.4%) women and men (45.9%), mostly retired from active employment (65.6%), with a mean age of 66.9 years (Table 8). The women were older and had a higher body mass index (BMI).

Surprisingly, almost one third (28.9%) of the patients had not been treated for their hypertension for at least 6 months when recruited into the LIFE study. Among those

Table 8 Selected Baseline Characteristics of LIFE Study Population

Variable	Total (n = 9194)	Men (n = 4224)	Women (n = 4970)
Age (yrs)	66.9 ± 7.0	66.1 ± 6.9	67.7 ± 7.0*
Body mass index (kg/m^2)	28.0 ± 4.8	27.6 ± 4.0	28.3 ± 5.3*
Retired (%)	65.5%	62.5%	68.2%*
Systolic BP (mm Hg)	174.4 ± 14.3	173.3 ± 14.5	175.4 ± 14.1
Diastolic BP (mm Hg)	97.8 ± 8.9	98.6 ± 8.8	97.1 ± 8.9*
FRS 5-year-event rate (%)	22.3 ± 9.5	28.5 ± 8.5	17.1 ± 6.7*

Values reflect mean ± standard deviation or percentages.

* Statistically significant difference between men and women, $P < 0.05$.

Abbreviations: *LIFE*, Losartan Intervention for Endpoint Reduction in Hypertension; *BP*, blood pressures; *FRS* Framingham Risk Score.

Table 9 Disease History for the Randomized LIFE Study Population

Disease	Total (n = 9194)	Men (n = 4224)	Women (n = 4970)
Cardiovascular system[1]			
Isolated systolic HT[2]	27.4%	24.0%	30.3%
Coronary heart disease	15.1%	18.4%	12.3%
Stroke and TIA	7.7%	8.7%	6.9%
Peripheral vascular disease	5.2%	5.3%	5.1%
Systolic murmur	3.7%	3.3%	4.1%
Atrial fibrillation	3.4%	4.4%	2.6%
Metabolic disorders			
Lipid disorders	18.0%	15.7%	20.0%
Obesity	2.7%	2.2%	3.2%
Endocrine disorders			
Non-insulin-dependent DM	10.3%	10.3%	10.4%
Hypothyroidism	4.1%	1.0%	6.7%
Insulin-dependent DM	2.0%	2.0%	1.9%

[1] Display limited to those diseases reported in 2.0% or more of total study population.
[2] Defined as systolic BP $\geq$ 160 mm Hg and diastolic BP < 95 mm Hg.
Abbreviations: *LIFE*, Losartan Intervention for Endpoint Reduction in Hypertension; *DM*, diabetes mellitus; *HT*, hypertension; *TIA*, transient ischemic attack; *BP*, blood pressure.

receiving antihypertensive medication at the time of recruitment, about half (55.7%) were receiving treatment with one drug and the remainder were being treated with two or more agents. Diuretics were taken by 27.5%, β-blockers by 26.7%, calcium channel blockers by 24.3%, and ACE inhibitors by 25.2%. Aspirin (21%) and postmenopausal hormone replacement therapy among women (18%) were the only concomitant drugs used by 10% or more of the study population. This finding is not unexpected, given the high cardiovascular disease comorbidity of the patients and the age of the women enrolled.

Table 10 Age and Race

	Men (n = 4224)	Women (n = 4970)
Age, years		
< 55	1.4	1.0
55–59	20.6	14.7
60–64	20.7	18.1
65–69	22.3	22.3
70–74	21.5	23.4
75–80	13.4	20.0
> 80	0.0	0.4
Race		
Caucasian	91.3	93.4
African-American	6.7	5.0
Hispanic-American	1.3	0.9
Asian	0.4	0.6
Other	0.2	0.1

Table 11 Biochemical Characteristics for the Randomized LIFE Study Population

Hemoglobin, g/100 mL	14.2 ± 1.2	14.8 ± 1.2	13.8 ± 1.0	< 0.001
Serum sodium, mmol/L	140.3 ± 2.6	140.3 ± 2.5	140.4 ± 2.6	0.022
Serum potassium, mmol/L	4.17 ± 0.40	4.20 ± 0.42	4.14 ± 0.38	< 0.001
Serum creatinine, μmol/L	86.9 ± 20.2	95.5 ± 19.7	79.6 ± 17.6	< 0.001
Serum uric acid, μmol/L	330 ± 78	360 ± 74	304 ± 72	< 0.001
Total cholesterol, mmol/L	6.04 ± 1.12	5.73 ± 1.06	6.31 ± 1.11	< 0.001
HDL cholesterol, mmol/L	1.49 ± 0.44	1.34 ± 0.37	1.62 ± 0.44	< 0.001
Total/HDL cholesterol ratio	4.34 ± 1.40	4.57 ± 1.44	4.15 ± 1.33	< 0.001
Serum glucose, mmol/L	6.02 ± 2.19	6.11 ± 2.23	5.95 ± 2.16	< 0.001

Abbreviation: *HDL*, high-density lipoprotein.

Self-reported alcohol and tobacco use among LIFE study participants are moderate or low; 32.1% of men and 57.6% of women report that they never use alcohol and 80.3% and 86.5%, respectively, reported that they do not smoke. About one half (51.8%) of participants reported exercising for more than 30 minutes at least twice a week (Table 12).

Despite reporting reasonably good health-related behavior, the patients in the LIFE study are, on average, overweight and have relatively high prevalences of diabetes mellitus, lipid disorders, and previously known coronary heart disease (Table 9). Being overweight is common in the LIFE population: 21.3% had a BMI of 30 to 35 kg/m^2, 5.4% had a BMI of 35 to 40 kg/m^2, and 1.9% had a BMI of 40 kg/m^2 or more at the time of randomization. More than one fourth (27.4%) have isolated systolic hypertension (systolic

Table 12 Alcohol Use, Tobacco Use, and Exercise

	Men (n = 4224)	Women (n = 4970)
Intake of alcohol, Drinks per week		
None	32.1	57.6
1–4	44.0	35.1
5–7	10.8	4.5
8–10	5.8	1.5
> 10	7.2	1.3
Tobacco use, Cigarettes/day		
Never	33.6	65.3
Ex-smoker	46.7	21.2
1–5	6.0	4.0
6–10	5.1	4.3
10–20	5.9	3.7
> 20	2.7	1.4
Exercise		
Never	17.9	25.4
≤ 30 min twice/week	25.0	27.2
> 30 min twice/week	56.9	47.4

BP ≥ 160 mm Hg and diastolic BP < 95 mm Hg), a condition associated with high cardiovascular risk (46), and women were more likely to have isolated systolic hypertension than men. The Framingham Risk Score indicates that participants in the LIFE study are at high risk for cardiovascular endpoints, with the 5-year probability of coronary mortal or morbid events equal to 22.3% (Table 8). Men had a higher Framingham Risk Score than women, although the predicted 5-year event rate attributable to factors other than gender was only moderately higher in men (19.2%) than in women (16.9%) ($P < 0.001$).

B. Baseline ECG/Echocardiographic Findings

All randomized patients in the LIFE study met the protocol-specified ECG criteria for LVH on the screening ECG. Two thirds (66%) of patients qualified based on the Cornell voltage QRS duration product formula, 21% qualified based on Sokolow-Lyon voltage, and 10% fulfilled both criteria.

As part of the LIFE study, a large substudy (including 964 patients, more than 10% of the total LIFE enrollment) is being undertaken to collect and analyze echocardiographic LV anatomic measurements (37). In this subset of subjects, echocardiograms are performed at study entry and at annual intervals thereafter. Centers were chosen to participate in this substudy based on an established expertise in quantitative echocardiography, with the goal of achieving approximately proportionate representation across the participating countries. Sonographers for each center underwent a training course to familiarize them with the standardized echocardiogram performance protocol to be used in the LIFE study. This protocol, which outlines the specific echocardiographic measurements obtained, is based on procedures used in previous studies (47, 48). Criteria to be used in LIFE are as follows: LVH was considered present if the ratio of LV mass to body surface area was above normal (that is, > 104 g/m^2 in women and> 116 g/m^2 in men) (47). Hypertrophy was considered concentric if LV relative wall thickness (posterior wall thickness/LV internal dimension) was above normal (that is, > 0.43) and eccentric if relative wall thickness was in the normal range (that is, ≤ 0.43).

Of the 964 participants in the LIFE echocardiography substudy, 59% were men, a larger proportion than in the overall LIFE study group (45.4%) predominantly because of the inclusion of centers that enrolled patients into the substudy from Veterans' Administration Hospitals in the United States and a center in Norway that recruited participants from the all-male Oslo Heart Study. The remaining demographic and baseline characteristics of participants in the LIFE echocardiography substudy were in general agreement with those of the larger LIFE study group (37) (Table 13)

Using LV mass/body surface area criteria to identify hypertrophy, abnormalities of LV geometry were found in 83% of women and 79% of men enrolled in the LIFE echocardiography substudy, with overall prevalences of 47% for eccentric LVH, 24% for concentric LVH, and 10% for concentric LVH remodeling. The distribution of LV geometric patterns was nearly identical in women and men. When LV mass/height$^{2.7}$ partition values of 46.79 g/m$^{2.7}$ in women and 49.29 g/m$^{2.7}$ in men were used, only 13% of the LIFE women and 17% of the LIFE men had normal LV geometry. Either concentric or eccentric LVH was present at baseline using echocardiography in 70% of the substudy participants by LV mass/body surface area criteria and in 76% of substudy subjects by LV mass/height criteria.

Additional preliminary analyses have shown high prevalences of LV systolic and diastolic dysfunction in LIFE patients. Measures of LV systolic or myocardial function,

Table 13 Selected Characteristics of Patients in the Echocardiographic Substudy

Variable	Echo patients (n = 964)
Age (yrs)	66.0 ± 7.0
Race, nonwhite (%)	16%
Height (cm)	169.4 ± 9.7
Weight (kg)	78.4
Body surface area (m^2)	1.89 ± 0.19
Body mass index (kg/m^2)	27.4 ± 4.7
Blood pressure (mm Hg)	176/98
Pulse	78 ± 19
Diabetes	11%
Coronary artery disease	13%
Stroke/transient ischemic attack	8%
Peripheral vascular disease	5%

or both, were depressed (below the second percentile in a reference population) in an appreciable minority of LIFE patients, ranging from 10% of those with normal LV geometry to 42% of those with concentric LVH (49). In addition, more than 80% of LIFE patients had abnormal diastolic filling patterns, predominantly because of impairment of early diastolic relaxation (50) (Table 14).

IV. DISCUSSION

The predominant goal of antihypertensive therapy is to reduce the risk of adverse cardiovascular events related to high BP. Available evidence suggests, however, that patients treated with current antihypertensive drugs still have a substantially higher risk of suffering hypertension-related fatal and nonfatal cardiovascular events than do matched normotensive individuals (51–53). Results of a meta-analysis of 17 controlled prevention trials in hypertension, comprising more than 40,000 middle-aged patients followed up for an average of 5 years, showed that the modest decrease in diastolic BP of 5 to 6 mm Hg in the intervention groups (mainly diuretics and β-blocker therapy) was associated with an approximate 40% decrease in stroke-related events, closely resembling the benefit pre-

Table 14 Echocardiographic Findings in Patients with LV Ejection Fraction > 60% (n = 333)

Variable	IVRT < 100 msec	IVRT > 100 msec	*P*
Left ventricular mass index	117.7 ± 23.5	119.5 ± 26.0	NS
Relative wall thickness	0.43 ± 0.005	0.45 ± 0.006	0.038
Midwall fractional shortening (%)	17 ± 1	16 ± 2	0.039
Circumferential end-systolic stress	140.3 ± 48.6	136.2 ± 39.7	NS
Stress-adjusted midwall shortening	99.40 ± 12.9	95.80 ± 13.1	0.024

Abbreviations: *LV*, left ventricular; *IVRT*, isovolumic relaxation time.

dicted from this degree of pressure reduction (54). The reduction in nonfatal and fatal coronary events associated with this same reduction in diastolic blood pressure, however, was much lower (16% to 21%) and fell short of that predicated for the observed change in arterial pressure. The suboptimal impact of current antihypertensive therapy on cardiovascular complications—in particular coronary events—may be the result, at least in part, of adverse metabolic effects of certain drug classes such as diuretics and β-blockers and an insufficient reversal of cardiovascular hypertrophy and vascular dysfunction (55).

Left ventricular hypertrophy is the most important risk indicator in hypertension. Blockade of the RAS system has been shown to be of cardinal importance for cardioprotection, and data suggest that ACE inhibitors are more effective in reversing LVH than traditional antihypertensive therapies (13–18). The LIFE study was designed to evaluate prospectively whether antihypertensive therapy that uniquely interrupts the RAS through selective inhibition of its primary effector hormone, angiotensin II, has a greater effect than conventional therapy on reversal of LVH, independent of any reduction in BP, and whether this activity is connected to a meaningful reduction in cardiovascular events.

By applying simple 12-lead ECG criteria for LVH, it has been feasible to identify a large group of high-risk hypertensive patients and then include from this population a total of 9194 patients, having an average 5-year likelihood of coronary heart disease of 22.3% by the Framingham Risk Score, for participation in the LIFE study. The use of a simple methodology such as the ECG for the analysis of LVH is a distinct characteristic of the LIFE study. Echocardiographic measurements in a subset of more than 10% of the randomized population confirmed that the ECG criteria used in the LIFE study identified hypertensive patients with a high prevalence of anatomical LVH.

The ability to enroll more than 9000 hypertensive patients drawn predominantly from primary health care centers supports the usefulness of using the cost-effective 12-lead ECG for identification of high-risk patients and demonstrates the feasibility of this approach in general practice. More than 33,000 ECGs were received from the investigators and more than 19,000 (57.8%) were approved by the ECG core laboratory (the number of ECGs evaluated by the investigators alone and not submitted to the ECG core center is unknown); an approval rate of 57.6% clearly indicates that most investigators were able to read the ECGs accurately, according to the study's criteria. Thus the feasibility of the approach used in the LIFE study to identify high-risk hypertensive patients will make the ultimate recommendations from this study possible to implement on a broad scale in clinical practice. Moreover, the randomized LIFE study population is representative of the hypertensive subjects with ECG-LVH in the age group under study, supporting the generalizability of the study findings to patients seen in clinical practice.

In conclusion, the LIFE study uses a unique approach to documenting improved cardiac care in hypertension through the use of rational pharmacological intervention targeted to blocking angiotensin II, an important growth factor of the RAS. By selecting high-risk hypertensive patients on the basis of target organ damage documented using the cost-effective technique of ECG, the study has the potential to define optimal drug therapy for reversing LVH. The LIFE study also has the unique potential of linking reversal of LVH to a reduction in adverse cardiovascular complications.

REFERENCES

1. Kannel WB, Gordon T, Offutt D. Left ventricular hypertrophy by electrocardiogram: prevalence, incidence and mortality in the Framingham Study. Ann Intern Med 1969; 71:89–105.

2. Dunn FG, McLenachan J, Isles CG, Brown I, Dargie HJ, Lever AF, Lorimer AR, Murray GD, Pringle SD, Robertson JW. Left ventricular hypertrophy and mortality in hypertension: an analysis of data form the Glasgow Blood Pressure Clinic. J Hypertens 1990; 8:775–782.
3. Savage DD, Drayer JIM, Henry WL, Mathews EC Jr, Ware JH, Gardin JM, Cohen ER, Epstein SE, Laragh JH. Echocardiographic assessment of cardiac anatomy and function in hypertensive subjects. Circulation 1979; 59:623–632.
4. Devereux RB, Pickering TG, Haschfield GA, Kleinert HD, Donby L, Clark L, Pregibon D, Jason M, Kleiner B, Borer JS, Laragh JH. Left ventricular hypertrophy in patients with hypertension: importance of blood pressure to regularly recurring stress. Circulation 1983; 68:470–476.
5. Levy D. Left ventricular hypertrophy. Epidemiological insights from the Framingham Heart Study. Drugs 1988; 35(suppl 5):1–5.
6. Koren MJ, Devereux RB, Casale PN, Savage DD, Laragh JH. Relation of left ventricular mass and geometry to morbidity and mortality in uncomplicated essential hypertension. Ann Intern Med 1991; 114:345–352.
7. Kannel WB. Prevalence and natural history of electrocardiographic left ventricular hypertrophy. Am J Med 1983; 75(suppl 3A):4–11.
8. Koren MJ, Ulin RJ, Laragh JH, Devereux RB. Reduction in left ventricular mass during treatment of essential hypertension is associated with improved prognosis. Am J Hypertens 1991; 4:1A.
9. Kannel WB, D'Agostino RB, Levy D, Belanger AJ. Prognostic significance of regression of left ventricular hypertrophy. Circulation 1988; 78(suppl II):II89.
10. Yurenev AP, Dyakonova HG, Novikov ID, Vitols A, Pahl L, Haynemann G, Wallrabe D, Tsifkova R, Romanovska L, Niderle P. Management of essential hypertension in patients with different degrees of left ventricular hypertrophy. Multicenter trial. Am J Hypertens 1992; 5: 182s–189s.
11. Muiesan ML, Salvetti M, Rizzoni D, Castellano M, Donato F, Agabiti-Rosei E. Association of change in left ventricular mass with prognosis during long-term antihypertensive treatment. J Hypertens 1995; 13:1091–1105.
12. Verdecchia P, Schillaci G, Borgioni C, Ciucci A, Gattobigio R, Zampi I, Reboldi G, Procellati C. Prognostic significance of serial changes in left ventricular mass in essential hypertension. Circulation 1998; 97:48–54.
13. Dahlöf B, Pennert K, Hansson L. Reversal of left ventricular hypertrophy in hypertensive patients—a meta-analysis of 109 treatment studies. Am J Hypertens 1992; 5:95–110.
14. Schmieder RE, Martus P, Klingbeil A. Reversal of left ventricular hypertrophy in essential hypertension. Meta-analysis of randomized double-blind studies. JAMA 1996; 275:1507–1513.
15. Dahlöf B, Herlitz H, Aurell M, Hansson L. Reversal of cardiovascular structural changes when treating essential hypertension: the importance of renin-angiotensin-aldosterone system. Am J Hypertens 1992; 5:900–901.
16. Agabiti-Rosei E, Ambrosioni E, Dal Palú C, Muiesan ML, Zanchetti A, on behalf of the RACE Study Group. ACE inhibitor ramipril is more effective than the β-blocker atenolol in reducing left ventricular mass in hypertension. Results of the RACE (ramipril cardioprotective evaluation) study. J Hypertens 1995; 13:1325–1334.
17. Roman MJ, Alderman MH, Pickering TG, Pini R, Keating JO, Sealy JE, Devereux RD. Differential effects of angiotensin converting enzyme inhibition and diuretic therapy on ambulatory blood pressure, left ventricular mass and vascular hypertrophy. Am J Hypertens 1998; 11: 387–396.
18. Julien J, Dufloux MA, Prasquer R, Chatellier G, Menard D, Plouin PF, Menard J, Corvol P. Effects of captopril and minoxidil on left ventricular hypertrophy in resistant hypertensive patients: a 6 month double-blind comparison. J Am Coll Cardiol 1990; 16:137–142.

19. Schelling P, Fischer H, Ganten D. Angiotensin and cell growth: a link to cardiovascular hypertrophy? J Hypertens 1991; 9:3–15.
20. Weber KT, Brilla CG. Pathological hypertrophy and cardiac interstitium. Fibrosis and the renin-angiotensin-aldosterone system. Circulation 1991; 83:1849–1865.
21. Dahlöf B. Structural cardiovascular changes in essential hypertension. Studies on the effects of antihypertensive therapy. Blood Press 1992; 1(suppl 6):1–75.
22. Julius S, Li Y, Brant D, Krause L, Taylor D. Quinapril, an angiotensin converting enzyme inhibitor, prevents cardiac hypertrophy during episodic hypertension. Hypertension 1991; 17: 1161–1166.
23. Linz W, Henning R, Schölkens BA. ACE inhibition and angiotensin II receptor antagonism on development and regression of cardiac hypertrophy in rats. J Hypertens 1991; 9(suppl 6): S400–401.
24. Urata H, Boehm KD, Philip A, Kinoshita A, Gabrovsek J, Bumpus FH, Husain A. Cellular localization and regional distribution of an angiotensin II-forming chymase in the heart. J Clin Invest 1993; 91:1269–1281.
25. Biollaz J, Brunner HR, Gavras I, Waeber B, Gavras H. Antihypertensive therapy with MK 421: angiotensin II-renin relationships to evaluate efficacy of converting enzyme blockade. J Cardiovasc Pharmacol 1982; 4:966–972.
26. Wong PC, Price WA Jr, Chiu AT, Duncia JV, Carini DJ, Wexler RR, Johnson AL, Timmermans PB. Non-peptide angiotensin II receptor antagonists. XI pharmacology of Exp 3174: an active metabolite of DuP753, an orally active antihypertensive agent. J Pharmacol Exper Ther 1990; 225:211–217.
27. McIntyre M, Caffe SE, Michalak RA, Reid JL. Losartan, an orally active angiotensin (AT_1) receptor antagonist: a review of its efficacy and safety in essential hypertension. Pharmacol Ther 1997; 74:181–194.
28. Mizuno K, Tani M, Hashimoto S, Niimura S, Sanada H, Watanabe H, Ohtsuki M, Fukuchi S. Effects of losartan, a nonpeptide angiotensin II receptor antagonist, on cardiac hypertrophy and the tissue angiotensin II content in spontaneously hypertensive rats. Life Sci 1992; 51: 367–374.
29. Oddie CJ, Dilley RJ, Bobik A. Long-term angiotensin II antagonism in spontaneously hypertensive rats: effects on blood pressure and cardiovascular amplifiers. Clin Exp Pharmacol Physiol 1992; 19:392–395.
30. Tedesco MA, Ratti G, Aquino D, Caccarale A, Acitorio M, Rocereto A, Cosimi R, Coppolino P, Iarussi D, Iacono A. The effectiveness and tolerability of losartan and effect on left ventricular mass in patients with essential hypertension. Cardiologia 1998; 43:53–59.
31. Tedesco MA, Ratti G, Aquino D, Limongelli G, Di Salvo G, Mennella S, Galzerano D, Iarussi, D, Iacono A. Effects of losartan on hypertension and left ventricular mass: a long-term study. J Hum Hypertens 1998; 12:505–510.
32. Cuspidi C, Lonati L, Sampieri L. Effects of losartan on blood pressure and left ventricular mass in essential hypertension. High Blood Pressure 1998; 7:11–15.
33. Pitt B, Segal R, Martinez FA, Meurers G, Cowley AJ, Thomas I, Deedwania PC, Ney DE, Snavely DB, Chang PI. Randomized trial of losartan versus captopril in patients over 65 with heart failure (Evaluation of Losartan in the Elderly Study, ELITE). Lancet 1997; 349:747–752.
34. Dahlöf B, Devereux R, de Faire U, Fyhrquist F, Hedner T, Ibsen H, Julius S, Kjeldsen S, Kristianson K, Lederballe-Pedersen O, Lindholm LH, Nieminen MS, Omvik P, Oparil S, Weld H, for the LIFE Study Group. The Losartan Intervention for Endpoint Reduction (LIFE) in Hypertension study: rationale, design, and methods. Am J Hypertens 1997; 10:705–713.
35. Dahlöf B, Devereux RB, Julius S, Kjeldsen SE, Beevers G, de Faire U, Fyhrquist F, Hedner T, Ibsen H, Kristianson K, Lederballe-Pedersen O, Lindholm LH, Nieminen MS, Omvik P, Oparil S, Wedel H, for the LIFE Study Group. Characteristics of 9194 patients with left ventricular hypertrophy. The LIFE Study. Hypertension 1998; 32:989–997.

36. Dahlöf B, Keller SE, Makris L, Goldberg AI, Sweet CS, Lim NY. Efficacy and tolerability of losartan potassium and atenolol in patients with mild to moderate essential hypertension. Am J Hypertens 1995; 8:578–583.
37. Devereux RB, Bella JN, Dahlöf B, Gerdts M, Niemenen M, Nielsen J, Papdemetriou V, for the LIFE Study Group. Left ventricular geometry and function in hypertensive patients with ECG left ventricular hypertrophy: the LIFE Trial (abstr). J Am Coll Cardiol 1998; 31 (2 suppl A):376A.
38. Molloy TJ, Okin PM, Devereux RB, Kligfield P. Electrocardiographic detection of left ventricular hypertrophy by the simple QRS voltage-duration product. Am J Coll Cardiol 1992; 20: 1180–1186.
39. Okin PM, Roman MJ, Devereux RB, Kligfield P. Gender differences and the electrocardiogram in left ventricular hypertrophy. Hypertension 1995; 25:242–249.
40. Okin PM, Roman MJ, Devereux RB, Kligfield P. Electrocardiographic identification of increased left ventricular mass by simple voltage duration products. Am J Coll Cardiol 1995; 25:417–423.
41. Casale PN, Devereux RB, Alonso DR, Campo E, Kligfield P. Improved sex-specific criteria of left ventricular hypertrophy for clinical and computer electrocardiogram interpretation: necropsy validation. Circulation 1987; 75:565–572.
42. Casale PN, Devereux RB, Kligfield P, Eisenberg RR, Miller DH, Chaudhary BS, Phillips MC. Electrocardiographic detection of left ventricular hypertrophy: development and prospective validation of improved criteria. J Am Coll Cardiol 1985; 6:572–580.
43. Schillaci G, Verdecchia P, Borgioni C, Ciucci A, Guerrieri M, Zampi I, Battistelli M, Bartoccini C, Porcellati C. Improved electrocardiographic diagnosis of left ventricular hypertrophy. Am J Cardiol 1995; 74:714–719.
44. Norman JE Jr, Levy D. Improved electrocardiographic detection of echocardiographic left ventricular hypertrophy: results of a correlated data base approach. J Am Coll Cardiol 1995; 25:1022–1029.
45. Lachin JM, Foulkes MA. Evaluation of sample size and power for analyses of survival with allowance for non-uniform patient entry, losses at follow-up, noncompliance and stratification. Biometrics 1986; 42:507–519.
46. SHEP Cooperative Research Group. Prevention of stroke by antihypertensive drug treatment in older persons with isolated systolic hypertension. Final results of the Systolic Hypertension in the Elderly Program (SHEP). JAMA 1991; 265:3255–3264.
47. Devereux RB, Dahlöf B, Levy D, Pfeffer MA. Comparison of enalapril versus nifedipine to decrease left ventricular hypertrophy in systemic hypertension (the PRESERVE trial). Am J Cardiol 1996; 78:61–65.
48. Devereux RB, Roman MJ, de Simone G, O'Grady MJ, Paranicas M, Yeh JL, Fabsitz RR, Howard BV. Relations of left ventricular mass to demographic and hemodynamic variables in American Indians: the Strong Heart Study. Circulation 1997; 96:1416–1423.
49. Wachtell K, Smith G, Gerdts E, Dahlöf B, Nieminen M, Papdemetriou V, Bella JN, Rokkedal J, Devereux RB. Left ventricular systolic function in hypertensive patients with ECG determined left ventricular hypertrophy: the LIFE Study (abstr). J Am Coll Cardiol 1998; 31: 523A.
50. Wachtell K, Papademetriou V, Smith G, Gerdts E, Nieminen M, Bella J, Rokkedal J, Devereux RB. Does isolated diastolic dysfunction exist in hypertensive patients with ECG defined LVH? (abstr). J Am Coll Cardiol 1998; 31:377A.
51. Lindholm L, Ejlertsson G, Schersten B. High risk of cerebro-cardiovascular morbidity in well-treated male hypertensives. Acta Med Scand 1984; 216:251–259.
52. Isles CG, Walker LM, Beevers DG. Mortality in patients of the Glasgow Blood Pressure Clinic. J Hypertens 1986; 4:141–156.
53. Samuelsson O, Wilhelmsen L, Andersson OK, Pennert K, Berglund G. Cardiovascular morbidity in relation to change in blood pressure and serum cholesterol levels in treated hypertension:

results from the Primary Prevention Trial in Göteborg, Sweden. JAMA 1987; 258:1768–1776.

54. MacMahon S, Rodgers A. The effects of antihypertensive treatment on vascular disease: reappraisal of the evidence. J Vasc Med Biol 1993; 4:265–271.
55. Dahlöf B. Regression of cardiovascular structural changes—a preventive strategy. Clin Exp Hypertens 1990;A12(5):877–896.

25

Prospective Collaborative Overviews of Major Randomized Trials of Blood-Pressure-Lowering Treatments

BRUCE NEAL and STEPHEN MacMAHON

University of Sydney, Sydney, New Zealand

I. BACKGROUND

Elevated blood pressure levels are clearly associated with the risks of stroke, coronary heart disease (CHD) (1–3), heart failure (4), and renal disease (5) in a variety of populations from both the western and eastern hemispheres. More recently, observational studies have shown blood pressure to be directly associated with the risks of recurrent stroke (6) and recurrent CHD events (7) among patients with a history of cardiovascular disease. Randomized trials have demonstrated the beneficial effects of blood pressure lowering treatments on the risks of stroke and CHD among patients with hypertension (8). Randomized trials have also demonstrated benefits of various drugs that lower blood pressure in several other patient groups, including those with CHD, congestive heart failure, and diabetic nephropathy. Several of these important trials are the subjects of earlier chapters in this book.

Although the evidence that blood pressure lowering reduces the risks of major cardiovascular disease is beyond question, there is much still to be learned about the effects of specific drug classes and of blood pressure lowering in high-risk patients without what has classically been defined as hypertension. At present, the majority of available data on the effects of blood pressure lowering on major cardiovascular outcomes in hypertensive patients has been provided by trials of diuretic- or beta-blocker-based regimens (9). The effects of angiotensin-converting enzyme (ACE) inhibitors, calcium antagonists, and other newer classes of agents on major cardiovascular outcomes remain substantially less certain. Similar uncertainty remains about the effects of blood pressure lowering with any agent among patients with other high-risk conditions, such as cerebrovascular disease, other vascular disease, or diabetes, particularly in the absence of what has usually been defined as hypertension.

II. ESTABLISHED EFFECTS OF BLOOD-PRESSURE-LOWERING TREATMENTS

A. Diuretic- or Beta-Blocker-Based Regimens

The combined results of previous randomized controlled trials of diuretic- or beta-blocker-based regimens, involving a total of about 47,000 patients with hypertension, have demonstrated that much of the epidemiologically expected benefit of the blood pressure reductions were achieved (9–11). A net reduction of 5 to 6 mm Hg in usual diastolic blood pressure was associated with a 38% (standard deviation [SD] 4) reduction in stroke risk and a 16% (SD 4) reduction in CHD risk. The proportional reductions in the risks of these events were broadly similar in patients with mild, moderate, or more severe hypertension, in older or younger patients, and in patients with or without a history of cerebrovascular disease. The size of the absolute benefits of treatment varied in direct proportion to the background level of risk (that is, patients at higher absolute risk of stroke or CHD experienced the largest absolute reduction in risk). Few data are available from these trials about the effects of treatment on heart failure or renal disease, although there have been reports of reduced heart failure risk from individual trials of diuretic-based regimens (12, 13).

Data from four trials provide direct randomized evidence about the comparative effects of diuretic- and beta-blocker-based regimens on the risks of stroke and CHD (14–17). Collectively, in these trials there was no detectable difference among the regimens in their effects on either outcome. However, although these studies involved a total of 24,000 patients (among whom about 300 strokes and 800 CHD events were observed), even in combination they lacked adequate statistical power to determine reliably any modest but potentially important treatment differences (for example, a 10% to 15% difference in the relative risk of CHD). Other data about the effects of beta-blockers are also available from trials among patients with CHD or heart failure. The results of these trials indicate that among patients with a history of myocardial infarction, beta-blockers reduce the risks both of reinfarction and cardiovascular death by about one fourth (18), and among patients with heart failure, they reduce the risk of cardiovascular death by about the same proportion (19). These effects of beta-blockers are somewhat larger than would be expected from the modest blood pressure reductions produced and may, therefore, partially reflect independent cardioprotective effects of beta-blocker drugs.

B. ACE Inhibitors

Comparatively few data are available about the effects of ACE inhibitors on the risks of stroke and CHD in patients with hypertension. One recently completed large-scale study compared the effects of captopril-based treatment with other regimens based on a diuretic or beta-blocker in patients with hypertension (20). Interpretation of the results of this study is complicated by a baseline difference in blood pressure levels between randomized groups that persisted during follow-up. Although there was no difference between groups in the incidence of CHD events, there were more strokes and fewer new cases of diabetes among patients assigned the ACE inhibitor. It is possible, however, that irregularities in the assignment of treatment, together with the unblinded study design, could have influenced the findings. Another recently completed trial compared the effects of ACE inhibitor-based and beta-blocker-based blood-pressure-lowering treatment in hypertensive patients with diabetes (21). This study observed no differences between groups in the incidence of stroke, CHD, total macrovascular events, or microvascular complications of diabetes. Two other small studies (22, 23) have reported ACE inhibitors to be superior to calcium antagonists in the prevention of major cardiovascular disease among patients with diabetes, but each of these recorded too few events to provide reliable evidence.

Other data from placebo-controlled trials of ACE inhibitors among patients with left ventricular dysfunction and patients with heart failure provide good evidence of reduced cardiovascular mortality and heart failure-related morbidity (24) and suggestive, but not definitive, evidence of a reduced risk of myocardial infarction (25). In addition, data also indicate that ACE inhibitors have a beneficial effect on the progression of renal disease in patients with diabetic nephropathy (26).

C. Calcium Antagonists

The results of one recently completed study (27) provide evidence of a significant reduction in stroke risk (of about 40% to 50%) among patients randomized to treatment with the calcium antagonist, nitrendipine. Similar results were reported from two other trials of nifedipine that used alternate assignment to active treatment or placebo instead of proper random assignment (28, 29). Too few CHD events were observed in any of these studies to draw reliable conclusions about the effects of calcium antagonists on the primary prevention of CHD in patients with hypertension.

Similarly, data from trials in patients with CHD provide no evidence of an overall effect of calcium antagonists on the risk of myocardial infarction (30, 31). Evidence is suggestive, but not definitive, of a reduced risk of myocardial infarction in patients treated with verapamil or diltiazem and an increased risk in patients treated with immediate-release nifedipine (32). More recent trials of long-acting dihydropyridine agents involving patients with heart failure have showed no clear evidence of an effect of calcium antagonists on overall mortality or morbidity (33, 34).

The effects of both calcium antagonists and ACE inhibitors on major noncardiovascular outcomes remain largely uncertain, although questions have been raised (primarily by the results of a few selected, nonrandomized, observational studies) about possible harmful effects of calcium antagonists on cancer and bleeding risks (32). The one large randomized trial of calcium antagonists that has been completed (27) recorded too few such events to provide reliable evidence about the effects of calcium antagonists on those outcomes. It has also been suggested that some calcium antagonists may have independent effects that reduce the benefits of blood-pressure-lowering for CHD (30). However, to date, the results from trials of newer agents in patients with CHD, left ventricular dysfunction, or heart failure suggest that any such independent effects, either beneficial or harmful, are unlikely to be large.

D. More Intensive Versus Less Intensive Blood Pressure Lowering

The Hypertension Detection and Follow-Up Program (HDFP) provided the first evidence that more intensive blood pressure lowering conferred greater benefits than less intensive treatment (35). That study demonstrated that a diuretic-based stepped-care regimen provided greater protection against cardiovascular events than did usual care. Two trials have recently provided more evidence about the effects of more intensive versus less intensive blood pressure lowering (36, 37). The Hypertension Optimal treatment (HOT) (36) study conducted among 18,790 individuals with uncomplicated hypertension showed no clear effect of more intensive treatment on the risks of stroke or CHD, although there was little separation of the blood pressure distributions between groups. The United Kingdom Prospective Diabetes Study (UKPDS 38) (37), conducted among 1148 patients with hypertension and type II diabetes, achieved more substantial separation of blood pressure distributions and observed a significantly lower risk of stroke in the group assigned more intensive blood pressure control. The overall risks of both macrovascular disease and microvascular disease were also reduced among those assigned more intensive therapy. Similar findings for macrovascular disease were observed in the subgroup with diabetes in the HOT study.

III. ONGOING AND PLANNED LARGE-SCALE TRIALS

In an effort to provide more reliable data with which to address the persisting uncertainties about the effects of blood pressure lowering treatments, a number of new randomized, controlled trials have been started over the past few years and others are currently being planned (38). These new trials fall into two main groups. First, trials comparing newer versus older drug classes in patients with high blood pressure, and second, trials comparing newer drug classes against an untreated (or less actively treated) control condition in patients with isolated systolic hypertension or a high-risk disease history (for example, established CHD, cerebrovascular disease, diabetes, or renal disease).

In comparison with the studies reported in the preceding chapters, many of these new trials are large—particularly some of those comparing newer and older agents. However, the most plausible differences between the effects of the different blood-pressure-lowering regimens being investigated in these studies are much smaller than the differences observed in trials comparing active treatment with inactive control. The most likely relative risk differences between different classes of blood-pressure-lowering agents on stroke or coronary heart disease may be 15% or less. The reliable detection of such differences requires randomized trials that record a thousand or more outcome events during the scheduled follow-up periods. Few of the ongoing or planned trials are likely to observe this number of events and, individually, are unlikely to resolve all the current uncertainties about the effects of different treatment regimens. For this reason, systematic overviews (or meta-analyses) in which data from the major ongoing or planned trials are combined may be useful in detecting any true differences that may exist.

IV. SYSTEMATIC OVERVIEWS OF ALL RELEVANT TRIALS

The combination of all relevant trial results in a systematic overview (or meta-analysis) will reduce random errors and biases (39) and, as a consequence, should provide more reliable information about the effects of individual treatment regimens than would any one study alone. Therefore, to ensure the identification of any moderate but important treatment effects or differences, the principal investigators of the ongoing randomized, controlled trials of blood-pressure-lowering treatments have agreed to collaborate in some prospectively planned overviews under the aegis of the World Health Organization—International Society of Hypertension (WHO-ISH) Liaison Committee. Specifically, two overviews are planned: one comparing newer versus older drug classes in patients with high blood pressure and the other comparing newer drug classes against an untreated (or less actively treated) control condition in patients with isolated systolic hypertension or a high-risk disease. These overviews should provide very reliable information about the effects of the main classes of blood-pressure-lowering agents on cardiovascular outcomes and will provide valuable information about the safety of the same agents for a number of other serious outcomes.

V. ADVANTAGES OF A PROSPECTIVE DESIGN USING INDIVIDUAL PATIENT DATA

A feature of the overviews planned by the WHO-ISH collaboration is that none of the trials to be included had reported results at the time the protocol for the project was finalized. The prospective nature of the overviews has therefore enabled the a priori specification of the principal research hypotheses and the criteria for study inclusion. In this way, retrospective outcome-dependent biases in the selection of questions for study and trials for inclusion are avoided. This does not preclude the investigation of other research questions, but the principal reports from the overviews will emphasize the prespecified analyses. The use of individual patient data in these overviews will also provide more information than has typically been available in overviews conducted using group data alone. Individual patient data will permit the conduct of more complex analyses (such as survival analyses to determine the evolution of any treatment differences over time) and will facilitate the investigation of the comparative effects of treatment in major patient subgroups. For several other treatments, including antiplatelet therapy in patients at risk of cardiovascular events (40–42) and adjuvant therapy in patients with breast cancer (43, 44), systematic overviews based on individual patient data have enabled the identification and characterization of small to moderate-sized treatment effects. These effects were not always accurately identified by individual studies but have proved to be of considerable importance in clinical management. Other treatments for which similar overviews are planned include antithrombotic treatments and cholesterol-lowering therapies (45).

VI. METHODS

A. Trial Eligibility

Trials are potentially eligible for inclusion in these overviews if they meet one of the following criteria: (a) randomization of patients between antihypertensive regimens based on different blood pressure lowering agents; (b) randomization of patients between a blood pressure lowering treatment and placebo (or other inactive control condition); or (c) randomization of patients between different blood pressure goals. In addition, eligible trials must have a planned minimum of 1000 patient-years of follow-up in each randomized group and must not have published or presented the main trial results before July 1995. Trials with factorial assignment of patients to other interventions, such as aspirin or cholesterol lowering, are eligible for inclusion, but trials in which any such additional randomized interventions are assigned jointly with the blood-pressure-lowering treatment are not eligible, as the effects of the blood-pressure-lowering treatments would be confounded by the effects of the other treatments.

B. Trial Identification

A registry has been established to identify all major ongoing or planned randomized trials of blood-pressure-lowering agents. Trials have been identified by a range of methods, including computer-aided literature searches, scrutiny of the reference lists of trial reports and review articles, scrutiny of abstracts and meeting proceedings, and by inquiry among colleagues, collaborators, and the manufactures of antihypertensive drugs. Determination of eligibility was based on a review of details of the study design provided to the secretariat. Studies identified subsequent to the preparation of this protocol will be added to the register, and the principal investigators will be invited to join the collaboration.

C. Data Collection

Both individual patient data and summary tabular data will be sought from each trial, as both are important for ensuring the accuracy of the overview analyses. Data requested for each participant will include baseline characteristics recorded at (or immediately before) randomization, selected measurements made during follow-up, and details of the occurrence of all predefined study outcomes during the scheduled follow-up period (Table 1). The individual patient data files obtained from each trial will be carefully checked for completeness of patient records, for balance of randomized group sizes (both overall and according to baseline prognostic categories), and for other indicators of possible anomalies. Summary tabular data to describe the number of patients allocated to each treatment

Table 1 Baseline, Follow-Up, and Outcome Data from Each Patient

Baseline (at or before randomization)	Follow-up (at annual, or similar intervals)	Outcomes (all events in each category recorded during scheduled follow-up period)
Patient identifier	Systolic blood pressure	Ischemic stroke
Date of randomization	Diastolic blood pressure	Cerebral hemorrhage
Treatment allocation	Weight	Subarachnoid hemorrhage
Date of birth/age	Serum cholesterol	Other stroke (including unknown)
Gender	Serum creatinine	Myocardial infarction
Ethnicity	Smoking status	Hospitalization for heart failure
Systolic blood pressure	Compliance	Hospitalization for renal disease
Diastolic blood pressure		Hospitalization or transfusion for noncerebral hemorrhage
Weight		Arterial revascularization procedure
Height		Major cancer (site-specific)
Smoking status		Admission to hospital for any other cause
Serum total cholesterol		Bone fracture
Serum creatinine		Death (cause-specific)
Regular aspirin/antiplatelet drug		Date for each event
Other BP-lowering drug		Date of last follow-up for fatal events
History of:		Date of last follow-up for nonfatal events
Hypertension		
Diabetes		
Left ventricular hypertrophy		
Heart failure		
Cerebrovascular disease		
Coronary heart disease		
Planned end of scheduled treatment and follow-up		

Abbreviation: *BP*, blood pressure.

group, the numbers who developed each of the primary study outcomes, and the absolute differences in blood pressure between the randomized groups at annual visits will also be sought from each trial. The internal consistency of the data will be confirmed by the direct comparison of analyses of the individual patient data with the summary data provided by each trial. Computer-generated reports on these consistency checks, and any queries arising, will be referred back, in confidence, to the collaborating investigator for review and resolution. This process should help to ensure that individual study results are correctly included in the overview and, hence, that the overview analyses are reliable.

D. Prespecified Study Outcomes

The study outcomes chosen for inclusion in these overviews represent the main cardiovascular disease outcomes likely to be affected by blood-pressure-lowering treatment regimens and the main noncardiovascular disease outcomes for which uncertainty has been expressed about the safety of some newer agents. The primary study outcomes for analysis in this collaborative overview are: nonfatal stroke or death from cerebrovascular disease (codes 430–438 in the 9th revision of the International Classification of Disease [ICD]); nonfatal myocardial infarction or death from CHD (ICD 410–414); heart failure causing death or requiring hospitalization (ICD 428); total cardiovascular deaths (ICD 396–459); total cardiovascular events (stroke, CHD events, heart failure, other cardiovascular death); and total mortality. The secondary study outcomes for analysis include: hemorrhagic stroke (ICD 431–432); ischemic stroke (ICD 433–434); death or hospitalization for renal disease (ICD 189, 403–404, 580–593); arterial revascularization procedure (ICD 36, 38.0, 38.1, 38.4); any bone fracture (ICD 800–829); death, hospitalization, or transfusion for any noncerebral hemorrhage (ICD 459, 578.9, but not 430–432); or major site-specific cancer (lung [ICD 162], large bowel [ICD 153–154], breast [ICD 174–175], or prostate [ICD 185]); and admission to hospital for any cause. Outcome data on serum creatinine levels at annual visits will also be analyzed.

E. Prespecified Study Comparisons

Two sets of primary comparisons have been prespecified (Table 2). The first concerns the overview of trials comparing regimens based on newer and older blood-pressure-lowering

Table 2 Prespecified Comparisons

Regimens comparing newer versus older blood pressure lowering drugs in patients with hypertension
Angiotensin-converting enzyme inhibitor versus diuretic or beta-blocker
Calcium antagonist versus diuretic or beta-blocker
Dihydropyridine calcium antagonist versus diuretic or beta-blocker
Verapamil or diltiazem versus diuretic or beta-blocker
Angiotensin-converting enzyme inhibitor versus calcium antagonist
Regimens comparing blood-pressure lowering versus control in high-risk patients and regimens comparing more intensive with less intensive blood-pressure lowering
Active versus placebo or other control
Angiotensin-converting enzyme inhibitor versus placebo
Calcium antagonist versus placebo
More intensive blood-pressure lowering versus less intensive blood-pressure lowering

treatments that produce similar blood pressure reductions. In this overview, the primary comparisons will be of (a) ACE inhibitor-based treatment versus diuretic- or beta-blocker-based treatment and (b) calcium antagonist-based treatment versus diuretic- or beta-blocker-based treatment. Separate analyses will also be conducted for the main subgroups of calcium antagonists. In addition, comparisons of ACE-inhibitor-based treatment and calcium-antagonist-based treatment will be performed.

In secondary analyses of this overview, tests of interaction will be performed to assess the associations of any treatment differences with the following patient characteristics: age, gender, diabetes, preexisting cardiovascular disease, baseline serum creatinine, baseline serum cholesterol, baseline systolic and diastolic blood pressure, and non-study blood pressure lowering drug treatment at entry. However, in the principal publications, the reporting of results for specific patient subgroups and for secondary outcomes will be restricted to those analyses for which the number of recorded events gives sufficient power to provide reasonably reliable results (for example, subgroups in which more than 1000 events were recorded would have reasonable power to detect a difference between treatment regimens of 20% or more).

The second set of primary comparisons concerns the overview of trials comparing blood pressure lowering regimens with an untreated or less actively treated control condition. In this overview, the primary comparisons will be of (a) ACE inhibitor-based treatment versus control and (b) calcium antagonist-based treatment versus control (with separate analyses conducted of the main subgroups of calcium antagonists). In addition, comparisons of more intensive and less intensive blood-pressure-lowering regimens will be made. Separate analyses will be conducted for patients with the following conditions: isolated systolic hypertension, coronary heart disease, cerebrovascular disease, renal disease, and diabetes.

For each of the prespecified primary comparisons of the effects of treatment regimens on primary study outcomes, the null hypothesis will be tested, namely, that there is no difference between regimens in their effects on outcome. In general, indirect nonrandomized comparisons between the results of the prespecified randomized comparisons described above will be avoided.

Additional research questions (for investigation in the subset of ongoing trials with results that remain blinded) may be formally added to an updated protocol at a recorded time. Comparisons of other new drug classes, such as alpha-blockers, angiotensin-II blockers, or vasopeptidase inhibitors will be conducted if sufficient trials of these agents are begun to warrant separate analyses.

F. Statistical Analyses

The principles that underlie such overviews of randomized trials and details of the statistical methods used for analysis are well established, have been described many times previously (43, 44), and are only briefly summarized here. The Mantel-Haenszel method for combining data from different studies will be used. In most of the trials that will contribute to this overview, results for particular outcomes of interest (for example, myocardial infarction or death from CHD) will be available separately for each participant for each year after randomization. Thus, for each trial a separate value can be calculated for each year of follow-up, and the sum of these separate values can be used to yield the log-rank test statistic for a year of event analysis in that trial. Separate log-rank test statistics for each trial can then be combined to produce an overview analysis of all trials. The main advantage of performing such an analysis is that pooled log-rank analyses can help to determine the time course over which any treatment differences evolve. Similarly, analyses combining the information from selected patient subgroups within separate trials will allow questions about the effects of treatment in major patient subgroups to be addressed. In interpreting subgroup results, emphasis will always be placed on the overall results, unless there is clear and consistent evidence of heterogeneity.

VII. RESULTS

A. Characteristics of the Eligible Trials

Thirty-seven trials that are ongoing or soon to start have been confirmed as being eligible for inclusion in the overview (Table 3). Agreement to participate has been confirmed by the principal investigators of 35 studies, and baseline data describing the trial design and characteristics of the study population have been obtained. These include 21 trials comparing different drug regimens and 21 trials comparing a treatment regimen with an untreated or less-treated control condition. Twenty of the trials are conducted exclusively in patients with hypertension, nine are conducted in patients selected on the basis of coronary disease or cerebrovascular disease, and seven in patients with renal disease or diabetes.

The total planned recruitment to these trials is 268,003 patients, the mean projected follow-up is 4.25 years, and the total projected patient-years of follow-up is 1,140,182. In the trials comparing different treatment regimens, 66,177 patients will be randomized between ACE inhibitor-based treatment and diuretic- or beta-blocker-based treatment, 42,888 between dihydropyridine calcium antagonist-based treatment and diuretic- or beta-blocker-based treatment, and 54,500 between verapamil or diltiazem calcium antagonist-based treatment and diuretic- or beta-blocker-based treatment. In the trials comparing a blood-pressure-lowering treatment with an untreated or less-treated control condition, the total number of patients planned is 75,295, of which 44,667 will be randomized between ACE inhibitor–based therapy and control, and 24,120 will be randomized between calcium antagonist–based therapy and control. In addition 20,790 patients will be randomized between regimens that aim to lower blood pressure more or less intensively.

B. Expected Numbers of Disease Events and Statistical Power

The first round of analyses is scheduled to be conducted in 1999 and the second in 2003. The selection of these dates was based on the projected availability of data and statistical power to detect plausible outcomes. Data from a total of 64,593 patients should be available in 1999 (patients contributing to comparisons of different treatment regimens and to comparisons of treatment versus no or less treatment). In 2003, data from all patients should be available. Estimates of the statistical power for the principal comparisons of treatment effects on stroke, major CHD events, and total cardiovascular events are given in Table 4. For comparisons between different treatment regimens, all calculations assume minimum detectable differences of 15% (relative risk = 0.85) for stroke, CHD, and total cardiovascular events. For comparisons between treatment and an untreated or less actively treated control condition, the calculations assume minimum detectable differences of 30% for stroke and 15% for CHD and total cardiovascular events. The estimates of statistical power are calculated with $\alpha = 0.05$. The estimated number of events for each study was derived in order of preference from a recent estimate provided by the collaborating

Table 3 Characteristics of Trials Identified as Eligible for Inclusion in Overviews

	Trial details						Patient characteristics				Estimated events	
									Entry blood pressure levels			
Acronym	Title	Ref no.	Patients (n)	Planned follow-up (years)	Randomized treatments (factorial assignments)	Completion date	Entry criteria	Age (years)	DBP	SBP	CHD	Stroke
AASK	African American Study of Kidney Disease and Hypertension	—	1200	5	ACE, beta, dCA (more, less)	2001	HBP + RD	18–70	≥95	any	144	72
ABCD	Appropriate Blood Pressure Control in Diabetes Trial	(46)	950	5	ACE, dCA	1998	DM	≥40≤74	any	No ISH	119	59
ACTION	A Coronary Disease Trial Investigating Outcome with Nifedipine GITS	(47)	6000	5	dCA, plac	2003	CAD	>34	none	None	918	333
ALLHAT	Antihypertensive therapy and lipid-lowering heart attack prevention trial	(48)	40000	6	ACE, alph, dCA, diur (chol, open)	2002	HBP + CVD risk	>55	>89<110	>139<180	2580	2790
ANBP2	Australian National Blood Pressure Study 2	(49)	6000	5	ACE, diur	2002	HBP	65–84	>89	>159	300	150
ASCOT	Anglo-Scandinavian Cardiac Outcomes Trial	—	18000	5	dCA ± ACE, beta ± diur (chol, plac)	2003	HBP + CVD risk	>39–79	>89	>139	1150	400
BENEDICT	Bergamo Nephrology Diabetes Complication Trial	—	2400	3	ACE, nCA, plac	2001	DM	>39	>89	>139	200	100
CAPPP	Captopril Prevention Project	(20)	10800	5	ACE, beta/diur	1998	HBP	25–66	>99	any	324	162
CLEVER	Chinese Lacidipine Event Reduction Trial	—	10000	3	dCA, plac	2002	HBP + CVD risk	50–79	95–115	160–210	200	400

CONVINCE	Controlled Onset Verapamil Investigation for Cardiovascular Endpoints	(50)	15000	5	nCA, beta/diur	2001	HBP + CVD risk	>54	>89<110	>139<190	1250	750
DIAB-HYCAR	Diabetes Hypertension Cardiovascular Morbidity-Mortality and Remipril	—	4000	3	ACE, plac	1999	DM + prot	>50	any	any	300	150
ELSA	European Lacidipine Study of Atherosclerosis	(51)	2251	4	dCA, beta	2000	HBP	45–75	>94<116	<149<211	89	44
EUROPA	European Trial on Reduction of Cardiac Events with Perindopril	—	10500	3	ACE, plac	2004	CAD	>18	any	any	964	350
HDS	Hypertension in Diabetes Study	(21)	1148	8.2	ACE, beta, open (ins, sul, diet)	1998	HBP + DM	25–75	>84	>149	244	122
HOPE	Heart Outcomes Prevention Evaluation Study	(52)	9541	4.7	ACE, plac (vit E, plac)	2000	CVD risk	>54	any	any	1200	550
HOT	Hypertension Optimal Treatment Trial	(36)	19196	3.5	more, less (asp, plac)	1997	HBP	50–80	>99<116	any	552	276
HYVET	Hypertension in the Very Elderly Trial	(53)	2100	5	ACE, diur, plac	2001	HBP	>80	>89<110	>159<220	683	341
IDNT	Irbesartan Diabetes Nephropathy Trial	—	1650	3	AIIA, dCA, plac	2000	DM + prot	30–70	>84	>134	124	62
INSIGHT	Int'l Nifedipine GITS Study Intervention as a Goal for Hypertension Therapy	(54)	6592	3	dCA, diur	1999	HBP + CVD risk	55–80	>94	>149	246	123
INVEST	International Verapamil/Trandolapril Study	(55)	27000	2	nCA, beta	2000	HBP + CAD	>49	None	None	581	268
LIFE	Losartan Intervention for Endpoint Reduction in Hypertension	(56)	9194	4	AIIA, beta	2001	HBP + LVH	55–80	95–115	160–200	693	347

Table 3 Continued

Acronym	Title	Trial details: Ref no.	Patients (n)	Planned follow-up (years)	Randomized treatments (factorial assignments)	Completion date	Patient characteristics: Entry criteria	Age (years)	Entry blood pressure levels: DBP	SBP	Estimated events: CHD	Stroke
NICS-EH	National Intervention Co-operative Study in Elderly Hypertensives	(57)	1000	5	dCA, diur	1997	HBP	>59	<115	$>159<220$	30	15
NORDIL	Nordic Diltazem Study	(58)	11000	5	nCA, beta/diur	2002	HBP	50–69	>99	any	360	180
PART2	Prevention of Atherosclerosis with Ramipril	—	617	4	ACE, plac	1998	athero	18–75	any	any	40	14
PEACE	Prevention of Events with Angiotensin Converting Enzyme Inhibition	—	8000	5	ACE, plac	—	CAD	>50	any	any	1224	444
PHYLLIS	Plaque Hypertension Lipid-Lowering Italian Study	(59)	450	3	ACE, plac (chol, plac)	2000	CIT	45–70	95–115	$>150<211$	7	4
PREVENT	Prospective Randomised Evaluation of Vascular Effects of Norvasc	—	825	5	dCA, plac	1997	ang CHD	30–80	any	any	20	6
PROGRESS	Perindopril Protection Against Recurrent Stroke Study	(60)	6000	5	ACE, plac	2000	Stroke or TIA	any	any	any	600	300
QUIET	Quinapril Ischaemia Event Trial	(61)	1750	3	ACE, plac	1996	ang CHD	18–75	any	any	500	350

RENAAL	Randomized Evaluation of NIDDM with the All Antagonist Losartan	—	1500	4	AIIA, plac	2002	DM	31–70	<110	<200	100	50
SCAT	Simvastatin/Enalapril Coronary Atherosclerosis Trial	(62)	460	5	ACE, plac (chol, plac)	1998	CAD	—	any	any	42	15
SCOPE	Study of Cognition and Prognosis in Elderly Patients with Hypertension	(63)	4000	2.5	AIIA, plac	2003	HBP	70–89	90–99	160–179	60	30
SHELL	Systolic Hypertension in the Elderly Lacidipine Long-Term Study	(64)	4800	3.5	dCA, diur	1999	HBP	>59	<95	>160<220	101	50
STOP-2	Swedish Trial in Old Patients with Hypertension	(65)	6628	4	ACE, beta/diur, dCA	1998	HBP	70–84	>104	>179	318	167
SYST-EUR	SYST-EUR Multicentre Trial	(27)	4695	1.6	dCA, plac	1997	ISH	>59	<95	160–119	500	250
VALUE*	Diovan Antihypertensive Long-term Use Evaluation	—	14400	6	AIIA, dCA	—	HBP + CVD risk	>49	<115	<210	1450	869
VHAS	Verapamil in Hypertension Atherosclerosis Study	(66)	1414	2	nCA, diur	1996	HBP	40–65	>94	>159	40	20

*Collaboration pending.

Abbreviations: *ACE*, angiotensin-converting enzyme inhibitor; *AIIA*, angiotensin II antagonist; *alph*, alpha blocker; *ang CHD*, angiographic coronary heart disease; *asp*, aspirin; *athero*, atherosclerosis; *beta*, beta blocker; *chol*, cholesterol lowering; *CIT*, carotid intimal thickness; *CVD*, cardiovascular disease; *dCA*, dihydropyridine calcium antagonist; *diur*, diuretic; *DM*, diabetes mellitus; *HBP*, high blood pressure; *ins*, insulin; *ISH*, isolated systolic hypertension; less, less intensive blood pressure lowering; *LVH*, left ventricular hypertrophy; *more*, more intensive blood pressure lowering; *nCA*, nondihydropyridine calcium antagonist; *open*, open control; *prot*, proteinuria; *RD*, renal disease; *sul*, sulfonyluria; *TIA*, transient ischemic attack; *vit E*, vitamin E.

Table 4 Estimates of Statistical Power* for Principal Prespecified Comparisons

Data available in 1999

		Estimated number of events			Estimated power (α = 0.05)		
Comparison	n	CHD	Stroke	CVD	CHD	Stroke	CVD
Newer vs older regimens							
ACE vs beta/diur	15,977	714	346	1169	55%	30%	78%
CA vs beta/diur	12,018	464	253	789	39%	22%	61%
dCA vs beta/diur	12,018	464	253	789	39%	22%	61%
nCA vs beta/diur	0	0	0	0	—	—	—
ACE vs CA	4419	213	112	358	19%	11%	31%
More vs less or none							
Active vs placebo/control	23,035	2342	1063	3746	98%	> 99%	> 99%
ACE vs placebo	17,157	2033	829	3148	96%	> 99%	> 99%
CA vs placebo	5520	225	200	468	20%	61%	40%
More vs less	18,790	205	288	542	18%	77%	60%

Data available in 2003

		Estimated number of events			Estimated power (α = 0.05)		
Comparison	n	CHD	Stroke	CVD	CHD	Stroke	CVD
Newer vs older regimens							
ACE vs beta/diur	66,177	4074	2773	7532	> 99%	99%	> 99%
CA vs beta/diur	97,388	4462	3219	3219	> 99%	99%	> 99%
dCA vs beta/diur	42,888	2231	2001	4655	96%	94%	> 99%
nCA vs beta/diur	54,500	2231	1218	3794	96%	78%	> 99%
ACE vs CA	24,779	1660	1469	3442	90%	86%	> 99%
More vs less or none							
Active vs placebo/control	75,295	6982	3940	12,014	> 99%	> 99%	> 99%
ACE vs placebo	44,667	5047	2691	8512	> 99%	> 99%	> 99%
CA vs placebo	24,120	1551	1037	2847	88%	> 99%	99%
More vs less	20,790	455	413	954	37%	91%	68%

*For comparisons between different treatment regimens, all calculations assume minimum detectable differences of 15% (relative risk = 0.85) for stroke, CHD, and total cardiovascular events. For comparisons between treatment and an untreated or less actively treated control condition, the calculations assume minimum detectable differences of 30% for stroke and 15% for CHD and total cardiovascular events.

Abbreviations: *ACE*, angiotensin-converting enzyme inhibitor; *beta*, beta blocker; *chol*, cholesterol lowering; *CIT*, carotid intimal thickness; *CVD*, cardiovascular disease; *dCA*, dihydropyridine calcium antagonist; *diur*, diuretic; less, less intensive blood pressure lowering; *more*, more intensive blood pressure lowering; *nCA*, nondihydropyridine calcium antagonist; *CHD*, nonfatal myocardial infarction plus death from coronary heart disease; *stroke*, nonfatal stroke plus death from cerebrovascular disease; *CVD*, 1.1 × (CHD plus stroke).

investigator, the original study sample size calculations or, in the absence of other information, an estimate based on the projected event rates of the most similar trials.

Overall the estimated number of events accrued will be about 10,000 strokes, 16,000 CHD events, and 29,000 cardiovascular events. These estimates are based on average event rates of 0.9% per annum for stroke, 1.5% per annum for CHD events, and 2.6%

per annum for total cardiovascular events (1.1 × sum of stroke and CHD events). These expected event rates are somewhat higher than those observed in the studies included in a previous overview of trials of antihypertensive therapy (0.6% pa for stroke and 0.8% pa for CHD events) (9), which may reflect the selective enrollment of higher risk patients in many of these studies (based on factors such as age, diabetes and a history of major cardiovascular disease).

By 2003, the available data should provide good power to detect modest differences in the frequency of each of the principal outcomes for the main treatment comparisons. By 1999, however, the power to assess such cause-specific treatment effects is likely to be suboptimal, and the principal focus of analyses at that time will be the combined outcome of total cardiovascular events for those comparisons for which there is reasonable statistical power to detect plausible treatment differences or effects.

VIII. SUMMARY

This project was initiated in 1995 as a collaboration between the principal investigators of all the major randomized trials of blood pressure lowering treatments ongoing at that time. With the commencement of new trials, the collaboration has expended to included representatives from as many eligible studies as possible. The principal objectives of the collaboration are to provide reliable data about the effects of newer classes of blood pressure lowering drugs on major causes of cardiovascular morbidity and mortality in a variety of patient groups at increased risk of cardiovascular disease events. This will be achieved through the conduct of overviews investigating the comparative effects of regimens based on newer and older classes of blood-pressure-lowering drugs and the effects of regimens based on newer drug classes in comparison with untreated or less-treated control conditions.

The combination of trial results in such overviews will reduce random errors and avoid biases in the selection of trials for inclusion and, as a consequence, should provide more reliable information about the effects of these drugs than would any one study alone. Separate analyses will be conducted for the main drug groups (principally, ACE inhibitors and calcium antagonists, with separate analyses of dihydropyridine agents and verapamil or diltiazem) and for the principal patient subgroups (in those with high blood pressure, CHD, cerebrovascular disease, renal disease, or diabetes). Thirty-seven trials of blood-pressure-lowering treatments have been identified as potentially eligible for inclusion in this project, and agreement to collaborate has been confirmed by the investigators from 35 trials. The eligible trials involve a projected total of about 268,000 patients, among whom a total of about 1.1 million patient-years of follow-up will be accrued on completion of all studies. The first round of analyses, based on data from about 65,000 patients, will be conducted in 1999.

ACKNOWLEDGMENTS

This project is conducted under the aegis of the WHO—ISH committee. Coordination of WHO-ISH collaboration has been funded in part by project and program grants provided by the Health Research Council of New Zealand and the National Health and Medical Research Council of Australia. The conduct of the project is overseen by a management committee comprising each of the collaborating principal investigators and representatives of the secretariat of the WHO-ISH Blood Pressure Lowering Treatment Trialists' Collaboration. Coordination of the project, including data management and statistical analysis, will be provided by the secretariat, which is based at the Institute for International Health at the University of Sydney, Australia.

REFERENCES

1. MacMahon S, Peto R, Cutler J, Collins R, Sortie P, Neaton J, Abbott R, Godwin J, Dyer A, Stamler J. Blood pressure, stroke, and coronery heart disease. Part I, prolonged differences in blood pressure: prospective observational studies corrected for the regression dilution bias. Lancet 1990; 335:765–774.
2. Prospective Studies Collaboration. Cholesterol, diastolic blood pressure, and stroke: 13,000 strokes in 450,000 people in 45 prospective cohorts. Lancet 1995; 346:1647–1653.
3. Eastern Stroke and Coronary Heart Disease Collaborative Research Group. Blood pressure, cholesterol and stroke in eastern Asia. Lancet 1996; 352:1801–1807.
4. Kannel WB, Castelli WP, McNamara PM, McKee PA, Feinleib M. Role of blood pressure in the development of congestive heart failure. N Engl J Med 1972; 287:781–787.
5. Kleg MJ, Whelton PK, Randall BL, Neaton JD, Brancati FL, Ford OE, Shulman NB, Stamler J. Blood pressure and end-stage renal disease in men. N Engl J Medicine 1996; 334:13–18.
6. Rodgers A, MacMahon S, Gamble G, Slattery J, Sandercock P, Warlow C, on behalf of the UKTIA Collaborative Group. Blood pressure and risk of stroke in patients with cerebrovascular disease. BMJ 1996; 313:147.
7. Flack J, Neaton J, Grimm R, Shih J, Cutler J, Ensrud K, MacMahon S, for the Multiple Risk Factor Intervention Trial Research Group. Blood pressure and mortality among men with prior myocardial infarction. Circulation 1995; 92:2437–2445.
8. MacMahon S, Neal B, Rodgers A. Blood pressure lowering for the primary and secondary prevention of coronary and cerebrovascular disease. Schweiz Med Wochenschr 1995; 125: 2479–2486.
9. MacMahon S, Rodgers A. The effects of antihypertensive treatment on vascular disease: reappraisal of the evidence in 1994. J Vasc Med Biol 1993; 4:265–271.
10. Collins R, Peto R, MacMahon S, Herbert P, Fiebach NH, Eberlein KA, Godwin J, Quizilbash N, Taylor JO, Hennekens CH. Blood pressure, stroke, and coronary heart disease. Part 2, short-term reductions in blood pressure: overview of randomised drug trials in their epidemiological context. Lancet 1990; 335:827–839.
11. Collins R, MacMahon S. Blood pressure, antihypertensive drug treatment and the risks of stroke and of coronary heart disease. Br Med Bull 1994; 50:272–298.
12. Kostis J, Davis B, Cutler J, Grimm R, Berge K, Cohen J, Lacy C, Perry H, Blaufox M, Wassertheil-Smoller S, Black H, Schron E, Berkson D, Curb J, Smith W, McDonald R, Applegate W. Prevention of heart failure by antihypertensive drug treatment in older persons with isolated systolic hypertension (ISH). SHEP Cooperative Research Group. JAMA 1997; 278:212–216.
13. Yusuf S, Thomas T, Abbott RD. Changes in hypertension treatment and in congestive heart failure mortality in the United States. Hypertension 1989; 3:74–79.
14. Medical Research Council Working Party. MRC trial of treatment of mild hypertension. Principal results. BMJ 1985; 291:97–104.
15. Medical Research Council Working Party. Medical Research Council trial of treatment of hypertension in older adults: principal results. BMJ 1992; 304:405–412.
16. The IPPPSH Collaborative Group. Cardiovascular risk and risk factors in a randomised trial of treatment based on the beta-blocker oxprenolol: the international prospective primary prevention study in hypertension (IPPPSH). J Hypertens 1985; 3:379–392.

17. Wilhelmsen L, Berglund G, Elmfeld D. Beta-blockers versus diuretics in hypertensive men. Main results from the HAPPHY trial. J Hypertens 1987; 5:561–576.
18. Yusuf S, Peto R, Lewis J, Collins R, Sleight P. Beta-blockade during and after myocardial infarction: an overview of the randomized trials. Prog Cardiovasc Dis 1985; 27:335–371.
19. Doughty RN, Rodgers A, Sharpe N, MacMahon S. Effects of beta-blocker therapy on mortality in patients with heart failure. A systematic overview of randomised controlled trials. Eur Heart J 1997; 18:560–565.
20. Hansson L, Lindholm L, Niskanen L, Lanke L, Hedner T, Niklason A, Luomanmaki K, Dahlof B, de Faire U, Morlin C, Kartberg B, Wester P, Bjorck J-E, Group for the CPPCS. Effect of angiotensin converting enzyme inhibition compared with conventional therapy on cardiovascular morbidity and mortality in hypertension: the Captopril Prevention Project (CAPPP) randomised trial. Lancet 1999; 353:611–616.
21. UK Prospective Diabetes Study Group. Efficacy of atenolol and captopril in reducing risk of macrovascular and microvascular complications in type 2 diabetes. BMJ 1998; 317:713–720.
22. Pahor M. The fosinopril amlodipine cardiovascular events trial (FACET) and new evidence on antihypertensive treatments in diabetics. Am J Hypertens 1998; 11(4) Part 2:245A.
23. Estacio R, Jeffers B, Hiatt W, Biggerstaff S, Gifford N, Schrier R. The effect of nisoldipine as compared with enalapril on cardiovascular outcomes in patients with non-insulin-dependent diabetes and hypertension. N Engl J Med 1998; 338:645–652.
24. Garg R, Yusuf S. Overview of randomized trials of angiotensin-converting enzyme inhibitors on mortality and morbidity in patients with heart failure. JAMA 1995; 273:1450–1456.
25. Lonn EM, Yusuf S, Jha P, Montague TJ, Teo KK, Benedict CR, Pitt B. Emerging role of angiotensin-converting enzyme inhibitors in cardiac and vascular protection. Circulation 1994; 90:2056–2067.
26. Lewis EJ, Hunsicker LG, Bain RP, Rohde RD. The effect of angiotensin converting enzyme inhibition on diabetic nephropathy. The Collaborative Study Group. N Engl J Med 1993; 329: 1456–1462.
27. Staessen J, Fagard R, Thijs L, Celis H, Arabidze G, Birkenhager W, Bulpitt C, de Leeuw P, Dollery C, Fletcher A, Forette F, Leonetti G, Nachev C, O'Brien E, Rosenfeld J, Rodicio J, Tuomilehto J, Zanchetti A, for the SYST-EUR Study Group. Randomised double-blind comparison of placebo and active treatment for older patients with isolated systolic hypertension. Lancet 1997; 350:757–764.
28. Liu L, Wang J, Gong L, Liu G, Staessen J, for the Systolic Hypertension in China (SYST-CHINA) Collaborative Group. Comparison of active treatment and placebo for older Chinese patients with isolated systolic hypertension. J Hypertens 1999. In press.
29. Gong L, Zhang W, Zhu J, 11 collaborating centres in the Shanghai area, Kong D, Page V, Ghadirian P, LeLorier J, Harnet P. Shanghai trial of nifedipine in the elderly (STONE). J Hypertens 1996; 14:1237–1245.
30. Held P, Yusuf S, Furberg C. Calcium channel blockers in acute myocardial infarction and unstable angina: an overview BMJ 1989; 229:1187–1192.
31. Yusuf S, Held P, Furberg C. Update of effects of calcium antagonists in myocardial infarction or angina in light of the Second Danish Verapamil Trial (DAVIT-II) and other recent studies. Am J Cardiol 1991; 67:1295–1297.
32. Ad Hoc Subcommittee of the Liaison Committee of the World Health Organisation and the International Society of Hypertension. Effects of calcium antagonists on the risks of coronary heart disease, cancer and bleeding. J Hypertens 1997; 15:105–115.
33. Cohn J, Ziesche S, Loss L, Anderson G, and the V-HeFT Study Group. Effect of felodipine on short-term exercise and neurohormone and long-term mortality in heart failure: results of V-Heft III. Circulation 1995; 92:1–143.
34. Packer M, O'Connor C, Ghali J, Pressler M, Carson P, Belkin R, Miller A, Neuberg G, Frid D, Wertheimer J, Cropp A, DeMets D, for the Prospective Randomized Amlodipine Survival

Evaluation Study Group. Effect of amlodipine on morbidity and mortality in severe chronic heart failure. N Engl J Med 1996; 335:1107–1114.
35. Hypertension Detection Follow up Program Cooperative Group. Five-year findings of the Hypertension Detection and Follow-up Program. I. Reduction in mortality in persons with high blood pressure, including mild hypertension. JAMA 1979; 242:2562–2571.
36. Hansson L, Zanchetti A, Carruthers S, Dahlof B, Elmfeldt D, Menard J, Julius S, Rahn K, Wedel H, Westerling S, for the HOT Study Group. Effects of intensive blood pressure lowering and low-dose aspirin in patients with hypertension: principal results of the hypertension optimal treatment (HOT) randomised trial. Lancet 1998; 351:1755–1762.
37. UK Prospective Diabetes Study Group. Tight blood pressure control and risk of macrovascular and microvascular complications in type 2 diabetes. BMJ 1998; 317:703–713.
38. World Health Organisation-International Society of Hypertension Blood Pressure Lowering Treatment Trialists' Collaboration. Protocol for prospective collaborative overviews of major randomized trials of blood pressure lowering treatments. J Hypertens 1998; 16:127–137.
39. Collins R, Gray R, Godwin J, Peto R. Avoidance of large biases and large random errors in the assessment of moderate treatment effects: the need for systematic overviews. Stat Med 1987; 6:245–250.
40. Antiplatelet Trialists Collaboration. Collaborative overview of randomised trials of antiplatelet therapy. II: Maintenance of vascular graft or arterial potency by antiplatelet therapy. BMJ 1994; 308:159–168.
41. Antiplatelet Trialists Collaboration. Collaborative overview of randomised trials of antiplatelet therapy. III: Reduction in venous thrombosis and pulmonary embolism by antiplatelet prophylaxis among surgical and medical patients. BMJ 1994; 308:235–246.
42. Antiplatelet Trialists' Collaboration. Collaborative overview of randomised trials of antiplatelet therapy. I: Prevention of death, myocardial infarction and stroke by prolonged antiplatelet therapy in various categories of patients. BMJ 1994; 308:81–106.
43. Early Breast Cancer Trialists' Collaborative Group. Treatment of early breast cancer. Vol. 1: Worldwide evidence 1985–1990.
44. Early Breast Cancer Trialists' Collaborative Group. Systematic treatment of early breast cancer by hormonal, cytotoxic or immune therapy: 133 randomised trials involving 31,000 recurrences and 24,000 deaths among 75,000 women. Lancet 1992; 339:1–15, 71–85.
45. Cholesterol Treatment Trialists' (CTT) Collaboration. Protocol for a prospective collaborative overview of all current and planned randomized trials of cholesterol treatment regimens. Am J Cardiol 1995; 75:1130–1134.
46. Schrier RW, Savage S. Appropriate blood pressure control in type II diabetes (ABCD trial): implications for complications. Am J Kidney Dis 1992; XX:653–657.
47. Lubsen J, P P-W. A 30,000 patient-years double-blind, placebo-controlled trial of nifedipine GITS in stable angina. Br J Clin Pract 1997; 51(suppl 88):23–26.
48. Davis B, Cutler J, Gordon D, Furberg C, Wright J, Cushman W, Grimm R, LaRosa J, Whelton P, Perry H, Alderman M, Ford C, Oparil S, Francis C, Proschan M, Pressel S, Black H, Hawkins C, for the ALLHAT Research Group. Rationale and design for the antihypertensive and lipid lowering treatment to prevent heart attack trial (ALLHAT). ALLHAT Research Group. Am J Hypertens 1996; 9:342–360.
49. Management committee on behalf of the High Blood Pressure Research Council of Australia. Australian comparative outcome trial of angiotensin converting enzyme inhibitor- and diuretic-based treatment of hypertension in the elderly (ANBP2): objectives and protocol. Clin Exp Pharmacol Physiol 1997; 24:188–192.
50. Black H, Elliott W, Neaton J, Grandits G, Grambsch P, Grimm R, Hansson L, Lacouciere Y, Muller J, Sleight P, Weber M, Whote W, Williams G, Wittes J, Zanchetti A, Fakouhi T. Rationale and design for the Controlled ONset Verapamil INvestigation of Cardiovascular Endpoints (CONVINCE) trial. Control Clin Trials 1998; 19(4):370–390.
51. Zanchetti A, on behalf of the ELSA Investigators. Prevalence of carotid atherosclerosis in

hypertension: preliminary data from the European Lacidipine Study on Atherosclerosis. Blood Press 1996; 5(suppl 4):30–35.
52. The HOPE Study Investigators. The HOPE (Heart Outcome Prevention Evaluation) Study: the design of a large, simple randomised trial of an angiotensin converting enzyme inhibitor (ramipril) and vitamin E in patients at high risk of cardiovascular events. Can J Cardiol 1996; 12:127–137.
53. Bulpitt C, Fletcher A, Amery A, Coope J, Grimley Evans J, Lightowlers S, O'Malley K, Palmer A, Potter J, Sever P, Staessen J, Swift C. The hypertension in the very elderly trial (HYVET). Drugs Aging 1994; 5:171–183.
54. Brown M, Castaigne A, Ruilope LM, Mancia G, Rosenthal T, de Leeuw PE, F. INSIGHT-international nifedipine GITS study intervention as a goal in hypertension treatment. J Human Hypertens 1996; 10(suppl 3):157S–160S.
55. Pepine C, Handberg-Thurmond E, Marks R, Conlon M, Cooper-DeHoff R, Volkers P, Zellig P, for the International Verapamil SR/Trandolapril study (INVEST) investigators. Rationale and design of the International Verapamil SR/Trandolapril study (INVEST): an Internet-based randomised trial in coronary heart disease patients with hypertension. J Am Coll Cardiol 1998; 32:1228–1237.
56. Dahlof B, Devereux R, de Faire U, Fyhrquist F, Hedner T, Ibsen H, Julius S, Kjeldsen S, Kristianson K, Lederballe-Pederson O, Lindholm L, Nieminen M, Omvik P, Oparil S, Wedel H, for the LIFE Study Group. The Losartan Intervention For Endpoint Reduction (LIFE) in Hypertension Study. Rationale, design, and methods. J Hypertens 1997; 10:705–713.
57. Kuramoto K, and the National Intervention Co-operative Study Group. Treatment of elderly hypertensives in Japan: national intervention co-operative study in elderly hypertensives. J Hypertens 1994; 12(suppl 6):S35–S40.
58. The NORDIL Group. The Nordic diltiazem study (NORDIL). A prospective intervention trial of calcium antagonist therapy in hypertension. Blood Press 1993; 2:312–321.
59. The PHYLLIS Project Group. Plaque hypertension lipid-lowering Italian study (PHYLLIS): a protocol for non-invasive evaluation of carotid atherosclerosis in hypercholesterolaemic hypertensive patients. J Hypertens 1993; 11(suppl 5):S314–S315.
60. PROGRESS Management Committee. Blood pressure lowering for the secondary prevention of stroke: rationale and design for PROGRESS. J Hypertens 1996; 14(suppl 2):S41–S46.
61. Lees R, Pitt B, Chan R, Holmvang G, Dinsmore RE, Campbell LW, Haber HE, Kliboner MI, Cashin Hemphill L. Baseline clinical and angiographic data in the Quinapril Ischaemic Event Trial (QUIET). Am J Cardiol 1996; 78:1011–1016.
62. Teo K, Burton J, Buller C, Plante S, Yokoyama S, Montague T. Rationale and design features of a clinical trial examining the effects of cholesterol lowering and angiotensin converting enzyme inhibition on coronary atherosclerosis. Can J Cardiol 1997; 13(6):591–599.
63. Hansson L, on behalf of the study on cognition and prognosis in the elderly (SCOPE) investigators. The study on cognition and prognosis in the elderly (SCOPE). Design and rationale. J Hypertens 1998; 16(suppl 2):246.
64. Malacco E, Gnemmi A, Romagnoli A, Coppini A, on behalf of the SHELL Study Group. Systolic hypertension in the elderly: long-term lacidipine treatment. J Cardiovasc Pharmacol 1994; 23(suppl 5):S62–S66.
65. Dahlof B, Hansson L, Lindholm L, Schersten B, Wester P, Ekbom T, Hedner T, de Faire U. STOP-Hypertension-2: a prospective intervention trial of "newer" versus "older" treatment alternatives in old patients with hypertension. Blood Press 1993; 2:136–141.
66. Zanchetti A, Magnani B, Dal Palu C, on behalf of the Verapamil Hypertension Atherosclerosis Study V. Atherosclerosis and calcium antagonists: the VHAS. J Human Hypertens 1992; 6(suppl 2):S45–S48.

Index

About the Editor

HENRY R. BLACK is Chairman of the Department of Preventive Medicine, the Charles J. and Margaret Roberts Professor of Preventive Medicine, Professor of Internal Medicine, Associate Vice President for Research, and Associate Dean for Clinical Research, Rush Medical College, Rush-Presbyterian-St. Luke's Medical Center, Chicago, Illinois. The author, coauthor, or coeditor of more than 220 journal articles, papers, book chapters, and books, Dr. Black is a Fellow of the American College of Physicians, the American College of Chest Physicians, the American Heart Association, the Society for Vascular Medicine and Biology, and the Council on Geriatric Cardiology, and a member of the American Society of Hypertension and the International Society of Nephrology, among others. He received the A.B. degree (1963) from Columbia College, New York, New York, and the M.D. degree (1967) from the New York University School of Medicine, New York.